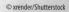

Contents

Editors and Contributing Authors   vi

Preface   vii

Acknowledgments   viii

CHAPTER 1   Principles of Cancer Chemotherapy   1

Introduction   1

The Role of Chemotherapy in the Treatment of Cancer   2

Principles of Combination Chemotherapy   3

CHAPTER 2   Chemotherapeutic and Biologic Drugs   5

CHAPTER 3   Guidelines for Chemotherapy and Dosing Modifications   421

CHAPTER 4   Common Chemotherapy Regimens in Clinical Practice   441

CHAPTER 5   Antiemetic Agents for the Treatment of Chemotherapy-Induced Nausea and Vomiting   589

Index   597

Editors

Edward Chu, MD
Professor of Medicine and Pharmacology & Chemical Biology
Chief, Division of Hematology-Oncology
Deputy Director
University of Pittsburgh Cancer Institute
University of Pittsburgh School of Medicine
Pittsburgh, PA

Vincent T. DeVita, Jr., MD
Amy and Joseph Perella Professor of Medicine
Professor of Epidemiology and Public Health
Yale University School of Medicine
New Haven, CT

Contributing Authors

M. Sitki Copur, MD
Adjunct Professor of Medicine
University of Nebraska
Medical Director, CHI Health St. Francis Cancer Treatment Center
Grand Island, NE

Dron Gauchan, MD
Adjunct Assistant Professor of Medicine
University of Nebraska
CHI Health St. Francis Cancer Treatment Center
Grand Island, NE

Laurie J. Harrold, MD
Staff Medical Oncologist
VA Pittsburgh Healthcare System
Pittsburgh, PA

Ryan Ramaekers, MD
Adjunct Assistant Professor of Medicine
University of Nebraska
CHI Health St. Francis Cancer Treatment Center
Grand Island, NE

Dawn E. Tiedemann, AOCN, APRN
Clinical Nurse Specialist
Hematology-Oncology Associates
Meriden, CT

PHYSICIANS'

CANCER
CHEMOTHERAPY
DRUG MANUAL

2017

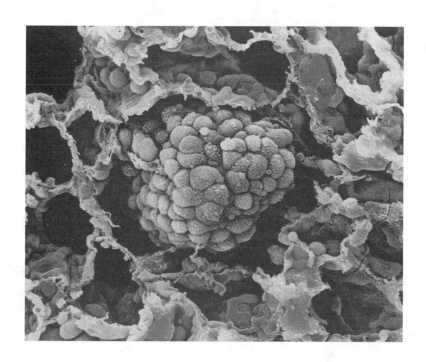

Other Jones & Bartlett Learning Oncology Titles

Breast Cancer Treatment by Focused Microwave Thermotherapy, Fenn
Cancer in Children and Adolescents, Carroll/Finlay
Cancer Nursing, 8e, Yarbro
Contemporary Issues in Breast Cancer: A Nursing Perspective, 2e, Hassey Dow
Dx/Rx: Brain Tumors, Quant
Dx/Rx: Breast Cancer, 2e, Lake
Dx/Rx: Cervical Cancer, 2e, Robison/Dizon
Dx/Rx: Colorectal Cancer, Holen/Chung
Dx/Rx: Genitourinary Oncology: Cancer of the Kidney, Bladder, and Testis, 2e, Galsky
Dx/Rx: Gynecologic Cancer, Dizon/Campos
Dx/Rx: Head and Neck Cancer, Hu et al.
Dx/Rx: Liver Cancer, Abou-Alfa/Ang
Dx/Rx: Lung Cancer, 2e, Azzoli
Dx/Rx: Leukemia, 2e, Burke
Dx/Rx: Lymphoma, Persky
Dx/Rx: Melanoma, Carvajal
Dx/Rx: Palliative Cancer Care, Malhotra/Moryl
Dx/Rx: Pancreatic Cancer, Lowery/O'Reilly
Dx/Rx: Prostate Cancer, 2e, Kampel
Dx/Rx: Upper Gastrointestinal Malignancies: Cancers of the Stomach and Esophagus, Shah
Genomic and Molecular Neuro-Oncology, Zhang/Fuller
Glioblastoma Multiforme, Markert et al.
Gynecologic Tumor Board: Clinical Cases in Diagnosis and Management of Cancer of the Female Reproductive System, Dizon/Abu-Rustum
Handbook of Breast Cancer Risk-Assessment, Vogel/Bevers
Handbook of Cancer Emergencies, Marinella
Handbook of Cancer Risk Assessment and Prevention, Colditz/Stein
Handbook of Radiation Oncology: Basic Principles and Clinical Protocols, Haffty/Wilson
How Cancer Works, Sompayrac
Management of Nausea and Vomiting in Cancer and Cancer Treatment, Hesketh
Medical and Psychosocial Care of the Care Survivor, Miller
Molecular Oncology of Breast Cancer, Ross/Hortobagyi
Molecular Oncology of Prostate Cancer, Ross/Foster
Pancreatic Cancer, Von Hoff/Evans/Hruban
Pediatric Stem Cell Transplantation, Mehta
Pocket Guide to Chemotherapy Protocols, 7e, Chu
Tarascon Pocket Oncologica, Marinella
The Cancer Book, Cooper
The Hospital for Sick Children Handbook of Supportive Care in Pediatric Oncology, Abla
The Johns Hopkins Breast Cancer Handbook for Health Care Professionals, Shockney/Tsangaris

For a complete list of our oncology titles, see www.jblearning.com/medicine/oncology.

PHYSICIANS'
CANCER
CHEMOTHERAPY
DRUG MANUAL
2017

Edward Chu, MD

Professor of Medicine and Pharmacology & Chemical Biology
Chief, Division of Hematology-Oncology
Deputy Director
University of Pittsburgh Cancer Institute
University of Pittsburgh School of Medicine
Pittsburgh, PA

Vincent T. DeVita, Jr., MD

Amy and Joseph Perella Professor of Medicine
Professor of Epidemiology and Public Health
Yale University School of Medicine
New Haven, CT

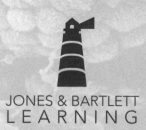

JONES & BARTLETT
LEARNING

World Headquarters
Jones & Bartlett Learning
5 Wall Street
Burlington, MA 01803
978-443-5000
info@jblearning.com
www.jblearning.com

Jones & Bartlett Learning books and products are available through most bookstores and online book-sellers. To contact Jones & Bartlett Learning directly, call 800-832-0034, fax 978-443-8000, or visit our website, www.jblearning.com.

Production Credits
Executive Editor: Nancy Anastasi Duffy
Marketing Manager: Lindsay White
Rights and Photo Research Coordinator: Wesley DeShano
Media Development Editor: Shannon Sheehan
Director of Vendor Management: Amy Rose
Manufacturing and Inventory Control Supervisor: Amy Bacus
Composition and Project Management: S4Carlisle Publishing Services
Cover Image: © Science Photo Library - MOREDUN ANIMAL HEALTH LTD/Brand X Pictures/Getty
Cover Design: Kristin E. Parker
Printing and Binding: Edward Brothers Malloy
Cover Printing: Edward Brothers Malloy

6048

Printed in the United States of America

20 19 18 17 16   10 9 8 7 6 5 4 3 2 1

Preface

The development of effective drugs for the treatment of cancer represents a significant achievement beginning with the discovery of the antimetabolites and alkylating agents in the 1940s and 1950s. The success of that effort can be attributed in large measure to the close collaboration and interaction between basic scientists, synthetic organic chemists, pharmacologists, and clinicians. This tradition continues to flourish, especially as we now enter the world of pharmacogenomics, genomics, and proteomics, and the rapid identification of new molecular targets for drug design and development.

In this, our 17th edition, we have condensed and summarized a wealth of information on chemotherapeutic and biologic agents in current clinical practice into a reference guide that presents essential information in a practical and readable format. The primary indications, drug doses and schedules, toxicities, and special considerations for each agent have been expanded and revised to take into account new information that has been gathered over the past year. In this edition, we have included 13 new agents that have all been approved by the FDA within the past year and have updated new indications for several previously approved agents.

This drug manual is divided into five chapters. *Chapter 1* gives a brief overview of the key principles of cancer chemotherapy and reviews the clinical settings where chemothcrapy is used. *Chapter 2* reviews individual chemotherapeutic and biologic agents that are in current clinical use; these agents are presented in alphabetical order according to their generic name. In this chapter, specific details are provided regarding drug classification and category, key mechanisms of action and resistance, critical aspects of clinical pharmacology and pharmacokinetics, clinical indications, special precautions and considerations, and toxicity. *Chapter 3* includes recommendations for dose modifications that are required in the setting of myelosuppression and/or liver and renal dysfunction. Relevant information is also provided highlighting the teratogenic potential of various agents. *Chapter 4* presents a review of the combination drug regimens and selected single-agent regimens for solid tumors and hematologic malignancies that are used commonly in daily clinical practice. This section is organized alphabetically by specific cancer type. Finally, *Chapter 5* reviews commonly used antiemetic agents and regimens used to treat chemotherapy-induced nausea and vomiting, which is a significant toxicity observed with many of the anticancer agents in current practice.

Our hope remains for this book to continue to serve as both an in-depth reference and an immediate source of practical information that can be used by physicians and other healthcare professionals actively involved in the daily care of cancer patients. This drug manual continues to be a work in progress, and our goal is to continue to provide new updates on an annual basis and to incorporate new drugs and treatment strategies that reflect the rapid advances in the field of cancer drug development.

Edward Chu, MD
Vincent T. DeVita, Jr., MD

Acknowledgments

This book represents the efforts of many dedicated people. It reflects my own personal and professional roots in the field of cancer pharmacology and cancer drug development. It also reaffirms the teaching and support of my colleagues and mentors at Brown University, the National Cancer Institute (NCI), and the Yale Cancer Center. In particular, Bruce Chabner, Paul Calabresi, Robert Parks, Joseph Bertino, and Vince DeVita have had a major influence on my development as a cancer pharmacologist and medical oncologist. While at the NCI, I was fortunate to have been trained under the careful tutelage of Carmen Allegra, Bob Wittes, and Bruce Chabner. At Yale, I was privileged to work with a group of extraordinarily talented individuals including Yung-chi Cheng, William Prusoff, Alan Sartorelli, and Vince DeVita, all of whom have graciously shared their scientific insights, wisdom, support, and friendship. I would also like to take this opportunity to thank my co-author, colleague, mentor, and friend, Vince DeVita, who recruited me to the Yale Cancer Center and who has been so tremendously supportive of my professional and personal career. Special thanks go to my colleagues at Jones & Bartlett Learning for giving me the opportunity to develop this book and for their continued encouragement, support, and patience throughout this entire process. I wish to thank my wife, Laurie Harrold, for her love and patience, for her insights as a practicing medical oncologist, and for her help in writing and reviewing various sections of this book. I would also like to thank my parents, Ming and Shih-Hsi Chu, for their constant love, support, and encouragement, and for instilling in me the desire, joy, and commitment to become a medical oncologist and cancer pharmacologist. Finally, this book is dedicated to my two dogs, Mika and Lexi, who are no longer with us, but who live in our hearts forever, and to our two new dogs, Rosie and Allie, and to my two beautiful children, Ashley and Joshua, who have brought me great joy and pride and who have shown me the true meaning of unconditional loyalty and love.

Edward Chu, MD

1

Principles of Cancer Chemotherapy

Vincent T. DeVita, Jr. and Edward Chu

Introduction

The development of chemotherapy in the 1950s and 1960s resulted in curative therapeutic strategies for patients with hematologic malignances and several types of
advanced solid tumors. These advances confirmed the principle that chemotherapy
could indeed cure cancer and provided the rationale for integrating chemotherapy
into combined-modality programs with surgery and radiation therapy in early stages
of disease to provide clinical benefit. Since its early days, the principal obstacles to the
clinical efficacy of chemotherapy have been toxicity to the normal tissues of the body
and the development of cellular drug resistance. The development and application of
molecular techniques to analyze gene expression of normal and malignant cells at the
level of DNA, RNA, and/or protein has greatly facilitated the identification of some
of the critical mechanisms through which chemotherapy exerts its antitumor effects
and activates the program of cell death. The newer advances in molecular diagnostics,
which now include next-generation sequencing, whole exome sequencing, and whole
genome sequencing, have provided important new insights into the molecular and
genetic events within cancer cells that can confer chemosensitivity to drug treatment
as well as having identified potential new therapeutic targets. This enhanced under-
standing of the molecular pathways by which chemotherapy and targeted therapies
exert their antitumor activity, and by which genetic alterations can result in resistance
to drug therapy, has provided the rational basis for developing innovative therapeutic
strategies.

1

The Role of Chemotherapy in the Treatment of Cancer

Chemotherapy is presently used in four main clinical settings: (1) primary induction treatment for advanced disease or for cancers for which there are no other effective treatment approaches; (2) neoadjuvant treatment for patients who present with localized disease, for whom local forms of therapy, such as surgery and/or radiation, are inadequate by themselves; (3) adjuvant treatment to local treatment modalities, including surgery and/or radiation therapy; and (4) direct instillation into sanctuary sites or by site-directed perfusion of specific regions of the body directly affected by the cancer.

Primary induction chemotherapy refers to drug therapy administered as the primary treatment for patients who present with advanced cancer for which no alternative treatment exists. This has been the main approach to treat patients with advanced, metastatic disease. In most cases, the goals of therapy are to palliate tumor-related symptoms, improve overall quality of life, and prolong time to tumor progression (TTP) and overall survival (OS). Cancer chemotherapy can be curative in a relatively small subset of patients who present with advanced disease. In adults, these potentially curable cancers include Hodgkin's and non-Hodgkin's lymphoma, germ cell cancer, acute leukemias, and choriocarcinoma, while the curable childhood cancers include acute lymphoblastic leukemia, Burkitt's lymphoma, Wilms' tumor, and embryonal rhabdomyosarcoma.

Neoadjuvant chemotherapy refers to the use of chemotherapy for patients who present with localized cancer for which alternative local therapies, such as surgery, exist but are less than completely effective. At present, neoadjuvant therapy is most often administered in the treatment of anal cancer, bladder cancer, breast cancer, esophageal cancer, laryngeal cancer, locally advanced non-small cell lung cancer (NSCLC), and osteogenic sarcoma. For diseases such as anal cancer, gastro-esophageal cancer, laryngeal cancer, and non-small cell lung cancer, optimal clinical benefit is usually derived when chemotherapy is administered with radiation therapy, either concurrently or sequentially.

One of the most important roles for cancer chemotherapy is in conjunction with local treatment modalities such as surgery and/or radiation therapy; this has been termed adjuvant chemotherapy. The development of disease recurrence, either locally or systemically, following surgery and/or radiation is mainly due to the spread of occult micrometastases. The goal of adjuvant therapy is, therefore, to reduce the incidence of both local and systemic recurrence and to improve the OS of patients. In general, chemotherapy regimens with clinical activity against advanced disease may have curative potential following surgical resection of the primary tumor, provided the appropriate dose and schedule are administered. It is now well established that adjuvant chemotherapy is effective in prolonging both disease-free survival (DFS) and OS in patients with breast cancer, colorectal cancer (CRC), gastric cancer, NSCLC, Wilms' tumor, and osteogenic sarcoma. Adjuvant chemotherapy is also recommended in patients with anaplastic astrocytomas. Patients with primary malignant melanoma at high risk of developing metastases derive benefit in terms of improved DFS and OS from adjuvant treatment with the biologic agent α-interferon, although this treatment must be given for 1 year's duration. The antihormonal agents tamoxifen, anastrozole, and letrozole are effective in the adjuvant therapy of postmenopausal women whose breast tumors express the estrogen receptor. However, they must be administered on a long-term basis, with treatment being given for 5 years. In support of the concept that prolonged duration of adjuvant therapy is associated with improved clinical benefit, recent studies have shown that imatinib adjuvant therapy for patients with surgically resected gastrointestinal stromal tumor (GIST) is more effective when given for 3 years as opposed to 1 year.

Principles of Combination Chemotherapy

With rare exceptions (e.g., choriocarcinoma and Burkitt's lymphoma), single drugs, at clinically tolerable doses, have been unable to cure cancer. In the 1960s and early 1970s, drug combination regimens were developed based on known biochemical actions of available anticancer drugs rather than on their clinical efficacy. Such regimens were, however, largely ineffective. The era of combination chemotherapy began when several active drugs from different classes became available for use in combination in the treatment of the acute leukemias and lymphomas. Following this initial success with hematologic malignancies, combination chemotherapy was subsequently extended to the treatment of solid tumors.

Combination chemotherapy with conventional cytotoxic agents accomplishes several key objectives not possible with single-agent therapy. First, it provides maximal cell kill within the range of toxicity tolerated by the host for each drug as long as dosing is not compromised. Second, it provides a broader range of interaction between drugs and tumor cells with different genetic abnormalities in a heterogeneous tumor population. Finally, it may prevent and/or slow the subsequent development of cellular drug resistance.

Certain principles have guided the selection of drugs in the most effective drug combinations, and they provide a paradigm for the development of new drug therapeutic regimens. First, only drugs known to be partially effective against the same tumor when used alone should be selected for use in combination. If available, drugs that produce some fraction of complete remission are preferred to those that produce only partial responses. Second, when several drugs of a class are available and are equally effective, a drug should be selected on the basis of toxicity that does not overlap with the toxicity of other drugs to be used in the combination. Although such selection leads to a wider range of side effects, it minimizes the risk of a potentially lethal effect caused by multiple insults to the same organ system by different drugs. Moreover, this approach allows dose intensity to be maximized. In addition, drugs should be used in their optimal dose and schedule, and drug combinations should be given at consistent intervals. The treatment-free interval between cycles should be the shortest possible time necessary for recovery of the most sensitive normal target tissue, which is usually the bone marrow. The biochemical, molecular, and pharmacologic mechanisms of interaction between the individual drugs in a given combination should be understood to allow for maximal effect. Finally, arbitrary reduction in the dose of an effective drug to allow for the addition of other, less-effective drugs may dramatically reduce the clinical activity of the most effective agent below the threshold of effectiveness and reduce the capacity of the combination regimen to cure disease in a given patient.

One final issue relates to the optimal duration of chemotherapy drug administration. Several randomized trials in the adjuvant treatment of breast cancer and CRC have shown that short-course treatment on the order of 6 months is as effective as long-course therapy (12 months). Studies are currently ongoing to determine whether a shorter course of 3 months of adjuvant chemotherapy will yield the same level of clinical benefit as 6 months of treatment of early-stage CRC. However, optimal duration may be dependent upon the particular tumor type, as it is now well-established that prolonged duration of adjuvant therapy in patients with surgically resected GIST results in improved clinical benefit. While progressive disease during chemotherapy is a clear indication to stop treatment in the advanced-disease setting, the optimal duration of chemotherapy for patients without disease progression has not been well defined. With the development of novel and more potent drug regimens, the potential risk of cumulative adverse events, such as cardiotoxicity secondary to the anthracyclines and neurotoxicity secondary to the taxanes and the platinum analogs, must also be factored in the decision-making process. There is, however, no evidence of clinical benefit in continuing therapy indefinitely until disease progression. A recent randomized study in metastatic CRC comparing continuous versus intermittent palliative chemotherapy showed that a policy of stopping and rechallenging with the same chemotherapy provides a reasonable treatment option for certain patients. Similar observations have been observed in the treatment of metastatic disease of other tumor types, including NSCLC, breast cancer, germ cell cancer, ovarian cancer, and small cell lung cancer (SCLC).

2

Chemotherapeutic and Biologic Drugs

Edward Chu, Ryan Ramaekers, Dron Gauchan,
Laurie J. Harrold, Dawn Tiedemann, and M. Sitki Copur

Abiraterone Acetate

TRADE NAME	Zytiga	CLASSIFICATION	Miscellaneous agent
CATEGORY	Hormonal agent	DRUG MANUFACTURER	Janssen Biotech, Johnson & Johnson

MECHANISM OF ACTION

- Prodrug of abiraterone.
- Selective inhibition of 17α-hydroxylase/C17, 20-lyase (CYP17). This enzyme is expressed in testicular, adrenal, and prostatic tumor tissues and is required for androgen biosynthesis.
- Inhibition of CYP17 leads to inhibition of the conversion of pregnenolone and progesterone to their 17α-hydroxy derivatives.
- Inhibition of CYP17 leads to inhibition of subsequent formation of dehydroepiandrosterone (DHEA) and androstenedione.
- Associated with a rebound increase in mineralocorticoid production by the adrenals.

MECHANISM OF RESISTANCE

- Upregulation of CYP17.
- Induction of androgen receptor (AR) and AR splice variants that result in ligand-independent AR transactivation.
- Expression of truncated androgen receptors.

ABSORPTION

Following oral administration, maximum drug levels are reached within 1.5–4 hours. Oral absorption is increased with food, and in particular, food with high fat content.

DISTRIBUTION

Highly protein bound (>99%) to albumin and α1-acid glycoprotein.

METABOLISM

Following oral administration, abiraterone acetate is rapidly hydrolyzed to abiraterone, the active metabolite. The two main circulating metabolites of abiraterone are abiraterone sulphate and N-oxide abiraterone sulphate, both of which are inactive. Nearly 90% of an administered dose is recovered in feces, while only 5% is eliminated in urine. The terminal half-life of abiraterone ranges from 5 to 14 hours, with a median half-life of 12 hours.

INDICATIONS

FDA-approved for use in combination with prednisone for the treatment of patients with metastatic, castration-resistant prostate cancer who have received prior chemotherapy containing docetaxel.

DOSAGE RANGE

Recommended dose is 1000 mg PO once daily in combination with prednisone 5 mg PO bid.

DRUG INTERACTIONS

- Use with caution in the presence of CYP2D6 substrates.
- Use with caution in the presence of CYP3A4 inhibitors and inducers.

SPECIAL CONSIDERATIONS

1. No dosage adjustment is necessary for patients with baseline mild hepatic impairment. In patients with moderate hepatic impairment (Child-Pugh Class B), reduce dose to 250 mg once daily. If elevations in ALT or AST >5 × ULN or total bilirubin >3 × ULN occur in patients, discontinue treatment. Avoid use in patients with severe hepatic impairment, as the drug has not been tested in this patient population.
2. No dosage adjustment is necessary for patients with renal impairment.
3. Abiraterone acetate should be taken on an empty stomach with no food being consumed for at least 2 hours before and for at least 1 hour after an oral dose. Tablets should be swallowed whole with water.
4. Closely monitor for adrenal insufficiency, especially if patients are withdrawn from prednisone, undergo a reduction in prednisone dose, or experience concurrent infection or stress.
5. Pregnancy category X. Breastfeeding should be avoided.

TOXICITY 1
Fatigue.

TOXICITY 2
Mild nausea and vomiting.

TOXICITY 3
Mild elevations in SGOT/SGPT.

TOXICITY 4
Hypertension.

TOXICITY 5
Peripheral edema.

TOXICITY 6
Hypokalemia.

TOXICITY 7
Arthralgias, myalgias, and muscle spasms.

TOXICITY 8
Hot flashes.

Ado-trastuzumab emtansine

DM1

MCC linker

Where n ~ 3.5
DM1/Mab

TRADE NAME	Kadcyla	CLASSIFICATION	Antibody-drug conjugate
CATEGORY	Biologic response modifier agent/ chemotherapy drug	DRUG MANUFACTURER	Genentech/ Roche

MECHANISM OF ACTION
- HER2-targeted antibody-drug conjugate that is made up of trastuzumab and the small-molecule microtubule inhibitor DM1.
- Upon binding to the HER2 receptor, ado-trastuzumab emtansine undergoes receptor-mediated internalization and lysosomal degradation, leading to intracellular release of the DM1 molecule.
- Binding of DM1 to tubulin leads to disruption of the microtubule network, resulting in cell-cycle arrest and apoptosis.
- Inhibits HER2 downstream signaling pathways.
- Immunologic-mediated mechanisms, such as antibody-dependent cell-mediated cytotoxicity (ADCC), may also be involved in antitumor activity.

MECHANISM OF RESISTANCE
None characterized to date.

ABSORPTION
Administered only via the intravenous (IV) route.

DISTRIBUTION
Extensive binding (93%) of ado-trastuzumab emtansine to plasma proteins.

METABOLISM
DM1 is metabolized by the liver microsomal enzymes CYP3A4/5. The median terminal half-life of ado-trastuzumab emtansine is on the order of 4 days.

INDICATIONS
1. FDA-approved for patients with HER2-positive metastatic breast cancer who have received prior treatment with trastuzumab and a taxane chemotherapy.
2. Patients should already have been treated for their metastatic breast cancer or have had their early-stage disease recur during or within 6 months after completion of adjuvant therapy.

DOSAGE RANGE
Recommended dose is 3.6 mg/kg IV every 3 weeks.

DRUG INTERACTIONS
None well characterized to date.

SPECIAL CONSIDERATIONS
1. Ado-trastuzumab emtansine can **NOT** be substituted for or with trastuzumab.
2. Baseline and periodic evaluations of left ventricular ejection fraction (LVEF) should be performed while on therapy. Treatment should be held if the LVEF drops <40% or is between 40%–45% with a 10% or greater absolute reduction from pretreatment baseline. Therapy should be permanently stopped if the LVEF function has not improved or has declined further. This is a black-box warning.
3. Monitor liver function tests (LFTs) and serum bilirubin levels closely as serious hepatotoxicity has been observed. This is a black-box warning.
4. Carefully monitor for infusion-related reactions, especially during the first infusion.
5. Monitor patients for pulmonary symptoms. Therapy should be held in patients presenting with new or progressive pulmonary symptoms and should be terminated in patients diagnosed with treatment-related pneumonitis or interstitial lung disease (ILD).
6. Closely monitor complete blood count (CBC) and specifically platelet counts.
7. HER2 testing using an FDA-approved diagnostic test to confirm the presence of HER2 protein overexpression or gene amplification is required for determining which patients should receive ado-trastuzumab emtansine therapy.
8. No formal guidelines are presently available for patients with hepatic dysfunction.
9. No dose adjustment is recommended for patients with mild-to-moderate renal dysfunction. Use with caution in patients with severe renal dysfunction.
10. Pregnancy category D. Breastfeeding should be avoided.

TOXICITY 1
Cardiac toxicity in the form of cardiomyopathy.

TOXICITY 2
Infusion-related reactions.

TOXICITY 3
Hepatotoxicity with transient elevations in LFTs. Severe drug-induced liver injury and hepatic encephalopathy have been reported rarely. Rare cases of nodular regenerative hyperplasia of the liver have also been reported.

TOXICITY 4
Myelosuppression with thrombocytopenia.

TOXICITY 5
Pulmonary toxicity presenting as cough, dyspnea, and infiltrates. Observed rarely in about 1% of patients.

TOXICITY 6
Neurotoxicity with peripheral sensory neuropathy.

TOXICITY 7
Asthenia, fatigue, and pyrexia.

Afatinib

TRADE NAME	Gilotrif	CLASSIFICATION	Signal transduction inhibitor
CATEGORY	Chemotherapy drug	DRUG MANUFACTURER	Boehringer Ingelheim

MECHANISM OF ACTION

- Potent and selective small-molecule inhibitor of the kinase domains of EGFR, HER2, and HER4, resulting in inhibition of autophosphorylation and inhibition of downstream ErbB signaling.
- Inhibition of the ErbB tyrosine kinases results in inhibition of critical mitogenic and antiapoptotic signals involved in proliferation, growth, invasion/metastasis, angiogenesis, and response to chemotherapy and/or radiation therapy.

MECHANISM OF RESISTANCE

- Mutations in ErbB tyrosine kinases leading to decreased binding affinity to afatinib.
- Presence of KRAS mutations.
- Presence of BRAF mutations.
- Activation/induction of alternative cellular signaling pathways such as PI3K/Akt, IGF-1R, and c-Met.
- Increased expression/activation of mTORC1 signaling pathway.

ABSORPTION

Oral bioavailability is on the order of 92%. Peak plasma drug levels are achieved in 2-5 hours after ingestion.

DISTRIBUTION

Extensive binding (95%) to plasma proteins. Steady-state drug levels are reached in approximately 8 days.

METABOLISM

Metabolism in the liver primarily by CYP3A4 microsomal enzymes. Elimination is mainly hepatic (85%) with excretion in the feces. Renal elimination of parent drug and its metabolites account for only about 4% of an administered dose. The terminal half-life of the parent drug is 37 hours.

INDICATIONS

FDA-approved as first-line treatment of metastatic non–small cell lung cancer (NSCLC) with EGFR exon 19 deletions or exon 21 (L858R) substitution mutations as detected by an FDA-approved test.

DOSAGE RANGE

Recommended dose is 40 mg/day PO.

DRUG INTERACTION 1

Phenytoin and other drugs that stimulate the liver microsomal CYP3A4 enzymes, including carbamazepine, rifampin, phenobarbital, and St. John's Wort—These drugs may increase the metabolism of afatinib, resulting in its inactivation.

DRUG INTERACTION 2

Drugs that inhibit the liver microsomal CYP3A4 enzymes, including ketoconazole, itraconazole, erythromycin, and clarithromycin—These drugs may decrease the metabolism of afatinib, resulting in increased drug levels and potentially increased toxicity.

DRUG INTERACTION 3

Warfarin—Patients receiving coumarin-derived anticoagulants should be closely monitored for alterations in their clotting parameters (PT and INR) and/or bleeding, as afatinib may inhibit the metabolism of warfarin by the liver P450 system. Dose of warfarin may require careful adjustment in the presence of afatinib therapy.

SPECIAL CONSIDERATIONS

1. Dose reduction is not recommended in patients with mild or moderate hepatic impairment. However, afatinib has not been studied in patients with severe hepatic dysfunction and should be used with caution in this setting.
2. Closely monitor patients for new or progressive pulmonary symptoms, including cough, dyspnea, and fever. Afatinib therapy should be interrupted pending further diagnostic evaluation.
3. In patients who develop a skin rash, topical antibiotics such as Cleocin (clindamycin) gel or erythromycin cream/gel or oral clindamycin, oral doxycycline, or oral minocycline may help.
4. Patients should be warned to avoid sunlight exposure.
5. Closely monitor in patients with a history of keratitis, ulcerative keratitis, or severe dry eye and in those who wear contact lenses.
6. Avoid Seville oranges, starfruit, pomelos, grapefruit, and grapefruit juice while on afatinib therapy.
7. Pregnancy category D. Breastfeeding should be avoided.

TOXICITY 1

Skin toxicity in the form of rash, erythema, and acneiform skin rash occurs in 90% of patients. Pruritus, dry skin, and nail bed changes are also observed. Grade 3 skin toxicity occurs in nearly 20% of patients, with bullous, blistering, and exfoliating lesions occurring rarely.

TOXICITY 2

Diarrhea is most common GI toxicity. Mild nausea/vomiting and mucositis.

TOXICITY 3

Pulmonary toxicity in the form of ILD manifested by increased cough, dyspnea, fever, and pulmonary infiltrates. Observed in 1.5% of patients, and incidence appears to be higher in Asian patients.

TOXICITY 4

Hepatic toxicity with mild-to-moderate elevations in serum transaminases. Usually transient and clinically asymptomatic.

TOXICITY 5

Fatigue, anorexia, and reduced appetite.

TOXICITY 6

Keratitis presenting as acute eye inflammation, lacrimation, light sensitivity, blurred vision, eye pain and/or red eye.

Albumin-Bound Paclitaxel

TRADE NAME	Abraxane	CLASSIFICATION	Taxane, antimicrotubule agent
CATEGORY	Chemotherapy drug	DRUG MANUFACTURER	Celgene

MECHANISM OF ACTION
- Albumin-bound form of paclitaxel with a mean particle size of about 130 nm. Selective binding of albumin-bound paclitaxel to specific albumin receptors present on tumor cells versus normal cells.
- Active moiety is paclitaxel, which is isolated from the bark of the Pacific yew tree, *Taxus brevifolia*.
- Cell cycle–specific, active in the mitosis (M) phase of the cell cycle.
- High-affinity binding to microtubules enhances tubulin polymerization. Normal dynamic process of microtubule network is inhibited, leading to inhibition of mitosis and cell division.

MECHANISM OF RESISTANCE
- Alterations in tubulin with decreased binding affinity for drug.
- Multidrug-resistant phenotype with increased expression of P170 glycoprotein. Results in enhanced drug efflux with decreased intracellular accumulation of drug. Cross-resistant to other natural products, including vinca alkaloids, anthracyclines, taxanes, and etoposide.

ABSORPTION
Administered by the IV route, as it is not orally bioavailable.

DISTRIBUTION
Distributes widely to all body tissues. Extensive binding (<90%) to plasma and cellular proteins.

METABOLISM
Paclitaxel is metabolized extensively by the hepatic P450 microsomal system. About 20% of the drug is excreted via fecal elimination. Less than 10% is eliminated as the parent form with the majority being eliminated as metabolites. Renal clearance is relatively minor with less than 1% of the drug cleared via the kidneys. The clearance of abraxane is 43% greater than paclitaxel, and the volume of distribution is about 50% higher than paclitaxel. Terminal elimination half-life is on the order of 27 hours.

INDICATIONS
1. FDA-approved for the treatment of breast cancer after failure of combination chemotherapy for metastatic disease or relapse within 6 months of adjuvant chemotherapy.

2. FDA-approved for the treatment of locally advanced or metastatic NSCLC, in combination with carboplatin, in patients who are not candidates for curative surgery or radiation therapy.
3. FDA-approved for the treatment of locally advanced or metastatic pancreatic cancer in combination with gemcitabine.

DOSAGE RANGE

1. Recommended dose for metastatic breast cancer is 260 mg/m^2 IV on day 1 every 21 days.
2. An alternative regimen is a weekly schedule of 125 mg/m^2 IV on days 1, 8, and 15 every 28 days.
3. Recommended dose for NSCLC is 100 mg/m^2 IV on days 1, 8, and 15 every 21 days.
4. Recommended dose for pancreatic cancer is 125 mg/m^2 IV on days 1, 8, and 15 every 28 days.

DRUG INTERACTIONS

None well characterized to date.

SPECIAL CONSIDERATIONS

1. Contraindicated in patients with baseline neutrophil counts <1500 cells/mm^3.
2. Closely monitor CBC with differential on a periodic basis.
3. Abraxane has not been studied in patients with renal dysfunction.
4. Use with caution in patients with abnormal liver function, as patients with abnormal liver function may be at higher risk for toxicity. The drug should **NOT** be given to patients with metastatic pancreatic cancer who have moderate to severe liver dysfunction. For diseases other than metastatic pancreatic cancer, dose reduction is recommended in patients with moderate or severe hepatic dysfunction.
5. In contrast to paclitaxel, no premedication is required to prevent hypersensitivity reactions prior to administration of abraxane.
6. Abraxane can **NOT** be substituted for or with other paclitaxel formulations, as the albumin form of paclitaxel may significantly alter the drug's clinical activity.
7. Closely monitor infusion site for infiltration during drug administration, as injection site reactions have been observed.
8. Use with caution when administering with known substrates or inhibitors of CYP2C8 and CYP3A4.
9. Pregnancy category D. Breastfeeding should be avoided.

TOXICITY 1

Myelosuppression with dose-limiting neutropenia and anemia. Thrombocytopenia relatively uncommon.

TOXICITY 2

Neurotoxicity mainly in the form of sensory neuropathy with numbness and paresthesias. Dose-dependent effect. In contrast to paclitaxel, abraxane-mediated neuropathy appears to be more readily reversible.

TOXICITY 3
Ocular and visual disturbances seen in 13% of patients, with severe cases seen in 1%.

TOXICITY 4
Asthenia, fatigue, and weakness.

TOXICITY 5
Alopecia with loss of total body hair.

TOXICITY 6
Nausea/vomiting, diarrhea, and mucositis are the main gastrointestinal (GI) toxicities. Mucositis is generally mild (seen in less than 10%). Mild-to-moderate nausea and vomiting, usually of brief duration.

TOXICITY 7
Transient elevations in serum transaminases, bilirubin, and alkaline phosphatase.

TOXICITY 8
Injection site reactions.

TOXICITY 9
Cardiac toxicity with chest pain, supraventricular tachycardia, hypertension, pulmonary embolus, peripheral edema, and rare cases of cardiac arrest.

Aldesleukin

TRADE NAMES	Interleukin-2, IL-2, Proleukin	CLASSIFICATION	Immunotherapy, cytokine
CATEGORY	Biologic response modifier agent	DRUG MANUFACTURER	Prometheus

MECHANISM OF ACTION
- Glycoprotein cytokine that functions as a T-cell growth factor.
- Biologic effect of interleukin-2 (IL-2) is mediated by specific binding to the interleukin-2 receptor (IL-2R).
- Precise mechanism by which IL-2 mediates its anticancer activity remains unknown but appears to require an intact immune system.
- Enhances lymphocyte mitogenesis and lymphocyte cytotoxicity.
- Induces lymphokine-activated (LAK) and natural killer (NK) cell activity.
- Induces interferon-γ production.

MECHANISM OF RESISTANCE
- Up to 75% of patients may develop anti–IL-2 antibodies.
- Increased expression of counter-regulatory factors, such as glucocorticoids, which act to reduce the efficacy of interleukin-2.

ABSORPTION
Not available for oral use and is administered only via the parenteral route. Peak plasma levels are achieved in 5 hours after subcutaneous (SC) administration.

DISTRIBUTION
After short IV infusion, high plasma concentrations of IL-2 are achieved followed by rapid distribution into the extravascular space.

METABOLISM
IL-2 is catabolized by renal tubular cells to amino acids. The major route of elimination is through the kidneys by both glomerular filtration and tubular secretion. The elimination half-life is 85 minutes.

INDICATIONS
1. Metastatic renal cell cancer.
2. Metastatic malignant melanoma.

DOSAGE RANGE
Renal cell cancer—600,000 IU/kg IV every 8 hours for a maximum of 14 doses. Following 9 days of rest, the schedule is repeated for another 14 doses, for a maximum of 28 doses per course.

DRUG INTERACTION 1
Corticosteroids—May decrease the antitumor efficacy of IL-2 due to its inhibitory effect on the immune system.

DRUG INTERACTION 2
Nonsteroidal anti-inflammatory drugs NSAIDs—May enhance the capillary leak syndrome observed with IL-2.

DRUG INTERACTION 3
Antihypertensives—IL-2 potentiates the effect of antihypertensive medications. For this reason, all antihypertensives should be stopped at least 24 hours before IL-2 treatment.

SPECIAL CONSIDERATIONS
1. Use with caution in patients with pre-existing cardiac, pulmonary, central nervous system (CNS), hepatic, and/or renal impairment as there is an increased risk for developing serious and sometimes fatal reactions.
2. Pretreatment evaluation should include CBC; serum chemistries, including LFTs, renal function, and electrolytes; pulmonary function tests (PFTs); and stress thallium.

3. Patients should be monitored closely throughout the entire treatment, including vital signs every 2–4 hours, strict input and output, and daily weights. Continuous cardiopulmonary monitoring is important during therapy.
4. Monitor for capillary leak syndrome (CLS), which begins almost immediately after initiation of therapy. Manifested by hypotension, peripheral edema, ascites, pleural and/or pericardial effusions, weight gain, and altered mental status.
5. Early administration of dopamine (1–5 mg/kg/min) in the setting of CLS may maintain perfusion to the kidneys and preserve renal function.
6. Use with caution in the presence of concurrent medications known to be nephrotoxic and hepatotoxic as IL-2 therapy is associated with both nephrotoxicity and hepatotoxicity.
7. Use with caution in patients with known autoimmune disease as treatment with IL-2 is associated with autoimmune thyroiditis leading to thyroid function impairment.
8. Allergic reactions have been reported in patients receiving iodine contrast media up to 4 months following IL-2 therapy.
9. Pregnancy category C. Breastfeeding should be avoided.

TOXICITY 1
Flu-like symptoms, including fever, chills, malaise, myalgias, and arthralgias. Observed in all patients.

TOXICITY 2
Vascular leak syndrome. Usual dose-limiting toxicity, characterized by weight gain, arrhythmias, tachycardia, hypotension, edema, oliguria and renal insufficiency, pleural effusions, and pulmonary congestion.

TOXICITY 3
Myelosuppression with anemia, thrombocytopenia, and neutropenia.

TOXICITY 4
Hepatotoxicity presenting as increases in serum bilirubin levels along with changes in serum transaminases. Usually reversible within 4–6 days after discontinuation of IL-2 therapy.

TOXICITY 5
Neurologic and neuropsychiatric findings can develop both acutely and chronically during treatment. Somnolence, delirium, and confusion are common but generally resolve after drug termination. Alterations in cognitive function and impaired memory more common with continuous infusion IL-2.

TOXICITY 6
Erythema, skin rash, urticaria, and generalized erythroderma may occur within a few days of starting therapy.

TOXICITY 7
Alterations in thyroid function, including hyperthyroidism and hypothyroidism.

Alectinib

TRADE NAMES	Alecensa	CLASSIFICATION	Signal transduction inhibitor
CATEGORY	Chemotherapy drug	DRUG MANUFACTURER	Genentech/Roche

MECHANISM OF ACTION

- Inhibits multiple receptor tyrosine kinases (RTKs), including anaplastic lymphoma kinase (ALK) and RET, which leads to inhibition of downstream signaling proteins, such as STAT3 and Akt.
- Pre-clinical studies show that it inhibits tumor cell lines that have ALK fusions, amplifications, or activating mutations. Major active metabolite of alectinib is M4, and it displays similar in vitro potency and activity as the parent drug.
- Retains activity in NSCLC tumors resistant to crizotinib.

MECHANISM OF RESISTANCE

None well characterized to date.

ABSORPTION

Rapidly absorbed after an oral dose with peak plasma levels achieved within 4 hours. Absolute oral bioavailability is approximately 37%. Food with a high fat content can significantly increase drug concentrations by up to 3-fold.

DISTRIBUTION

Extensive binding of alectinib and M4 metabolite (>99%) to plasma proteins.

METABOLISM

Metabolized in the liver primarily by CYP3A4 microsomal enzymes with formation of the major active metabolite M4. Elimination is mainly hepatic with excretion in feces (98%) with 84% as unchanged parent drug and 6% as M4 metabolite. Renal elimination is relatively minor with <0.5% of an administered dose being recovered in the urine. Steady-state drug levels of parent alectinib and the M4 metabolite are achieved in approximately 7 days. The terminal half-life of alectinib is approximately 33 hours and 31 hours for the M4 metabolite.

INDICATIONS
FDA-approved for the treatment of patients with ALK-positive metastatic NSCLC who have progressed on or are intolerant to crizotinib.

DOSAGE RANGE
Recommended dose is 600 mg PO daily.

DRUG INTERACTION 1
Drugs such as ketoconazole, itraconazole, erythromycin, clarithromycin, atazanavir, indinavir, nefazodone, nelfinavir, ritonavir, saquinavir, telithromycin, and voriconazole may decrease the rate of metabolism of alectinib, resulting in increased drug levels and potentially increased toxicity.

DRUG INTERACTION 2
Drugs such as rifampin, phenytoin, phenobarbital, carbamazepine, and St. John's Wort may increase the rate of metabolism of alectinib, resulting in its inactivation.

SPECIAL CONSIDERATIONS
1. Use with caution in patients with hepatic dysfunction, as alectinib is eliminated mainly via the liver.
2. No dose adjustment is needed for patients with mild hepatic dysfunction. However, the drug has not been evaluated in patients with moderate to severe hepatic dysfunction.
3. No dose reduction is needed for patients with mild or moderate renal dysfunction. However, the drug has not been evaluated in patients with severe renal dysfunction or end-stage renal disease.
4. Patients receiving alectinib along with oral warfarin anticoagulant therapy should have their coagulation parameters (PT and INR) monitored frequently.
5. Monitor LFTs and serum bilirubin every 2 weeks for the first 2 months of treatment and then periodically, as alectinib may cause hepatotoxicity. More frequent testing is required in patients who develop LFT elevations. May need to suspend, dose-reduce, or permanently stop alectinib with the development of drug-induced hepatotoxicity.
6. Closely monitor patients for new or progressive pulmonary symptoms, including cough, dyspnea, and fever.
7. Closely monitor heart rate and blood pressure for evidence of bradycardia.
8. Monitor CPK levels every 2 weeks during the first month of treatment and in patients with unexplained muscle pain, tenderness, or weakness.
9. ALK testing using an FDA-approved test is required to confirm the presence of ALK-positive NSCLC for determining which patients should receive alectinib therapy.
10. Pregnancy category D. Breastfeeding should be avoided.

TOXICITY 1

Hepatotoxicity with elevations in serum transaminases (SGOT, SGPT).

TOXICITY 2

Nausea/vomiting, constipation, diarrhea, and abdominal pain are the most common GI side effects.

TOXICITY 3

Pulmonary toxicity with increased cough, dyspnea, fever, and pulmonary infiltrates.

TOXICITY 4

Constitutional side effects with fatigue, asthenia, and anorexia.

TOXICITY 5

Bradycardia.

TOXICITY 6

Myalgia or musculoskeletal pain with CPK elevation.

TOXICITY 7

Skin rash.

Alemtuzumab

TRADE NAME	Campath	**CLASSIFICATION**	Monoclonal antibody
CATEGORY	Biologic response modifier agent	**DRUG MANUFACTURER**	Genzyme

MECHANISM OF ACTION

- Recombinant humanized monoclonal antibody (Campath-1H) directed against the 21–28 kDa cell-surface glycoprotein CD52 that is expressed on most normal and malignant B and T lymphocytes, NK cells, monocytes, and macrophages.
- CD52 antigen is not expressed on the surface of hematopoietic stem cells and mature plasma cells.
- Immunologic mechanisms involved in antitumor activity, including ADCC and/or complement-mediated cell lysis.

MECHANISM OF RESISTANCE
None yet defined.

ABSORPTION
Alemtuzumab is given only by the IV route.

DISTRIBUTION
Peak and trough levels rise during the first few weeks of therapy and approach steady-state levels by week 6. However, there is marked variability, and drug levels correlate roughly with the number of circulating CD52+ B cells.

METABOLISM
Metabolism has not been extensively characterized. Half-life is on the order of 12 days with minimal clearance by the liver and kidneys.

INDICATIONS
1. Relapsed and/or refractory B-cell chronic lymphocytic leukemia (B-CLL)—Indicated in patients who have been treated with alkylating agents and who have failed fludarabine therapy.
2. T-cell prolymphocytic leukemia—Clinical activity in patients who failed first-line therapy.

DOSAGE RANGE
Recommended dose is 30 mg/day IV three times per week for a maximum of 12 weeks.

DRUG INTERACTIONS
None known.

SPECIAL CONSIDERATIONS
1. Contraindicated in patients with active systemic infections, underlying immunodeficiency (HIV-positive, AIDS, etc.), or known type I hypersensitivity or anaphylactic reactions to alemtuzumab or any of its components.
2. Patients should be premedicated with acetaminophen, 650 mg PO, and diphenhydramine, 50 mg PO, 30 minutes before drug infusion to reduce the incidence of infusion-related reactions.
3. Alemtuzumab should be initiated at a dose of 3 mg, administered daily as a 2-hour IV infusion. When this daily dose of 3 mg is tolerated, the daily dose can then be increased to 10 mg. Once the 10-mg daily dose is tolerated, the maintenance dose of 30 mg daily can then be initiated. This maintenance dose of 30 mg/day is administered three times each week on alternate days (Monday, Wednesday, and Friday) for a maximum of 12 weeks. Dose escalation to the 30-mg daily dose usually can be accomplished within 7 days. Alemtuzumab should **NOT** be given by IV push or bolus.

4. Monitor closely for infusion-related events, which usually occur within the first 30–60 minutes after the start of the infusion and most commonly during the first week of therapy. Pulse, blood pressure, and oral temperature should be measured every 15–30 minutes. Immediate institution of diphenhydramine (50 mg IV), acetaminophen (625 mg PO), hydrocortisone (200 mg IV), and/or vasopressors may be required. Resuscitation equipment should be readily available at bedside.

5. Patients should be placed on anti-infective prophylaxis upon initiation of therapy to reduce the risk of serious opportunistic infections. This should include Bactrim DS, 1 tablet PO bid three times per week, and famciclovir or equivalent, 250 mg PO bid. Fluconazole may also be included in the regimen to reduce the incidence of fungal infections. If a serious infection occurs while on therapy, alemtuzumab should be stopped immediately and only reinitiated following the complete resolution of the underlying infection.

6. Monitor CBC and platelet counts on a weekly basis during alemtuzumab therapy. Treatment should be stopped for severe hematologic toxicity or in any patient with evidence of autoimmune anemia and/ or thrombocytopenia.

7. Most significant antitumor effects of alemtuzumab are observed in peripheral blood, bone marrow, and spleen. Tumor cells usually cleared from blood within 1–2 weeks of initiation of therapy, while normalization in bone marrow may take up to 6–12 weeks. Lymph nodes, especially those that are large and bulky, seem to be less responsive to therapy.

8. Pregnancy category C. Should be given to a pregnant woman only if clearly indicated. Breastfeeding should be avoided during treatment and for at least 3 months following the last dose of drug.

TOXICITY 1

Infusion-related symptoms, including fever, chills, nausea and vomiting, urticaria, skin rash, fatigue, headache, diarrhea, dyspnea, and/or hypotension. Usually occur within the first week of initiation of therapy.

TOXICITY 2

Significant immunosuppressive agent with an increased incidence of opportunistic infections, including *Pneumocystis jiroveci* (formerly *carinii*), cytomegalovirus (CMV), herpes zoster, *Candida, Cryptococcus*, and *Listeria* meningitis. Prophylaxis with anti-infective agents is indicated as outlined above. Recovery of CD4 and CD8 counts is slow and may take over 1 year to return to normal.

TOXICITY 3

Myelosuppression with neutropenia most common, but anemia and thrombocytopenia also observed. In rare instances, pancytopenia with marrow hypoplasia occurs, which can be fatal.

Altretamine

TRADE NAMES	Hexalen, Hexamethylmelamine, HMM	CLASSIFICATION	Nonclassic alkylating agent
CATEGORY	Chemotherapy drug	DRUG MANUFACTURER	MGI Pharma

MECHANISM OF ACTION
- Triazine derivative that requires biochemical activation in the liver for its antitumor activity.
- Exact mechanism(s) of action unclear but appears to act like an alkylating agent. Forms cross-links with DNA, resulting in inhibition of DNA synthesis and function.
- May also inhibit RNA synthesis.

MECHANISM OF RESISTANCE
- Mechanisms of resistance have not been well characterized.
- Does not exhibit cross-resistance to other classic alkylating agents and does not exhibit multidrug-resistant phenotype.

ABSORPTION
Oral absorption is extremely variable secondary to extensive first-pass metabolism in the liver. Peak plasma levels are achieved 0.5–3 hours after an oral dose.

DISTRIBUTION
Widely distributed throughout the body, with highest concentrations found in tissues with high fat content. About 90% of drug is bound to plasma proteins.

METABOLISM
Extensively metabolized in the liver by the microsomal P450 system. Less than 1% of parent compound is excreted in urine. About 60% of drug is eliminated in urine as demethylated metabolites (pentamethylmelamine and tetramethylmelamine) within the first 24 hours. The terminal elimination half-life is on the order of 4–10 hours.

INDICATIONS
Ovarian cancer—Active in advanced disease and in persistent and/or recurrent tumors following first-line therapy with a cisplatin- and/or alkylating agent–based regimen.

DOSAGE RANGE

Usual dose is 260 mg/m²/day PO for either 14 or 21 days on a 28-day schedule. Total daily dose is given in four divided doses after meals and bedtime.

DRUG INTERACTION 1

Cimetidine—Cimetidine increases the half-life and subsequent toxicity of altretamine. In contrast, ranitidine does not affect drug metabolism.

DRUG INTERACTION 2

Phenobarbital—Phenobarbital may decrease the half-life and toxicity of altretamine.

DRUG INTERACTION 3

Monoamine oxidase (MAO) inhibitors—Concurrent use of MAO inhibitors with altretamine may result in significant orthostatic hypotension.

SPECIAL CONSIDERATIONS

1. Closely monitor patient for signs of neurologic toxicity.
2. Vitamin B6 (pyridoxine) may be used to decrease the incidence and severity of neurologic toxicity. However, antitumor activity may be compromised with vitamin B6 treatment.
3. Pregnancy category D. Breastfeeding should be avoided.

TOXICITY 1

Nausea and vomiting. Usually mild to moderate, observed in 30% of patients, and worsens with increasing cumulative doses of drug.

TOXICITY 2

Myelosuppression. Dose-limiting toxicity. Leukocyte and platelet nadirs occur at 3–4 weeks with recovery by day 28. Anemia occurs in 20% of patients.

TOXICITY 3

Neurotoxicity in the form of somnolence, mood changes, lethargy, depression, agitation, hallucinations, and peripheral neuropathy. Observed in about 25% of patients.

TOXICITY 4

Hypersensitivity, skin rash.

TOXICITY 5

Elevations in LFTs, mainly alkaline phosphatase.

TOXICITY 6

Flu-like syndrome in the form of fever, malaise, arthralgias, and myalgias.

TOXICITY 7

Abdominal cramps and diarrhea are occasionally observed.

Aminoglutethimide

TRADE NAME	Cytadren	CLASSIFICATION	Adrenal steroid inhibitor
CATEGORY	Hormonal agent	DRUG MANUFACTURER	Novartis

MECHANISM OF ACTION
- Nonsteroidal inhibitor of corticosteroid biosynthesis.
- Produces a chemical adrenalectomy with a decreased synthesis of estrogens, androgens, glucocorticoids, and mineralocorticoids.

ABSORPTION
Excellent bioavailability via the oral route. Peak plasma concentrations occur within 1–1.5 hours after ingestion.

DISTRIBUTION
Approximately 25% of the drug is bound to plasma proteins. Significant reduction in distribution with prolonged treatment.

METABOLISM
Metabolized in the liver by the cytochrome P450 system with N-acetylaminoglutethimide being the major metabolite. Metabolism is under genetic control, and acetylator status of patients is important. About 40%–50% of the drug is excreted unchanged in the urine. Initial half-life of drug is about 13 hours but decreases to 7 hours with chronic treatment, suggesting that the drug may accelerate its own rate of degradation.

INDICATIONS
1. Breast cancer—Hormone-responsive, advanced disease.
2. Prostate cancer—Hormone-responsive, advanced disease.

DOSAGE RANGE
Usual dose is 250 mg PO qid (1000 mg total).

DRUG INTERACTION 1
Warfarin, phenytoin, phenobarbital, theophylline, medroxyprogesterone, and digoxin—Aminoglutethimide enhances the metabolism of warfarin, phenytoin, phenobarbital, theophylline, medroxyprogesterone, and digoxin, thereby decreasing their clinical activity.

DRUG INTERACTION 2
Dexamethasone—Aminoglutethimide enhances the metabolism of dexamethasone but not hydrocortisone.

SPECIAL CONSIDERATIONS
1. Administer hydrocortisone along with aminoglutethimide to prevent adrenal insufficiency. The use of higher doses during the initial 2 weeks of therapy reduces the frequency of adverse events. For example, start at 100 mg PO daily for the first 2 weeks, then 40 mg PO daily in divided doses. Higher doses of steroid replacement may be required under conditions of stress such as surgery, trauma, or acute infection.
2. Closely monitor patient for signs and symptoms of hypothyroidism. Monitor thyroid function tests on a regular basis.
3. Monitor for signs and symptoms of orthostatic hypotension. May need to add fludrocortisone (Florinef) 0.1–0.2 mg PO qd.
4. Monitor patient for signs of somnolence and lethargy. Severe cases may warrant immediate discontinuation of drug.
5. Discontinue drug if skin rash persists for more than 1 week.
6. Pregnancy category D. Breastfeeding should be avoided.

TOXICITY 1
Maculopapular skin rash. Usually seen in the first week of therapy. Self-limited with resolution in 5–7 days, and discontinuation of therapy not necessary.

TOXICITY 2
Fatigue, lethargy, and somnolence. Occur in 40% of patients, and onset is within the first week of therapy. Dizziness, nystagmus, and ataxia are less common (10% of patients).

TOXICITY 3
Mild nausea and vomiting.

TOXICITY 4
Hypothyroidism.

TOXICITY 5
Adrenal insufficiency. Occurs in the absence of hydrocortisone replacement. Presents as postural hypotension, hyponatremia, and hyperkalemia.

TOXICITY 6
Myelosuppression. Leukopenia and thrombocytopenia rarely occur.

Anastrozole

TRADE NAME	Arimidex	**CLASSIFICATION**	Nonsteroidal aromatase inhibitor
CATEGORY	Hormonal agent	**DRUG MANUFACTURER**	AstraZeneca

MECHANISM OF ACTION
- Potent and selective nonsteroidal inhibitor of aromatase.
- Inhibits the synthesis of estrogens by inhibiting the conversion of adrenal androgens (androstenedione and testosterone) to estrogens (estrone, estrone sulfate, and estradiol). Serum estradiol levels are suppressed by 90% within 14 days, and nearly completely suppressed after 6 weeks of therapy.
- No inhibitory effect on adrenal corticosteroid or aldosterone biosynthesis.

MECHANISM OF RESISTANCE
- Decreased expression of estrogen receptors (ER).
- Mutations in the ER leading to decreased binding affinity to anastrozole.
- Overexpression of growth factor receptors, such as EGFR, HER2/neu, IGF-1R, or TGF-β that counteract the inhibitory effects of anastrozole.
- Presence of ESR1 mutations.

ABSORPTION
Excellent bioavailability via the oral route, with 85% of a dose absorbed within 2 hours of ingestion. Absorption is not affected by food.

DISTRIBUTION
Widely distributed throughout the body. About 40% of drug is bound to plasma proteins.

METABOLISM
Extensively metabolized in the liver (up to 85%) by N-dealkylation, hydroxylation, and glucuronidation, to inactive forms. Half-life of drug is about 50 hours. Steady-state levels of drug are achieved after 7 days of a once-daily administration. The major route of elimination is fecal, with renal excretion accounting for only 10% of drug clearance.

INDICATIONS

1. Metastatic breast cancer—FDA-approved for the first-line treatment of postmenopausal women with hormone-receptor positive or hormone-receptor unknown disease.
2. Metastatic breast cancer—Postmenopausal women with hormone-receptor positive, advanced disease, and progression while on tamoxifen therapy.
3. Adjuvant treatment of postmenopausal women with hormone-receptor positive, early-stage breast cancer; FDA-approved.

DOSAGE RANGE

1. Metastatic breast cancer—Recommended dose is 1 mg PO qd for both first-and second-line therapy.
2. Early-stage breast cancer—Recommended dose is 1 mg PO qd for adjuvant therapy. The optimal duration of therapy is unknown. In the ATAC trial, anastrozole was given for 5 years.

DRUG INTERACTIONS

None well characterized.

SPECIAL CONSIDERATIONS

1. No dose adjustments are required for patients with either hepatic or renal dysfunction.
2. Caution patients about the risk of hot flashes.
3. No need for glucocorticoid and/or mineralocorticoid replacement.
4. Closely monitor women with osteoporosis or at risk of osteoporosis by performing bone densitometry at the start of therapy and at regular intervals. Treatment or prophylaxis for osteoporosis should be initiated when appropriate.
5. Pregnancy category D. Breastfeeding should be avoided.

TOXICITY 1

Asthenia is most common toxicity and occurs in up to 20% of patients.

TOXICITY 2

Mild nausea and vomiting. Constipation or diarrhea can also occur.

TOXICITY 3

Hot flashes. Occur in 10% of patients.

TOXICITY 4

Dry, scaling skin rash.

TOXICITY 5

Arthralgias occur in 10%–15% of patients involving hands, knees, hips, lower back, and shoulders. Early morning stiffness is usual presentation.

TOXICITY 6

Headache.

TOXICITY 7
Peripheral edema in 7% of patients.

TOXICITY 8
Flu-like syndrome in the form of fever, malaise, and myalgias.

Arsenic trioxide (As_2O_3)

TRADE NAME	Trisenox	**CLASSIFICATION**	Natural product
CATEGORY	Chemotherapy and differentiating agent	**DRUG MANUFACTURER**	Cephalon, Teva

MECHANISM OF ACTION
- Precise mechanism of action has not been fully elucidated.
- Induces differentiation of acute promyelocytic leukemic cells by degrading the chimeric PML/RAR-α protein, resulting in release of the maturation block at the promyelocyte stage of myelocyte differentiation.
- Induces apoptosis through a mitochondrial-dependent pathway, resulting in release of cytochrome C and subsequent caspase activation.
- Direct antiproliferative activity by arresting cells at either the G1-S or G2-M checkpoints.
- Inhibits the process of angiogenesis through apoptosis of endothelial cells and/or inhibition of production of critical angiogenic factors, including vascular endothelial growth factor.

MECHANISM OF RESISTANCE
None well characterized to date.

ABSORPTION
Arsenic trioxide is given only by the IV route.

DISTRIBUTION
Widely distributes in liver, kidneys, heart, lung, hair, nails, and skin.

METABOLISM
The clinical pharmacology of arsenic trioxide has not been well characterized. Metabolism occurs via reduction of pentavalent arsenic to trivalent arsenic and methylation reactions mediated by methyltransferase enzymes that occur primarily in the liver. However, the methyltransferases appear to be distinct from the liver microsomal P450 system. The methylated trivalent arsenic metabolite is excreted mainly in the urine.

INDICATIONS

Acute promyelocytic leukemia (APL)—FDA-approved for induction of remission and consolidation in patients with APL who are refractory to or have relapsed following first-line therapy with all-trans retinoic acid (ATRA) and anthracycline-based chemotherapy and whose APL is characterized by the presence of the t(15;17) translocation or PML/RAR-α gene expression.

DOSAGE RANGE

- Induction therapy—0.15 mg/kg/day IV for a maximum of 60 days.
- Consolidation therapy—Should be initiated 3 weeks after completion of induction treatment and only in those patients who achieve a complete bone marrow remission. The recommended dosage is 0.15 mg/ kg/day IV for 5 days/week for a total of 5 weeks.

DRUG INTERACTION 1

Medications that can prolong the QT interval such as antiarrhythmics—Increased risk of prolongation of the QT interval and subsequent arrhythmias when arsenic trioxide is administered concomitantly.

DRUG INTERACTION 2

Amphotericin B—Increased risk of prolonged QT interval and torsades de pointes ventricular arrhythmia in patients receiving amphotericin and induction therapy with arsenic trioxide.

SPECIAL CONSIDERATIONS

1. Contraindicated in patients who are hypersensitive to arsenic.
2. Use with caution in patients who are on agents that prolong the QT interval, in those who have a history of Torsades de Pointes, pre-existing QT interval prolongation, untreated sinus node dysfunction, high-degree atrioventricular block, or in those who may be severely dehydrated or malnourished at baseline.
3. Use with caution in patients with renal impairment as renal excretion is the main route of elimination of arsenic.
4. Before initiation of therapy, all patients should have a baseline electrocardiogram (ECG) performed and serum electrolytes, calcium, magnesium, blood urea nitrogen (BUN), and creatinine should be evaluated. Any pre-existing electrolyte abnormalities should be corrected before starting therapy.
5. Serum electrolytes and magnesium should be closely monitored during therapy. Serum potassium concentrations should be maintained above 4 mEq/L and magnesium concentrations above 1.8 mg/dL.
6. Therapy should be stopped when the QT interval >500 milliseconds and only resumed when the QT interval drops to below 460 milliseconds, all electrolyte abnormalities are corrected, and cardiac monitoring shows no evidence of arrhythmias.
7. Monitor closely for new-onset fever, dyspnea, weight gain, abnormal respiratory symptoms and/or physical findings, or chest X-ray abnormalities, because 30% of patients will develop the APL

differentiation syndrome. This syndrome can be fatal, and high-dose steroids with dexamethasone 10 mg IV bid should be started immediately and continued for 3–5 days. While this syndrome more commonly occurs with median baseline white blood cells of 5000 mm^3, it can occur in the absence of leukocytosis. In most cases, therapy can be resumed once the syndrome has completely resolved.

8. Monitor CBC every other day and bone marrow cytology every 10 days during induction therapy.
9. Pregnancy category D. Breastfeeding should be avoided as arsenic is excreted in breast milk.

TOXICITY 1
Fatigue.

TOXICITY 2
Prolonged QT interval (>500 msec) on ECG seen in 40%–50% of patients. Does not usually increase upon repeat exposure to arsenic trioxide, and QT interval returns to baseline following termination of therapy. Torsades de Pointes ventricular arrhythmia and/or complete AV block can be observed in this setting.

TOXICITY 3
APL differentiation syndrome. Occurs in about 30% of patients and is characterized by fever, dyspnea, skin rash, fluid retention and weight gain, pleural and/or pericardial effusions. This syndrome is identical to the retinoic acid syndrome observed with retinoid therapy.

TOXICITY 4
Leukocytosis is observed in 50%–60% of patients with a gradual increase in white blood cells (WBCs) that peaks between 2 and 3 weeks after starting therapy. Usually resolves spontaneously without treatment and/or complications.

TOXICITY 5
Light-headedness most commonly observed during drug infusion.

TOXICITY 6
Mild nausea and vomiting, abdominal pain, and diarrhea.

TOXICITY 7
Musculoskeletal pain.

TOXICITY 8
Mild hyperglycemia.

TOXICITY 9
Peripheral neuropathy.

TOXICITY 10
Carcinogen and teratogen.

Asparaginase

TRADE NAMES	Elspar, L-Asparaginase	**CLASSIFICATION**	Enzyme
CATEGORY	Chemotherapy drug	**DRUG MANUFACTURER**	Merck

MECHANISM OF ACTION
- Purified from *Escherichia coli* and/or *Erwinia chrysanthemi*.
- Tumor cells lack asparagine synthetase and thus require exogenous sources of L-asparagine.
- L-Asparaginase hydrolyzes circulating L-asparagine to aspartic acid and ammonia.
- Depletion of the essential amino acid L-asparagine results in rapid inhibition of protein synthesis. Cytotoxicity of drug correlates well with inhibition of protein synthesis.

MECHANISM OF RESISTANCE
- Increased expression of the L-asparagine synthetase gene, which facilitates the cellular production of L-asparagine from endogenous sources.
- Formation of antibodies against L-asparaginase, resulting in inhibition of function.

ABSORPTION
L-Asparaginase is not orally bioavailable.

DISTRIBUTION
Remains in the vascular compartment after IV administration. After intramuscular (IM) injection, peak plasma levels are reached within 14–24 hours. Peak plasma levels after IM injection are 50% lower than those achieved with IV injection. Plasma protein binding is on the order of 30%. The apparent volume of distribution is about 70%–80% of the plasma volume. Cerebrospinal fluid (CSF) penetration is negligible (<1% of plasma level).

METABOLISM
Metabolism is not well characterized. Minimal urinary and/or biliary excretion occurs. Plasma half-life depends on formulation of drug; 40–50 hours for *E. coli*–derived L-asparaginase and 3–5 days for polyethylene glycol (PEG)-asparaginase.

INDICATIONS
Acute lymphocytic leukemia.

DOSAGE RANGE
1. Dose varies depending on specific regimens. L-Asparaginase is given at a dose of 6000–10,000 IU/m^2 IM every 3 days for a total of nine doses. Treatment with L-asparaginase is started after completion of other chemotherapy drugs used in the induction therapy of acute lymphoblastic leukemia (vincristine, prednisone, and doxorubicin).

2. L-Asparaginase is given less commonly as a single agent at a dose of 200 IU/kg IV for 28 consecutive days.

DRUG INTERACTION 1

Methotrexate—L-Asparaginase can inhibit the cytotoxic effects of methotrexate and thus rescue from methotrexate antitumor activity and host toxicity. It is recommended that these drugs be administered 24 hours apart.

DRUG INTERACTION 2

Vincristine—L-Asparaginase inhibits the clearance of vincristine, resulting in increased host toxicity, especially neurotoxicity. Vincristine should be administered 12–24 hours before L-asparaginase.

SPECIAL CONSIDERATIONS

1. An intradermal skin test dose of 2 IU should be performed before the initial administration of L-asparaginase or whenever the dose is being repeated more than 1 week from the immediately previous one. The patient should be observed for at least 1 hour before the full dose is given. A negative dermal test does not completely rule out the possibility of an allergic reaction.
2. Monitor patient for allergic reactions and/or anaphylaxis. Contraindicated in patients with a prior history of anaphylactic reaction. L-Asparaginase isolated from the Erwinia species may be tried in patients previously treated with E. coli asparaginase, but allergic reactions may still occur.
3. L-Asparaginase is a contact irritant in both powder and solution forms. The drug must be handled and administered with caution.
4. Induction treatment of acute lymphoblastic leukemia with L-asparaginase may induce rapid lysis of blast cells. Prophylaxis against tumor lysis syndrome with vigorous IV hydration, urinary alkalinization, and allopurinol is recommended for all patients.
5. Contraindicated in patients with either active pancreatitis or a history of pancreatitis. If pancreatitis develops while on therapy, L-asparaginase should be stopped immediately.
6. Close monitoring of LFTs, amylase, coagulation tests, and fibrinogen levels.
7. L-Asparaginase can interfere with thyroid function tests. This effect is probably due to a marked reduction in serum concentration of thyroxine-binding globulin, which is observed within 2 days after the first dose. Levels of thyroxine-binding globulin return to normal within 4 weeks of the last dose.
8. Pregnancy category C. Breastfeeding should be avoided.

TOXICITY 1

Hypersensitivity reaction. Occurs in up to 25% of patients. Mild form manifested by skin rash and urticaria. Anaphylactic reaction may be life-threatening and presents as bronchospasm, respiratory distress, and hypotension. Resuscitation drugs and equipment should be readily available at bedside before drug treatment.

TOXICITY 2

Fever, chills, nausea, and vomiting. Acute reaction observed in about two-thirds of patients.

TOXICITY 3

Mild elevation in LFTs, including serum bilirubin, alkaline phosphatase, and SGOT. Common and usually transient. Liver biopsy reveals fatty changes.

TOXICITY 4

Increased risk of both bleeding and clotting. Alterations in clotting with decreased levels of clotting factors, including fibrinogen, factors IX and XI, antithrombin III, proteins C and S, plasminogen, and α-2-antiplasmin. Observed in over 50% of patients.

TOXICITY 5

Pancreatitis develops in up to 10% of patients. Usually manifested as transient increase in serum amylase levels with quick resolution upon cessation of therapy.

TOXICITY 6

Neurologic toxicity, including lethargy, confusion, agitation, hallucinations, and/ or coma. These side effects may require treatment discontinuation. Severe neurotoxicity resembles ammonia toxicity.

TOXICITY 7

Myelosuppression is mild and rarely observed.

TOXICITY 8

Decreased serum levels of insulin, lipoproteins, and albumin.

TOXICITY 9

Renal toxicity. Usually mild and manifested by mild elevations in BUN and creatinine, proteinuria, and elevated serum acid levels.

Atezolizumab

TRADE NAMES	Tecentriq	CLASSIFICATION	Monoclonal antibody
CATEGORY	Immune checkpoint inhibitor	DRUG MANUFACTURER	Genentech/ Roche

MECHANISM OF ACTION

- Humanized IgG4 antibody that binds to the PD-L1 ligand expressed on tumor cells an/or tumor infiltrating cells, which then blocks the interaction between the PD-L1 ligand and the PD-1 and B7.1 receptors found on T cells and antigen presenting cells.
- Blockade of the PD-1 pathway-mediated immune checkpoint overcomes immune escape mechanisms and enhances T-cell immune response, leading to T-cell activation and proliferation.

MECHANISM OF RESISTANCE

- Increased expression and/or activity of other immune checkpoint pathways.
- Increased expression of other immune escape mechanisms.

DISTRIBUTION

Distribution in body is not well characterized. Steady-state levels are achieved by 6-9 weeks.

METABOLISM

Metabolism of atezolizumab has not been extensively characterized. The terminal half-life is on the order of 27 days.

INDICATIONS

FDA-approved for locally advanced or metastatic bladder cancer who have disease progression during or following platinum-based chemotherapy or who have disease progression within 12 months of neoadjuvant or adjuvant therapy with platinum-based chemotherapy.

DOSAGE RANGE

Recommended dose is 1200 mg IV every 3 weeks.

DRUG INTERACTIONS

None well characterized to date.

SPECIAL CONSIDERATIONS

1. Atezolizumab can result in significant immune-mediated adverse reactions due to T-cell activation and proliferation. These immune-mediated reactions may involve any organ system, with the most common reactions being pneumonitis, hepatitis, colitis, hypophysitis, pancreatitis, neurological disorders, and adrenal and thyroid dysfunction.
2. Atezolizumab should be withheld for any of the following:
   - Grade 2 pneumonitis
   - Grade 2 or 3 colitis
   - SGOT/SGPT >3×ULN and up to 5×ULN or total bilirubin >1.5×ULN and up to 3×ULN
   - Symptomatic hypophysitis, adrenal insufficiency, hypothyroidism, hyperthyroidism, or grade ¾ hyperglycemia
   - Grade 2 ocular inflammatory toxicity
   - Grade 2 or 3 pancreatitis or grade 3 or 4 increases in serum amylase or lipase levels
   - Grade 3 or 4 infection
   - Grade 2 infusion-related reactions
   - Grade 3 skin rash
3. Atezolizumab should be permanently discontinued for any of the following:
   - Grade 3 or 4 pneumonitis
   - SGOT/SGPT >5×ULN or total bilirubin >3×ULN

- Grade 4 diarrhea or colitis
- Grade 4 hypophysitis
- Myasthenic syndrome/myasthenia gravis, Guillain-Barré or meningoencephalitis (all grades)
- Grade 3 or 4 ocular inflammatory toxicity
- Grade 4 or any grade of recurrent pancreatitis
- Grade 3 or 4 infusion-related reactions
- Grade 4 skin rash

4. The first infusion should be administered over 60 minutes. If the first infusion is well-tolerated, all subsequent infusions may be delivered over 30 minutes.
5. Monitor for symptoms and signs of infection.
6. Monitor thyroid and adrenal function prior to and during therapy.
7. Dose modification is not needed for patients with renal dysfunction.
8. Dose modification is not needed for patients with mild hepatic dysfunction. Atezolizumab has not been studied in patients with moderate or severe hepatic dysfunction.
9. Pregnancy category D.

TOXICITY 1
Colitis with diarrhea and abdominal pain.

TOXICITY 2
Pneumonitis with dyspnea and cough.

TOXICITY 3
GI side effects with nausea/vomiting; dry mouth; hepatitis with elevations in SGOT/SGPT, alkaline phosphatase, and serum bilirubin.

TOXICITY 4
Immune-related endocrinopathies, including hypophysitis, thyroid disorders, adrenal insufficiency, and diabetes

TOXICITY 5
Pancreatitis.

TOXICITY 6
Immune-related neurologic disorders, including myasthenic syndrome/myasthenia gravis, Guillan-Barré, or meningo-encephalitis.

TOXICITY 7
Hyperglycemia.

TOXICITY 8
Infections with sepsis, herpes encephalitis, and mycobacterial infections. All-grade infections in up to 38% of patients and >grade 3 infections seen in 11% of patients with urinary tract infections being the most common cause of >grade 3 infections.

TOXICITY 9
Infusion-related reactions.

TOXICITY 10
Ocular toxicity.

TOXICITY 11
Maculopapular skin rash, erythema, dermatitis, and pruritus.

TOXICITY 12
Fatigue, anorexia, and asthenia.

Axitinib

TRADE NAMES	Inlyta, AG-13736	CLASSIFICATION	Signal transduction inhibitor
CATEGORY	Chemotherapy drug	DRUG MANUFACTURER	Pfizer

MECHANISM OF ACTION
- Small-molecule inhibitor of the ATP-binding domains of VEGFR-1, VEGFR-2, and VEGFR-3 tyrosine kinases.
- Shows limited effects on platelet-derived growth factor (PDGFR) and c-Kit (CD117).
- Interferes with processes involved in tumor growth and proliferation, metastasis, and angiogenesis.

MECHANISM OF RESISTANCE
- Mechanisms of resistance have not been well characterized.
- Increased expression of VEGFR-1, VEGFR-2, and VEGFR-3.

ABSORPTION
Rapid oral absorption when given with food with a mean absolute bioavailability of approximately 60%. Peak plasma concentrations are reached 2 to 6 hours after oral ingestion, and steady state is achieved within 2 to 3 days of dosing.

DISTRIBUTION
Volume of distribution is 160 L. Extensively bound (>99%) to albumin and to α1-acid glycoprotein.

METABOLISM

Metabolism is primarily in the liver by CYP3A4 and CYP3A5 enzymes and to a lesser extent by CYP1A2, CYP2C19, and UGT1A1. Sulfoxide and N-glucuronide metabolites are significantly less potent against VEGFR-2 compared to parent drug. Hepatobiliary excretion is the main pathway of drug elimination. Approximately 40% is eliminated in feces, of which 12% as unchanged drug, and 23% in the urine as metabolites. The terminal half-life is 2 to 5 hours.

INDICATIONS

FDA-approved for the treatment of advanced renal cell carcinoma after failure of one prior systemic therapy.

DOSAGE RANGE

Recommended starting dose is 5 mg PO bid. Dose can be increased or decreased based on tolerability or safety. Dose increase—If dose is tolerated for at least 2 consecutive weeks, dose can be increased to 7 mg PO bid, then up to 10 mg PO bid. Dose reduction—To minimize the risk of adverse events, the dose can be decreased to 3 mg PO bid, then to 2 mg PO bid.

DRUG INTERACTION 1

Drugs such as ketoconazole, itraconazole, erythromycin, clarithromycin, atazanavir, indinavir, nefazodone, nelfinavir, ritonavir, saquinavir, telithromycin, and voriconazole may decrease the rate of metabolism of axitinib, resulting in increased drug levels and potentially increased toxicity.

DRUG INTERACTION 2

Drugs such as rifampin, phenytoin, phenobarbital, carbamazepine, and St. John's Wort may increase the rate of metabolism of axitinib, resulting in its inactivation.

DRUG INTERACTION 3

Proton pump inhibitors, H2-receptor inhibitors, and antacids—Drugs that alter the pH of the upper GI tract may alter axitinib solubility, thereby reducing drug bioavailability and decreasing systemic drug exposure.

SPECIAL CONSIDERATIONS

1. No dose adjustment is needed for patients with CrCl > 15 mL/min. However, caution should be used in patients with end-stage renal disease.
2. Dose adjustment is not required in patients with mild hepatic impairment. The dose of axitinib should be reduced by 50% in patients with moderate impairment (Child-Pugh Class B). Axitinib has not been studied in patients with severe hepatic impairment (Child-Pugh Class C).
3. Axitinib should be taken approximately 12 hours apart with or without food and should be taken with water.
4. Patients should be warned of the increased risk of arterial thromboembolic events, including myocardial ischemia and stroke.

5. Patients should be warned of the increased risk of venous thromboembolic events, including deep vein thrombosis (DVT) and pulmonary embolism (PE).
6. Blood pressure should be well controlled prior to starting axitinib therapy. Closely monitor blood pressure while on therapy and treat as needed with standard oral antihypertensive medication.
7. Axinitib therapy should be stopped at least 24 hours prior to scheduled surgery.
8. Closely monitor thyroid function tests and thyroid-stimulating hormone (TSH), as axitinib therapy results in hypothyroidism.
9. Closely monitor LFTs and serum bilirubin while on therapy.
10. Avoid Seville oranges, starfruit, pomelos, grapefruit, and grapefruit products while on therapy.
11. Pregnancy category D. Breastfeeding should be avoided.

TOXICITY 1
Hypertension occurs in 40% of patients and usually within the first month of treatment.

TOXICITY 2
Increased risk of arterial and venous thromboembolic events.

TOXICITY 3
Bleeding complications.

TOXICITY 4
GI perforations and wound-healing complications.

TOXICITY 5
Diarrhea, nausea/vomiting, and constipation.

TOXICITY 6
Proteinuria develops in up to 10% of patients.

TOXICITY 7
Hypothyroidism.

TOXICITY 8
Elevations in SGOT/SGPT and serum bilirubin.

TOXICITY 9
Reversible posterior leukoencephalopathy syndrome (RPLS) occurs rarely (<1%) and presents with headache, seizure, lethargy, confusion, blindness, and other visual disturbances.

Azacitidine

(chemical structure diagram)

TRADE NAME	Vidaza	CLASSIFICATION	Antimetabolite, hypomethylating agent
CATEGORY	Chemotherapy drug	DRUG MANUFACTURER	Celgene

MECHANISM OF ACTION
- Cytidine analog.
- Cell cycle–specific with activity in the S-phase.
- Requires activation to the nucleotide metabolite azacitidine triphosphate.
- Incorporation of azacitidine triphosphate into RNA, resulting in inhibition of RNA processing and function.
- Incorporation of azacitidine triphosphate into DNA, resulting in inhibition of DNA methyltransferases, which then leads to a loss of DNA methylation and gene reactivation. Aberrantly silenced genes, such as tumor suppressor genes, are reactivated and expressed.

MECHANISM OF RESISTANCE
None well characterized to date.

ABSORPTION
Not available for oral use and is administered via the SC and IV route. The bioavailability of SC azacitidine is 89% relative to IV azacitidine.

DISTRIBUTION
The distribution in humans has not been fully characterized. Does cross blood-brain barrier.

METABOLISM
The precise route of elimination and metabolic fate of azacitidine is not well characterized in humans. In vitro studies suggest that azacitidine may be metabolized by the liver. One of the elimination pathways is via deamination by cytidine deaminase, found principally in the liver but also in plasma, granulocytes, intestinal epithelium, and peripheral tissues. Urinary excretion is the main route of elimination of the parent drug and its metabolites. The half-lives of azacitidine and its metabolites are approximately 4 hours.

INDICATIONS

FDA-approved for treatment of patients with myelodysplastic syndromes (MDS), including refractory anemia, refractory anemia with ringed sideroblasts, refractory anemia with excess blasts, refractory anemia with excess blasts in transformation, and chronic myelomonocytic leukemia.

DOSAGE RANGE

Recommended dose is 75 mg/m^2 SC or IV daily for 7 days. Cycles should be repeated every 4 weeks.

DRUG INTERACTIONS

None characterized to date.

SPECIAL CONSIDERATIONS

1. Patients should be treated for a minimum of four cycles, as it may take longer than four cycles for clinical benefit.
2. Patients should be pretreated with effective antiemetics to prevent nausea/vomiting.
3. Monitor complete blood counts on a regular basis during therapy.
4. Use with caution in patients with underlying kidney dysfunction. If unexplained elevations in BUN or serum creatinine occur, the next cycle should be delayed, and the subsequent dose should be reduced by 50%. If unexplained reductions in serum bicarbonate levels to <20 mEq/L occur, the subsequent dose should be reduced by 50%.
5. Pregnancy category D. Breastfeeding should be avoided.

TOXICITY 1

Myelosuppression with neutropenia and thrombocytopenia.

TOXICITY 2

Fatigue and anorexia.

TOXICITY 3

GI toxicity in the form of nausea/vomiting, constipation, and abdominal pain.

TOXICITY 4

Renal toxicity with elevations in serum creatinine, renal tubular acidosis, and hypokalemia.

TOXICITY 5

Peripheral edema.

Belinostat

TRADE NAMES	Beleodaq, PXD101	CLASSIFICATION	Histone deacetylase (HDAC) inhibitor
CATEGORY	Chemotherapy drug	DRUG MANUFACTURER	Spectrum Pharmaceuticals

MECHANISM OF ACTION
- Potent inhibitor of class I, II, and IV histone deacetylase enzymes.
- Inhibition of HDAC activity leads to accumulation of acetyl groups on the histone lysine residues, resulting in open chromatin structure and transcriptional activation.
- HDAC inhibition activates differentiation, inhibits the cell cycle, and induces cell cycle arrest and apoptosis.
- Preferential cytotoxicity towards tumor cells compared to normal cells.
- In vivo, exhibits stimulation of the immune system and blockage of angiogenesis.

MECHANISM OF RESISTANCE
None well characterized to date.

DISTRIBUTION
Belinostat has limited body tissue distribution. Approximately 92.9%–95.8% of drug is bound to plasma proteins. Plasma levels are achieved 4 hours after ingestion.

METABOLISM
Extensively metabolized in the liver by hepatic UGT1A1 with the belinostat glucuronide being the main metabolite. Also undergoes metabolism by CYP2A6, CYP2C9, and CYP3A4 enzymes to form belinostat amide and belinostat acid metabolites. Approximately 40% of belinostat is excreted renally with less than 2% of the dose recovered unchanged in urine. All major metabolites are excreted in urine within the first 24 hours after dose administration. The elimination half-life is on the order of 1 hour.

INDICATIONS
FDA-approved for the treatment of patients with relapsed or refractory peripheral T-cell lymphoma (PTCL).

DOSAGE RANGE
Recommended dose is 1000 mg/m² IV on days 1 through 5 with cycles repeated every 21 days.

DRUG INTERACTION 1
Atazanavir—Avoid concomitant administration of belinostat with atazanavir, a strong UGT1A1 inhibitor. Concomitant administration with atanazavir may increase belinostat exposure.

DRUG INTERACTION 2
Gemfibrozil—Avoid concomitant administration with gemfibrozil, a UGT1A1 inhibitor.

SPECIAL CONSIDERATIONS
1. Use with caution in patients with hepatic impairment, and especially in those with moderate and severe hepatic impairment, as belinostat has not been used in these settings.
2. Belinostat can be used safely in patients with CrCL >39 mL/min. Use with caution in patients whose CrCl <39 mL/min as the drug has not been sufficiently studied in this setting, and dose reduction may be required.
3. Serious and sometimes fatal infections, including pneumonia and sepsis, have occurred. Patients with a history of extensive or intensive chemotherapy may be at higher risk of life-threatening infections.
4. Closely monitor CBCs during therapy.
5. Monitor patients with advanced stage disease and/or high tumor burden as belinostat therapy can result in tumor lysis syndrome.
6. Fatal hepatotoxicity and liver function test abnormalities may occur. Monitor liver function tests before treatment and before the start of each cycle. Interrupt and/or adjust dosage until recovery, or permanently discontinue based on the severity of the hepatic toxicity.
7. Monitor ECG with QTc measurement at baseline and periodically during therapy as QTc prolongation has been observed, albeit not as frequently as with vorinostat and romidepsin.
8. Patients with the UGT1A1*28 allele are at increased risk for developing side effects, given the importance of UGT1A1 in drug metabolism. In this setting, the starting dose of belinostat should be reduced to 750 mg/m².
9. Pregnancy category D.

TOXICITY 1
Nausea/vomiting and diarrhea are the most common GI toxicities.

TOXICITY 2
Myelosuppression with thrombocytopenia and anemia more common than neutropenia.

TOXICITY 3
Fatigue and anorexia.

TOXICITY 4
Hepatotoxicity.

TOXICITY 5
Tumor lysis syndrome.

TOXICITY 6
Increased risk of infections.

TOXICITY 7
QTc prolongation.

Bendamustine

TRADE NAME	Treanda	**CLASSIFICATION**	Alkylating agent
CATEGORY	Chemotherapy drug	**DRUG MANUFACTURER**	Cephalon, Teva

MECHANISM OF ACTION

- Bifunctional alkylating agent consisting of a purine benzimidazole ring and a nitrogen mustard moiety.
- Forms cross-links with DNA resulting in single- and double-strand breaks and inhibition of DNA synthesis and function.
- Inhibits mitotic checkpoints and induces mitotic catastrophe, leading to cell death.
- Cell cycle–nonspecific. Active in all phases of the cell cycle.

MECHANISM OF RESISTANCE

- Increased activity of DNA repair enzymes.
- Increased expression of sulfhydryl proteins, including glutathione and glutathione-related enzymes.
- Cross-resistance between bendamustine and other alkylating agents is only partial.

ABSORPTION

High oral bioavailability on the order of 90%. No oral formulation is currently available, and as such, it is administered only by the IV route.

DISTRIBUTION

Bendamustine is highly protein bound (>95%), mainly to albumin. Protein binding is not affected by age or low serum albumin levels.

METABOLISM

Metabolized in the liver via hydrolysis to both active and inactive forms. Two active minor metabolites, M3 and M4, are mainly formed by CYP1A2 enzymes. Parent drug and its metabolites are eliminated to a large extent by the kidneys, and 45% of the parent drug is excreted in urine. The elimination half-life of the parent compound is approximately 40 minutes.

INDICATIONS

1. FDA-approved for the treatment of chronic lymphocytic leukemia (CLL).
2. FDA-approved for the treatment of indolent B-cell non-Hodgkin's lymphoma that has progressed during or within 6 months of treatment with rituximab or a rituximab-containing regimen.

DOSAGE RANGE

1. CLL treatment-naïve—100 mg/m^2 IV on days 1 and 2 every 28 days. May give up to a total of six cycles.
2. Non-Hodgkin's lymphoma—120 mg/m^2 IV on days 1 and 2 every 21 days. May give up to a total of eight cycles.

DRUG INTERACTIONS

Inhibitors or inducers of CYP1A2—Concurrent use of bendamustine with CYP1A2 inhibitors (ciprofloxacin, fluvoxamine) or CYP1A2 inducers (omeprazole, smoking) may alter bendamustine metabolism and subsequent drug levels.

SPECIAL CONSIDERATIONS

1. Use with caution in patients with mild or moderate renal impairment.
2. Bendamustine should not be used in patients with CrCl <40 mL/min.
3. Use with caution in patients with mild hepatic impairment. Should not be used in setting of moderate (SGOT or SGPT 2.5–10 × ULN and total bilirubin 1.5–3 × ULN) or severe (total bilirubin >3 × ULN) hepatic impairment.
4. Monitor for tumor lysis syndrome, especially within the first treatment cycle. Consider using allopurinol during the first 1 to 2 weeks of bendamustine therapy in patients at high risk.
5. Closely monitor CBCs on a periodic basis. Treatment delays and/or dose reduction may be warranted. Prior to starting the next cycle of therapy, the ANC should be ≥1000/mm^3 and the platelet count ≥75,000/mm^3.
6. Closely monitor for hypersensitivity infusion reactions, and discontinuation of therapy should be considered in patients who experience grade 3 or 4 infusion reactions.
7. Bendamustine therapy should be held or discontinued in the setting of severe or progressive skin reactions.
8. Pregnancy category D. Breastfeeding should be avoided.

TOXICITY 1
Myelosuppression with neutropenia and thrombocytopenia is dose-limiting and may warrant treatment delay or dose reduction.

TOXICITY 2
Mild nausea and vomiting.

TOXICITY 3
Hypersensitivity reactions presenting with fever, chills, pruritus, and rash. Anaphylactoid and severe anaphylactic reactions have occurred rarely.

TOXICITY 4
Pyrexia, fatigue, and asthenia.

TOXICITY 5
Tumor lysis syndrome typically occurs within the first treatment cycle and in high-risk patients.

TOXICITY 6
Skin rash, toxic skin reactions, and bullous exanthema occur in <10% of patients.

Bevacizumab

TRADE NAME	Avastin	CLASSIFICATION	Monoclonal antibody, anti-VEGF antibody
CATEGORY	Biologic response modifier agent	DRUG MANUFACTURER	Genentech/Roche

MECHANISM OF ACTION
- Recombinant humanized monoclonal antibody directed against the vascular endothelial growth factor (VEGF). Binds to all isoforms of VEGF-A. VEGF is a pro-angiogenic growth factor that is overexpressed in a wide range of solid human cancers, including colorectal cancer.
- Precise mechanism(s) of action remains unknown.
- Binding of VEGF prevents its subsequent interaction with VEGF receptors (VEGFR) on the surface of endothelial cells and tumors, and in so doing, results in inhibition of VEGFR-mediated signaling.
- Inhibits formation of new blood vessels in primary tumor and metastatic tumors.
- Inhibits tumor blood vessel permeability and reduces interstitial tumoral pressures, and in so doing, may enhance blood flow delivery within tumor.

- Restores antitumor response by enhancing dendritic cell function.
- Immunologic mechanisms may also be involved in antitumor activity, and they include recruitment of ADCC and/or complement-mediated cell lysis.

MECHANISM OF RESISTANCE

- Increased expression of pro-angiogenic factor ligands, such as PlGF, bFGF, and hepatocyte growth factor (HGF).
- Recruitment of bone marrow–derived cells, which circumvents the requirement of VEGF signaling and restores neovascularization and tumor angiogenesis.
- Increased pericyte coverage of the tumor vasculature, which serves to support its integrity and reduces the need for VEGF-mediated survival signaling.
- Activation and enhancement of invasion and metastasis to provide access to normal tissue vasculature without obligate neovascularization.

DISTRIBUTION

Distribution in body is not well characterized. The predicted time to reach steady-state levels is on the order of 100 days.

METABOLISM

Metabolism of bevacizumab has not been extensively characterized. Peripheral half-life is on the order of 17–21 days with minimal clearance by the liver or kidneys. Tissue half-life has not been well characterized.

INDICATIONS

1. Metastatic colorectal cancer—FDA-approved for use in combination with any intravenous 5-fluorouracil (5-FU)–based chemotherapy in first-line therapy.
2. Metastatic colorectal cancer—FDA-approved for use in the second-line setting in combination with fluoropyrimidine-based chemotherapy after progression on first-line treatment that includes bevacizumab.
3. NSCLC—FDA-approved for non-squamous NSCLC in combination with carboplatin/paclitaxel.
4. Glioblastoma—FDA-approved as a single agent for glioblastoma with progressive disease following prior therapy.
5. Renal cell cancer—FDA-approved in combination with interferon-α for metastatic renal cell cancer.
6. Cervical cancer—FDA-approved in combination with cisplatin/paclitaxel or paclitaxel/topotecan for metastatic or recurrent cervical cancer.
7. Ovarian, fallopian tube, or primary peritoneal cancer—FDA-approved in combination with paclitaxel, pegylated liposomal doxorubicin, or topotecan for platinum-resistant recurrent disease.

DOSAGE RANGE

1. Recommended dose for the first-line treatment of advanced colorectal cancer is 5 mg/kg IV in combination with intravenous 5-FU–based chemotherapy on an every-2-week schedule.

2. Recommended dose for the second-line treatment of advanced colorectal cancer in combination with FOLFOX-4 is 10 mg/kg IV on an every-2-week schedule.
3. Can also be administered at 7.5 mg/kg IV every 3 weeks when used in combination with capecitabine-based regimens for advanced colorectal cancer.
4. Recommended dose for advanced NSCLC is 15 mg/kg IV every 3 weeks with carboplatin/paclitaxel.
5. Recommended dose for glioblastoma is 10 mg/kg IV every 2 weeks.
6. Recommended dose for renal cell cancer is 10 mg/kg IV every 2 weeks with interferon-α.
7. Recommended dose for cervical cancer is 15 mg/kg every 3 weeks with cisplatin/paclitaxel or paclitaxel/topotecan.
8. Recommended dose for ovarian, fallopian tube, or primary peritoneal cancer is 10 mg/kg every 2 weeks with paclitaxel, pegylated liposomal doxorubicin, or weekly topotecan or 15 mg/kg every 3 weeks with topotecan given every 3 weeks.

DRUG INTERACTIONS
None well characterized to date.

SPECIAL CONSIDERATIONS
1. Patients should be warned of the increased risk of arterial thromboembolic events, including myocardial infarction and stroke. Risk factors are age ≥65 years and history of angina, stroke, and prior arterial thromboembolic events. This represents a black-box warning.
2. Patients should be warned of the potential for serious and, in some cases, fatal hemorrhage resulting from hemoptysis in patients with NSCLC. These events have been mainly observed in patients with a central, cavitary, and/or necrotic lesion involving the pulmonary vasculature and have occurred suddenly. Patients with recent hemoptysis (≥1/2 tsp of red blood) should not receive bevacizumab. This represents a black-box warning.
3. Bevacizumab treatment can result in the development of GI perforations, which in some cases has resulted in death. This event represents a black-box warning for the drug. Use with caution in patients who have undergone recent surgical and/or invasive procedures. Bevacizumab should be given at least 28 days after any surgical and/or invasive intervention.
4. Bevacizumab treatment can result in the development of wound dehiscence, which in some cases can be fatal. This represents a black-box warning. Use with caution in patients who have undergone recent surgical and/or invasive procedures. Bevacizumab should be given at least 28 days after any surgical and/or invasive intervention.
5. Carefully monitor for infusion-related symptoms. May need to treat with diphenhydramine (Benadryl) and acetaminophen.
6. Use with caution in patients with uncontrolled hypertension as bevacizumab can result in grade 3 hypertension in about 10% of patients.

Should be permanently discontinued in patients who develop hypertensive crisis. In most cases, however, hypertension is well-managed by increasing the dose of the antihypertensive medication and/or with the addition of another antihypertensive medication.

7. Bevacizumab should be terminated in patients who develop the nephrotic syndrome. Therapy should be interrupted for proteinuria ≥2 grams/24 hours and resumed when <2 grams/24 hours.

8. Bevacizumab treatment can result in RPLS, as manifested by headache, seizure, lethargy, confusion, blindness and other visual side effects, as well as other neurologic disturbances. This syndrome can occur from 16 hours to 1 year after initiation of therapy, and usually resolves or improves within days, and magnetic resonance imaging is necessary to confirm the diagnosis.

9. There are no recommended dose reductions for bevacizumab. In the setting of adverse events, bevacizumab should be discontinued or temporarily interrupted.

10. Pregnancy category B.

TOXICITY 1
Gastrointestinal perforations and wound healing complications.

TOXICITY 2
Bleeding complications with epistaxis being most commonly observed. Serious, life-threatening pulmonary hemorrhage occurs in rare cases in patients with NSCLC, as outlined previously in Special Considerations.

TOXICITY 3
Increased risk of arterial thromboembolic events, including myocardial infarction, angina, and stroke. There is also an increased incidence of venous thromboembolic events.

TOXICITY 4
Hypertension occurs in 5–18%. Usually well controlled with oral antihypertensive medication.

TOXICITY 5
Proteinuria with nephrotic syndrome <1%.

TOXICITY 6
Infusion-related symptoms with fever, chills, urticaria, flushing, fatigue, headache, bronchospasm, dyspnea, angioedema, and hypotension. Infusion reactions occur in <3% of patients and severe reactions occur in 0.2% of patients.

TOXICITY 7
CNS events with dizziness and depression. RPLS occurs rarely (incidence of <0.1%) and presents with headache, seizure, lethargy, confusion, blindness, and other visual disturbances.

B

Bexarotene

TRADE NAME	Targretin	CLASSIFICATION	Retinoid
CATEGORY	Differentiating agent	DRUG MANUFACTURER	Eisai

MECHANISM OF ACTION
- Selectively binds and activates retinoid X receptors (RXRs).
- RXRs form heterodimers with various other receptors, including retinoic acid receptors (RARs), vitamin D receptors, and thyroid receptors. Once activated, these receptors function as transcription factors, which then regulate the expression of various genes involved in controlling cell differentiation, growth, and proliferation.
- Precise mechanism by which bexarotene exerts its antitumor activity in cutaneous T-cell lymphoma (CTCL) remains unknown.

ABSORPTION
Well absorbed by the GI tract. Peak plasma levels observed 2 hours after oral administration.

DISTRIBUTION
Distribution is not well characterized. Highly bound to plasma proteins (>99%).

METABOLISM
Extensive metabolism occurs in the liver via the cytochrome P450 system to both active and inactive metabolites. Both parent drug and its metabolites are eliminated primarily through the hepatobiliary system and in feces. Renal clearance is minimal, accounting for <1%. The elimination half-life is about 7 hours.

INDICATIONS
Treatment of cutaneous manifestations of CTCL in patients who are refractory to at least one prior systemic therapy.

DOSAGE RANGE
Recommended initial dose is 300 mg/m^2/day PO. Should be taken as a single dose with food.

DRUG INTERACTION 1
Gemfibrozil—Gemfibrozil inhibits metabolism of bexarotene by the liver P450 system, resulting in increased plasma concentrations. Concurrent administration of gemfibrozil with bexarotene is not recommended.

DRUG INTERACTION 2

Inhibitors of cytochrome P450 system—Drugs that inhibit the liver P450 system, such as ketoconazole, itraconazole, and erythromycin, may cause an increase in plasma concentrations of bexarotene.

DRUG INTERACTION 3

Inducers of cytochrome P450 system—Drugs that induce the liver P450 system, such as rifampin, phenytoin, and phenobarbital, may cause a reduction in plasma bexarotene concentrations.

SPECIAL CONSIDERATIONS

1. Use with caution in patients with abnormal liver function. Monitor liver function tests at baseline and during therapy. Treatment should be discontinued when LFTs are three-fold higher than the upper limit of normal (ULN).
2. Use with caution in diabetic patients who are on insulin, agents enhancing insulin secretion, or insulin sensitizers, as bexarotene therapy can enhance their effects, resulting in hypoglycemia.
3. Use with caution in patients with history of lipid disorders, as significant alterations in lipid profile are observed with bexarotene therapy. Lipid profile should be obtained at baseline, weekly until the lipid response is established, and at 8-week intervals.
4. Thyroid function tests should be obtained at baseline and during therapy, as bexarotene is associated with hypothyroidism.
5. Use with caution in patients with known hypersensitivity to retinoids.
6. Patients should be advised to limit vitamin A supplementation to <1500 IU/day to avoid potential additive toxic effects with bexarotene.
7. Patients should be advised to avoid exposure to sunlight, as bexarotene is associated with photosensitivity.
8. Patients who experience new-onset visual difficulties should have an ophthalmologic evaluation, as bexarotene is associated with retinal complications, development of new cataracts, and/or worsening of pre-existing cataracts.
9. Pregnancy category X. Must not be given to a pregnant woman or to a woman who intends to become pregnant. If a woman becomes pregnant while on therapy, bexarotene must be stopped immediately.

TOXICITY 1

Hypertriglyceridemia and hypercholesterolemia are common. Reversible upon dose reduction, cessation of therapy, or when antilipemic therapy is begun (gemfibrozil is not recommended, see Drug Interaction 1).

TOXICITY 2

Hypothyroidism develops in 50% of patients.

TOXICITY 3

Headache and asthenia.

TOXICITY 4
Myelosuppression with leukopenia more common than anemia.

TOXICITY 5
Nausea, abdominal pain, and diarrhea.

TOXICITY 6
Skin rash, dry skin, and rarely alopecia.

TOXICITY 7
Dry eyes, conjunctivitis, blepharitis, cataracts, corneal lesions, and visual field defects.

Bicalutamide

$C_{18}H_{14}N_2O_4F_4S$

TRADE NAME	Casodex	CLASSIFICATION	Antiandrogen
CATEGORY	Hormonal drug	DRUG MANUFACTURER	AstraZeneca

MECHANISM OF ACTION
- Nonsteroidal antiandrogen agent that binds to androgen receptor and inhibits androgen uptake as well as inhibiting androgen binding in the nuclei of androgen-sensitive prostate cancer cells.
- Affinity to androgen receptor is four-fold greater than flutamide.

MECHANISM OF RESISTANCE
- Decreased expression of androgen receptor.
- Mutation in androgen receptor leading to decreased binding affinity to bicalutamide.

ABSORPTION
Well absorbed by the GI tract. Peak plasma levels observed 1–2 hours after oral administration. Absorption is not affected by food.

DISTRIBUTION

Distribution is not well characterized. Extensively bound to plasma proteins (96%).

METABOLISM

Extensive metabolism occurs in the liver via oxidation and glucuronidation by cytochrome P450 enzymes to inactive metabolites. Both parent drug and its metabolites are cleared in urine and feces. The elimination half-life is long, on the order of several days.

INDICATIONS

Stage D2 metastatic prostate cancer.

DOSAGE RANGE

Recommended dose is 50 mg PO once daily, either alone or in combination with a luteinizing hormone–releasing hormone (LHRH) analog.

DRUG INTERACTIONS

Warfarin—Bicalutamide can displace warfarin from its protein-binding sites, leading to increased anticoagulant effect. Coagulation parameters (PT and INR) must be followed closely, and dose adjustments may be needed.

SPECIAL CONSIDERATIONS

1. Use with caution in patients with abnormal liver function. Monitor LFTs at baseline and during therapy.
2. Caution patients about the potential for hot flashes. Consider the use of clonidine 0.1–0.2 mg PO daily, megestrol acetate 20 mg PO bid, or soy tablets 1 tablet PO tid for prevention and/or treatment.
3. Instruct patients on the potential risk of altered sexual function and impotence.
4. Pregnancy category D. Breastfeeding should be avoided.

TOXICITY 1

Hot flashes, decreased libido, impotence, gynecomastia, nipple pain, and galactorrhea. Occur in 50% of patients.

TOXICITY 2

Constipation observed in 10% of patients. Nausea, vomiting, and diarrhea occur rarely.

TOXICITY 3

Transient elevations in serum transaminases are rare.

B

Bleomycin

TRADE NAME	Blenoxane	CLASSIFICATION	Antitumor antibiotic
CATEGORY	Chemotherapy drug	DRUG MANUFACTURER	Bristol-Myers Squibb

MECHANISM OF ACTION
- Small peptide with a molecular weight of 1500.
- Contains a DNA-binding region and an iron-binding region at opposite ends of the molecule.
- Iron is absolutely necessary as a cofactor for free-radical generation and bleomycin's cytotoxic activity.
- Cytotoxic effects result from the generation of activated oxygen free radical species, which causes single-and double-strand DNA breaks and eventual cell death.

MECHANISM OF RESISTANCE
- Increased expression of DNA repair enzymes, resulting in enhanced repair of DNA damage.
- Decreased drug accumulation through altered uptake of drug.

ABSORPTION
Oral bioavailability of bleomycin is poor. After IM administration, peak levels are obtained in about 60 minutes but reach only one-third the levels achieved after an IV dose. When administered in the intrapleural space for the treatment of malignant pleural effusion (pleurodesis), approximately 45%–50% of the drug is absorbed into the systemic circulation.

DISTRIBUTION
Distributes into intra-and extracellular fluid. Less than 10% of drug bound to plasma proteins.

METABOLISM

After IV administration, there is a rapid, biphasic disappearance from the circulation. The terminal half-life is approximately 3 hours in patients with normal renal function. Bleomycin is rapidly inactivated in tissues, especially the liver and kidney, by the enzyme bleomycin hydrolase. Elimination of bleomycin is primarily via the kidneys, with 50%–70% of an administered dose being excreted unchanged in urine. Patients with impaired renal function may experience increased drug accumulation and are at risk for increased toxicity. Dose reductions are required in the presence of renal dysfunction.

INDICATIONS

1. Hodgkin's and non-Hodgkin's lymphoma.
2. Germ cell tumors.
3. Head and neck cancer.
4. Squamous cell carcinomas of the skin, cervix, and vulva.
5. Sclerosing agent for malignant pleural effusion and ascites.

DOSAGE RANGE

1. Hodgkin's lymphoma—10 units/m^2 IV on days 1 and 15 every 28 days, as part of the ABVD regimen.
2. Testicular cancer—30 units IV on days 2, 9, and 16 every 21 days, as part of the PEB regimen.
3. Intracavitary instillation into pleural space—60 units/m^2.

DRUG INTERACTION 1

Oxygen—High concentrations of oxygen may enhance the pulmonary toxicity of bleomycin. FIO$_2$ should be maintained at no higher than 25% when possible.

DRUG INTERACTION 2

Cisplatin—Cisplatin decreases renal clearance of bleomycin and, in so doing, may lead to higher drug levels, resulting in greater toxicity.

DRUG INTERACTION 3

Radiation therapy—Radiation therapy enhances the pulmonary toxicity of bleomycin.

DRUG INTERACTION 4

Brentuximab—Co-administration of bleomycin and brentuximab may increase the risk of pulmonary toxicity. As such, the concomitant use of these two agents is contraindicated.

SPECIAL CONSIDERATIONS

1. PFTs with special focus on DLCO and vital capacity should be obtained at baseline and before each cycle of therapy. A decrease of >15% in PFTs should mandate the immediate discontinuation of bleomycin, even in the absence of clinical symptoms. Increased risk of pulmonary toxicity when cumulative dose >400 units.
2. Chest X-ray should be obtained at baseline and before each cycle of therapy to monitor for evidence of infiltrates and/or interstitial lung findings.

3. Monitor for clinical signs of pulmonary dysfunction, including shortness of breath, dyspnea, decreased O_2 saturation, and decreased lung expansion.

4. Use with caution in patients with impaired renal function because drug clearance may be reduced. Doses should be reduced in the presence of renal dysfunction. Baseline CrCl should be obtained, and renal status should be monitored before each cycle.

5. Patients with lymphoma may be at increased risk for developing an anaphylactic reaction. This complication can be immediate or delayed. An anaphylaxis kit that includes epinephrine, antihistamines, and corticosteroids should be readily available at bedside during bleomycin administration.

6. Premedicate patients with acetaminophen 30 minutes before administration of drug and every 6 hours for 24 hours if fever and chills are noted.

7. Patients undergoing surgery must inform the surgeon and anesthesiologist of prior treatment with bleomycin. High concentrations of forced inspiratory oxygen (FIO_2) at the time of surgery may enhance the pulmonary toxicity of bleomycin.

TOXICITY 1
Skin reactions are the most common side effects and include erythema, hyperpigmentation of the skin, striae, and vesiculation. Skin peeling, thickening of the skin and nail beds, hyperkeratosis, and ulceration can also occur. These manifestations usually occur when the cumulative dose has reached 150–200 units.

TOXICITY 2
Pulmonary toxicity is dose-limiting. Occurs in 10% of patients. Usually presents as pneumonitis with cough, dyspnea, dry inspiratory crackles, and infiltrates on chest X-ray. Increased incidence in patients >70 years of age and with cumulative doses >400 units. Rarely progresses to pulmonary fibrosis but can be fatal in about 1% of patients. PFTs are the most sensitive approach to follow, with specific focus on DLCO and vital capacity. A decrease of 15% or more in the PFTs should mandate immediate stoppage of the drug.

TOXICITY 3
Hypersensitivity reaction in the form of fever and chills observed in up to 25% of patients. True anaphylactoid reactions are rare but more common in patients with lymphoma.

TOXICITY 4
Vascular events, including myocardial infarction, stroke, and Raynaud's phenomenon, are rarely reported.

TOXICITY 5
Myelosuppression is relatively mild.

Blinatumomab

TRADE NAME	Blincyto	CLASSIFICATION	Monoclonal antibody
CATEGORY	Biologic response modifier agent	DRUG MANUFACTURER	Amgen

MECHANISM OF ACTION

- Bispecific T-cell engaging (BiTE) antibody that binds to CD19 expressed on precursor B-cells and CD3 expressed on the surface of T-cells. This antibody lacks the constant region of common monoclonal antibodies.
- This binding causes cytotoxic T-cells to be physically linked to malignant CD19-positive B cells and triggers the signaling cascade leading to the upregulation of cell adhesion molecules, production of cytolytic proteins, release of inflammatory cytokines, proliferation of T-cells ultimately resulting in lysis of CD19-positive B cells.
- CD19 is expressed on all stages of B-lineage acute lymphocytic leukemia (ALL), across all Non-Hodgkin's lymphoma subtypes, and in CLL.
- Mechanism of action differs from that of conventional monoclonal antibodies, which uses antibody-dependent cellular cytotoxicity and engages natural killer T-cells, macrophages, and neutrophils to cause tumor cell death.

ABSORPTION

Blinatumomab is given only by the IV route.

DISTRIBUTION

Following continuous intravenous infusion, steady-state serum concentrations are achieved within one day and remain stable over time.

METABOLISM

The metabolism of blinatumomab has not been well characterized. As with other antibodies, it is assumed that blinatumumab is degraded to small peptides and amino acids via catabolic pathways. The mean elimination half-life is approximately 2 hours.

INDICATIONS

1. FDA-approved for the treatment of adult patients with relapsed and/or refractory Philadelphia chromosome-negative, B-cell precursor ALL.
2. FDA-approved for the treatment of pediatric patients with relapsed and/or refractory Philadelphia chromosome-negative, B-cell precursor ALL.

DOSAGE RANGE

A single cycle of therapy consists of 28 days of continuous IV infusion followed by a 14-day drug-free interval (total of 42 days).

For patients > 45 kg, the recommended dose for cycle 1 is 9 µg/day on days 1-7 and then 28 µg/day continuous IV Infusion on days 8-28, followed by a 14-day treatment-free interval. For subsequent cycles, the dose is 28 µg/day on days 1-28 followed by a 14-day break.

For patients < 45 kg, the recommended dose for cycle 1 is 5 µg/m^2/day on days 1-7 and then 15 µg/m^2/day on days 8-28, followed by a 14-day treatment-free interval. For subsequent cycles, the dose is 15 µg/m^2/day on days 1-28 followed by a 14-day break.

DRUG INTERACTIONS

None well characterized to date.

SPECIAL CONSIDERATIONS

1. Hospitalization is recommended for the first 9 days of the first cycle of therapy and for the first 2 days of the second cycle.
2. Adult patients should be premedicated with 20 mg dexamethasone 1 hour prior to the first dose of therapy of each cycle, prior to a step dose (cycle 1, day 8), and when restarting an infusion after an interruption of more than 4 hours. Pediatric patients should be premedicated with 5 mg/m^2 dexamethasone up to a maximum of 20 mg prior to the first dose of therapy in the first cycle, prior to a step dose (cycle 1, day 8), and when restarting an infusion after an interruption of more than 4 hours.
3. Monitor for infusion-related events, which may be clinically indistinguishable from the manifestations of Cytokine Release Syndrome (CRS) with life-threatening or fatal consequences.
4. Monitor for CRS, which presents as fever, headache, nausea/vomiting, elevations in serum transaminases and increased serum bilirubin, and hypotension. In some cases, disseminated intravascular coagulation (DIC), capillary leak syndrome (CLS), and hemophagocytic lymphohistiocytosis/macrophage activation syndrome (HLH/MAS) have been reported as part of CRS.
5. Monitor for neurologic toxicity, presenting as encephalopathy, convulsions, speech disorders, disturbances in consciousness, confusion and disorientation, and coordination and balance disorders. The median time to onset of any neurological toxicity is 7 days.
6. Cranial magnetic resonance imaging (MRI) changes showing leukoencephalopathy have been observed, especially in patients with prior treatment with cranial irradiation and chemotherapy (including systemic high-dose methotrexate or intrathecal cytarabine). The clinical significance of these imaging changes is unknown.
7. Monitor for signs and symptoms of infection as blinatumomab therapy is associated with an increased risk of pneumonia, bacteremia, sepsis, opportunistic infection, and catheter-site infections.

8. Monitor CBCs closely while on therapy.
9. Monitor for tumor lysis syndrome, especially in patients with high numbers of circulating cells (>25,000/mm^3) or high tumor burden. Appropriate measures should be taken to prevent the development of tumor lysis syndrome while receiving blinatumumab therapy.
10. Patients should be advised against performing activities that require mental alertness, including operating heavy machinery and driving.
11. Closely monitor therapy in older patients (>65) as they experience a higher rate of neurological toxicities, including cognitive disorder, encephalopathy, confusion, and serious infections.
12. Monitor serum transaminases and serum bilirubin at baseline and periodically during therapy. Treatment should be stopped if the serum transaminases rise to >5×ULN or if bilirubin rises to >3×ULN. No dose modification is needed for patients with baseline CrCl > 30 mL/min. There is currently no information available for patients with CrCL <30 mL/min or for patients on hemodialysis.
13. Pregnancy category C. Breast-feeding should be avoided.

TOXICITY 1
Infusion-related symptoms

TOXICITY 2
Cytokine release syndrome (CRS).

TOXICITY 3
Tumor lysis syndrome characterized by hyperkalemia, hyperuricemia, hyperphosphatemia, hypocalcemia, and renal insufficiency. Usually occurs within the first 12–24 hours of treatment. Risk is increased in patients with high numbers of circulating malignant cells (>25,000/mm^3) and/or high tumor burden.

TOXICITY 4
Neurological toxicities with encephalopathy, seizures, speech disorders, confusion, balance disorders. Leukoencephalopathy with MRI changes can also be observed in rare cases.

TOXICITY 5
Myelosuppression with neutropenia, anemia, and thrombocytopenia.

TOXICITY 6
Increased risk of bacterial, fungal, viral, and opportunistic infections.

TOXICITY 7
GI toxicity in the form of nausea/vomiting, abdominal pain, diarrhea, constipation, and elevations in serum transaminases and serum bilirubin.

B

Bortezomib

TRADE NAME	Velcade	CLASSIFICATION	Proteasome inhibitor
CATEGORY	Chemotherapy drug	DRUG MANUFACTURER	Millennium: The Takeda Oncology Company

MECHANISM OF ACTION
- Reversible inhibitor of the 26S proteasome.
- The 26S proteasome is a large protein complex that degrades ubiquinated proteins. This pathway plays an essential role in regulating the intracellular concentrations of various cellular proteins.
- Inhibition of the 26S proteasome prevents the targeted proteolysis of ubiquinated proteins, and disruption of this normal pathway can affect multiple signaling pathways within the cell, leading to cell death.
- Results in downregulation of the NF-κB pathway. NF-κB is a transcription factor that stimulates the production of various growth factors, including IL-6, cell adhesion molecules, and antiapoptotic proteins, all of which contribute to cell growth and chemoresistance. Inhibition of the NF-κB pathway by bortezomib leads to inhibition of cell growth and restores chemosensitivity.

MECHANISM OF RESISTANCE
- Activation of NF-κB pathway via proteasome-independent mechanisms.
- Mutations in the proteasome β5 subunit (PSMB5) gene leading to overexpression of PSMB5 protein.
- Increased expression of the multidrug-resistant gene with elevated P170 protein levels, which leads to increased drug efflux and decreased intracellular drug accumulation.

ABSORPTION
Bortezomib is given by the intravenous and subcutaneous routes. Total systemic exposure is equivalent for intravenous and subcutaneous administration.

DISTRIBUTION
Volume of distribution not well characterized. About 80% of drug bound to plasma proteins.

METABOLISM

Bortezomib has a mean elimination half-life of 76 to 108 hours upon multiple dosing with the 1.3 mg/m^2 dose. It is metabolized by the liver cytochrome P450 system. The major metabolic pathway is deboronation, forming two deboronated metabolites. The deboronated metabolites are inactive as 26S proteasome inhibitors. Elimination pathways for bortezomib have not been well characterized.

INDICATIONS

1. FDA-approved for the treatment of multiple myeloma.
2. FDA-approved for the treatment of mantle cell lymphoma after at least one prior therapy.

DOSAGE RANGE

Recommended dose for relapsed multiple myeloma and mantle cell lymphoma is 1.3 mg/m^2 administered by IV or SC twice weekly for 2 weeks (on days 1, 4, 8, and 11) followed by a 10-day rest period (days 12–21).

DRUG INTERACTION 1

Ketoconazole and other CYP3A4 inhibitors—Co-administration of ketoconazole and other CYP3A4 inhibitors may decrease the metabolism of bortezomib, resulting in increased drug levels and potentially increased toxicity.

DRUG INTERACTION 2

CYP3A4 inducers—Co-administration of bortezomib with potent CYP3A4 inducers, such as rifampin, may increase the metabolism of bortezomib, resulting in decreased drug levels.

DRUG INTERACTION 3

St. John's wort may alter the metabolism of bortezomib, resulting in decreased drug levels.

SPECIAL CONSIDERATIONS

1. Contraindicated in patients with hypersensitivity to boron, bortezomib, and/or mannitol.
2. Use with caution in patients with impaired liver function, because drug metabolism and/or clearance may be reduced. Patients with mild hepatic impairment do not require dose modification. However, patients with moderate to severe hepatic impairment should be started at a reduced dose of 0.7 mg/m^2 in the first cycle. Depending on patient tolerability, the dose can be either increased to 1.0 mg/m^2 or further reduced to 0.5 mg/m^2 in subsequent cycles.
3. The pharmacokinetics of bortezomib are not influenced by the degree of renal impairment. Therefore, dosing adjustments of bortezomib are not necessary for patients with renal insufficiency. Since dialysis may reduce bortezomib concentrations, the drug should be administered after the dialysis procedure.

4. Use with caution in patients with a history of syncope, patients who are on antihypertensive medications, and patients who are dehydrated, because bortezomib can cause orthostatic hypotension.

5. Bortezomib should be withheld at the onset of any grade 3 non-hematologic toxicity, excluding neuropathy, or any grade 4 hematologic toxicities. After symptoms have resolved, therapy can be restarted with a 25% dose reduction. With respect to neuropathy, the dose of bortezomib should be reduced to 1.0 mg/m^2 with grade 1 peripheral neuropathy with pain or grade 2 peripheral neuropathy. In the presence of grade 2 neurotoxicity, therapy should be withheld until symptoms have resolved and restarted at a dose of 0.7 mg/m^2 along with changing the treatment schedule to once per week. In the presence of grade 4 neurotoxicity, therapy should be discontinued.

6. The use of SC bortezomib may be considered in patients with pre-existing neuropathy or in those at high risk of developing peripheral neuropathy.

7. Patients should avoid taking green tea products and supplements, as they have been shown to block the clinical efficacy of bortezomib.

8. Patients should avoid taking St. John's wort, as it has been shown to increase the metabolism of bortezomib, leading to lower effective drug levels.

9. Pregnancy category D. Breastfeeding should be avoided.

TOXICITY 1
Fatigue, malaise, and generalized weakness. Usually observed during the first and second cycles of therapy.

TOXICITY 2
GI toxicity in the form of nausea/vomiting and diarrhea.

TOXICITY 3
Myelosuppression with thrombocytopenia and neutropenia.

TOXICITY 4
Peripheral sensory neuropathy, although a mixed sensorimotor neuropathy has also been observed. Symptoms may improve and/or return to baseline upon discontinuation of bortezomib.

TOXICITY 5
Fever (>38°C) in up to 40% of patients.

TOXICITY 6
Orthostatic hypotension in up to 12% of patients.

TOXICITY 7
Congestive heart failure (CHF) and new onset of reduced LVEF. Rare cases of QT-interval prolongation.

TOXICITY 8
Pulmonary toxicity in the form of pneumonitis, interstitial pneumonia, lung infiltrates, and acute respiratory distress syndrome (ARDS). Pulmonary hypertension has also been reported.

TOXICITY 9
Reversible posterior leukoencephalopathy syndrome (RPLS) is a rare event and presents with headache, seizure, lethargy, confusion, blindness, and other visual disturbances.

Bosutinib

TRADE NAME	Bosulif, SKI-606	**CLASSIFICATION**	Signal transduction inhibitor
CATEGORY	Chemotherapy drug	**DRUG MANUFACTURER**	Pfizer

MECHANISM OF ACTION
- Potent inhibitor of the Bcr-Abl tyrosine kinase. Retains activity in 16 of 18 imatinib-resistant Bcr-Abl mutations.
- Does not have activity against T315I or V299L Bcr-Abl mutations.
- Potent inhibitor of the Src family (Src, Lyn, and Hck) kinases. Src family kinases (SFK) are involved in cancer cell adhesion, migration, invasion, proliferation, differentiation, and survival.

MECHANISM OF RESISTANCE
Single-point mutations, either T315I or V299L, within the ATP-binding pocket of the Abl tyrosine kinase.

ABSORPTION
Well absorbed following oral administration, with peak plasma concentrations at 4 to 6 hours. Administration of a high-fat meal results in higher drug concentrations.

DISTRIBUTION
Exhibits extensive plasma protein binding (96%).

METABOLISM
Metabolized in the liver primarily by CYP3A4 microsomal enzymes with all of the metabolites inactive. Approximately 91% and 3% of an administered dose of drug is eliminated in the feces and urine, respectively. The mean elimination half-life is 22.5 hours.

INDICATIONS
1. FDA-approved for the treatment of adult patients with chronic-, accelerated-, or blast-phase Philadelphia chromosome–positive (Ph+) CML with resistance or intolerance to prior therapy.
2. Active as first-line therapy for chronic-phase Ph+ CML.

DOSAGE RANGE
1. Recommended dose is 500 mg PO once daily with food.
2. Consider dose escalation to 600 mg PO once daily with food in patients who do not reach complete hematological response (CHR) by week 8 or a complete cytogenetic response (CCyR) by week 12.

DRUG INTERACTIONS
1. Concomitant use of CYP3A inhibitors, such as ketoconazole, voriconazole, posaconazole, clarithromycin, fluconazole, erythromycin, diltiazem, aprepitant, verapamil, grapefruit juice, and ciprofloxacin, can decrease the metabolism of bosutinib, resulting in increased plasma drug concentrations.
2. Drugs that are moderate or strong CYP3A inducers, such as rifampin, phenytoin, carbamazepine, St. John's wort, and phenobarbital, can increase the metabolism of bosutinib resulting in decreased plasma drug concentration.
3. Proton pump inhibitors, such as lansoprazole, can decrease plasma concentrations of bosutinib.
4. Drugs that are P-glycoprotein substrates, such as digoxin, may have higher plasma concentrations when taken with bosutinib.

SPECIAL CONSIDERATIONS
1. Important to carefully review patient's list of medications as bosutinib has several potential drug–drug interactions.
2. Monitor CBC weekly during the first month and then monthly thereafter.
3. Monitor liver function on a monthly basis for the first 3 months and periodically thereafter.
4. The dose of bosutinib should be reduced to 200 mg PO daily in the presence of pre-existing mild, moderate, and severe hepatic dysfunction.
5. The dose of bosutinib should be reduced to 300 mg PO daily in the presence of severe renal dysfunction (CrCl <30 mL/min). No dose reduction is needed in the presence of mild-to-moderate renal impairment.
6. Bosutinib should be taken with food, and drug tablets should not be crushed.

7. Avoid concomitant use of proton pump inhibitors (PPIs) while on bosutinib therapy. Consider using short-acting antacids or H2 blockers instead of PPIs.
8. Be cautious of potential for fluid retention that can manifest as pericardial effusion, pleural effusion, pulmonary edema, or peripheral edema.
9. Avoid Seville oranges, starfruit, pomelos, grapefruit juice, grapefruit products, and St. John's wort while on therapy.
10. Pregnancy category D. Breastfeeding should be avoided.

TOXICITY 1
Gastrointestinal toxicity is common, presenting as diarrhea in more than 80%, nausea/vomiting, and abdominal pain.

TOXICITY 2
Myelosuppression with thrombocytopenia, anemia, and neutropenia.

TOXICITY 3
Skin rash occurs in about one-third of patients and is associated with pruritus.

TOXICITY 4
Elevation of serum transaminases (SGOT/SGPT), usually within the first 3 months of therapy.

TOXICITY 5
Fluid retention manifesting as peripheral edema, pericardial effusion, pleural effusion, or pulmonary edema.

TOXICITY 6
Fatigue and asthenia.

Brentuximab

TRADE NAMES	Adcetris, SGN-35	CLASSIFICATION	Monoclonal antibody
CATEGORY	Biologic response modifier agent	DRUG MANUFACTURER	Seattle Genetics and Millennium: The Takeda Oncology Company

MECHANISM OF ACTION
- Brentuximab is a CD30-directed antibody-drug conjugate (ADC) that is made up of three components: (1) chimeric IgG1 antibody cAC10, specific for CD30; (2) microtubule-disrupting agent monomethyl auristatin E (MMAE); and (3) protease-cleavable linker that covalently attaches MMAE to cAC10. Approximately four molecules of MMAE are conjugated to each antibody molecule.

- Targets the CD30 antigen, a cell surface protein expressed on the surface of Hodgkin's Reed-Sternberg cells and on anaplastic large-cell lymphomas (ALCLs), embryonal carcinomas, and select subtypes of B-cell–derived, non-Hodgkin's lymphomas and mature T-cell lymphomas. Normal expression of CD30 is highly restricted to a relatively small population of activated B cells and T cells and a small portion of eosinophils.
- Binding of the ADC to CD30-expressing cells is followed by internalization of the ADC–CD30 complex with subsequent release of MMAE via proteolytic cleavage.
- MMAE inhibits the microtubule network within the tumor cell, resulting in cell cycle arrest at the G2/M interphase and apoptotic death.
- Chimeric antibody mediates complement-dependent cell lysis (CDCC) in the presence of human complement and antibody-dependent cellular cytotoxicity (ADCC) with human effector cells.

MECHANISM OF RESISTANCE
None well characterized to date.

ABSORPTION
Brentuximab is given only by the IV route.

DISTRIBUTION
Median time to maximum drug concentration occurs immediately after infusion for the antibody-drug conjugate and approximately 2 to 3 days after infusion for MMAE. Steady-state blood levels for both the antibody-drug conjugate and MMAE are reached in 21 days.

METABOLISM
Only a small fraction of MMAE released from brentuximab is metabolized, which is mediated by CYP3A4 and CYP3A5. Approximately 25% of the total MMAE administered as part of the ADC infusion was recovered in feces and urine over a 1-week period, with 70% being recovered in feces. The terminal half-life estimates of the antibody-drug conjugate and MMAE are 4 to 6 days and 3 to 4 days, respectively.

INDICATIONS
1. FDA-approved for patients with Hodgkin's lymphoma after failure of autologous stem cell transplant (ASCT) or after failure of at least two prior multiagent chemotherapy regimens in patients who are not ASCT candidates.
2. FDA-approved as post-autologous stem cell transplant consolidation for patients with Hodgkin's lymphoma at high risk for relapse or progression.
3. FDA-approved for patients with anaplastic large-cell lymphoma after failure of at least one prior multiagent chemotherapy regimen.

DOSAGE RANGE
Recommended dose is 1.8 mg/kg IV every 3 weeks.

DRUG INTERACTIONS

Bleomycin—Co-administration of brentuximab with bleomycin may increase the risk of pulmonary toxicity. As such, the concomitant use of these two agents is contraindicated.

SPECIAL CONSIDERATIONS

1. Patients should be premedicated with acetaminophen and diphen-hydramine to reduce the incidence of infusion-related reactions.
2. Monitor for infusion-related events, which usually occur 30–120 minutes after the start of the first infusion. Infusion should be immediately stopped if signs or symptoms of an allergic reaction are observed. Immediate institution of diphenhydramine, acetaminophen, corticosteroids, IV fluids, and/or vasopressors may be necessary. Resuscitation equipment should be readily available at bedside.
3. Monitor for tumor lysis syndrome, especially in patients with rapidly proliferating disease and high tumor burden.
4. Monitor CBCs at regular intervals during therapy.
5. Consider the diagnosis of progressive multifocal leukoencephalopathy (PML) in patients who present with new onset or changes in pre-existing neurological signs or symptoms. This represents a black-box warning.
6. Patients should not receive live, attenuated vaccines while on brentuximab therapy. In patients who have recently been vaccinated, brentuximab therapy should not be initiated for least 2 weeks.
7. Pregnancy category C. Breastfeeding should be avoided.

TOXICITY 1

Infusion-related symptoms, including fever, chills, urticaria, flushing, fatigue, headache, bronchospasm, rhinitis, dyspnea, angioedema, nausea, and/or hypotension.

TOXICITY 2

Tumor lysis syndrome. Characterized by hyperkalemia, hyperuricemia, hyperphosphatemia, hypocalcemia, and renal insufficiency. Usually occurs within the first 12–24 hours of treatment. Risk is increased in patients with rapidly proliferating tumor and/or high tumor burden.

TOXICITY 3

Myelosuppression with neutropenia and anemia being most commonly observed.

TOXICITY 4

Peripheral sensory neuropathy is the most common neurologic side effect.

TOXICITY 5

Progressive multifocal leukoencephalopathy (PML).

TOXICITY 6
Skin reactions, including rash, pruritus, and Stevens-Johnson syndrome.

TOXICITY 7
Mild nausea/vomiting and diarrhea are the most common GI side effects.

Busulfan

$$CH_3 - \overset{\overset{O}{\|}}{\underset{\underset{O}{\|}}{S}} - O - CH_2CH_2CH_2CH_2O - \overset{\overset{O}{\|}}{\underset{\underset{O}{\|}}{S}} - CH_3$$

TRADE NAMES	Myleran, Busulfex	CLASSIFICATION	Alkylating agent
CATEGORY	Chemotherapy drug	DRUG MANUFACTURER	GlaxoSmithKline

MECHANISM OF ACTION
- Methanesulfonate-type bifunctional alkylating agent.
- Interacts with cellular thiol groups and nucleic acids to form DNA–DNA and DNA–protein cross-links. Cross-linking of DNA results in inhibition of DNA synthesis and function.
- Cell cycle–nonspecific, active in all phases of the cell cycle.

MECHANISM OF RESISTANCE
- Decreased cellular uptake of drug.
- Increased intracellular thiol content due to glutathione or glutathione-related enzymes.
- Enhanced activity of DNA repair enzymes.

ABSORPTION
Excellent oral bioavailability with peak levels in serum occurring within 2–4 hours after administration. About 30% of drug is bound to plasma proteins.

DISTRIBUTION
Distributes rapidly in plasma with broad tissue distribution. Crosses the blood-brain barrier and also crosses the placental barrier.

METABOLISM
Metabolized primarily in the liver by the cytochrome P450 system. Metabolites, including sulfoxane, 3-hydroxysulfoxane, and methanesulfonic acid, are excreted in urine, with 50%–60% excreted within 48 hours. Metabolism may be influenced by circadian rhythm with higher clearance rates observed in the evening, especially in younger patients. The terminal half-life is 2.5 hours.

INDICATIONS

1. Chronic myelogenous leukemia (CML) (standard dose).
2. Bone marrow/stem cell transplantation for refractory leukemia, lymphoma (high dose). Use in combination with cyclophosphamide as conditioning regimen prior to allogeneic stem cell transplantation for CML.

DOSAGE RANGE

1. CML—Usual dose for remission induction is 4–8 mg/day PO. Dosing on a weight basis is 1.8 mg/m^2/day. Maintenance dose is usually 1–3 mg/day PO.
2. Transplant setting—4 mg/kg/day IV for 4 days to a total dose of 16 mg/kg.

DRUG INTERACTION 1

Acetaminophen—Acetaminophen may decrease busulfan metabolism in the liver when given 72 hours before busulfan, resulting in enhanced toxicity.

DRUG INTERACTION 2

Itraconazole—Itraconazole reduces busulfan metabolism by up to 20%.

DRUG INTERACTION 3

Phenobarbital and phenytoin—Phenobarbital and phenytoin increase busulfan metabolism in the liver by inducing the activity of the liver microsomal system.

SPECIAL CONSIDERATIONS

1. Monitor CBC while on therapy. When the total WBC count has declined to approximately 15,000/mm^3, busulfan should be withheld until the nadir is reached and the counts begin to rise above this level. A decrease in the WBC count may not be seen during the first 10–15 days of therapy, and it may continue to fall for more than 1 month even after the drug has been stopped.
2. Monitor patients for pulmonary symptoms as busulfan can cause interstitial pneumonitis.
3. Ingestion of busulfan on an empty stomach may decrease the risk of nausea and vomiting.
4. Pregnancy category D. Breastfeeding should be avoided.

TOXICITY 1

Myelosuppression with pancytopenia is dose-limiting toxicity.

TOXICITY 2

Nausea/vomiting and diarrhea are common (>80% of patients) but generally mild with standard doses. Anorexia is also frequently observed.

TOXICITY 3

Mucositis is dose-related and may require interruption of therapy in some instances.

TOXICITY 4

Hyperpigmentation of skin, especially in hand creases and nail beds. Skin rash and pruritus also observed.

TOXICITY 5

Impotence, male sterility, amenorrhea, ovarian suppression, menopause, and infertility.

TOXICITY 6

Pulmonary symptoms, including cough, dyspnea, and fever, can be seen after long-term therapy. Interstitial pulmonary fibrosis, referred to as "busulfan lung," is a rare but severe side effect of therapy. May occur 1–10 years after discontinuation of therapy.

TOXICITY 7

Adrenal insufficiency occurs rarely.

TOXICITY 8

Hepatotoxicity with elevations in LFTs. Hepatoveno-occlusive disease is observed with high doses of busulfan used in transplant setting.

TOXICITY 9

Insomnia, anxiety, dizziness, and depression are the most common neurologic side effects. Seizures can occur, usually with high-dose therapy.

TOXICITY 10

Increased risk of secondary malignancies, especially acute myelogenous leukemia, with long-term chronic use.

Cabazitaxel

TRADE NAMES	Jevtana	CLASSIFICATION	Taxane, antimi-crotubule agent
CATEGORY	Chemotherapy drug	DRUG MANUFACTURER	Sanofi-Aventis

MECHANISM OF ACTION
- Semisynthetic taxane prepared with a precursor extracted from yew needles.
- Binds to tubulin and promotes its assembly into microtubules while simultaneously inhibiting disassembly. This effect leads to stabilization of microtubules, which results in the inhibition of mitotic and interphase cellular functions.
- Cell cycle–specific agent with activity in the mitotic (M) phase.

MECHANISM OF RESISTANCE
- Alterations in tubulin with decreased affinity for drug.
- Unlike other taxanes, cabazitaxel is a poor substrate for the multidrug resistance P-glycoprotein efflux pump and may be useful for treating multidrug-resistant tumors.

ABSORPTION
Cabazitaxel is given only by the IV route. It is poorly soluble and not orally bioavailable.

DISTRIBUTION
Cabazitaxel distributes widely to all body tissues and penetrates the blood-brain barrier. Extensive binding (89%–92%) to plasma proteins.

METABOLISM
Metabolized extensively in the liver (>95%), mainly by the CYP3A4/5 isoenzymes (80%–90%), and to a lesser extent by CYP2C8. Approximately 20 cabazitaxel metabolites are formed in the liver. Only about 24% is eliminated as the parent form, with the majority (76%) of an administered dose being eliminated as metabolites. Renal clearance is minimal with less than 4% of the drug cleared by the kidneys. Prolonged terminal half-life is about 77 hours. After a 1-hour infusion, approximately 80% of an administered dose is eliminated within 2 weeks.

INDICATIONS

FDA-approved for the treatment of patients with hormone-refractory, metastatic prostate cancer previously treated with a docetaxel-containing treatment regimen.

DOSAGE RANGE

Recommended dose is 25 mg/m^2 as a 1-hour infusion every 3 weeks in combination with oral prednisone 10 mg administered daily throughout cabazitaxel treatment.

DRUG INTERACTION 1

Concomitant administration of CYP3A4 inhibitors such as ketoconazole, itraconazole, clarithromycin, atazanavir, indinavir, nefazodone, nelfinavir, ritonavir, saquinavir, telithromycin, and voriconazole may reduce cabazitaxel metabolism, resulting in increased plasma drug concentrations.

DRUG INTERACTION 2

Concomitant administration of CYP3A4 inducers such as phenytoin, carbamazepine, rifampin, phenobarbital, and St. John's Wort may enhance cabazitaxel metabolism, resulting in decreased plasma drug concentrations and potentially reduced clinical activity.

SPECIAL CONSIDERATIONS

1. Contraindicated in patients with history of severe hypersensitivity reactions to cabazitaxel or to other drugs formulated with polysorbate 80.
2. Closely monitor CBCs on a weekly basis during cycle 1 and before each treatment cycle thereafter. Contraindicated in patients with severe neutropenia (i.e., ANC < 1500 cells/mm^3). Neutropenia prophylaxis should be considered in patients with high-risk clinical features (age >65, poor performance status, poor nutritional status, extensive prior radiation, other serious comorbid illnesses, or previous episodes of febrile neutropenia).
3. Patients should receive premedication with IV doses of an antihistamine, corticosteroid, and an H2-antagonist to prevent the incidence of hypersensitivity reactions.
4. Patients with a history of severe hypersensitivity reactions should **NOT** be rechallenged with cabazitaxel.
5. Contraindicated in patients with hepatic dysfunction (total bilirubin = ULN, AST and/or ALT = 1.5 × ULN). Use with caution in patients with abnormal liver function, as they are at higher risk for life-threatening toxicities.
6. Use with caution in patients with severe renal impairment and/or end-stage renal disease. No differences in cabazitaxel clearance have been observed in patients with mild or moderate renal impairment.
7. Pregnancy category D. Breastfeeding should be avoided.

TOXICITY 1

Myelosuppression with dose-limiting neutropenia. Thrombocytopenia and anemia are also observed.

TOXICITY 2

Hypersensitivity reaction characterized by generalized skin rash, flushing, erythema, hypotension, dyspnea, and/or bronchospasm. Usually occurs within the first few minutes of infusion and more frequently with the first and second infusions.

TOXICITY 3

Diarrhea, nausea/vomiting, constipation, abdominal pain, dysgeusia, and loss of appetite are the main GI side effects.

TOXICITY 4

Fatigue and asthenia.

TOXICITY 5

Neurotoxicity, mainly in the form of peripheral neuropathy, dizziness, and headache.

TOXICITY 6

Myalgias and arthralgias.

TOXICITY 7

Cardiac toxicity in the form of arrhythmias, hypotension, and peripheral edema.

TOXICITY 8

Alopecia occurs in 10% of patients.

TOXICITY 9

Hematuria and dysuria. Renal failure is a rare event.

Cabozantinib

TRADE NAME	Cometriq	CLASSIFICATION	Signal transduction inhibitor
CATEGORY	Chemotherapy drug	DRUG MANUFACTURER	Exilixis

MECHANISM OF ACTION

- Small-molecule inhibitor of tyrosine kinases associated with RET, MET, VEGFR-1, VEGFR-2, VEGFR-3, Kit, Flt-3, Axl, and Tie-2.
- Inhibition of the various receptor tyrosine kinases results in inhibition of critical signaling pathways involved in proliferation, growth, invasion/metastasis, angiogenesis, and maintenance of the tumor microenvironment.

MECHANISM OF RESISTANCE

None well characterized to date.

ABSORPTION

Oral absorption results in peak plasma concentrations at 2–6 hours, and is increased by food with a high fat content.

DISTRIBUTION

Extensive binding to plasma proteins (>99.7%). With daily dosing, steady-state blood levels are achieved in about 15 days.

METABOLISM

Cabozantinib is metabolized in the liver primarily by CYP3A4 enzymes. Approximately 80% of an administered dose is recovered, with 54% in feces and 27% in urine. The terminal half-life is on the order of 80–90 hours.

INDICATIONS

1. FDA-approved for the treatment of progressive, metastatic medullary thyroid cancer.
2. FDA-approved for the treatment of advanced renal cell cancer following prior anti-angiogenic therapy.

DOSAGE RANGE

1. Medullary thyroid cancer—Recommended dose is 140 mg PO daily.
2. Renal cell cancer—Recommended dose is 60 mg PO daily.

DRUG INTERACTIONS

- Drugs that stimulate liver microsomal CYP3A4 enzymes, including phenytoin, carbamazepine, rifampin, phenobarbital, and St. John's wort, may increase the metabolism of cabozantinib, resulting in its inactivation.
- Drugs that inhibit liver microsomal CYP3A4 enzymes, including ketoconazole, itraconazole, erythromycin, and clarithromycin, may reduce the metabolism of cabozantinib, resulting in increased drug levels and potentially increased toxicity.

SPECIAL CONSIDERATIONS

1. Patients should be instructed not to eat for at least 2 hours before and at least 1 hour after taking cabozantinib.
2. Use is not recommended in patients with moderate-to-severe hepatic dysfunction.

3. Dose adjustment of cabozantinib is not recommended for patients with mild-to-moderate renal dysfunction. However, the drug has not been studied in the setting of severe renal impairment, and for this reason, cabozantinib is not recommended in the setting of severe renal dysfunction.
4. Monitor for new GI signs and symptoms, as GI perforations and fistulas can occur. This is a black-box warning.
5. Monitor blood pressure closely while on therapy. Use with caution in patients with uncontrolled hypertension.
6. Monitor patients for signs and symptoms of bleeding as severe, sometimes fatal hemorrhage can occur. Do not use in patients with a recent history of hemorrhage or hemoptysis. This is a black-box warning.
7. Cabozantinib therapy should be discontinued in patients who develop arterial thromboembolic events, including myocardial infarction (MI), cerebrovascular accident (CVA).
8. Routinely monitor urinary protein levels by urine dipstick analysis. Therapy should be discontinued for patients who develop nephrotic syndrome.
9. An oral examination should be performed prior to initiation of therapy and periodically while on therapy. Patients should be advised to practice good oral hygiene. Cabozantinib should be held for at least 28 days prior to any invasive dental procedure.
10. Dose modification is recommended in patients who experience the hand-foot syndrome.
11. Cabozantinib therapy should be discontinued in patients who develop the neurologic RPLS syndrome.
12. Cabozantinib tablets can **NOT** be substituted with cabozantinib capsules.
13. Pregnancy category D. Breastfeeding should be avoided.

TOXICITY 1
Mild-to-moderate skin reactions with rash, dry skin, alopecia, erythema, changes in hair color, and hyperkeratosis. Hand-foot syndrome occurs in up to 50% of patients with grade 3/4 severity in 15% of patients.

TOXICITY 2
Diarrhea, nausea/vomiting, and mucositis are the most common GI side effects.

TOXICITY 3
Fatigue and asthenia.

TOXICITY 4
Hypertension.

TOXICITY 5
Bleeding complications, which in some cases, can be fatal.

TOXICITY 6
Osteonecrosis of the jaw, presenting as jaw pain, osteomyelitis, osteitis, bone erosion, and toothache.

TOXICITY 7
Proteinuria.

TOXICITY 8
RPLS with seizures, headache, visual disturbances, confusion, or altered mental function.

TOXICITY 9
Hepatotoxicity with elevations in SGOT, SGPT, and alkaline phosphatase.

Capecitabine

TRADE NAME	Xeloda	CLASSIFICATION	Antimetabolite
CATEGORY	Chemotherapy drug	DRUG MANUFACTURER	Roche

MECHANISM OF ACTION
- Fluoropyrimidine carbamate prodrug form of 5-FU. Capecitabine itself is inactive.
- Activation to cytotoxic forms is a complex process that involves three successive enzymatic steps. Metabolized in liver to

5'-deoxy-5-fluorocytidine (5'-DFCR) by the carboxylesterase enzyme and then to 5'-DFUR by cytidine deaminase (found in liver and in tumor tissues). Subsequently converted to 5-FU by the enzyme thymidine phosphorylase, which is expressed in higher levels in tumor versus normal tissue.
- Inhibition of the target enzyme thymidylate synthase (TS) by the 5-FU metabolite FdUMP.
- Incorporation of 5-FU metabolite FUTP into RNA resulting in alterations in RNA processing and/or mRNA translation.
- Incorporation of 5-FU metabolite FdUTP into DNA resulting in inhibition of DNA synthesis and function.
- Inhibition of TS leads to accumulation of dUMP and subsequent misincorporation of dUTP into DNA, resulting in inhibition of DNA synthesis and function.

MECHANISM OF RESISTANCE
- Increased expression of thymidylate synthase.
- Decreased levels of reduced folate substrate 5,10-methylenetetrahydrofolate.
- Decreased incorporation of 5-FU into RNA.
- Decreased incorporation of 5-FU into DNA.
- Increased activity of DNA repair enzymes, uracil glycosylase and dUTPase.
- Decreased expression of mismatch repair enzymes (hMLH1, hMSH2).
- Increased salvage of physiologic nucleosides, including thymidine.
- Increased expression of dihydropyrimidine dehydrogenase.
- Alterations in TS with decreased binding affinity of enzyme for FdUMP.

ABSORPTION
Capecitabine is readily absorbed by the GI tract. Peak plasma levels are reached in 1.5 hours, while peak 5-FU levels are achieved at 2 hours after oral administration. The rate and extent of absorption are reduced by food.

DISTRIBUTION
Plasma protein binding of capecitabine and its metabolites is less than 60%. Primarily bound to albumin (35%).

METABOLISM
Capecitabine undergoes extensive enzymatic metabolism to 5-FU. After being absorbed as an intact molecule from the GI tract, it undergoes an initial hydrolysis reaction in the liver catalyzed by carboxylesterase to 5'-DFCR. In the next step, 5'-DFCR is converted in the liver and other tissues to 5'-DFUR by the enzyme cytidine deaminase. Finally, 5'-DFUR is converted to 5-FU by the enzyme thymidine phosphorylase in tumor tissue as well as in normal tissues expressing this enzyme. Selective accumulation of 5-FU within tumor tissue (colorectal) versus normal tissue (colon) (3.2×) and plasma (21×) has been demonstrated in a population of colorectal cancer patients requiring definitive surgical resection who received capecitabine preoperatively.

Catabolism accounts for >85% of drug metabolism. Dihydropyrimidine dehydrogenase (DPD) is the main enzyme responsible for the catabolism of 5-FU, and it is present in liver and extrahepatic tissues such as GI mucosa, WBCs, and the kidneys. Greater than 90% of an administered dose of drug and its metabolites is cleared in the urine. The major metabolite excreted in urine is α-fluoro-β-alanine (FBAL). About 3% of the administered dose is excreted in urine as unchanged drug. The elimination half-life of capecitabine and capecitabine metabolites is on the order of 45–60 minutes.

INDICATIONS

1. Metastatic breast cancer—FDA-approved when used in combination with docetaxel for the treatment of patients with metastatic breast cancer after failure of prior anthracycline-containing chemotherapy.
2. Metastatic breast cancer—FDA-approved as monotherapy in patients refractory to both paclitaxel- and anthracycline-based chemotherapy or when anthracycline therapy is contraindicated.
3. Metastatic colorectal cancer—FDA-approved as first-line therapy when fluoropyrimidine therapy alone is preferred.
4. Stage III colon cancer—FDA-approved as adjuvant therapy when fluoropyrimidine therapy alone is preferred.
5. Clinical activity in gastric cancer, gastroesophageal cancer, and other GI cancers.

DOSAGE RANGE

1. Recommended dose is 1250 mg/m^2 PO bid (morning and evening) for 2 weeks with 1 week rest. For combination therapy (capecitabine in combination with docetaxel) with docetaxel being dosed at 75 mg/m^2 day 1 of a 21-day cycle.
2. May decrease dose of capecitabine to 850–1000 mg/m^2 bid on days 1–14 to reduce risk of toxicity without compromising efficacy (see section Special Considerations [8]).
3. An alternative dosing schedule for capecitabine monotherapy is 1250–1500 mg/m^2 PO bid for 1 week on and 1 week off. This schedule appears to be well tolerated, with no compromise in clinical efficacy.
4. Capecitabine should be used at lower doses (850–1000 mg/m^2 bid on days 1–14) when used in combination with other cytotoxic agents, such as oxaliplatin.

DRUG INTERACTION 1

Capecitabine-warfarin interaction—Patients receiving concomitant capecitabine and oral coumarin-derivative anticoagulant therapy should have their coagulation parameters (PT and INR) monitored frequently in order to adjust the anticoagulant dose accordingly. A clinically important capecitabine-warfarin drug interaction has been documented. Altered coagulation parameters and/or bleeding, including death, have been reported in patients taking capecitabine concomitantly with coumarin-derivative anticoagulants such as warfarin and phenprocoumon. Postmarketing reports have shown clinically significant increases in PT and INR in patients who were stabilized on anticoagulants at the time capecitabine was introduced. These events occurred within several days and up to several months after initiating capecitabine therapy and, in a few cases, within 1 month after stopping capecitabine. These events occurred in patients with and without liver metastases. Age >60 and a diagnosis of cancer independently predispose patients to an increased risk of coagulopathy.

DRUG INTERACTION 2

Aluminum hydroxide, magnesium hydroxide—Concomitant use of aluminum hydroxide– or magnesium hydroxide–containing antacids may increase the bioavailability of capecitabine by 16%–35%.

DRUG INTERACTION 3

Phenytoin—Capecitabine may increase phenytoin blood levels and subsequent phenytoin toxicity. Dose adjustment of phenytoin may be necessary.

DRUG INTERACTION 4

Leucovorin—Leucovorin enhances the antitumor activity and toxicity of capecitabine.

SPECIAL CONSIDERATIONS

1. Capecitabine should be taken with a glass of water within 30 minutes after a meal.
2. Contraindicated in patients with known hypersensitivity to 5-FU.
3. Contraindicated in patients with known dihydropyrimidine dehydrogenase (DPD) deficiency.
4. No dose adjustments are necessary in patients with mild-to-moderate liver dysfunction. However, patients should be closely monitored.
5. In the setting of moderate renal dysfunction (baseline CrCl, 30–50 mL/min), a 25% dose reduction is recommended. Patients should be closely monitored as they may be at greater risk for increased toxicity. Contraindicated in patients with severe renal impairment (CrCl <30 mL/min).
6. Patients should be monitored for diarrhea and its associated sequelae, including dehydration, fluid imbalance, and infection. Elderly patients (>80 years of age) are especially vulnerable to the GI toxicity of capecitabine. Moderate-to-severe diarrhea (> grade 2) is an indication to interrupt therapy immediately. Subsequent doses should be reduced accordingly.
7. Drug therapy should be stopped immediately in the presence of grades 2 to 4 hyperbilirubinemia until complete resolution or a decrease in intensity to grade 1.
8. Drug therapy should be stopped immediately in the presence of grades 2 or higher adverse events until complete resolution or a decrease in intensity to grade 1. Treatment should continue at 75% of the initial starting dose for grades 2 or 3 toxicity. For grade 4 toxicities, if the physician chooses to continue treatment, treatment should continue at 50% of the initial starting dose.
9. Patients who experience unexpected, severe grade 3 or 4 myelosuppression, GI toxicity, and/or neurologic toxicity upon initiation of therapy may have an underlying deficiency in dihydropyrimidine dehydrogenase. Therapy must be

discontinued immediately, and further testing to identify the presence of this pharmacogenetic syndrome should be considered.

10. Vitamin B6 (pyridoxine, 50 mg PO bid) may be used to prevent and/ or reduce the incidence and severity of hand-foot syndrome. Dose may be increased to 100 mg PO bid if symptoms do not resolve within 3–4 days.

11. Celecoxib at a dose of 200 mg PO bid may be effective in preventing and/or reducing the incidence and severity of hand-foot syndrome. A low-dose nicotine patch has also been found to be effective in this setting.

12. In patients with the hand-foot syndrome, the affected skin should be well hydrated using a bland and mild moisturizer. Instruct patients to soak affected hands and feet in cool to tepid water for 10 minutes, then apply petroleum jelly onto the wet skin. The use of lanolin-containing salves or ointments such as Bag Balm emollient may help.

13. Diltiazem can prevent capecitabine-induced coronary vasospasm and chest pain and may allow patients to continue to receive capecitabine.

14. Pregnancy category D. Breastfeeding should be avoided.

TOXICITY 1
Diarrhea is dose-limiting, observed in up to 55% of patients. Similar to GI toxicity observed with continuous infusion 5-FU. Mucositis, loss of appetite, dehydration also noted.

TOXICITY 2
Hand-foot syndrome (palmar-plantar erythrodysesthesia). Severe hand-foot syndrome is seen in 15%–20% of patients. Characterized by tingling, numbness, pain, erythema, dryness, rash, swelling, increased pigmentation, and/or pruritus of the hands and feet. Similar to dermatologic toxicity observed with continuous infusion 5-FU.

TOXICITY 3
Nausea and vomiting occur in 15%–53% of patients.

TOXICITY 4
Elevations in serum bilirubin (20%–40%), alkaline phosphatase, and hepatic transaminases (SGOT, SGPT). Usually transient and clinically asymptomatic.

TOXICITY 5
Myelosuppression is observed less frequently than with IV 5-FU. Leukopenia more common than thrombocytopenia.

TOXICITY 6
Neurologic toxicity manifested by confusion, cerebellar ataxia, and rarely encephalopathy.

TOXICITY 7
Cardiac symptoms of chest pain, ECG changes, and serum enzyme elevation. Rare event but increased risk in patients with prior history of ischemic heart disease.

TOXICITY 8
Tear-duct stenosis, acute and chronic conjunctivitis.

Carboplatin

TRADE NAME	Paraplatin, CBDCA	**CLASSIFICATION**	Platinum analog
CATEGORY	Chemotherapy drug	**DRUG MANUFACTURER**	Bristol-Myers Squibb

MECHANISM OF ACTION
- Covalently binds to DNA with preferential binding to the N-7 position of guanine and adenine.
- Reacts with two different sites on DNA to produce cross-links, either intrastrand (>90%) or interstrand (<5%). Formation of DNA adducts results in inhibition of DNA synthesis and function as well as inhibition of transcription.
- Binding to nuclear and cytoplasmic proteins may result in cytotoxic effects.
- Cell cycle–nonspecific agent.

MECHANISM OF RESISTANCE
- Reduced accumulation of carboplatin due to alterations in cellular transport.
- Increased inactivation by thiol-containing proteins such as glutathione and glutathione-related enzymes.
- Enhanced DNA repair enzyme activity (e.g., ERCC-1).
- Deficiency in mismatch repair (MMR) enzymes (e.g., hMLH1, hMSH2).

ABSORPTION
Not absorbed by the oral route.

DISTRIBUTION
Widely distributed in body tissues. Crosses the blood-brain barrier and enters the CSF. Does not bind to plasma proteins and has an apparent volume of distribution of 16 L.

METABOLISM

Carboplatin does not undergo significant metabolism. As observed with cisplatin, carboplatin undergoes aquation reaction in the presence of low concentrations of chloride. This reaction is 100-fold slower with carboplatin when compared to cisplatin. Carboplatin is extensively cleared by the kidneys, with about 60%–70% of drug excreted in urine within 24 hours. The elimination of carboplatin is slower than that of cisplatin, with a terminal half-life of 2–6 hours.

INDICATIONS

1. Ovarian cancer.
2. Germ cell tumors.
3. Head and neck cancer.
4. Small cell lung cancer (SCLC) and NSCLC.
5. Bladder cancer.
6. Relapsed and refractory acute leukemia.
7. Endometrial cancer.

DOSAGE RANGE

1. Dose of carboplatin is usually calculated to a target area under the curve (AUC) based on the glomerular filtration rate (GFR).
2. Calvert formula is used to calculate dose—Total dose (mg) = (target AUC) × (GFR + 25). Note: Dose is in mg **NOT** mg/m^2.
3. Target AUC is usually between 5 and 7 mg/mL/min for previously untreated patients. In previously treated patients, lower AUCs (between 4 and 6 mg/mL/min) are recommended. AUCs >7 are not associated with improved response rates.
4. Bone marrow/stem cell transplant setting—Doses up to 1600 mg/m^2 divided over several days.

DRUG INTERACTION 1

Myelosuppressive agents—Increased risk of myelosuppression when carboplatin is combined with other myelosuppressive drugs.

DRUG INTERACTION 2

Paclitaxel—Carboplatin should be administered after paclitaxel when carboplatin and paclitaxel are used in combination. This sequence prevents delayed paclitaxel excretion, which results in increased paclitaxel drug levels and potentially increased host toxicity.

SPECIAL CONSIDERATIONS

1. Use with caution in patients with abnormal renal function. Dose reduction is required in the setting of renal dysfunction. Baseline CrCl must be obtained. Renal status must be closely monitored during therapy.
2. Although carboplatin is not as emetogenic as cisplatin, pretreatment with antiemetic agents is strongly recommended.

3. Avoid needles or IV administration sets containing aluminum because precipitation of drug may occur.
4. Contraindicated in patients with a history of severe allergic reactions to cisplatin, other platinum compounds, mannitol.
5. In contrast to cisplatin, IV hydration pretreatment and post-treatment are not necessary. However, patients should still be instructed to maintain adequate oral hydration.
6. Hemodialysis clears carboplatin at 25% of the rate of renal clearance. Peritoneal dialysis is unable to remove carboplatin.
7. Risk of hypersensitivity reactions increases from 1% to 27% in patients receiving more than seven courses of carboplatin-based therapy. For such patients, a 0.02-mL intradermal injection of an undiluted aliquot of their planned carboplatin dose can be administered 1 hour before each cycle of carboplatin. This skin test identifies patients in whom carboplatin may be safely administered.
8. Pregnancy category D. Breastfeeding should be avoided.

TOXICITY 1
Myelosuppression is significant and dose-limiting. Dose-dependent, cumulative toxicity is more severe in elderly patients. Thrombocytopenia is most commonly observed, with nadir by day 21.

TOXICITY 2
Nausea and vomiting. Delayed nausea and vomiting can also occur, albeit rarely. Significantly less emetogenic than cisplatin.

TOXICITY 3
Renal toxicity. Significantly less common than with cisplatin and rarely symptomatic.

TOXICITY 4
Peripheral neuropathy is observed in less than 10% of patients. Patients older than 65 years and/or previously treated with cisplatin may be at higher risk for developing neurologic toxicity.

TOXICITY 5
Mild and reversible elevation of liver enzymes, particularly alkaline phosphatase and SGOT.

TOXICITY 6
Allergic reaction. Can occur within a few minutes of starting therapy. Presents mainly as skin rash, urticaria, and pruritus. Bronchospasm and hypotension are uncommon.

TOXICITY 7
Alopecia is uncommon.

C

Carfilzomib

TRADE NAMES	Kyprolis	CLASSIFICATION	Proteasome inhibitor
CATEGORY	Chemotherapy drug	DRUG MANUFACTURER	Onyx

MECHANISM OF ACTION
- Tetrapeptide epoxyketone proteasome inhibitor of the 26S proteasome.
- Binds to the N-terminal threonine-containing active sites of the 20S proteasome, the proteolytic core within the 26S proteasome.
- The 26S proteasome is a large protein complex that degrades ubiquinated proteins. This pathway plays an essential role in regulating the intracellular concentrations of various cellular proteins.
- Inhibition of the 26S proteasome prevents the targeted proteolysis of ubiquinated proteins, and disruption of this normal pathway can affect multiple signaling pathways within the cell, leading to cell death.
- Results in downregulation of the NF-κB pathway. NF-κB is a transcription factor that stimulates the production of various growth factors, including IL-6, cell adhesion molecules, and antiapoptotic proteins, all of which contribute to cell growth and chemoresistance.
- Can overcome resistance to bortezomib.
- Displays *in vitro* growth inhibitory activity in both solid tumors and hematologic malignancy cancer cells.

MECHANISM OF RESISTANCE
Increased expression of the multidrug-resistant gene with elevated P170 protein, leading to increased drug efflux and decreased intracellular accumulation.

ABSORPTION
Carfilzomib is given only by the IV route.

DISTRIBUTION
Mean steady-state volume of distribution is 28 L. Based on *in vitro* testing, about 97% of drug bound to plasma proteins.

METABOLISM
Carfilzomib is rapidly and extensively metabolized by peptidase cleavage and epoxide hydrolysis. The metabolites have no documented antitumor activity. Liver P450-mediated mechanisms play a relatively minor role in drug metabolism. Carfilzomib is rapidly cleared with a half-life of about 1 hour on day 1 of cycle 1.

INDICATIONS
1. FDA-approved for the treatment of patients with multiple myeloma who have received at least two prior therapies, including bortezomib and an immunomodulatory therapy.
2. FDA-approved in combination with lenalidomide and dexamethasone as second-line treatment for patients with multiple myeloma.

DOSAGE RANGE
Recommended dose for cycle 1 is 20 mg/m^2/day and if tolerated, the dose can be increased to 27 mg/m^2/day for cycle 2 and all subsequent cycles. Carfilzomib is administered by IV on 2 consecutive days each week for 3 weeks (days 1, 2, 8, 9, 15, and 16) followed by a 12-day rest period (days 17–28).

DRUG INTERACTIONS
None have been well characterized to date.

SPECIAL CONSIDERATIONS
1. Closely monitor for cardiac complications. Patients with prior history of MI in the preceding 6 months, congestive heart failure (CHF), and conduction system abnormalities not controlled by medication may be at increased risk for cardiac complications.
2. Closely monitor pulmonary status given the risk of pulmonary arterial hypertension and pulmonary complications.
3. Monitor for infusion-related events, which can occur immediately following or up to 24 hours after drug dministration. Premedication with dexamethasone 4 mg PO or IV prior to all doses of carfilzomib during cycle 1 and prior to all doses during the first cycle of dose escalation has been shown to reduce the incidence and severity of infusion reactions.
4. Patients should be well hydrated prior to drug administration to reduce the risk of renal toxicity.
5. Patients with high tumor burden are at increased risk for developing tumor lysis syndrome.
6. Monitor CBCs routinely as carfilzomib therapy is associated with thrombocytopenia, with nadirs occurring at around day 8 of each 28-day cycle.
7. Monitor LFTs on a routine basis as hepatotoxicity and rare cases of hepatic failure have been reported with carfilzomib.
8. Pregnancy category D. Breastfeeding should be avoided.

TOXICITY 1
Fatigue and generalized weakness.

TOXICITY 2
Cardiac toxicity with CHF, MI, and rare cases of cardiac arrest.

TOXICITY 3
Myelosuppression with thrombocytopenia, neutropenia, and anemia.

TOXICITY 4
Pulmonary arterial hypertension. Rare event observed in 2% of patients.

TOXICITY 5
Pulmonary toxicity presenting as dyspnea in up to 35% of patients.

TOXICITY 6
Hepatotoxicity with elevations in serum transaminases (SGOT, SGPT). Drug-induced hepatotoxicity with fatal outcomes has been reported.

TOXICITY 7
Fever (>38°C) is relatively common.

TOXICITY 8
Orthostatic hypotension.

Carmustine

$$Cl - CH_2 - CH_2 - N - \overset{\overset{\displaystyle O}{\|}}{C} - NH - CH_2 - CH_2 - Cl$$
$$|$$
$$NO$$

TRADE NAME	BCNU, Bischloro-ethylnitrosourea	**CLASSIFICATION**	Alkylating agent
CATEGORY	Chemotherapy drug	**DRUG MANUFACTURER**	Bristol-Myers Squibb

MECHANISM OF ACTION
- Nitrosourea analog.
- Cell cycle–nonspecific.
- Chloroethyl metabolites interfere with the synthesis of DNA, RNA, and protein.

MECHANISM OF RESISTANCE
- Decreased cellular uptake of drug.
- Increased intracellular thiol content due to glutathione or glutathione-related enzymes.
- Enhanced activity of DNA repair enzymes.

ABSORPTION
Not absorbed via the oral route.

DISTRIBUTION
Lipid-soluble drug with broad tissue distribution. Crosses the blood-brain barrier, reaching concentrations >50% of those in plasma.

METABOLISM
After IV infusion, carmustine is rapidly taken up into tissues and degraded. Extensively metabolized in the liver. Approximately 60%–70% of drug is excreted in urine in its metabolite form, while 10% is excreted as respiratory CO_2. Short serum half-life of only 15–20 minutes.

INDICATIONS
1. Brain tumors—Glioblastoma multiforme, brain stem glioma, medulloblastoma, astrocytoma, and ependymoma.
2. Hodgkin's lymphoma.
3. Non-Hodgkin's lymphoma.
4. Multiple myeloma.
5. Glioblastoma multiforme—Implantable BCNU-impregnated wafer (Gliadel).

DOSAGE RANGE
1. Usual dose is 200 mg/m^2 IV every 6 weeks. Dose can sometimes be divided over 2 days.
2. Higher doses (450–600 mg/m^2) are used with stem cell rescue.
3. Implantable BCNU-impregnated wafers–Up to eight wafers are placed into the surgical resection site after excision of the primary brain tumor.

DRUG INTERACTION 1
Cimetidine—Cimetidine enhances the toxicity of carmustine.

DRUG INTERACTION 2
Amphotericin B—Amphotericin B enhances the cellular uptake of carmustine, thus resulting in increased toxicity, including renal toxicity.

DRUG INTERACTION 3
Digoxin—Carmustine may decrease the plasma levels of digoxin.

DRUG INTERACTION 4
Phenytoin—Carmustine may decrease the plasma levels of phenytoin.

SPECIAL CONSIDERATIONS
1. Administer carmustine slowly over a period of 1–2 hours to avoid intense pain and/or burning at the site of injection. Strategies to decrease pain and/or burning include diluting the drug, slowing the rate of administration, or placing ice above the IV injection site.
2. Monitor CBC while on therapy. Repeated cycles should not be given before 6 weeks, given the delayed and potentially cumulative myelosuppressive effects of carmustine.

3. PFTs should be obtained at baseline and monitored periodically during therapy. There is an increased risk of pulmonary toxicity in patients with a baseline forced vital capacity (FVC) or DLCO below 70% of predicted.
4. Pregnancy category D. Breastfeeding should be avoided.

TOXICITY 1
Myelosuppression is dose-limiting. Nadir typically occurs at 4–6 weeks.

TOXICITY 2
Nausea and vomiting may occur within 2 hours after a dose of drug and can last for up to 4–6 hours.

TOXICITY 3
Facial flushing and a burning sensation at the IV injection site. Skin contact with drug may cause brownish discoloration and pain.

TOXICITY 4
Hepatotoxicity with transient elevations in serum transaminases develops in up to 90% of patients within 1 week of therapy. With high-dose therapy, hepatic veno-occlusive disease may be observed in 5%–20% of patients.

TOXICITY 5
Impotence, male sterility, amenorrhea, ovarian suppression, menopause, and infertility. Gynecomastia is occasionally observed.

TOXICITY 6
Pulmonary toxicity is uncommon at low doses. At cumulative doses greater than 1400 mg/m^2, ILD and pulmonary fibrosis in the form of an insidious cough, dyspnea, pulmonary infiltrates, and/or respiratory failure may develop.

TOXICITY 7
Renal toxicity is uncommon at total cumulative doses < 1000 mg/m^2.

TOXICITY 8
Increased risk of secondary malignancies, especially acute myelogenous leukemia and myelodysplasia.

Ceritinib

TRADE NAMES	Zykadia	CLASSIFICATION	Signal transduction inhibitor
CATEGORY	Chemotherapy drug	DRUG MANUFACTURER	Novartis

MECHANISM OF ACTION
- Inhibits multiple receptor tyrosine kinases (RTKs), including anaplastic lymphoma kinase (ALK), insulin-like growth factor-1 receptor (IGF-1R), insulin receptor, and ROS1, which results in inhibition of tumor growth, tumor angiogenesis, and metastasis.
- Retains activity in NSCLC tumors resistant to crizotinib, including ALK mutations at L1196M, G1269A, I1171T, and S1206Y. However, it does not overcome resistance to G1202R or F1174C mutations.

MECHANISM OF RESISTANCE
- Not well characterized to date.

ABSORPTION
Rapidly absorbed after an oral dose with peak plasma levels achieved within 4–6 hours. Absolute oral bioavailability has not yet been determined. Food with a high fat content can significantly increase drug concentrations by up to 50%–73%.

DISTRIBUTION
Extensive binding (97%) to plasma proteins.

METABOLISM
Metabolized in the liver primarily by CYP3A4 microsomal enzymes. Elimination is mainly hepatic with excretion in feces (92%) with nearly 70% as unchanged parent drug. Renal elimination is relatively minor with only 1.3% of an administered dose being recovered in the urine. Steady-state drug levels are achieved in approximately 15 days. The terminal half-life of ceritinib is approximately 40 hours.

INDICATIONS
FDA-approved for the treatment of patients with ALK-positive metastatic NSCLC who have progressed on or are intolerant to crizotinib.

DOSAGE RANGE
Recommended dose is 750 mg PO daily.

DRUG INTERACTION 1
Drugs such as ketoconazole, itraconazole, erythromycin, clarithromycin, atazanavir, indinavir, nefazodone, nelfinavir, ritonavir, saquinavir, telithromycin, and voriconazole may decrease the rate of metabolism of ceritinib, resulting in increased drug levels and potentially increased toxicity.

DRUG INTERACTION 2
Drugs such as rifampin, phenytoin, phenobarbital, carbamazepine, and St. John's wort may increase the rate of metabolism of ceritinib, resulting in its inactivation.

SPECIAL CONSIDERATIONS

1. Use with caution in patients with hepatic dysfunction, as ceritinib is eliminated mainly via the liver.
2. No dose adjustment is needed for patients with mild hepatic dysfunction. However, the drug has not been evaluated in patients with moderate to severe hepatic dysfunction.
3. Patients receiving ceritinib along with oral warfarin anticoagulant therapy should have their coagulation parameters (PT and INR) monitored frequently as elevations in INR and bleeding events have been observed.
4. Closely monitor LFTs and serum bilirubin on a monthly basis and as clinically indicated, as ceritinib may cause hepatotoxicity. More frequent testing is required in patients who develop LFT elevations. May need to suspend, dose-reduce, or permanently stop ceritinib with the development of drug-induced hepatotoxicity.
5. Closely monitor patients for new or progressive pulmonary symptoms, including cough, dyspnea, and fever.
6. Closely monitor blood sugar levels, especially in diabetic patients or in those on steroids.
7. Baseline and periodic evaluations of ECG and electrolyte status should be performed while on therapy. Use with caution in patients at risk of developing QT prolongation, including hypokalemia, hypomagnesemia, congenital long QT syndrome, patients taking antiarrhythmic medications or any other drugs that may cause QT prolongation.
8. ALK testing using an FDA-approved test is required to confirm the presence of ALK-positive NSCLC for determining which patients should receive ceritinib therapy.
9. Ceritinib should be taken on an empty stomach and should not be taken within 2 hours of a meal.
10. Avoid the concomitant use of proton pump inhibitors, H2-receptor inhibitors, and antacids as these drugs may alter the pH of the upper GI tract, which could change ceritinib solubility, leading to reduced drug bioavailability and decreased systemic drug exposure.
11. Avoid Seville oranges, starfruit, pomelos, grapefruit, and grapefruit products while on ceritinib therapy.
12. Pregnancy category D. Breastfeeding should be avoided.

TOXICITY 1
Hepatotoxicity with elevations in serum transaminases (SGOT, SGPT).

TOXICITY 2
Nausea/vomiting, diarrhea, and abdominal pain are the most common GI side effects.

TOXICITY 3
Pulmonary toxicity with increased cough, dyspnea, fever, and pulmonary infiltrates.

TOXICITY 4
Constitutional side effects with fatigue, asthenia, and anorexia.

TOXICITY 5
Cardiac toxicity with QTc prolongation and sinus bradycardia.

TOXICITY 6
Hyperglycemia.

TOXICITY 7
Skin rash.

Cetuximab

TRADE NAME	Erbitux	CLASSIFICATION	Monoclonal antibody, anti-EGFR antibody
CATEGORY	Biologic response modifier agent	DRUG MANUFACTURER	Bristol-Myers Squibb and ImClone/Eli Lilly

MECHANISM OF ACTION
- Recombinant chimeric IgG1 monoclonal antibody directed against the epidermal growth factor receptor (EGFR). EGFR is overexpressed in a broad range of human solid tumors, including colorectal cancer, head and neck cancer, NSCLC, pancreatic cancer, and breast cancer.
- Precise mechanism(s) of action remains unknown.
- Binds with nearly 10-fold higher affinity to EGFR than normal ligands EGF and TGF-α, which then results in inhibition of EGFR. Prevents both homodimerization and heterodimerization of the EGFR, which leads to inhibition of autophosphorylation and inhibition of EGFR signaling.
- Inhibition of the EGFR signaling pathway results in inhibition of critical mitogenic and antiapoptotic signals involved in proliferation, growth, invasion/metastasis, and angiogenesis.
- Inhibition of the EGFR pathway enhances the response to chemotherapy and/or radiation therapy.
- Immunologic mechanisms may also be involved in antitumor activity, and they include recruitment of ADCC and/or complement-mediated cell lysis.

MECHANISM OF RESISTANCE
- Mutations in EGFR leading to decreased binding affinity to cetuximab.
- Decreased expression of EGFR.
- Increased expression of TGF-α ligand.
- Presence of KRAS mutations, which mainly occur in codons 12 and 13.
- Presence of BRAF mutations.
- Presence of NRAS mutations.
- Increased expression of HER2 through gene amplification.

- Increased HER3 expression.
- Activation/induction of alternative cellular signaling pathways, such as PI3K/Akt and IGF-1R.

DISTRIBUTION
Distribution in the body is not well characterized.

METABOLISM
Metabolism of cetuximab has not been extensively characterized. Half-life is on the order of 5–7 days.

INDICATIONS
1. FDA-approved for the treatment of EGFR-expressing mCRC in combination with irinotecan in irinotecan-refractory disease or as monotherapy in patients who are deemed to be irinotecan-intolerant. The use of cetuximab is not recommended for the treatment of mCRC with KRAS mutations.
2. Approved in Europe in combination with cytotoxic chemotherapy in the front-line treatment of wild-type KRAS mCRC. FDA-approved in combination with FOLFIRI in the front-line treatment of wild-type KRAS mCRC.
3. Head and neck cancer—FDA-approved for use in combination with radiation therapy for the treatment of locally or regionally advanced squamous cell cancer of the head and neck.
4. Head and neck cancer—FDA-approved for use in combination with platinum-based therapy with 5-FU for the treatment of recurrent locoregional disease or metastatic squamous cell cancer of the head and neck.
5. Head and neck cancer—FDA-approved as monotherapy for the treatment of recurrent or metastatic squamous cell cancer of the head and neck progressing after platinum-based therapy.

DOSAGE RANGE
1. Loading dose of 400 mg/m^2 IV administered over 120 minutes, followed by maintenance dose of 250 mg/m^2 IV given on a weekly basis.
2. An alternative dosing schedule is 500 mg/m^2 IV every 2 weeks with no need for a loading dose.

DRUG INTERACTIONS
None well characterized to date.

SPECIAL CONSIDERATIONS
1. Cetuximab should be used with caution in patients with known hypersensitivity to murine proteins and/or any individual components.
2. The level of EGFR expression does not accurately predict for cetuximab clinical activity. As such, EGFR testing should not be required for the clinical use of cetuximab.

3. Extended KRAS and NRAS testing should be performed in all patients being considered for cetuximab therapy. Only patients with wild-type KRAS and NRAS should be treated with cetuximab either as monotherapy or in combination with cytotoxic chemotherapy.
4. Development of skin toxicity appears to be a surrogate marker for cetuximab clinical activity.
5. Use with caution in patients with underlying ILD as these patients are at increased risk for developing worsening of their ILD.
6. In patients who develop a skin rash, topical antibiotics such as clindamycin gel or erythromycin cream or either oral clindamycin, oral doxycycline, or oral minocycline may help. Patients should be warned to avoid sunlight exposure.
7. About 90% of patients experience severe infusion reactions with the first infusion despite the use of prophylactic antihistamine therapy. However, some patients may experience infusion reactions with later infusions.
8. Electrolyte status should be closely monitored, especially serum magnesium levels, as hypomagnesemia has been observed with cetuximab treatment.
9. Pregnancy category C. Breastfeeding should be avoided.

TOXICITY 1
Infusion-related symptoms with fever, chills, urticaria, flushing, fatigue, headache, bronchospasm, dyspnea, angioedema, and hypotension. Occurs in 40%–50% of patients, although severe reactions occur in less than 1%. Usually mild-to-moderate in severity and observed most commonly with administration of the first infusion.

TOXICITY 2
Pruritus, dry skin with mainly a pustular, acneiform skin rash. Presents mainly on the face, neck region, and upper trunk. Improves with continued treatment and resolves upon cessation of therapy.

TOXICITY 3
Pulmonary toxicity in the form of ILD manifested by increased cough, dyspnea, and pulmonary infiltrates. Observed in less than 1% of patients and more frequent in patients with underlying pulmonary disease.

TOXICITY 4
Hypomagnesemia.

TOXICITY 5
Asthenia and generalized malaise observed in nearly 50% of patients.

TOXICITY 6
Paronychial inflammation with swelling of the lateral nail folds of the toes and fingers. Occurs with prolonged use.

Chlorambucil

$$Cl-N-\bigcirc-CH_2CH_2CH_2CO_2H$$

TRADE NAME	Leukeran	**CLASSIFICATION**	Alkylating agent
CATEGORY	Chemotherapy drug	**DRUG MANUFACTURER**	GlaxoSmithKline

MECHANISM OF ACTION
- Aromatic analog of nitrogen mustard.
- Functions as a bifunctional alkylating agent.
- Forms cross-links with DNA resulting in inhibition of DNA synthesis and function.
- Cell cycle–nonspecific. Active in all phases of the cell cycle.

MECHANISM OF RESISTANCE
- Decreased cellular uptake of drug.
- Increased activity of DNA repair enzymes.
- Increased expression of sulfhydryl proteins, including glutathione and glutathione-related enzymes.

ABSORPTION
Oral bioavailability is approximately 75% when taken with food. Maximum plasma levels are achieved within 1–2 hours after oral administration. Extensively bound to plasma proteins.

DISTRIBUTION
Distribution of chlorambucil has not been well studied.

METABOLISM
Metabolized extensively by the liver cytochrome P450 system to both active and inactive forms. Parent drug and its metabolites are eliminated by the kidneys, and 60% of drug metabolites are excreted in urine within 24 hours. The terminal elimination half-life is 1.5–2.5 hours for the parent drug and about 2.5–4 hours for drug metabolites.

INDICATIONS
1. Chronic lymphocytic leukemia (CLL).
2. Non-Hodgkin's lymphoma.
3. Hodgkin's lymphoma.
4. Waldenstrom's macroglobulinemia.

DOSAGE RANGE

CLL—0.1–0.2 mg/kg PO daily for 3–6 weeks as required. This dose is for initiation of therapy. For maintenance therapy, a dose of 2–4 mg PO daily is recommended.

DRUG INTERACTIONS

Phenobarbital, phenytoin, and other drugs that stimulate the liver P450 system— Concurrent use of chlorambucil with these drugs may increase its metabolic activation, leading to increased formation of toxic metabolites.

SPECIAL CONSIDERATIONS

1. Careful review of patient's medication list is required.
2. Contraindicated within 1 month of radiation and/or cytotoxic therapy, recent smallpox vaccine, and seizure history.
3. Use with caution when combined with allopurinol or colchicine as drug-induced hyperuricemia may be exacerbated.
4. Closely monitor CBCs. Discontinuation of chlorambucil is not necessary at the first sign of a reduction in the WBCs. However, fall may continue for 10 days or more after the last dose.
5. Therapy should be discontinued promptly if generalized skin rash develops as this side effect may rapidly progress to erythema multiforme, toxic epidermal necrolysis, or Stevens-Johnson syndrome.
6. Pregnancy category D. Breastfeeding should be avoided.

TOXICITY 1

Myelosuppression is dose-limiting. Leukopenia and thrombocytopenia observed equally, with delayed and prolonged nadir occurring 25–30 days and recovery by 40–45 days. Usually reversible, but irreversible bone marrow failure can occur.

TOXICITY 2

Mild nausea and vomiting are common.

TOXICITY 3

Hyperuricemia.

TOXICITY 4

Pulmonary fibrosis and pneumonitis are dose-related and potentially life-threatening. Relatively rare event.

TOXICITY 5

Seizures. Children with nephrotic syndrome and patients receiving large cumulative doses are at increased risk. Patients with a history of seizure disorder may be especially prone to seizures.

TOXICITY 6

Skin rash, urticaria on face, scalp, and trunk with spread to legs seen in the early stages of therapy. Stevens-Johnson syndrome and toxic epidermal neurolysis are rare events.

TOXICITY 7
Amenorrhea, oligospermia/azoospermia, and sterility.

TOXICITY 8
Increased risk of secondary malignancies, including acute myelogenous leukemia.

Cisplatin

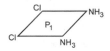

TRADE NAME	CDDP, Platinol	CLASSIFICATION	Platinum analog
CATEGORY	Chemotherapy drug	DRUG MANUFACTURER	Bristol-Myers Squibb

MECHANISM OF ACTION
- Covalently binds to DNA with preferential binding to the N-7 position of guanine and adenine.
- Reacts with two different sites on DNA to produce cross-links, either intrastrand (>90%) or interstrand (<5%). Formation of DNA adducts results in inhibition of DNA synthesis and function as well as inhibition of transcription.
- Binding to nuclear and cytoplasmic proteins may result in cytotoxic effects.

d(GpG) adduct

H_3N NH_3
Pt
5′ — G — G — 3′
3′ — C — C — 5′

d(ApG) adduct

H_3N NH_3
Pt
5′ — A — G — 3′
3′ — T — C — 5′

d(GpXpG) adduct

H_3N NH_3
Pt
5′ — G — X — G — 3′
3′ — C — X — C — 5′

Interstrand cross-link

H_3N NH_3
Pt
— G — C —
— C — G —

MECHANISM OF RESISTANCE
- Increased inactivation by thiol-containing proteins such as glutathione and glutathione-related enzymes.
- Increased DNA repair enzyme activity (e.g., ERCC-1).
- Deficiency in mismatch repair enzymes (e.g., hMHL1, hMSH2).
- Decreased drug accumulation due to alterations in cellular transport.

ABSORPTION
Not absorbed orally. Systemic absorption is rapid and complete after intraperitoneal (IP) administration.

DISTRIBUTION
Widely distributed to all tissues, with highest concentrations in the liver and kidneys. Less than 10% remaining in the plasma 1 hour after infusion.

METABOLISM
Plasma concentrations of cisplatin decay rapidly, with a half-life of approximately 20–30 minutes following bolus administration. Within the cytoplasm of the cell, low concentrations of chloride (4 mM) favor the aquation reaction whereby the chloride atom is replaced by a water molecule, resulting in a highly reactive species. Platinum clearance from plasma proceeds slowly after the first 2 hours due to covalent binding with serum proteins, such as albumin, transferrin, and γ-globulin. Approximately 10%–40% of a given dose of cisplatin is excreted in the urine in 24 hours, with 35%–50% being excreted in the urine after 5 days of administration. Approximately 15% of the drug is excreted unchanged.

INDICATIONS
1. Testicular cancer.
2. Ovarian cancer.
3. Bladder cancer.
4. Head and neck cancer.
5. Esophageal cancer.
6. SCLC and NSCLC.
7. Non-Hodgkin's lymphoma.
8. Trophoblastic neoplasms.

DOSAGE RANGE
1. Ovarian cancer—75 mg/m^2 IV on day 1 every 21 days as part of the cisplatin/paclitaxel regimen, and 100 mg/m^2 on day 1 every 21 days as part of the cisplatin/cyclophosphamide regimen.
2. Testicular cancer—20 mg/m^2 IV on days 1–5 every 21 days as part of the PEB regimen.
3. NSCLC—60–100 mg/m^2 IV on day 1 every 21 days as part of the cisplatin/etoposide or cisplatin/gemcitabine regimens.
4. Head and neck cancer—20 mg/m^2/day IV continuous infusion for 4 days.

DRUG INTERACTION 1

Phenytoin—Cisplatin decreases pharmacologic effect of phenytoin. For this reason, phenytoin dose may need to be increased with concurrent use with cisplatin.

DRUG INTERACTION 2

Amifostine, mesna—The nephrotoxic effect of cisplatin is inactivated by amifostine and mesna.

DRUG INTERACTION 3

Aminoglycosides, amphotericin B, other nephrotoxic agents—Increased renal toxicity with concurrent use of cisplatin and aminoglycosides, amphotericin B, and/or other nephrotoxic agents.

DRUG INTERACTION 4

Etoposide, methotrexate, ifosfamide, bleomycin—Cisplatin reduces the renal clearance of etoposide, methotrexate, ifosfamide, and bleomycin, resulting in the increased accumulation of each of these drugs.

DRUG INTERACTION 5

Etoposide—Cisplatin may enhance the antitumor activity of etoposide.

DRUG INTERACTION 6

Radiation therapy—Cisplatin acts as a radiosensitizing agent.

DRUG INTERACTION 7

Paclitaxel—Cisplatin should be administered after paclitaxel when cisplatin and paclitaxel are used in combination. This sequence prevents delayed paclitaxel excretion and increased toxicity.

DRUG INTERACTION 8

Aminoglycosides, furosemide—Risk of ototoxicity is increased when cisplatin is combined with aminoglycosides and loop diuretics such as furosemide.

SPECIAL CONSIDERATIONS

1. Contraindicated in patients with known hypersensitivity to cisplatin or other platinum analogs.
2. Use with caution in patients with abnormal renal function. Dose of drug must be reduced in the setting of renal dysfunction. Creatinine clearance should be obtained at baseline and before each cycle of therapy. Carefully monitor renal function (BUN and creatinine) as well as serum electrolytes (Na, Mg, Ca, K) during treatment.
3. Fluid status of patient is critical. Patients must be hydrated before, during, and post-drug administration. Usual approach is to give at least 1 liter before and 1 liter post-drug treatment of 0.9% sodium chloride with 20 mEq of KCl. With higher doses of drug, more aggressive hydration should be considered, with at least 2 liters of fluid administered before

drug. In this setting, urine output should be greater than 100 mL/hr. Furosemide diuresis may be used after every 2 liters of fluid.

4. Use with caution in patients with hearing impairment or pre-existing peripheral neuropathy. Baseline audiology exam and periodic evaluation during therapy are recommended to monitor the effects of drug on hearing. Contraindicated in patients with pre-existing hearing deficit.

5. Cisplatin is a potent level 5 emetogenic agent. Give antiemetic premedication to prevent cisplatin-induced nausea and vomiting. Prophylaxis against delayed emesis (>24 hours after the drug administration) is also recommended. A combination of a 5-HT3 antagonist (e.g., ondansetron or granisetron) and dexamethasone is standard therapy for prevention of nausea and vomiting.

6. Avoid aluminum needles when administering the drug because precipitate may form, resulting in decreased potency.

7. Cisplatin is inactivated in the presence of alkaline solutions containing sodium bicarbonate.

TOXICITY 1

Nephrotoxicity. Dose-limiting toxicity in up to 35%–40% of patients. Effects on renal function are dose-related and usually observed at 10–20 days after therapy. Generally reversible. Electrolyte abnormalities, mainly hypomagnesemia, hypocalcemia, and hypokalemia, are common. Hyperuricemia rarely occurs.

TOXICITY 2

Nausea and vomiting. Two forms are observed: acute (within the first 24 hours) and delayed (>24 hours). Early form begins within 1 hour of starting cisplatin therapy and may last for 8–12 hours. The delayed form can present 3–5 days after drug administration.

TOXICITY 3

Myelosuppression occurs in 25%–30% of patients, with WBCs, platelets, and RBCs equally affected. Neutropenia and thrombocytopenia are more pronounced at higher doses. Coombs-positive hemolytic anemia rarely observed.

TOXICITY 4

Neurotoxicity usually in the form of peripheral sensory neuropathy. Paresthesias and numbness in a classic stocking-glove pattern. Tends to occur after several cycles of therapy and risk increases with cumulative doses. Loss of motor function, focal encephalopathy, and seizures also observed. Neurologic effects may be irreversible.

TOXICITY 5

Ototoxicity with high-frequency hearing loss and tinnitus.

TOXICITY 6

Hypersensitivity reactions consisting of facial edema, wheezing, bronchospasm, and hypotension. Usually occur within a few minutes of drug administration.

TOXICITY 7
Ocular toxicity manifested as optic neuritis, papilledema, and cerebral blindness. Altered color perception may be observed in rare cases.

TOXICITY 8
Transient elevation in LFTs, mainly SGOT and serum bilirubin.

TOXICITY 9
Metallic taste of foods and loss of appetite.

TOXICITY 10
Vascular events, including myocardial infarction, arteritis, cerebrovascular accidents, and thrombotic microangiopathy. Raynaud's phenomenon has been reported.

TOXICITY 11
Azoospermia, impotence, and sterility.

TOXICITY 12
Alopecia.

TOXICITY 13
Syndrome of inappropriate antidiuretic hormone secretion (SIADH).

Cladribine

TRADE NAME	2-Chlorodeoxyadenosine, 2-CdA, Leustatin	**CLASSIFICATION**	Antimetabolite
CATEGORY	Chemotherapy drug	**DRUG MANUFACTURER**	Ortho Biotech

MECHANISM OF ACTION
- Purine deoxyadenosine analog with high specificity for lymphoid cells.
- Presence of the 2-chloro group on adenine ring renders cladribine resistant to breakdown by adenosine deaminase.

- Antitumor activity against both dividing and resting cells.
- Metabolized intracellularly to 5′-triphosphate form (Cld-ATP), which is the presumed active species.
- Triphosphate metabolite incorporates into DNA resulting in inhibition of DNA chain extension and inhibition of DNA synthesis and function.
- Inhibition of ribonucleotide reductase.
- Depletes nicotine adenine dinucleotide (NAD) concentration, resulting in depletion of ATP.
- Induction of apoptosis (programmed cell death).

MECHANISM OF RESISTANCE
- Decreased expression of the activating enzyme deoxycytidine kinase resulting in decreased formation of cytotoxic cladribine metabolites.
- Increased expression of 5′-nucleotidase, which dephosphorylates cladribine nucleotide metabolites Cld-AMP and Cld-ATP.

ABSORPTION
Oral absorption is variable with about 50% oral bioavailability. Nearly 100% of drug is bioavailable after SC injection.

DISTRIBUTION
Widely distributed throughout the body. About 20% of drug is bound to plasma proteins. Crosses the blood-brain barrier, but CSF concentrations reach only 25% of those in plasma.

METABOLISM
Extensively metabolized intracellularly to nucleotide metabolite forms. Intracellular concentrations of phosphorylated metabolites exceed those in plasma by several hundred-fold. Terminal half-life is on the order of 5–7 hours. Cleared by the kidneys via a cation organic carrier system. Renal clearance is approximately 50%, with 20%–35% of drug eliminated unchanged.

INDICATIONS
1. Hairy cell leukemia.
2. Chronic lymphocytic leukemia.
3. Non-Hodgkin's lymphoma (low-grade).

DOSAGE RANGE
Usual dose is 0.09 mg/kg/day IV via continuous infusion for 7 days. One course is usually administered. If patient does not respond to one course, it is unlikely that a response will be seen with a second course of therapy.

DRUG INTERACTIONS
None known.

SPECIAL CONSIDERATIONS
1. Use with caution in patients with abnormal renal function.
2. Closely monitor for signs of infection. Patients are at increased risk for opportunistic infections, including herpes, fungus, and *Pneumocystis jiroveci*.

3. Closely monitor for signs of tumor lysis syndrome. Increased risk in patients with a high tumor cell burden.
4. Allopurinol should be given before initiation of therapy to prevent hyperuricemia.
5. Pregnancy category D. Breastfeeding should be avoided.

TOXICITY 1

Myelosuppression is dose-limiting toxicity. Neutropenia more commonly observed than anemia or thrombocytopenia. Leukocyte nadir occurs at 7–14 days, with recovery in 3–4 weeks.

TOXICITY 2

Immunosuppression. Decrease in CD4 and CD8 cells occurs in most patients. Increased risk of opportunistic infections, including fungus, herpes, and *Pneumocystis jiroveci*. Complete recovery of CD4 counts to normal may take up to 40 months.

TOXICITY 3

Fever occurs in 40%–50% of patients. Most likely due to release of pyrogens and/or cytokines from tumor cells. Associated with fatigue, malaise, myalgias, arthralgias, and chills. Incidence decreases with continued therapy.

TOXICITY 4

Mild nausea and vomiting observed in less than 30% of patients.

TOXICITY 5

Tumor lysis syndrome. Rare event, most often in the setting of high tumor cell burden.

TOXICITY 6

Skin reaction at the site of injection.

Clofarabine

TRADE NAMES	Clolar	CLASSIFICATION	Antimetabolite
CATEGORY	Chemotherapy drug	DRUG MANUFACTURER	Genzyme

MECHANISM OF ACTION

- Purine deoxyadenosine nucleoside analog.
- Presence of the 2-fluoro group on the sugar ring renders clofarabine resistant to breakdown by adenosine deaminase.
- Cell cycle–specific with activity in the S-phase.
- Requires intracellular activation to the cytotoxic triphosphate nucleotide metabolite.
- Incorporation of clofarabine triphosphate into DNA resulting in chain termination and inhibition of DNA synthesis and function.
- Clofarabine triphosphate inhibits DNA polymerases α, β, and γ, which, in turn, interferes with DNA synthesis, DNA repair, and DNA chain elongation.
- Clofarabine triphosphate disrupts the mitochondrial membrane, leading to release of cytochrome C and the induction of apoptosis.
- Inhibits the enzyme ribonucleotide reductase, resulting in decreased levels of essential deoxyribonucleotides for DNA synthesis and function.

MECHANISM OF RESISTANCE

- Decreased activation of drug through decreased expression of the anabolic enzyme deoxycytidine kinase.
- Decreased transport of drug into cells.
- Increased expression of cytidine triphosphate (CTP) synthetase activity, resulting in increased concentrations of competing physiologic nucleotide substrate dCTP.

ABSORPTION

Not absorbed via the oral route.

DISTRIBUTION

Approximately 50% bound to plasma proteins, primarily to albumin.

METABOLISM

Extensively metabolized intracellularly to nucleotide metabolite forms. Clofarabine has high affinity for the activating enzyme deoxycytidine kinase and is a more efficient substrate for this enzyme than the normal substrate deoxycytidine. Renal clearance is approximately 50%–60%. The pathways of non-renal elimination remain unknown. The terminal elimination half-life is on the order of 5 hours.

INDICATIONS

FDA-approved for the treatment of pediatric patients 1–21 years of age with relapsed or refractory acute lymphoblastic leukemia after at least two prior regimens.

C

DOSAGE RANGE
Recommended dose is 52 mg/m^2 IV over 2 hours daily for 5 days every 2–6 weeks.

DRUG INTERACTIONS
None well characterized to date.

SPECIAL CONSIDERATIONS
1. Use with caution in patients with abnormal liver and/or renal function. Closely monitor liver and renal function during therapy.
2. As clofarabine is excreted mainly by the kidneys, drugs with known renal toxicity should be avoided during the 5 days of drug treatment.
3. Concomitant use of medications known to cause liver toxicity should be avoided.
4. Patients should be closely monitored for evidence of tumor lysis syndrome and systemic inflammatory response syndrome (SIRS)/capillary leak syndrome, which result from rapid reduction in peripheral leukemic cells following drug treatment. The use of hydrocortisone 100 mg/m^2 IV on days 1–3 may prevent the development of SIRS or capillary leak.
5. Pregnancy category D. Breastfeeding should be avoided.

TOXICITY 1
Myelosuppression is dose-limiting with neutropenia, anemia, and thrombocytopenia.

TOXICITY 2
Capillary leak syndrome/SIRS with tachypnea, tachycardia, pulmonary edema, and hypotension. Pericardial effusion observed in up to 35% of patients, but usually minimal to small and not hemodynamically significant.

TOXICITY 3
Nausea/vomiting and diarrhea are most common GI side effects.

TOXICITY 4
Hepatic dysfunction with elevation of serum transaminases and bilirubin. Usually occur within 1 week and reversible with resolution in 14 days.

TOXICITY 5
Increased risk of opportunistic infections, including fungal, viral, and bacterial infections.

TOXICITY 6
Renal toxicity with elevation in serum creatinine observed in up to 10% of patients.

TOXICITY 7
Cardiac toxicity as manifested by left ventricular dysfunction and tachycardia.

Cobimetinib

TRADE NAME	Cotellic	**CLASSIFICATION**	Signal transduction inhibitor
CATEGORY	Chemotherapy drug	**DRUG MANUFACTURER**	Genentech/Roche

MECHANISM OF ACTION
- Reversible inhibitor of mitogen-activated extracellular signal-regulated kinase 1 (MEK1) and kinase 2 (MEK2).
- Results in inhibition of downstream regulators of the extracellular signal-regulated kinase (ERK) pathway, leading to inhibition of cellular proliferation.
- Inhibits growth of BRAF-V600 mutation-positive melanoma, such as V600E and V600K.

MECHANISM OF RESISTANCE
None well-characterized to date.

ABSORPTION
Oral bioavailability is on the order of 46%. Peak plasma drug concentrations are achieved in 2.4 hours after oral ingestion. Food with a high fat content does not affect C_{max} and AUC. Steady-state blood levels are achieved in 9 days.

DISTRIBUTION
Extensive binding (95%) of cobimetinib to plasma proteins.

METABOLISM
Metabolized mainly via CYP3A oxidation and UGT2B7 glucuronidation in the liver. Elimination is hepatic with 76% of an administered dose excreted in feces (6.6% as parent drug), with renal elimination accounting for only about 18% of an administered dose (1.6% as parent drug). The median terminal half-life of cobimetinib is 44 hours.

INDICATIONS
FDA-approved for unresectable or metastatic melanoma with a BRAF-V600E or V600K mutation in combination with vemurafenib.

DOSAGE RANGE
Recommended dose is 60 mg PO daily for 21 days on a 28-day cycle. Can be taken with or without food.

DRUG INTERACTION 1
Phenytoin and other drugs that stimulate the liver microsomal CYP3A4 enzymes, including carbamazepine, rifampin, phenobarbital, and St. John's wort—These drugs may increase the metabolism of cobimetinib, resulting in its inactivation.

DRUG INTERACTION 2
Drugs that inhibit the liver microsomal CYP3A4 enzymes, including ketoconazole, itraconazole, erythromycin, and clarithromycin—These drugs may decrease the metabolism of cobimetinib, resulting in increased drug levels and potentially increased toxicity.

DRUG INTERACTION 3
Warfarin—Patients receiving coumarin-derived anticoagulants should be closely monitored for alterations in their clotting parameters (PT and INR) and/or bleeding, as cobimetinib may inhibit the metabolism of warfarin by the liver P450 system. Dose of warfarin may require careful adjustment in the presence of cobimetinib therapy.

SPECIAL CONSIDERATIONS
1. Baseline and periodic evaluations of LVEF, at 1 month after treatment initiation and every 3 months thereafter, should be performed while on therapy. The median time to first onset of LVEF reduction is 4 months. Treatment should be held if the absolute LVEF drops by 10% from pretreatment baseline. Therapy should be permanently stopped for symptomatic cardiomyopathy or persistent, asymptomatic LVEF dysfunction that does not resolve within 4 weeks.
2. Patients should be warned about the possibility of visual disturbances.
3. Careful eye exams should be done at baseline and with any new visual changes to rule out the possibility of serous retinopathy or retinal vein occlusion.
4. Monitor patients for symptoms and signs of bleeding.
5. Monitor patients for an increased risk of new primary cancers, both cutaneous and non-cutaneous, while on therapy and for up to 6 months following the last dose of cobimetinib.
6. Monitor patients for skin reactions.
7. Monitor liver function tests periodically during therapy.
8. Monitor patients for skin reactions. The median time to grade 3 or 4 skin toxicity was 11 days.
9. Patients should be educated to avoid sun exposure.
10. Baseline and periodic CPK levels while on therapy as rhabdomyolysis has been observed with cobimetinib therapy.

11. BRAF testing using an FDA-approved diagnostic test to confirm the presence of the BRAF-V600E or V600K mutations is required for determining which patients should receive cobimetinib therapy.
12. No dose adjustment is needed for patients with mild hepatic dysfunction. Caution should be used in patients with moderate or severe hepatic dysfunction.
13. No dose adjustment is needed for patients with mild or moderate renal dysfunction. Use with caution in patients with severe renal dysfunction.
14. Pregnancy category D. Breastfeeding should be avoided.

TOXICITY 1
Cardiac toxicity in the form of cardiomyopathy.

TOXICITY 2
Ocular side effects, including impaired vision, serous retinopathy, retinal detachment, and retinal vein occlusion.

TOXICITY 3
GI toxicity with diarrhea, nausea/vomiting, and mucositis.

TOXICITY 4
Skin toxicity with rash, dermatitis, acneiform rash, hand-foot syndrome, erythema, pruritus, and paronychia. Severe skin toxicity observed in 12% of patients.

TOXICITY 3
Hepatotoxicity

TOXICITY 4
Increased risk of bleeding with GI hemorrhage, reproductive hemorrhage, and hematuria being most commonly observed.

TOXICITY 5
Increased risk of cutaneous squamous cell cancer, keratoacanthoma, and basal cell cancer.

TOXICITY 6
Rhabdomyolysis. Occurs in 14% of patients.

TOXICITY 7
Photosensitivity.

TOXICITY 8
Hypertension.

Crizotinib

TRADE NAMES	Xalkori	CLASSIFICATION	Signal transduction inhibitor
CATEGORY	Chemotherapy drug	DRUG MANUFACTURER	Pfizer

MECHANISM OF ACTION
- Inhibits multiple receptor tyrosine kinases (RTKs), including ALK, hepatocyte growth factor receptor (c-Met), and recepteur d'origine nantais (RON), which results in inhibition of tumor growth, tumor angiogenesis, and metastasis.

MECHANISM OF RESISTANCE
- Mutations in the ALK kinase domain.
- Mutations in EGFR.
- Activation of non-ALK oncogenic pathways.

ABSORPTION
Rapidly absorbed after an oral dose with peak plasma levels achieved within 4–6 hours. Oral bioavailability on the order of 40%–60%. Food with a high fat content reduces oral bioavailability by up to 15%.

DISTRIBUTION
Extensive binding (90%) to plasma proteins. Steady-state drug concentrations are reached in 15 days.

METABOLISM
Metabolized in the liver primarily by CYP3A4 and CYP3A5 microsomal enzymes. Elimination is hepatic with excretion in feces (~60%), with renal elimination accounting for 20% of an administered dose. Unchanged crizotinib represents approximately 50% of an administered dose in feces and about 2% in urine. The terminal half-life of crizotinib is approximately 40 hours.

INDICATIONS

1. FDA-approved for the treatment of locally advanced or metastatic NSCLC that is ALK–positive as detected by an FDA-approved test.
2. FDA-approved for the treatment of patients with metastatic NSCLC whose tumors are ROS1-positive.

DOSAGE RANGE

Recommended dose is 250 mg PO bid.

DRUG INTERACTION 1

Drugs such as ketoconazole, itraconazole, erythromycin, clarithromycin, atazanavir, indinavir, nefazodone, nelfinavir, ritonavir, saquinavir, telithromycin, and voriconazole may decrease the rate of metabolism of crizotinib, resulting in increased drug levels and potentially increased toxicity.

DRUG INTERACTION 2

Drugs such as rifampin, phenytoin, phenobarbital, carbamazepine, and St. John's wort may increase the rate of metabolism of crizotinib, resulting in its inactivation.

DRUG INTERACTION 3

Proton pump inhibitors, H2-receptor inhibitors, and antacids—Drugs that alter the pH of the upper GI tract may alter crizotinib solubility, thereby reducing drug bioavailability and decreasing systemic drug exposure.

SPECIAL CONSIDERATIONS

1. Use with caution in patients with hepatic dysfunction, as crizotinib has not been studied in this setting.
2. Dose reduction to 250 mg PO once daily in patients with severe renal dysfunction (CrCl<30 mL/min) not requiring dialysis.
3. Patients should be advised against performing activities that require mental alertness, including operating machinery and driving.
4. Patients receiving crizotinib along with oral warfarin anticoagulant therapy should have their coagulation parameters (PT and INR) monitored frequently, as elevations in INR and bleeding events have been observed.
5. Closely monitor LFTs and serum bilirubin on a monthly basis and as clinically indicated, as crizotinib may cause life-threatening and/or fatal hepatotoxicity. More frequent testing is required in patients who develop LFT elevations. May need to suspend, dose-reduce, or permanently stop crizotinib with the development of drug-induced hepatotoxicity.
6. Closely monitor patients for new or progressive pulmonary symptoms, including cough, dyspnea, and fever.
7. Patients should be aware of potential visual changes, including blurry vision, photosensitivity, and flashes/floaters. Careful eye exam should be performed in the setting of new or worsening floaters and/ or photopsia to rule out the presence of retinal detachment.
8. Baseline and periodic evaluations of ECG and electrolyte status should be performed while on therapy. Use with caution in patients at risk of developing QT prolongation, including hypokalemia, hypomagnesemia, congenital long QT syndrome, patients taking antiarrhythmic medications or any other drugs that may cause QT prolongation.

9. ALK testing using an FDA-approved test is required to confirm the presence of ALK-positive NSCLC for determining which patients should receive crizotinib therapy.
10. Avoid Seville oranges, starfruit, pomelos, grapefruit, and grapefruit juice while on crizotinib therapy.
11. Pregnancy category D. Breastfeeding should be avoided.

TOXICITY 1

Hepatotoxicity with elevations in serum transaminases (SGOT, SGPT). Drug-induced hepatotoxicity with fatal outcomes have been reported.

TOXICITY 2

Nausea/vomiting and diarrhea are the most common GI side effects.

TOXICITY 3

Pulmonary toxicity with increased cough, dyspnea, fever, and pulmonary infiltrates.

TOXICITY 4

Constitutional side effects with fatigue, asthenia, and anorexia.

TOXICITY 5

Cardiac toxicity with QTc prolongation and sinus bradycardia.

TOXICITY 6

Visual side effects, including diplopia, blurry vision, visual field defects, floaters/flashes, visual brightness, and reduced visual acuity.

TOXICITY 7

Peripheral sensory and/or motor neuropathy have been reported in up to 10% of patients.

Cyclophosphamide

TRADE NAME	Cytoxan, CTX	CLASSIFICATION	Alkylating agent
CATEGORY	Chemotherapy drug	DRUG MANUFACTURER	Bristol-Myers Squibb

MECHANISM OF ACTION
- Inactive in its parent form.
- Activated by the liver cytochrome P450 microsomal system to the cytotoxic metabolites phosphoramide mustard and acrolein.
- Cyclophosphamide metabolites form cross-links with DNA, resulting in inhibition of DNA synthesis and function.
- Cell cycle–nonspecific agent, active in all phases of the cell cycle.

MECHANISM OF RESISTANCE
- Decreased cellular uptake of drug.
- Decreased expression of drug-activating enzymes of the liver P450 system.
- Increased expression of sulfhydryl proteins including glutathione and glutathione-associated enzymes.
- Increased expression of aldehyde dehydrogenase resulting in enhanced enzymatic detoxification of drug.
- Enhanced activity of DNA repair enzymes.

ABSORPTION
Well absorbed by the GI tract with a bioavailability of nearly 90%.

DISTRIBUTION
Distributed throughout the body, including brain and CSF. Also distributed in milk and saliva. Minimal binding of parent drug to plasma proteins; however, about 60% of the phosphoramide mustard metabolite is bound to plasma proteins.

METABOLISM
Extensively metabolized in the liver by the cytochrome P450 system to both active and inactive forms. The active forms are 4-hydroxycyclophosphamide, phosphoramide mustard, and acrolein. Parent drug and its metabolites are eliminated exclusively in urine. The elimination half-life ranges from 4 to 6 hours.

INDICATIONS
1. Breast cancer.
2. Non-Hodgkin's lymphoma.
3. Chronic lymphocytic leukemia.
4. Ovarian cancer.
5. Bone and soft tissue sarcoma.
6. Rhabdomyosarcoma.
7. Neuroblastoma and Wilms' tumor.

DOSAGE RANGE
1. Breast cancer—When given orally, the usual dose is 100 mg/m^2 PO on days 1–14 given every 28 days. When administered IV, the usual dose is 600 mg/m^2 given every 21 days as part of the AC or CMF regimens.
2. Non-Hodgkin's lymphoma—Usual dose is 400–600 mg/m^2 IV on day 1 every 21 days, as part of the CVP regimen, and 750 mg/m^2 on day 1 every 21 days, as part of the CHOP regimen.
3. High-dose bone marrow transplantation—Usual dose in the setting of bone marrow transplantation is 60 mg/kg IV for 2 days.

C

DRUG INTERACTION 1
Phenobarbital, phenytoin, and other drugs that stimulate the liver P450 system—Increase the rate of metabolic activation of cyclophosphamide to its cytotoxic metabolites.

DRUG INTERACTION 2
Anticoagulants—Cyclophosphamide increases the effect of anticoagulants, and thus the dose of anticoagulants may need to be decreased depending on the coagulation parameters, PT/INR.

DRUG INTERACTION 3
Digoxin—Cyclophosphamide decreases the plasma levels of digoxin by activating its metabolism in the liver.

DRUG INTERACTION 4
Doxorubicin—Cyclophosphamide may increase the risk of doxorubicin-induced cardiotoxicity.

SPECIAL CONSIDERATIONS
1. Use with caution in patients with abnormal renal function. Dose should be reduced in the setting of renal dysfunction. CrCl should be obtained at baseline and before each cycle of therapy.
2. Administer oral form of drug during the daytime.
3. Encourage fluid intake of at least 2–3 L/day to reduce the risk of hemorrhagic cystitis. High-dose therapy requires administration of IV fluids for hydration.
4. Encourage patients to empty bladder several times daily (on average, every 2 hours) to reduce the risk of bladder toxicity.
5. Pregnancy category D. Breastfeeding should be avoided.

TOXICITY 1
Myelosuppression is dose-limiting. Mainly leukopenia with nadir occurring at 7–14 days with recovery by day 21. Thrombocytopenia may occur, usually with high-dose therapy.

TOXICITY 2
Bladder toxicity in the form of hemorrhagic cystitis, dysuria, and increased urinary frequency occurs in 5%–10% of patients. Time of onset is variable and may begin within 24 hours of therapy or may be delayed for up to several weeks. Usually reversible upon discontinuation of drug. Uroprotection with mesna and hydration must be used with high-dose therapy to prevent bladder toxicity.

TOXICITY 3
Nausea and vomiting. Usually dose-related, occurs within 2–4 hours of therapy, and may last up to 24 hours. Anorexia is fairly common.

TOXICITY 4
Alopecia generally starting 2–3 weeks after starting therapy. Skin and nails may become hyperpigmented.

TOXICITY 5
Amenorrhea with ovarian failure. Sterility may be permanent.

TOXICITY 6
Cardiotoxicity is observed with high-dose therapy.

TOXICITY 7
Increased risk of secondary malignancies, including acute myelogenous leukemia and bladder cancer, especially in patients with chronic hemorrhagic cystitis.

TOXICITY 8
Immunosuppression with an increased risk of infections.

TOXICITY 9
SIADH.

TOXICITY 10
Hypersensitivity reaction with rhinitis and irritation of the nose and throat. Usually self-resolving in 1–3 days, but steroids and/or diphenhydramine may be required.

Cytarabine

TRADE NAME	Cytosine arabinoside, Ara-C	CLASSIFICATION	Antimetabolite
CATEGORY	Chemotherapy drug	DRUG MANUFACTURER	Bedford Laboratories

MECHANISM OF ACTION

- Deoxycytidine analog originally isolated from the sponge *Cryptotethya crypta*.
- Cell cycle–specific with activity in the S-phase.
- Requires intracellular activation to the nucleotide metabolite ara-CTP. Antitumor activity of cytarabine is determined by a balance between intracellular activation and degradation and the subsequent formation of cytotoxic ara-CTP metabolites.
- Incorporation of ara-CTP into DNA resulting in chain termination and inhibition of DNA synthesis and function.
- Ara-CTP inhibits several DNA polymerases α, β, and γ, which then interferes with DNA synthesis, DNA repair, and DNA chain elongation.
- Ara-CTP inhibits ribonucleotide reductase, resulting in decreased levels of essential deoxyribonucleotides required for DNA synthesis and function.

MECHANISM OF RESISTANCE

- Decreased activation of drug through decreased expression of the anabolic enzyme deoxycytidine kinase.
- Increased breakdown of drug by the catabolic enzymes, cytidine deaminase and deoxycytidylate (dCMP) deaminase.
- Decreased nucleoside transport of drug into cells.
- Increased expression of CTP synthetase activity resulting in increased concentrations of competing physiologic nucleotide substrate dCTP.

ABSORPTION

Poor oral bioavailability (<20%) as a result of extensive deamination within the GI tract.

DISTRIBUTION

Rapidly cleared from the bloodstream after IV administration. Distributes rapidly into tissues and total body water. Crosses the blood-brain barrier with CSF levels reaching 20%–40% of those in plasma. Binding to plasma proteins has not been well characterized.

METABOLISM

Undergoes extensive metabolism, with approximately 70%–80% of drug being recovered in the urine as the ara-U metabolite within 24 hours. Deamination occurs in liver, plasma, and peripheral tissues. The principal enzyme involved in drug catabolism is cytidine deaminase, which converts ara-C into the inactive metabolite ara-U. dCMP deaminase converts ara-CMP into ara-UMP, and this represents an additional catabolic pathway of the drug. The terminal elimination half-life is 2–6 hours. The half-life of ara-C in CSF is somewhat longer, ranging from 2 to 11 hours, due to the relatively low activity of cytidine deaminase present in CSF.

INDICATIONS
1. Acute myelogenous leukemia.
2. Acute lymphocytic leukemia.
3. Chronic myelogenous leukemia.
4. Leptomeningeal carcinomatosis.
5. Non-Hodgkin's lymphoma.

DOSAGE RANGE
Several different doses and schedules have been used:
1. Standard dose—100 mg/m^2/day IV on days 1–7 as a continuous IV infusion, in combination with an anthracycline as induction chemotherapy for AML.
2. High-dose—1.5–3.0 g/m^2 IV q 12 hours for 3 days as a high-dose, intensification regimen for AML.
3. SC—20 mg/m^2 SC for 10 days per month for 6 months, associated with IFN-α for treatment of CML.
4. Intrathecal—10–30 mg intrathecal (IT) up to three times weekly in the treatment of leptomeningeal carcinomatosis secondary to leukemia or lymphoma.

DRUG INTERACTION 1
Gentamicin—Cytarabine antagonizes the efficacy of gentamicin.

DRUG INTERACTION 2
5-Fluorocytosine—Cytarabine inhibits the efficacy of 5-fluorocytosine by preventing its cellular uptake.

DRUG INTERACTION 3
Digoxin—Cytarabine decreases the oral bioavailability of digoxin, thereby decreasing its efficacy. Digoxin levels should be monitored closely while on therapy.

DRUG INTERACTION 4
Alkylating agents, cisplatin, and ionizing radiation—Cytarabine enhances the cytotoxicity of various alkylating agents (cyclophosphamide, carmustine), cisplatin, and ionizing radiation by inhibiting DNA repair mechanisms. Concurrent use of high-dose cytarabine and cisplatin may increase risk of ototoxicity.

DRUG INTERACTION 5
Methotrexate—Pretreatment with methotrexate enhances the formation of ara-CTP metabolites, resulting in enhanced cytotoxicity.

DRUG INTERACTION 6
Fludarabine, hydroxyurea—Pretreatment with fludarabine and/or hydroxyurea potentiates the cytotoxicity of cytarabine by enhancing the formation of cytotoxic ara-CTP metabolites.

DRUG INTERACTION 7
GM-CSF, interleukin-3—Cytokines including GM-CSF and interleukin-3 enhance cytarabine-mediated apoptosis mechanisms.

DRUG INTERACTION 8
L-Asparaginase—Increased risk of pancreatitis when L-asparaginase is given before cytarabine.

SPECIAL CONSIDERATIONS
1. Monitor CBCs on a regular basis during therapy.
2. Use with caution in patients with abnormal liver and/or renal function. Dose modification should be considered in this setting as patients are at increased risk for toxicity. Monitor hepatic and renal function during therapy.
3. Alkalinization of the urine (pH > 7.0), allopurinol, and vigorous IV hydration are recommended to prevent tumor lysis syndrome in patients with acute myelogenous leukemia.
4. High-dose therapy should be administered over a 1- to 2-hour period.
5. Conjunctivitis is observed with high-dose therapy as the drug is excreted in tears. Patients should be treated with hydrocortisone eye drops (2 drops OU qid for 10 days) on the night before the start of therapy.
6. Pregnancy category D. Breastfeeding should be avoided.

TOXICITY 1
Myelosuppression is dose-limiting. Leukopenia and thrombocytopenia are common. Nadir usually occurs by days 7–10, with recovery by days 14–21. Megaloblastic anemia has also been observed.

TOXICITY 2
Nausea and vomiting. Mild-to-moderate emetogenic agent with increased severity observed with high-dose therapy. Anorexia, diarrhea, and mucositis usually occur 7–10 days after therapy.

TOXICITY 3
Cerebellar ataxia, lethargy, and confusion. Neurotoxicity develops in up to 10% of patients. Onset usually 5 days after drug treatment and lasts up to 1 week. In most cases, CNS toxicities are mild and reversible. Risk factors for neurotoxicity include high-dose therapy, age older than 40, and abnormal renal and/or liver function.

TOXICITY 4
Transient hepatic dysfunction with elevation of serum transaminases and bilirubin. Most often associated with high-dose therapy.

TOXICITY 5
Acute pancreatitis.

TOXICITY 6
Ara-C syndrome. Described in pediatric patients and represents an allergic reaction to cytarabine. Characterized by fever, myalgia, malaise, bone pain, maculopapular skin rash, conjunctivitis, and occasional chest pain. Usually occurs within 12 hours of drug infusion. Steroids appear to be effective in treating and/or preventing the onset of this syndrome.

TOXICITY 7
Pulmonary complications include non-cardiogenic pulmonary edema, acute respiratory distress, and *Streptococcus viridans* pneumonia. Observed with high-dose therapy.

TOXICITY 8
Erythema of skin, alopecia, and hidradenitis are usually mild and self-limited. Hand-foot syndrome observed rarely with high-dose therapy.

TOXICITY 9
Conjunctivitis and keratitis. Usually associated with high-dose regimens.

TOXICITY 10
Seizures, alterations in mental status, and fever may be observed within the first 24 hours after IT administration.

D

Dabrafenib

TRADE NAMES	Tafinlar	CLASSIFICATION	Signal transduction inhibitor
CATEGORY	Chemotherapy drug	DRUG MANUFACTURER	GlaxoSmithKline

MECHANISM OF ACTION
- Inhibits mutant forms of BRAF serine-threonine kinase, including BRAF-V600E, which results in constitutive activation of microtubule-associated protein kinase (MAPK) signaling.
- Inhibits wild-type BRAF and CRAF kinases. This inhibitory activity against wild-type BRAF is in sharp contrast to vemurafenib.

MECHANISM OF RESISTANCE
- Increased expression of MAPK signaling.
- Activation/induction of alternative cellular signaling pathways, such as FGFR, EGFR, and PI3K/Akt.
- Reactivation of Ras/Raf signaling.

ABSORPTION
High oral bioavailability on the order of 95%. The time to peak drug concentrations is 2 hours. Food with a high fat content reduces both C_{max} and AUC.

DISTRIBUTION
Extensive binding (>99%) of dabrafenib to plasma proteins.

METABOLISM
Metabolized in the liver primarily by CYP2C8 and CYP3A4 microsomal enzymes to produce the hydroxy-dabrafenib metabolite, which is further metabolized by CYP3A4 to the carboxy-dabrafenib metabolite. The hydroxy metabolite as well as other metabolites may have clinical activity. Elimination is hepatic with excretion in feces (~70%), with renal elimination accounting for about 25% of the administered dose. The median terminal half-life of dabrafenib is approximately 8 hours.

INDICATIONS
1. FDA-approved as a single agent for unresectable or metastatic melanoma with BRAF-V600E mutation as determined by an FDA-approved diagnostic test.

2. FDA-approved in combination with trametinib for unresectable or metastatic melanoma with BRAF-V600E mutation as determined by an FDA-approved diagnostic test.
3. Not recommended for wild-type BRAF melanoma.

DOSAGE RANGE

Recommended dose is 150 mg PO bid. Should be taken at least 1 hour before or at least 2 hours after a meal.

DRUG INTERACTION 1

Drugs such as ketoconazole, itraconazole, erythromycin, clarithromycin, atazanavir, indinavir, nefazodone, nelfinavir, ritonavir, saquinavir, telithromycin, and voriconazole may decrease the rate of metabolism of dabrafenib, resulting in increased drug levels and potentially increased toxicity.

DRUG INTERACTION 2

Drugs such as rifampin, phenytoin, phenobarbital, carbamazepine, and St. John's wort may increase the rate of metabolism of dabrafenib, resulting in its inactivation.

DRUG INTERACTION 3

Warfarin—Dabrafenib may alter the anticoagulant effect of warfarin by prolonging the PT and INR. Coagulation parameters (PT and INR) need to be closely monitored and dose of warfarin may require adjustment.

SPECIAL CONSIDERATIONS

1. Careful skin exams should be done at baseline, every 2 months while on therapy, and for up to 6 months following discontinuation of therapy given the increased incidence of cutaneous squamous cell cancers and keratoacanthomas.
2. Closely monitor body temperature as dabrafenib can cause febrile drug reactions. Dabrafenib should be withheld for fevers >101.3, and patients should be carefully evaluated for infection.
3. Monitor serum glucose levels in patients with diabetes or hyperglycemia.
4. Monitor patients for eye reactions, including uveitis and iritis.
5. BRAF testing using an FDA-approved diagnostic test to confirm the presence of the BRAF-V600E mutation is required for determining which patients should receive dabrafenib therapy.
6. No dose adjustment is needed for patients with mild hepatic dysfunction and in those with mild-to-moderate renal dysfunction. However, caution should be used in patients with moderate-to-severe hepatic dysfunction and in those with severe renal dysfunction.
7. Avoid Seville oranges, pomelos, starfruit, grapefruit, and grapefruit products while on dabrafenib therapy.
8. Pregnancy category D. Breastfeeding should be avoided.

TOXICITY 1

Cutaneous squamous cell cancers and keratoacanthomas occur in up to 10% of patients. Usually occurs within 6–8 weeks of starting therapy.

TOXICITY 2
Skin reactions, including hyperkeratosis, hand-foot syndrome, and rash.

TOXICITY 3
Fever.

TOXICITY 4
Hyperglycemia.

TOXICITY 5
Arthralgias and myalgias.

TOXICITY 6
Opthalmologic side effects, including uveitis, iritis, and photophobia.

TOXICITY 7
Constipation is the most common GI side effect.

TOXICITY 8
Fatigue.

Dacarbazine

TRADE NAME	DIC, DTIC-dome, Imidazole Carboxamide	CLASSIFICATION	Nonclassic alkylating agent
CATEGORY	Chemotherapy drug	DRUG MANUFACTURER	Ben Venue Laboratories, Bayer

MECHANISM OF ACTION
- Cell cycle–nonspecific drug.
- Initially developed as a purine antimetabolite, but its antitumor activity is not mediated via inhibition of purine biosynthesis.
- Metabolic activation is required for antitumor activity.
- While the precise mechanism of cytotoxicity is unclear, this drug methylates nucleic acids and inhibits DNA, RNA, and protein synthesis.

MECHANISM OF RESISTANCE

Increased activity of DNA repair enzymes such as O6-alkylguanine-DNA alkyltransferase (AGAT).

ABSORPTION

Slow and variable oral absorption. For this reason, IV administration is preferred.

DISTRIBUTION

Volume of distribution exceeds total body water content, and drug is widely distributed in body tissues. About 20% of drug is loosely bound to plasma proteins.

METABOLISM

Metabolized in the liver by the microsomal P450 system to active metabolites (MTIC, AIC). The elimination half-life of the drug is 5 hours. About 40%–50% of the parent drug is excreted unchanged in urine within 6 hours, and tubular secretion appears to predominate. No specific guidelines for dacarbazine dosing in the setting of hepatic and/or renal dysfunction. However, dose modification should be considered in patients with moderate to severe hepatic and/or renal dysfunction.

INDICATIONS

1. Metastatic malignant melanoma.
2. Hodgkin's lymphoma.
3. Soft tissue sarcomas.
4. Neuroblastoma.

DOSAGE RANGE

1. Hodgkin's lymphoma—375 mg/m^2 IV on days 1 and 15 every 28 days, as part of the ABVD regimen.
2. Melanoma—220 mg/m^2 IV on days 1–3 and days 22–24 every 6 weeks, as part of the Dartmouth regimen. As a single agent, 250 mg/m^2 IV for 5 days or 800–1000 mg/m^2 IV every 3 weeks.

DRUG INTERACTION 1

Heparin, lidocaine, and hydrocortisone—Incompatible with dacarbazine.

DRUG INTERACTION 2

Phenytoin, phenobarbital—Decreased efficacy of dacarbazine when administered with phenytoin and phenobarbital as these drugs induce dacarbazine metabolism by the liver P450 system.

SPECIAL CONSIDERATIONS

1. Dacarbazine is a potent vesicant, and it should be carefully administered to avoid the risk of extravasation.
2. Dacarbazine is a highly emetogenic agent. Use aggressive antiemetics before drug administration to decrease risk of nausea and vomiting.
3. Patients should avoid sun exposure for several days after dacarbazine therapy.
4. Pregnancy category C. Breastfeeding should be avoided.

TOXICITY 1

Myelosuppression is dose-limiting toxicity. Leukopenia and thrombocytopenia are equally likely, with nadir occurring at 21–25 days.

TOXICITY 2

Nausea and vomiting can be severe, usually occurring within 1–3 hours and lasting for up to 12 hours. Aggressive antiemetic therapy strongly recommended. Anorexia is common, but diarrhea occurs rarely.

TOXICITY 3

Flu-like syndrome in the form of fever, chills, malaise, myalgias, and arthralgias. May last for several days after therapy.

TOXICITY 4

Pain and/or burning at the site of injection.

TOXICITY 5

CNS toxicity in the form of paresthesias, neuropathies, ataxia, lethargy, headache, confusion, and seizures.

TOXICITY 6

Increased risk of photosensitivity.

TOXICITY 7

Teratogenic, mutagenic, and carcinogenic.

Dactinomycin-D

TRADE NAME	Actinomycin-D, Cosmegen	CLASSIFICATION	Antitumor antibiotic
CATEGORY	Chemotherapy drug	DRUG MANUFACTURER	Merck

MECHANISM OF ACTION
- Product of the *Streptomyces* species.
- Consists of a tricyclic phenoxazone chromophore, which is linked to two short, identical cyclic polypeptides.
- Chromophore moiety preferentially binds to guanine-cytidine base pairs. Binding to single- and double-stranded DNA results in inhibition of DNA synthesis and function.
- Formation of oxygen free radicals results in single- and double-stranded DNA breaks and subsequent inhibition of DNA synthesis and function.
- Inhibition of RNA and protein synthesis may also contribute to the cytotoxic effects.

MECHANISM OF RESISTANCE
- Reduced cellular uptake of drug, resulting in decreased intracellular drug accumulation.
- Increased expression of the multidrug-resistant gene with elevated P170 protein levels leads to increased drug efflux and decreased intracellular drug accumulation.

ABSORPTION
Poor oral bioavailability and is administered only via the IV route.

DISTRIBUTION
After an IV bolus injection, dactinomycin rapidly disappears from the circulation in about 2 minutes. Concentrates in nucleated blood cells. Does not cross the blood-brain barrier. Appears to be highly bound to plasma proteins.

METABOLISM
Clinical pharmacology is not well characterized. Metabolized only to small extent. Most of drug is eliminated in unchanged form by biliary (50%) and renal (20%) excretion. Terminal elimination half-life ranges from 30 to 40 hours.

INDICATIONS
1. Wilms' tumor.
2. Rhabdomyosarcoma.
3. Germ cell tumors.
4. Gestational trophoblastic disease.
5. Ewing's sarcoma.

DOSAGE RANGE
1. Adults—0.4–0.45 mg/m^2 IV on days 1–5 every 2–3 weeks.
2. Children—0.015 mg/kg/day (up to a maximum dose of 0.5 mg/day) IV on days 1–5 over a period of 16–45 weeks depending on the specific regimen.

DRUG INTERACTIONS
None well characterized.

SPECIAL CONSIDERATIONS

1. Administer drug slowly by IV push to avoid extravasation.
2. Contraindicated in patients actively infected with chickenpox or herpes zoster as generalized infection may result in death.
3. Use with caution in patients either previously treated with radiation therapy or currently receiving radiation therapy. Increased risk of radiation-recall skin reaction.
4. Patients should be cautioned against sun exposure while on therapy.
5. Pregnancy category C. May be excreted in breast milk. Breastfeeding should be avoided.

TOXICITY 1

Myelosuppression is dose-limiting and can be severe. Neutropenia and thrombocytopenia equally observed. Nadir occurs at days 8–14 after administration.

TOXICITY 2

Nausea and vomiting. Onset within the first 2 hours of therapy, lasts for up to 24 hours, and may be severe.

TOXICITY 3

Mucositis and/or diarrhea. Usually occurs within 5–7 days and can be severe.

TOXICITY 4

Alopecia is common.

TOXICITY 5

Hyperpigmentation of skin, erythema, and increased sensitivity to sunlight. Radiation-recall reaction with erythema and desquamation of skin observed with prior or concurrent radiation therapy.

TOXICITY 6

Potent vesicant. Tissue damage occurs with extravasation of drug.

TOXICITY 7

Elevation of serum transaminases in less than 15% of patients. Dose- and schedule-dependent. Hepatoveno-occlusive disease observed rarely with higher doses and daily schedule.

Daratumumab

TRADE NAME	Darzalex	**CLASSIFICATION**	Monoclonal antibody
CATEGORY	Biologic response modifier agent	**DRUG MANUFACTURER**	Janssen Pharmaceutical and Johnson & Johnson

MECHANISM OF ACTION
- Daratumumab is an IgG1κ human monoclonal antibody directed against CD38. CD38 is a cell surface glycoprotein that is highly expressed on multiple myeloma cells, yet expressed at low levels on normal lymphoid and myeloid cells.
- Daratumumab inhibits the growth of CD38 expressing tumor cells by inducing apoptosis directly through Fc-mediated crosslinking as well as by immune-mediated tumor cell lysis through complement-dependent cytotoxicity (CDCC), antibody-dependent cell-mediated cytotoxicity (ADCC), and antibody-dependent cellular phagocytosis.
- Myeloid-derived suppressor cells (MDSCs) and regulatory T cells are sensitive to daratumumab-mediated cell lysis.

MECHANISM OF RESISTANCE
None well characterized to date.

ABSORPTION
Administered only by the intravenous route.

DISTRIBUTION
The mean volume of distribution is 4.7 L. Steady state is achieved by 5 months into the every 4-week dosing schedule

METABOLISM
The mean terminal half-life is approximately 18 days.

INDICATIONS
FDA-approved for patients with multiple myeloma who have received at least three prior lines of therapy, including a proteasome inhibitor and an immunomodulatory agent or who are double-refractory to a proteasome inhibitor and an immunomodulatory agent.

DOSAGE RANGE
Recommended dose is 16 mg/kg on a weekly basis for weeks 1-8, then every 2 weeks for weeks 9-24, and finally every 4 weeks from week 25 onwards until disease progression.

DRUG INTERACTION
No known significant interactions have been characterized to date.

SPECIAL CONSIDERATIONS
1. Daratumumab should be administered by infusion IV at the appropriate infusion rate. Consider increasing infusion rate only in the absence of infusion reactions. Please see package insert for specific details on the appropriate infusion rate.
2. Approximately 50% of infusion reactions occur with the first infusion, and nearly all reactions occur during the infusion or within 4 hours of completing the infusion.
3. Premedication with antihistamines (diphenhydramine 25-50 mg PO or IV), antipyretics (acetaminophen 650-1000 mg), and corticosteroids (methylprednisolone 100 mg or equivalent dose of an intermediate-acting or long-acting steroid) is required to reduce the risk of infusion reactions. Interrupt the infusion for any reaction and manage as appropriate. Administer daratumumab in a clinical facility with immediate access to resuscitative measures (e.g., glucocorticoids, epinephrine, bronchodilators, and/or oxygen).
4. Administer oral corticosteroids (20 mg methylprednisolone) on the first and second day after all infusions to reduce the risk of delayed infusion reactions. For patients with chronic obstructive pulmonary disease, consider short- and long-acting bronchodilators and inhaled corticosteroids.
5. Blood transfusion centers should be informed that a patient has received daratumumab, as this drug can bind to CD38 on red blood cells. This binding may result in a positive indirect antiglobulin test (Coombs test), and this effect may persist for up to 6 months after the last infusion.
6. Patients should be typed and screened for red blood cell transfusions prior to starting daratumumab therapy.
7. Daratumumab may interfere with an accurate assessment of the myeloma response as the drug may be detected on serum protein electrophoresis and immunofixation assays that are used to monitor for endogenous M-protein levels.
8. No dose adjustments are recommended for patients with renal dysfunction.
9. No dose adjustments are recommended for patients with mild hepatic dysfunction. However, the drug has not been studied in the setting of moderate or severe hepatic dysfunction.
10. Closely monitor CBCs on a periodic basis.
11. Prophylaxis for herpes zoster virus re-activation is recommended.
12. Pregnancy category not assigned.

TOXICITY 1
Meylosuppression with neutropenia, thrombocytopenia, and anemia.

TOXICITY 2
Infusion reactions, which present with bronchospasm, cough, wheezing, dyspnea, laryngeal edema, and hypertension.

TOXICITY 3:
Nasal congestion and allergic rhinitis.

TOXICITY 4:
Fatigue, reduced appetite, headache.

TOXICITY 5:
Arthralgias, musculoskeletal chest pain, and back pain.

TOXICITY 6:
Increased risk of infections, including URI, nasopharyngitis, and pneumonia. Reactivation of herpes zoster virus has been reported in 3% of patients.

TOXICITY 7:
GI side effects with mild nausea/vomiting, diarrhea, and constipation.

Dasatinib

TRADE NAMES	Sprycel, BMS-354825	CLASSIFICATION	Signal transduction inhibitor
CATEGORY	Chemotherapy drug	DRUG MANUFACTURER	Bristol-Meyers Squibb

MECHANISM OF ACTION
- Potent inhibitor of the Bcr-Abl kinase and Src family of kinases (Src, Lck, Yes, Fyn), c-Kit, and PDGFR-β.
- Differs from imatinib in that it binds to the active and inactive conformations of the Abl kinase domain and overcomes imatinib resistance resulting from Bcr-Abl mutations.

MECHANISM OF RESISTANCE
Single point mutation within the ATP-binding pocket of the Abl tyrosine kinase (T3151).

ABSORPTION
Dasatinib has good oral bioavailability. Rapidly absorbed following oral administration. Peak plasma concentrations are observed between 30 minutes and 6 hours of oral ingestion.

DISTRIBUTION
Extensive distribution in the extravascular space. Binding of parent drug and its active metabolite to plasma proteins in the range of 90%–95%.

METABOLISM
Metabolized in the liver primarily by CYP3A4 liver microsomal enzymes. Other liver P450 enzymes, such as UGT, play a relatively minor role in metabolism. Approximately 85% of an administered dose is eliminated in feces within 10 days. The terminal half-life of the parent drug is in the order of 4–6 hours.

INDICATIONS
1. FDA-approved for the treatment of adults with chronic phase (CP), accelerated phase (AP), or myeloid or lymphoid blast (MB or LB) phase CML with resistance or intolerance to imatinib.
2. FDA-approved for the treatment of adults with Ph+ ALL with resistance or intolerance to prior therapy.
3. FDA-approved in the front-line treatment of patients with chronic phase CML.

DOSAGE RANGE
1. Recommended dose is 70 mg PO bid.
2. An alternative starting dose is 100 mg PO once daily in patients with chronic-phase CML resistant or intolerant to prior therapy including imatinib.

DRUG INTERACTION 1
Dasatinib is an inhibitor of CYP3A4 and may decrease the metabolic clearance of drugs that are metabolized by CYP3A4.

DRUG INTERACTION 2
Drugs such as ketoconazole, itraconazole, erythromycin, and clarithromycin decrease the rate of metabolism of dasatinib, resulting in increased drug levels and potentially increased toxicity.

DRUG INTERACTION 3
Drugs such as rifampin, phenytoin, phenobarbital, carbamazepine, and St. John's wort increase the rate of metabolism of dasatinib, resulting in its inactivation.

DRUG INTERACTION 4
Solubility of dasatinib is pH-dependent. In the presence of famotidine, PPIs, and/or antacids, dasatinib concentrations are reduced.

SPECIAL CONSIDERATIONS

1. Oral dasatinib tablets can be taken with or without food, but must not be crushed or cut.
2. Important to review patient's list of medications as dasatinib has several potential drug–drug interactions.
3. Patients should be warned about not taking the herbal medicine St. John's Wort while on dasatinib therapy.
4. Monitor CBC on a weekly basis for the first 2 months and periodically thereafter.
5. Use with caution when patients are on aspirin, NSAIDs, or anticoagulation as there is an increased risk of bleeding.
6. Closely monitor electrolyte status, especially calcium and phosphate levels, as oral calcium supplementation may be required.
7. Sexually active patients on dasatinib therapy should use adequate contraception.
8. Avoid Seville oranges, starfruit, pomelos, grapefruit, and grapefruit juice while on dasatinib therapy.
9. Patients should be closely monitored for depressive symptoms and suicide ideation while on therapy.
10. Pregnancy category D. Breastfeeding should be avoided.

TOXICITY 1

Myelosuppression with thrombocytopenia, neutropenia, and anemia.

TOXICITY 2

Bleeding complications in up to 40% of patients resulting from platelet dysfunction.

TOXICITY 3

Fluid retention occurs in 50% of patients, with peripheral edema and pleural effusions. Usually mild-to-moderate in severity.

TOXICITY 4

GI toxicity in the form of diarrhea, nausea/vomiting, and abdominal pain.

TOXICITY 5

Fatigue, asthenia, and anorexia.

TOXICITY 6

Elevations in serum transaminases and/or bilirubin.

TOXICITY 7

Hypocalcemia and hypophosphatemia.

TOXICITY 8

Cardiac toxicity in the form of heart failure and QTc prolongation. Occurs rarely (3%–4%). Pulmonary hypertension can also occur (5%).

TOXICITY 9

Insomnia, depression, and suicidal ideation.

Daunorubicin

TRADE NAME	Daunomycin, Cerubidine, Rubidomycin	CLASSIFICATION	Antitumor antibiotic
CATEGORY	Chemotherapy drug	DRUG MANUFACTURER	Ben Venue and Bedford Laboratories

MECHANISM OF ACTION
- Cell cycle–nonspecific agent.
- Intercalates into DNA resulting in inhibition of DNA synthesis and function.
- Inhibits transcription through inhibition of DNA-dependent RNA polymerase.
- Inhibits topoisomerase II by forming a cleavable complex with DNA and topoisomerase II to create uncompensated DNA helix torsional tension, leading to eventual DNA breaks.
- Formation of cytotoxic oxygen free radicals results in single- and double-stranded DNA breaks with inhibition of DNA synthesis and function.

MECHANISM OF RESISTANCE
- Increased expression of the multidrug-resistant gene with elevated P170 levels, which leads to increased drug efflux and decreased intracellular drug accumulation.
- Decreased expression of topoisomerase II.
- Mutation in topoisomerase II with decreased binding affinity to drug.
- Increased expression of sulfhydryl proteins, including glutathione and glutathione-dependent enzymes.

ABSORPTION
Daunorubicin is not absorbed orally.

DISTRIBUTION
Significantly more lipid-soluble than doxorubicin. Widely distributed to tissues with high concentrations in heart, liver, lungs, kidneys, and spleen. Does not cross the blood-brain barrier. Extensively binds to plasma proteins (60%–70%).

METABOLISM

Metabolism in the liver with formation of one of its primary metabolites, daunorubicinol, which has antitumor activity. Parent compound and its metabolites are excreted mainly through the hepatobiliary system into feces. Renal clearance accounts for only 10%–20% of drug elimination. The half-life of the parent drug is 20 hours, while the half-life of the daunorubicinol metabolite is 30–40 hours.

INDICATIONS

1. Acute myelogenous leukemia—Remission induction and relapse.
2. Acute lymphoblastic leukemia—Remission induction and relapse.

DOSAGE RANGE

1. AML—45 mg/m^2 IV on days 1–3 of the first course of induction therapy and on days 1 and 2 on subsequent courses. Used in combination with continuous infusion ara-C.
2. ALL—45 mg/m^2 IV on days 1–3 in combination with vincristine, prednisone, and L-asparaginase.
3. Single agent—40 mg/m^2 IV every 2 weeks.

DRUG INTERACTION 1

Dexamethasone, heparin—Daunorubicin is incompatible with dexamethasone and heparin, as a precipitate will form.

DRUG INTERACTION 2

Dexrazoxane—Cardiotoxic effects of daunorubicin are inhibited by the iron-chelating agent dexrazoxane (ICRF-187, Zinecard).

SPECIAL CONSIDERATIONS

1. Use with caution in patients with abnormal liver function. Dose reduction is required in the setting of liver dysfunction.
2. Because daunorubicin is a vesicant, administer slowly over 60 minutes with a rapidly flowing IV. Careful administration of the drug, usually through a central venous catheter, is necessary as the drug is a strong vesicant. Close monitoring is necessary to avoid extravasation. If extravasation is suspected, immediately stop infusion, withdraw fluid, elevate extremity, and apply ice to involved site. May administer local steroids. In severe cases, consult a plastic surgeon.
3. Monitor cardiac function before (baseline) and periodically during therapy with either multigated acquisition (MUGA) radionuclide scan or echocardiogram to assess LVEF. Risk of cardiotoxicity is higher in patients >70 years of age, in patients with prior history of hypertension or pre-existing heart disease, and in patients previously treated with anthracyclines or prior radiation therapy to the chest. Cumulative doses of >550 mg/m^2 are associated with increased risk for cardiotoxicity.
4. Use with caution in patients previously treated with radiation therapy as daunorubicin can cause a radiation-recall skin reaction.

5. Patients should be cautioned to avoid sun exposure and to wear sun protection when outside.
6. Patients should be warned about the potential for red-orange discoloration of urine that may occur for 1–2 days after drug administration.
7. Pregnancy category D. Breastfeeding should be avoided.

TOXICITY 1
Myelosuppression. Dose-limiting toxicity with leukopenia being more common than thrombocytopenia. Nadir occurs at 10–14 days with recovery by day 21.

TOXICITY 2
Nausea and vomiting. Usually mild, occurring in 50% of patients within 1–2 hours of treatment.

TOXICITY 3
Mucositis and diarrhea are common within the first week of treatment but not dose-limiting.

TOXICITY 4
Cardiotoxicity. Acute form presents within the first 2–3 days as arrhythmias and/or conduction abnormalities, ECG changes, pericarditis, and/or myocarditis. Usually transient and mostly asymptomatic.

Chronic form associated with a dose-dependent, dilated cardiomyopathy and congestive heart failure. Incidence increases with cumulative doses greater than 550 mg/m^2.

TOXICITY 5
Strong vesicant. Extravasation can lead to tissue necrosis and chemical thrombophlebitis at the injection site.

TOXICITY 6
Hyperpigmentation of nails, rarely skin rash, and urticaria. Radiation-recall skin reaction can occur at prior sites of irradiation. Increased hypersensitivity to sunlight.

TOXICITY 7
Alopecia is universal. Usually reversible within 5–7 weeks after termination of treatment.

TOXICITY 8
Red-orange discoloration of urine. Lasts 1–2 days after drug administration.

Daunorubicin liposome

TRADE NAME	DaunoXome	CLASSIFICATION	Antitumor antibiotic
CATEGORY	Chemotherapy drug	DRUG MANUFACTURER	Diatos

MECHANISM OF ACTION

- Liposomal encapsulation of daunorubicin.
- Protected from chemical and enzymatic degradation, displays reduced plasma protein binding, and shows decreased uptake in normal tissues when compared to parent compound, daunorubicin.
- Penetrates tumor tissue into which daunorubicin is released, possibly through increased permeability of tumor neovasculature to liposome particles.
- Cell cycle–nonspecific agent.
- Intercalates into DNA resulting in inhibition of DNA synthesis and function.
- Inhibits transcription through inhibition of DNA-dependent RNA polymerase.
- Inhibits topoisomerase II by forming a cleavable complex with DNA and topoisomerase II to create uncompensated DNA helix torsional tension, leading to eventual DNA breaks.
- Formation of oxygen free radicals results in single- and double-stranded DNA breaks with subsequent inhibition of DNA synthesis and function.

MECHANISM OF RESISTANCE

- Increased expression of the multidrug-resistant gene with elevated P170 levels. This leads to increased drug efflux and decreased intracellular drug accumulation.
- Decreased expression of topoisomerase II.
- Mutation in topoisomerase II with decreased binding affinity to drug.
- Increased expression of sulfhydryl proteins, including glutathione and glutathione-dependent enzymes.

ABSORPTION

Daunorubicin liposome is not absorbed orally.

DISTRIBUTION

Small, steady-state volume of distribution (6 L) in contrast to the parent drug, daunorubicin. Distribution is limited mainly to the intravascular compartment. Does not cross the blood-brain barrier. Minimal binding to plasma proteins.

METABOLISM

Metabolism in the liver but the primary metabolite, daunorubicinol, is present only in low concentrations. Cleared from plasma at 17 mL/min in contrast to daunorubicin, which is cleared at 240 mL/min. Elimination half-life is about 4–5 hours, far shorter than that of daunorubicin.

INDICATIONS

HIV-associated, advanced Kaposi's sarcoma—First-line therapy.

DOSAGE RANGE

Usual dose is 40 mg/m^2 IV every 2 weeks.

DRUG INTERACTIONS

None known.

SPECIAL CONSIDERATIONS

1. Use with caution in patients with abnormal liver function. Dose reduction is required in the setting of liver dysfunction.
2. Because the parent drug, daunorubicin, is a vesicant, administer slowly over 60 minutes with a rapidly flowing IV. Careful monitoring is necessary to avoid extravasation. If extravasation is suspected, immediately stop infusion, withdraw fluid, elevate extremity, and apply ice to involved site. May administer local steroids. In severe cases, consult a plastic surgeon.
3. Monitor cardiac function before (baseline) and periodically during therapy with either MUGA radionuclide scan or echocardiogram to assess LVEF. Risk of cardiotoxicity is higher in patients >70 years of age, in patients with prior history of hypertension or pre-existing heart disease, and in patients previously treated with anthracyclines or prior radiation therapy to the chest. Cumulative doses of >320 mg/m^2 are associated with increased risk for cardiotoxicity.
4. Patients may develop back pain, flushing, and chest tightness during the first 5 minutes of infusion. These symptoms are probably related to the lipid component of liposomal daunorubicin. Infusion should be discontinued until symptoms resolve and then resumed at a slower rate.
5. Pregnancy category D. Breastfeeding should be avoided.

TOXICITY 1

Myelosuppression. Dose-limiting toxicity with neutropenia being moderate to severe.

TOXICITY 2

Nausea and vomiting. Occur in 50% of patients and are usually mild.

TOXICITY 3

Mucositis and diarrhea are common but not dose-limiting.

TOXICITY 4

Cardiotoxicity. Acute form presents within the first 2–3 days as arrhythmias and/or conduction abnormalities, ECG changes, pericarditis, and/or myocarditis. Usually transient and mostly asymptomatic.

Chronic form associated with a dose-dependent, dilated cardiomyopathy associated with congestive heart failure. Incidence increases when cumulative doses are greater than 320 mg/m^2.

TOXICITY 5

Infusion-related reaction. Occurs within the first 5 minutes of infusion and manifested by back pain, flushing, and tightness in chest and throat. Observed in about 15% of patients and usually with the first infusion. Improves upon termination of infusion and typically does not recur upon reinstitution at a slower infusion rate.

TOXICITY 6

Vesicant. Extravasation can lead to tissue necrosis and chemical thrombophlebitis at the site of injection.

TOXICITY 7

Hyperpigmentation of nails, rarely skin rash, and urticaria. Radiation-recall skin reaction can occur at prior sites of irradiation. Increased hypersensitivity to sunlight.

TOXICITY 8

Alopecia. Lower incidence than its parent compound, daunorubicin.

Decitabine

TRADE NAMES	5-Aza-2'-deoxycytidine, Dacogen	CLASSIFICATION	Antimetabolite
CATEGORY	Antineoplastic agent, hypomethylating agent	DRUG MANUFACTURER	Eisai

MECHANISM OF ACTION

- Deoxycytidine analog.
- Cell cycle–specific with activity in the S-phase.
- Requires activation to the nucleotide metabolite decitabine triphosphate.
- Incorporation of decitabine triphosphate into DNA, results in inhibition of DNA methyltransferases, which then leads to loss of DNA methylation and gene reactivation. Aberrantly silenced genes, such as tumor suppressor genes, are reactivated and expressed.

MECHANISM OF RESISTANCE
None well characterized to date.

ABSORPTION
Administered only by the IV route.

DISTRIBUTION
Distribution in humans has not been fully characterized. Drug crosses blood-brain barrier. Plasma protein binding of decitabine is negligible.

METABOLISM
The precise route of elimination and metabolic fate of decitabine is not known in humans. One of the elimination pathways is via deamination by cytidine deaminase, found principally in the liver but also in plasma, granulocytes, intestinal epithelium, and peripheral tissues.

INDICATIONS
FDA-approved for treatment of patients with myelodysplastic syndromes (MDS), including previously treated and untreated, de novo, and secondary MDS of all French-American-British subtypes (refractory anemia, refractory anemia with ringed sideroblasts, refractory anemia with excess blasts, refractory anemia with excess blasts in transformation, and chronic myelomonocytic leukemia), and intermediate-1, intermediate-2, and high-risk International Prognostic Scoring System groups.

DOSAGE RANGE
1. Recommended dose is 15 mg/m^2 continuous infusion IV over 3 hours repeated every 8 hours for 3 days. Cycles should be repeated every 6 weeks.
2. An alternative schedule is 20 mg/m^2 IV over 1 hour daily for 5 days given every 28 days.

DRUG INTERACTIONS
None well characterized to date.

SPECIAL CONSIDERATIONS
1. Patients should be treated for a minimum of four cycles. In some cases, a complete or partial response may take longer than four cycles.
2. Monitor CBC on a regular basis during therapy. See prescribing information for recommendations regarding dose adjustments.
3. Decitabine therapy should not be resumed if serum creatinine ≥2 mg/dL, SGPT and/or total bilirubin two times upper limit of normal (ULN), and in the presence of active or uncontrolled infection.
4. Use with caution in patients with underlying liver and/or kidney dysfunction.
5. Pregnancy category D. Breastfeeding should be avoided.

TOXICITY 1
Myelosuppression with pancytopenia is dose-limiting.

TOXICITY 2
Fatigue and anorexia.

TOXICITY 3
GI toxicity in the form of nausea/vomiting, constipation, and abdominal pain.

TOXICITY 4
Hyperbilirubinemia.

TOXICITY 5
Peripheral edema.

Degarelix

TRADE NAME	Firmagon	CLASSIFICATION	GnRH antagonist
CATEGORY	Hormonal agent	DRUG MANUFACTURER	Ferring

MECHANISM OF ACTION
Binds immediately and reversibly to GnRH receptors of the pituitary gland, which leads to inhibition of luteinizing hormone (LH) and follicle stimulating hormone (FSH) production. Causes a rapid and sustained suppression of testosterone without the initial surge that is observed with LHRH agonist therapy.

ABSORPTION
Not orally absorbed because of extensive proteolysis in the hepatobiliary system. Forms a depot upon subcutaneous administration from which degarelix is released into the circulation.

DISTRIBUTION
Distribution throughout total body water. Approximately 90% of degarelix is bound to plasma proteins.

METABOLISM
Metabolism occurs mainly via hydrolysis with excretion of peptide fragments in feces. Approximately 70%–80% is eliminated in feces while the remaining 20%–30% is eliminated in urine. The elimination half-life is approximately 53 days.

INDICATIONS
Advanced prostate cancer.

DOSAGE RANGE
Administer 240 mg SC as a starting dose and then 80 mg SC every 28 days.

DRUG INTERACTIONS
None well characterized.

SPECIAL CONSIDERATIONS
1. Initiation of treatment with degarelix does not induce a transient tumor flare in contrast to LHRH agonists, such as goserelin and leuprolide.
2. Serum testosterone levels decrease to castrate levels within 3 days of initiation of therapy.
3. Use with caution in patients with congenital long QT syndrome, electrolyte abnormalities, CHF, and in patients on antiarrhythmic medications, such as quinidine, procainamide, amiodarone, or sotalol, as long-term androgen deprivation therapy prolongs the QT interval.
4. Pregnancy category X. Breastfeeding should be avoided.

TOXICITY 1
Hot flashes with decreased libido and impotence.

TOXICITY 2
Local discomfort at the site of injection with erythema, swelling, and/or induration.

TOXICITY 3
Weight gain.

TOXICITY 4
Mild elevations in serum transaminases.

TOXICITY 5
Fatigue.

Denileukin diftitox

TRADE NAMES	Ontak, DAB389	CLASSIFICATION	Immunotherapy
CATEGORY	Biologic response modifier agent	DRUG MANUFACTURER	Eisai

MECHANISM OF ACTION
- Recombinant fusion protein composed of amino acid sequences of human interleukin-2 (IL-2) and the enzymatic and translocation domains of diphtheria toxin.
- Specifically binds to the CD25 component of the IL-2 receptor and then internalized via endocytosis.
- Upon release of diphtheria toxin into cytosol, cellular protein synthesis is inhibited, and cell death via apoptosis occurs.

ABSORPTION
Not available for oral use and is administered only via the IV route.

DISTRIBUTION
Volume of distribution is similar to that of circulating blood, and the initial distribution half-life is approximately 2–5 minutes.

METABOLISM
Metabolized primarily via catabolism by proteolytic degradation pathways. The elimination half-life is 70–80 minutes.

INDICATIONS
Persistent or recurrent cutaneous T-cell lymphoma in which the malignant cells express the CD25 component of the IL-2 receptor.

DOSAGE RANGE
Recommended dose is 9 or 18 mg/kg/day IV on days 1–5 every 21 days.

DRUG INTERACTIONS
None known.

SPECIAL CONSIDERATIONS
1. Expression of CD25 on tumor skin biopsy must be confirmed before administration of denileukin diftitox. A testing service is available and can be reached by calling 1-800-964-5836.
2. Contraindicated in patients with a known hypersensitivity to denileukin diftitox or any of its components, including IL-2 and diphtheria toxin.
3. Use with caution in patients with pre-existing cardiac and pulmonary disease, as they are at increased risk for developing serious and sometimes fatal reactions.

4. Resuscitative equipment and medications, including IV antihistamines, corticosteroids, and epinephrine should be readily available at bedside prior to treatment.
5. Monitor serum albumin at baseline and during therapy. Low serum albumin levels place patient at increased risk for vascular leak syndrome. Delay administration of denileukin until the serum albumin is 3 g/dL.
6. Patients should be monitored closely throughout the entire treatment, including vital signs, pre-and post-infusion weights, and evidence of peripheral edema.
7. Premedication with acetaminophen, NSAIDs, and antihistamines can help to reduce the incidence and severity of hypersensitivity reactions.
8. Pregnancy category C. Breastfeeding should be avoided.

TOXICITY 1
Flu-like symptoms with fever, chills, asthenia, myalgias, arthralgias, and headache. Usually mild, transient, and easily manageable.

TOXICITY 2
Hypersensitivity reaction manifested by hypotension, back pain, dyspnea, skin rash, chest pain or tightness, tachycardia, dysphagia, and rarely anaphylaxis. Observed in nearly 70% of patients during or within the first 24 hours of drug infusion.

TOXICITY 3
Vascular leak syndrome characterized by hypotension, edema, and/or hypoalbuminemia. Usually self-limited process. Pre-existing low serum albumin (<3 g/dL) predisposes patients to this syndrome.

TOXICITY 4
Diarrhea may be delayed with prolonged duration. Anorexia along with nausea and vomiting also observed.

TOXICITY 5
Myelosuppression is uncommon with anemia occurring more frequently than neutropenia.

TOXICITY 6
Hepatotoxicity with elevations in serum transaminases and hypoalbuminemia (albumin <2.3 g/dL) in 15%–20% of patients. Usually occurs during the first course and resolves within 2 weeks of stopping therapy.

Docetaxel

TRADE NAME	Taxotere	**CLASSIFICATION**	Taxane, antimicrotubule agent
CATEGORY	Chemotherapy drug	**DRUG MANUFACTURER**	Sanofi-Aventis

MECHANISM OF ACTION
- Semisynthetic taxane. Derived from the needles of the European yew tree.
- High-affinity binding to microtubules enhances tubulin polymerization. Normal dynamic process of microtubule network is inhibited, leading to inhibition of mitosis and cell division.
- Cell cycle–specific agent with activity in the mitotic (M) phase.

MECHANISM OF RESISTANCE
- Alterations in tubulin with decreased affinity for drug.
- Multidrug-resistant (MDR-1) phenotype with increased expression of P170 glycoprotein. Results in enhanced drug efflux with decreased intracellular accumulation of drug. Cross-resistant to other natural products, including vinca alkaloids, anthracyclines, taxanes, and etoposide.

ABSORPTION
Not administered orally.

DISTRIBUTION
Distributes widely to all body tissues. Extensive binding (>90%) to plasma and cellular proteins.

METABOLISM
Extensively metabolized by the hepatic P450 microsomal system. About 75% of drug is excreted via fecal elimination. Less than 10% is eliminated as the parent compound with the majority being eliminated as metabolites. Renal clearance is relatively minor with less than 10% of drug clearance via the kidneys. Plasma elimination is tri-exponential with a terminal half-life of 11 hours.

INDICATIONS

1. Breast cancer—FDA-approved for the treatment of locally advanced or metastatic breast cancer after failure of prior chemotherapy.
2. Breast cancer—FDA-approved in combination with doxorubicin and cyclophosphamide for adjuvant treatment of patients with node-positive breast cancer.
3. NSCLC—FDA-approved for locally advanced or metastatic disease after failure of prior platinum-based chemotherapy.
4. NSCLC—FDA-approved in combination with cisplatin for treatment of patients with locally advanced or metastatic disease who have not previously received chemotherapy.
5. Prostate cancer—FDA-approved in combination with prednisone for androgen-independent (hormone-refractory) metastatic prostate cancer.
6. Gastric cancer—FDA-approved in combination with cisplatin and 5-fluorouracil (5-FU) for advanced gastric cancer, including adenocarcinoma of the gastroesophageal junction, in patients who have not received prior chemotherapy.
7. Head and neck cancer—FDA-approved for use in combination with cisplatin and 5-FU for induction treatment of patients with inoperable, locally advanced disease.
8. SCLC.
9. Refractory ovarian cancer.
10. Bladder cancer.

DOSAGE RANGE

1. Metastatic breast cancer—60, 75, and 100 mg/m^2 IV every 3 weeks or 35–40 mg/m^2 IV weekly for 3 weeks with 1-week rest.
2. Breast cancer—75 mg/m^2 IV every 3 weeks in combination with cyclophosphamide and doxorubicin for adjuvant therapy.
3. NSCLC—75 mg/m^2 IV every 3 weeks or 35–40 mg/m^2 IV weekly for 3 weeks with 1-week rest after platinum-based chemotherapy.
4. NSCLC—75 mg/m^2 IV every 3 weeks in combination with cisplatin in patients who have not received prior chemotherapy.
5. Metastatic prostate cancer—75 mg/m^2 IV every 3 weeks in combination with prednisone.
6. Advanced gastric cancer—75 mg/m^2 IV every 3 weeks in combination with cisplatin and 5-FU.
7. Head and neck cancer—75 mg/m^2 IV every 3 weeks in combination with cisplatin and 5-FU for induction therapy of locally advanced disease.

DRUG INTERACTION 1

Radiation therapy—Docetaxel acts as a radiosensitizing agent.

DRUG INTERACTION 2

Inhibitors and/or activators of the liver cytochrome P450 CYP3A4 enzyme system—Concurrent use with drugs such as cyclosporine, ketoconazole, and erythromycin may affect docetaxel metabolism and its subsequent antitumor and toxic effects.

SPECIAL CONSIDERATIONS

1. Use with caution in patients with abnormal liver function. Patients with abnormal liver function are at significantly higher risk for toxicity, including treatment-related mortality.
2. Closely monitor CBCs; docetaxel therapy should not be given to patients with neutrophil counts of <1500 cells/mm^3.
3. Patients should receive steroid premedication to reduce the incidence and severity of fluid retention and hypersensitivity reactions. Give dexamethasone 8 mg PO bid for 3 days beginning 1 day before drug administration.
4. Closely monitor patients for allergic and/or hypersensitivity reactions, which are related to the polysorbate 80 vehicle in which the drug is formulated. Usually occur with the first and second treatments. Emergency equipment, including Ambu bag, ECG machine, fluids, pressors, and other drugs for resuscitation, must be at bedside before initiation of treatment.
5. Contraindicated in patients with known hypersensitivity reactions to docetaxel and/or polysorbate 80.
6. Use only glass, polypropylene bottles, or polypropylene or polyolefin plastic bags for drug infusion. Administer only through polyethylene-lined administration sets.
7. Monitor patient's weight, measure daily input and output, and evaluate for peripheral edema.
8. Pregnancy category D. Breastfeeding should be avoided.

TOXICITY 1

Myelosuppression. Neutropenia is dose-limiting, with nadir at days 7–10 and recovery by day 14. Thrombocytopenia and anemia are also observed.

TOXICITY 2

Hypersensitivity reactions with generalized skin rash, erythema, hypotension, dyspnea, and/or bronchospasm. Usually occur within the first 2–3 minutes of an infusion and almost always within the first 10 minutes. Most frequently observed with first or second treatments. Usually prevented by premedication with steroid; overall incidence decreased to less than 3%. When it occurs during drug infusion, treat with hydrocortisone IV, diphenhydramine 50 mg IV, and/or cimetidine 300 mg IV.

TOXICITY 3

Fluid retention syndrome. Presents as weight gain, peripheral and/or generalized edema, pleural effusion, and ascites. Incidence increases with total doses >400 mg/m^2. Occurs in about 50% of patients.

TOXICITY 4

Maculopapular skin rash and dry, itchy skin. Most commonly affects forearms and hands. Brown discoloration of fingernails may occur. Observed in up to 50% of patients usually within 1 week after therapy.

TOXICITY 5

Alopecia occurs in up to 80% of patients.

TOXICITY 6

Mucositis and/or diarrhea seen in 40% of patients. Mild-to-moderate nausea and vomiting, usually of brief duration.

TOXICITY 7

Peripheral neuropathy is less commonly observed with docetaxel than with paclitaxel.

TOXICITY 8

Generalized fatigue and asthenia are common, occurring in 60%–70% of patients. Arthralgias and myalgias also observed.

TOXICITY 9

Reversible elevations in serum transaminases, alkaline phosphatase, and bilirubin.

TOXICITY 10

Vesicant. Phlebitis and/or swelling can be seen at the injection site.

Doxorubicin

TRADE NAMES	Adriamycin, Hydroxydaunorubicin	**CLASSIFICATION**	Antitumor antibiotic
CATEGORY	Chemotherapy drug	**DRUG MANUFACTURER**	Bedford Laboratories

MECHANISM OF ACTION

- Anthracycline antibiotic isolated from *Streptomyces* species.
- Intercalates into DNA, resulting in inhibition of DNA synthesis and function.
- Inhibits transcription through inhibition of DNA-dependent RNA polymerase.

- Inhibits topoisomerase II by forming a cleavable complex with DNA and topoisomerase II to create uncompensated DNA helix torsional tension, leading to eventual DNA breaks.
- Formation of cytotoxic oxygen free radicals results in single- and double-stranded DNA breaks with subsequent inhibition of DNA synthesis and function.

MECHANISM OF RESISTANCE

- Increased expression of the multidrug-resistant gene with elevated P170 levels, which leads to increased drug efflux and decreased intracellular drug accumulation.
- Decreased expression of topoisomerase II.
- Mutation in topoisomerase II with decreased binding affinity to doxorubicin.
- Increased expression of sulfhydryl proteins, including glutathione and glutathione-dependent proteins.

ABSORPTION

Not absorbed orally.

DISTRIBUTION

Widely distributed to tissues. Does not cross the blood-brain barrier. About 75% of doxorubicin and its metabolites are bound to plasma proteins.

METABOLISM

Metabolized extensively in the liver to the active hydroxylated metabolite, doxorubicinol. About 40%–50% of drug is eliminated via biliary excretion in feces. Less than 10% of drug is cleared by the kidneys. Prolonged terminal half-life of 20–48 hours.

INDICATIONS

1. Breast cancer.
2. Hodgkin's and non-Hodgkin's lymphoma.
3. Soft tissue sarcoma.
4. Ovarian cancer.
5. SCLC and NSCLC.
6. Bladder cancer.
7. Thyroid cancer.
8. Hepatoma.
9. Gastric cancer.
10. Wilms' tumor.
11. Neuroblastoma.
12. Acute lymphoblastic leukemia.

DOSAGE RANGE

1. Single agent—60–75 mg/m^2 IV every 3 weeks.
2. Single agent—15–20 mg/m^2 IV weekly.
3. Combination therapy—45–60 mg/m^2 every 3 weeks.
4. Continuous infusion—60–90 mg/m^2 IV over 96 hours.

DRUG INTERACTION 1
Dexamethasone, 5-FU, heparin—Doxorubicin is incompatible with dexamethasone, 5-FU, and heparin, as concurrent use will lead to precipitate formation.

DRUG INTERACTION 2
Dexrazoxane—The cardiotoxic effects of doxorubicin are inhibited by the iron-chelating agent dexrazoxane.

DRUG INTERACTION 3
Cyclophosphamide—Increased risk of hemorrhagic cystitis and cardiotoxicity when doxorubicin is given with cyclophosphamide. Important to be able to distinguish between hemorrhagic cystitis and the normal red-orange urine observed with doxorubicin therapy.

DRUG INTERACTION 4
Phenobarbital, phenytoin—Increased plasma clearance of doxorubicin when given concurrently with barbiturates and/or phenytoin.

DRUG INTERACTION 5
Trastuzumab, mitomycin-C—Increased risk of cardiotoxicity when doxorubicin is given with trastuzumab or mitomycin-C.

DRUG INTERACTION 6
6-Mercaptopurine—Increased risk of hepatotoxicity when doxorubicin is given with 6-mercaptopurine.

SPECIAL CONSIDERATIONS
1. Use with caution in patients with abnormal liver function. Dose reduction is required in the setting of liver dysfunction.
2. Because doxorubicin is a strong vesicant, administer slowly with a rapidly flowing IV. Avoid using veins over joints or in extremities with compromised venous and/or lymphatic drainage. Use of a central venous catheter is recommended for patients with difficult venous access and mandatory for prolonged infusions. Careful monitoring is necessary to avoid extravasation. If extravasation is suspected, immediately stop infusion, withdraw fluid, elevate extremity, and apply ice to involved site. May administer local steroids. In severe cases, consult a plastic surgeon.
3. Monitor cardiac function before (baseline) and periodically during therapy with either MUGA radionuclide scan or echocardiogram to assess LVEF. Risk of cardiotoxicity is higher in patients >70 years of age, in patients with prior history of hypertension or pre-existing heart disease, in patients previously treated with anthracyclines, or in patients with prior radiation therapy to the chest. Cumulative doses of >450 mg/m^2 are associated with increased risk for cardiotoxicity.
4. Risk of cardiotoxicity is decreased with weekly or continuous infusion schedules. Use of the iron-chelating agent dexrazoxane (ICRF-187) is also effective at reducing the development of cardiotoxicity.

5. Use with caution in patients previously treated with radiation therapy as doxorubicin can cause radiation-recall skin reaction. Increased risk of skin toxicity when doxorubicin is given concurrently with radiation therapy.
6. Patients should be cautioned to avoid sun exposure and to wear sun protection when outside.
7. Patients should be warned about the potential for red-orange discoloration of urine for 1–2 days after drug administration.
8. Pregnancy category D. Breastfeeding should be avoided.

TOXICITY 1

Myelosuppression. Dose-limiting toxicity with leukopenia more common than thrombocytopenia or anemia. Nadir usually occurs at days 10–14 with full recovery by day 21.

TOXICITY 2

Nausea and vomiting. Usually mild, occurring in 50% of patients within the first 1–2 hours of treatment.

TOXICITY 3

Mucositis and diarrhea. Common but not dose-limiting.

TOXICITY 4

Cardiotoxicity. Acute form presents within the first 2–3 days as arrhythmias and/or conduction abnormalities, ECG changes, pericarditis, and/or myocarditis. Usually transient and mostly asymptomatic and not dose-related.

Chronic form results in a dose-dependent, dilated cardiomyopathy associated with congestive heart failure. Risk increases when cumulative doses are greater than 450 mg/m^2.

TOXICITY 5

Strong vesicant. Extravasation can lead to tissue necrosis and chemical thrombophlebitis at the site of injection.

TOXICITY 6

Hyperpigmentation of nails, rarely skin rash, and urticaria. Radiation-recall skin reaction can occur at prior sites of irradiation. Increased hypersensitivity to sunlight.

TOXICITY 7

Alopecia. Universal but usually reversible within 3 months after termination of treatment.

TOXICITY 8

Red-orange discoloration of urine. Usually occurs within 1–2 days after drug administration.

TOXICITY 9

Allergic, hypersensitivity reactions are rare.

D

Doxorubicin liposome

TRADE NAME	Doxil	CLASSIFICATION	Antitumor antibiotic
CATEGORY	Chemotherapy drug	DRUG MANUFACTURER	Janssen, Sun Pharma

MECHANISM OF ACTION
- Liposomal encapsulation of doxorubicin.
- Protected from chemical and enzymatic degradation, reduced plasma protein binding, and decreased uptake in normal tissues.
- Penetrates tumor tissue into which doxorubicin is released.
- Intercalates into DNA, resulting in inhibition of DNA synthesis and function.
- Inhibits transcription through inhibition of DNA-dependent RNA polymerase.
- Inhibits topoisomerase II by forming a cleavable complex with DNA and topoisomerase II. This creates uncompensated DNA helix torsional tension, leading to eventual DNA breaks.
- Formation of cytotoxic oxygen free radicals results in single- and double-stranded DNA breaks and subsequent inhibition of DNA synthesis and function.

MECHANISM OF RESISTANCE
- Increased expression of the multidrug-resistant gene with elevated P170 protein levels, which leads to increased drug efflux and decreased intracellular drug accumulation.
- Decreased expression of topoisomerase II.
- Mutation in topoisomerase II with decreased binding affinity to drug.
- Increased expression of sulfhydryl proteins, including glutathione and glutathione-dependent proteins.

ABSORPTION
Liposomal doxorubicin is not absorbed orally.

DISTRIBUTION
Mainly confined to the intravascular compartment. In contrast to parent drug, doxorubicin, which has a large V_d (700–1100 L/m^2), liposomal doxorubicin has a small V_d (2 L/m^2). Does not cross the blood-brain barrier. Binding to plasma proteins has not been well characterized.

METABOLISM
Plasma clearance of liposomal doxorubicin is slower than that of doxorubicin, resulting in AUCs that are significantly greater than an equivalent dose of doxorubicin. Prolonged terminal half-life of about 55 hours.

INDICATIONS
1. AIDS-related Kaposi's sarcoma—Used in patients with disease that has progressed on prior combination chemotherapy and/or in patients who are intolerant to such therapy.
2. Ovarian cancer—Metastatic disease refractory to both paclitaxel and platinum-based chemotherapy regimens.
3. Multiple myeloma—FDA-approved in combination with bortezomib in patients who have not previously received bortezomib and who have received at least one prior therapy.

DOSAGE RANGE
1. Kaposi's sarcoma—20 mg/m^2 IV every 21 days.
2. Ovarian cancer—50 mg/m^2 IV every 28 days.
3. Multiple myeloma—30 mg/m^2 IV on day 4 after bortezomib, which is administered at 1.3 mg/m^2 IV on days 1, 4, 8, and 11 every 21 days.

DRUG INTERACTIONS
None well characterized to date.

SPECIAL CONSIDERATIONS
1. Liposomal doxorubicin should **NOT** be substituted for doxorubicin and should be used only where indicated.
2. Use with caution in patients with abnormal liver function. Dose reduction is required in the setting of liver dysfunction.
3. Infusions of liposomal doxorubicin should be given at an initial rate of 1 mg/min over a period of at least 30 minutes to avoid the risk of infusion-associated reactions. This reaction is thought to be related to the lipid component of liposomal doxorubicin. In the event of such a reaction, with flushing, dyspnea, or facial swelling, the infusion should be stopped immediately. If symptoms are minor, can restart infusion at 50% the initial rate. Patients should not be rechallenged in the face of a severe hypersensitivity reaction.
4. Careful monitoring is necessary to avoid extravasation. If extravasation is suspected, immediately stop infusion, withdraw fluid, elevate extremity, and apply ice to involved site. May administer local steroids. In severe cases, consult a plastic surgeon.
5. Monitor cardiac function before (baseline) and periodically during therapy with either MUGA radionuclide scan or echocardiogram to assess LVEF. Risk of cardiotoxicity is higher in patients >70 years of age, in patients with prior history of hypertension or pre-existing heart disease, in patients previously treated with anthracyclines, or in patients with prior radiation therapy to the chest.
6. Monitor CBC weekly while on therapy.
7. Patients should be cautioned about the risk of hand-foot syndrome.
8. Patients should be warned about the potential for red-orange discoloration of urine for 1–2 days after drug administration.
9. Pregnancy category D. Breastfeeding should be avoided.

TOXICITY 1

Myelosuppression. Dose-limiting toxicity with leukopenia more common than thrombocytopenia or anemia. Nadir usually occurs at days 10–14, with full recovery by day 21.

TOXICITY 2

Nausea and vomiting. Usually mild, occurring in 20% of patients.

TOXICITY 3

Mucositis and diarrhea. Common but not dose-limiting.

TOXICITY 4

Cardiotoxicity. Acute form presents within the first 2–3 days as arrhythmias and/or conduction abnormalities, ECG changes, pericarditis and/or myocarditis. Usually transient and mostly asymptomatic, and not dose-related.

Chronic form results in a dose-dependent dilated cardiomyopathy associated with congestive heart failure.

TOXICITY 5

Skin toxicity manifested as the hand-foot syndrome with skin rash, swelling, erythema, pain, and/or desquamation. Usually mild with onset at 5–6 weeks after the start of treatment. May require subsequent dose reduction. More commonly observed in ovarian cancer patients (37%) than in those with Kaposi's sarcoma (5%).

TOXICITY 6

Hyperpigmentation of nails, skin rash, and urticaria. Radiation-recall skin reaction can occur at prior sites of irradiation.

TOXICITY 7

Alopecia. Common but generally reversible within 3 months after termination of treatment.

TOXICITY 8

Infusion reaction with flushing, dyspnea, facial swelling, headache, back pain, tightness in the chest and throat, and/or hypotension. Occurs in about 5%–10% of patients, usually with the first treatment. Upon stopping the infusion, resolves within several hours to a day.

TOXICITY 9

Red-orange discoloration of urine. Usually occurs within 1–2 days after drug administration.

Enzalutamide

TRADE NAME	Xtandi	CLASSIFICATION	Antiandrogen
CATEGORY	Hormonal agent	DRUG MANUFACTURER	Astellas/Medivation

MECHANISM OF ACTION
- Pure androgen receptor (AR) antagonist that acts on different steps in the androgen receptor signaling pathway.
- Competitively inhibits androgen binding to ARs and by inhibiting AR nuclear translocation and co-activator recruitment of the ligand-receptor complex.
- Inhibits the androgen-AR pathway at the receptor and post-receptor ligand binding level.
- The N-desmethyl enzalutamide metabolite exhibits similar antitumor activity to enzalutamide.

MECHANISM OF RESISTANCE
- Androgen receptor gene rearrangement, promoting synthesis of constitutively active truncated androgen receptor splice variants that lack the androgen receptor ligand-binding domain.
- Resistance may also be mediated by NF-κB2/p52 via activation of androgen receptor and splice variants.
- Decreased expression of androgen receptor.
- Mutation in androgen receptor leading to decreased binding affinity to enzalutamide.

ABSORPTION
Rapidly absorbed following oral administration. Peak plasma levels observed 0.5–3 hours after oral ingestion. Steady-state drug levels achieved by day 28 following daily dosing. Co-administration with food does not alter the extent of absorption.

DISTRIBUTION
The mean apparent volume of distribution after a single oral dose is 110 L (29% CV). Extensive binding (97%–98%) to plasma proteins, primarily albumin. N-desmethyl enzalutamide metabolite also exhibits extensive binding to plasma proteins (95%).

METABOLISM

Following oral administration, the major metabolites are enzalutamide, N-desmethyl enzalutamide, and an inactive carboxylic acid metabolite. In vitro, human CYP2C8 and CYP3A4 are responsible for the metabolism of this drug. CYP2C8 is primarily responsible for the formation of the active metabolite N-dimethyl enzalutamide. Primarily eliminated by hepatic metabolism.

INDICATIONS

1. FDA-approved for the treatment of metastatic castration-resistant prostate cancer in patients who have received prior chemotherapy containing docetaxel.
2. FDA-approved for first-line treatment of metastatic castration-resistant prostate cancer.

DOSAGE RANGE

1. Recommended dose is 160 mg PO once daily.

DRUG INTERACTIONS

1. Co-administration with strong CYP2C8 inhibitors, such as gemfibrozil, increases the plasma drug concentrations of both enzalutamide and N-desmethyl enzalutamide.
2. Co-administration with strong or moderate CYP2C8 inducers (e.g., rifampin) may alter the plasma exposure of enzalutamide.
3. Co-administration with strong CYP3A4 inhibitors (e.g., itraconazole) may increase the plasma drug concentration of enzalutamide and N-desmethyl enzalutamide.
4. Co-administration with strong CYP3A4 inducers (e.g., carbamazepine, phenobarbital, phenytoin, rifabutin, rifampin, rifapentine), and moderate CYP3A4 inducers (e.g., bosentan, efavirenz, etravirine, modafinil, nafcillin) and St. John's Wort may decrease the plasma drug concentration of enzalutamide.

SPECIAL CONSIDERATIONS

1. No initial dosage adjustment is necessary for patients with mild-to-moderate renal impairment. The drug has not been tested in patients with severe renal impairment (CrCL <30 mL/min) or end-stage renal disease.
2. No initial dosage adjustment is necessary for patients with mild or moderate hepatic impairment. Patients with severe baseline hepatic impairment (Child-Pugh Class C) have not been evaluated.
3. Closely monitor patients for seizure activity. It remains unclear which patients are at increased risk for developing seizures.
4. Pregnancy category X. Enzalutamide can cause fetal harm when administered to a pregnant woman. It is contraindicated in women who are or may become pregnant while receiving the drug.

TOXICITY 1

Asthenia/fatigue occurs in 50% of patients.

TOXICITY 2

Musculoskeletal adverse events occur including back pain, arthralgia, musculoskeletal pain, muscle weakness, musculoskeletal stiffness, and nonpathologic bone fractures.

TOXICITY 3

Diarrhea occurs in about 20% of patients and is usually mild.

TOXICITY 4

Hot flashes occur in 20% of patients.

TOXICITY 5

Peripheral edema.

TOXICITY 6

Seizures occur rarely in <1% of patients, which usually resolve upon discontinuation of therapy.

Epirubicin

TRADE NAMES	4 Epi-doxorubicin, Ellence	CLASSIFICATION	Antitumor antibiotic
CATEGORY	Chemotherapy drug	DRUG MANUFACTURER	Pfizer

MECHANISM OF ACTION

- Anthracycline derivative of doxorubicin.
- Intercalates into DNA, which results in inhibition of DNA synthesis and function.
- Inhibits topoisomerase II by forming a cleavable complex with topoisomerase II and DNA.
- Formation of cytotoxic oxygen free radicals, which can cause single- and double-stranded DNA breaks.

MECHANISM OF RESISTANCE

- Increased expression of the multidrug-resistant gene with enhanced drug efflux. This results in decreased intracellular drug accumulation.
- Decreased expression of topoisomerase II.
- Mutation in topoisomerase II with decreased binding affinity to drug.
- Increased expression of glutathione and glutathione-associated enzymes.

ABSORPTION

Not orally bioavailable.

DISTRIBUTION

Rapid and extensive distribution to formed blood elements and to body tissues. Does not cross the blood-brain barrier. Epirubicin is extensively bound (about 80%) to plasma proteins. Peak plasma levels are achieved immediately.

METABOLISM

Extensive metabolism by the liver microsomal P450 system. Both active (epirubicinol) and inactive metabolites are formed. Elimination is mainly through the hepatobiliary route. Renal clearance accounts for only 20% of drug elimination. The half-life is approximately 30–38 hours for the parent compound and 20–31 hours for the epirubicinol metabolite.

INDICATIONS

1. Breast cancer—FDA-approved as part of adjuvant therapy in women with axillary node involvement following resection of primary breast cancer.
2. Metastatic breast cancer.
3. Gastric cancer—Active in the treatment of metastatic disease as well as early-stage disease.

DOSAGE RANGE

1. Usual dose is 100–120 mg/m^2 IV every 3 weeks.
2. In heavily pretreated patients, consider starting at lower dose of 75–90 mg/m^2 IV every 3 weeks.
3. Alternative schedule is 12–25 mg/m^2 IV on a weekly basis.

DRUG INTERACTION 1

Heparin—Epirubicin is incompatible with heparin as a precipitate will form.

DRUG INTERACTION 2

5-FU, cyclophosphamide—Increased risk of myelosuppression when epirubicin is used in combination with 5-FU and cyclophosphamide.

DRUG INTERACTION 3

Cimetidine—Cimetidine decreases the AUC of epirubicin by 50% and should be discontinued upon initiation of epirubicin therapy.

SPECIAL CONSIDERATIONS

1. Use with caution in patients with abnormal liver function. Dose modification should be considered in patients with liver dysfunction.
2. Use with caution in patients with severe renal impairment. Dose should be reduced by at least 50% when serum creatinine >5 mg/dL.
3. Use with caution in elderly patients as they are at increased risk for developing toxicity.
4. Careful monitoring of drug administration is necessary to avoid extravasation. If extravasation is suspected, stop infusion immediately, withdraw fluid, elevate arm, and apply ice to site. In severe cases, consult plastic surgeon.
5. Monitor cardiac function before (baseline) and periodically during therapy with either MUGA radionuclide scan or echocardiogram to assess LVEF. Risk of cardiotoxicity is higher in elderly patients >70 years of age, in patients with prior history of hypertension or pre-existing heart disease, in patients previously treated with anthracyclines, or in patients with prior radiation therapy to the chest. In patients with no prior history of anthracycline therapy, cumulative doses of 900 mg/m^2 are associated with increased risk for cardiotoxicity.
6. Epirubicin may be administered on a weekly schedule to decrease the risk of cardiotoxicity.
7. Monitor weekly CBC while on therapy.
8. Use with caution in patients previously treated with radiation therapy as epirubicin may induce a radiation-recall reaction.
9. Patients may experience red-orange discoloration of urine for 24 hours after drug administration.
10. Pregnancy category D. Breastfeeding should be avoided.

TOXICITY 1

Myelosuppression. Dose-limiting toxicity with leukopenia more common than thrombocytopenia. Nadir typically occurs 8–14 days after treatment, with recovery of counts by day 21. Risk of myelosuppression greater in elderly patients and in those previously treated with chemotherapy and/or radiation therapy.

TOXICITY 2

Mild nausea and vomiting. Occur less frequently than with doxorubicin.

TOXICITY 3

Mucositis and diarrhea. Dose-dependent, common, and generally mild.

TOXICITY 4

Cardiotoxicity. Cardiac effects are similar to but less severe than those of doxorubicin. Acute toxicity presents as rhythm or conduction disturbances, chest pain, and myopericarditis syndrome that typically occurs within the first 24–48 hours of drug administration. Transient and mostly asymptomatic, not dose-related.

Chronic form of cardiotoxicity presents as a dilated cardiomyopathy with congestive heart failure. Risk of congestive heart failure increases significantly with cumulative doses >900 mg/m^2. Continuous infusion and weekly schedules are associated with decreased risk of cardiotoxicity. Dexrazoxane may be helpful in preventing epirubicin-mediated cardiotoxicity.

TOXICITY 5
Alopecia. Onset within 10 days of initiation of therapy and regrowth of hair upon termination of treatment. Occurs much less commonly than with doxorubicin, being observed in only 25%–50% of patients.

TOXICITY 6
Potent vesicant. Extravasation can lead to tissue injury, inflammation, and chemical thrombophlebitis at the site of injection.

TOXICITY 7
Skin rash, flushing, hyperpigmentation of skin and nails, and photosensitivity. Radiation-recall skin reaction can occur at previous sites of irradiation.

TOXICITY 8
Red-orange discoloration of urine for 24 hours after drug administration.

Eribulin

TRADE NAME	Halaven	CLASSIFICATION	Nontaxane, antimicrotubule agent
CATEGORY	Chemotherapy drug	DRUG MANUFACTURER	Eisai

MECHANISM OF ACTION
- Synthetic analog of halichondrin B, a product isolated from the marine sponge *Halichondria okadai*.

- Potent antimicrotubule agent, with a novel mechanism that is distinct from other known antimicrotubule agents.
- Cell cycle–specific as it leads to a block in the G2-M phase of the cell cycle.
- Inhibits microtubule growth by sequestering tubulin in nonproductive aggregates with no effect on microtubule shortening.
- Maintains activity in various taxane-resistant tumor cell lines.

MECHANISM OF RESISTANCE

- None well characterized to date.
- Appears to be less susceptible to multidrug resistance P-glycoprotein efflux pump. As such, it may be used in treating multidrug-resistant tumors.

ABSORPTION

Administered only by the IV route.

DISTRIBUTION

Rapidly and extensively distributed with a mean volume of distribution of 43–114 L/m^2. Variable binding to plasma proteins that ranges from 49%–65%.

METABOLISM

No major eribulin metabolites have been identified. Elimination occurs primarily via the hepatobiliary route as parent drug in feces (82%), with only a small amount of drug excreted in the urine (9%). The mean elimination half-life is approximately 40 hours.

INDICATIONS

1. FDA-approved for the treatment of patients with metastatic breast cancer who have previously received at least two chemotherapeutic regimens for the treatment of metastatic disease. Prior therapy should have included an anthracycline and a taxane in either the adjuvant or metastatic setting.
2. FDA-approved for the treatment of patients with unresectable or metastatic liposarcoma who have received a prior anthracycline-containing regimen.

DOSAGE RANGE

Recommended dose is 1.4 mg/m^2 IV on days 1 and 8 of a 21-day cycle.

DRUG INTERACTIONS

Drugs that are associated with QT prolongation—Arsenic trioxide, astemizole, bepridil, certain phenothiazines (chlorpromazine, mesoridazine, and thioridazine), chloroquine, clarithromycin, Class IA antiarrhythmics (disopyramide, procainamide, quinidine), Class III antiarrhythmics (amiodarone, bretylium, dofetilide, ibutilide, sotalol), dextromethorphan, droperidol, erythromycin, grepafloxacin, halofantrine, haloperidol, methadone, pentamidine, posaconazole, saquinavir, sparfloxacin, terfenadine, and troleandomycin.

SPECIAL CONSIDERATIONS

1. Use with caution in patients with moderate renal impairment (CrCl 30–50 mL/min). In this setting, a lower starting dose of 1.1 mg/m^2 is recommended. The safety of this drug is not known in patients with severe renal impairment (CrCl <30 mL/min).
2. Use with caution in patients with mild hepatic impairment (Child-Pugh A). In this setting, a lower starting dose of 1.1 mg/m^2 is recommended. In patients with moderate hepatic impairment (Child-Pugh B), a dose of 0.7 mg/m^2 is recommended. The drug has not been studied in patients with severe hepatic impairment (Child-Pugh C).
3. Closely monitor CBCs on a periodic basis.
4. Monitor ECG with QTc measurement at baseline and periodically during therapy, as QTc prolongation has been observed. Use with caution in patients with a history of CHF, bradyarrhythmias, concomitant use of drugs that prolong QT interval, congenital QT syndrome, and electrolyte abnormalities (hypokalemia and hypomagnesemia).
5. Pregnancy category D. Breastfeeding should be avoided.

TOXICITY 1

Myelosuppression with dose-limiting neutropenia. Thrombocytopenia and anemia observed are observed at a much lower extent.

TOXICITY 2

Fatigue, asthenia, and anorexia.

TOXICITY 3

GI side effects in the form of nausea/vomiting, mucositis, diarrhea, dyspepsia, and dry mouth.

TOXICITY 4

Peripheral neuropathy.

TOXICITY 5

QTc prolongation occurs rarely.

Erlotinib

| **TRADE NAMES** | Tarceva, OSI-774 | **CLASSIFICATION** | Signal transduction inhibitor |
| **CATEGORY** | Chemotherapy drug | **DRUG MANUFACTURER** | OSI, Genentech/Roche |

MECHANISM OF ACTION

- Potent and selective small-molecule inhibitor of the EGFR tyrosine kinase, resulting in inhibition of EGFR autophosphorylation and inhibition of EGFR signaling.
- Inhibition of the EGFR tyrosine kinase results in inhibition of critical mitogenic and antiapoptotic signals involved in proliferation, growth, metastasis, angiogenesis, and response to chemotherapy and/or radiation therapy.
- Active in the absence or presence of EGFR–activating mutations, although activity appears to be higher in tumors that express EGFR–activating mutations.

MECHANISM OF RESISTANCE

- Mutations in the EGFR tyrosine kinase leading to decreased binding affinity to erlotinib.
- Presence of KRAS mutations.
- Presence of BRAF mutations.
- Activation/induction of alternative cellular signaling pathways such as PI3K/Akt and IGF-1R.
- Increased expression of HER2 through gene amplification.
- Increased expression of c-Met through gene amplification.
- Increased expression of NF-κB signaling pathway.

ABSORPTION

Oral bioavailability is approximately 60% and is increased by food to almost 100%.

DISTRIBUTION

Extensive binding (90%) to plasma proteins, including albumin and α1-acid glycoprotein, and extensive tissue distribution. Peak plasma levels are achieved 4 hours after ingestion. Steady-state drug concentrations are reached in 7–8 days.

METABOLISM

Metabolism in the liver primarily by the CYP3A4 microsomal enzyme and by CYP1A2 to a lesser extent. Elimination is mainly hepatic with excretion in the feces, and renal elimination of parent drug and its metabolites account for only about 8% of an administered dose. Following a 100 mg oral dose, 91% of the dose was recovered: 83% in feces (1% of the dose as intact parent) and 8% in urine (0.3%) of the dose as intact parent. The terminal half-life of the parent drug is 36 hours.

INDICATIONS
1. FDA-approved as first-line treatment of metastatic NSCLC with EGFR exon 19 deletions or exon 21 (L858R) substitution mutations.
2. FDA-approved as monotherapy for the treatment of locally advanced or metastatic NSCLC after failure of at least one prior chemotherapy regimen.
3. FDA-approved as maintenance treatment of patients with locally advanced or metastatic NSCLC whose disease has not progressed after four cycles of platinum-based first-line chemotherapy.
4. FDA-approved in combination with gemcitabine for the first-line treatment of patients with locally advanced unresectable or metastatic pancreatic cancer.

DOSAGE RANGE
1. NSCLC—Recommended dose is 150 mg/day PO.
2. Pancreatic cancer—Recommended dose is 100 mg/day PO in combination with gemcitabine.

DRUG INTERACTION 1
Phenytoin and other drugs that stimulate the liver microsomal CYP3A4 enzymes, including carbamazepine, rifampin, phenobarbital, and St. John's wort—These drugs may increase the metabolism of erlotinib, resulting in its inactivation.

DRUG INTERACTION 2
Drugs that inhibit the liver microsomal CYP3A4 enzymes, including ketoconazole, itraconazole, erythromycin, and clarithromycin—These drugs may decrease the metabolism of erlotinib, resulting in increased drug levels and potentially increased toxicity.

DRUG INTERACTION 3
Warfarin—Patients receiving coumarin-derived anticoagulants should be closely monitored for alterations in their clotting parameters (PT and INR) and/or bleeding, as erlotinib may inhibit the metabolism of warfarin by the liver P450 system. Dose of warfarin may require careful adjustment in the presence of erlotinib therapy.

SPECIAL CONSIDERATIONS
1. Use with caution in patients with hepatic impairment, and dose reduction and/or interruption should be considered.
2. Nonsmokers and patients with EGFR-positive tumors are more sensitive to erlotinib therapy.
3. Erlotinib should not be used in combination with platinum-based chemotherapy as there is no evidence of clinical benefit.
4. Closely monitor patients for new or progressive pulmonary symptoms, including cough, dyspnea, and fever. Erlotinib therapy should be interrupted pending further diagnostic evaluation.

5. Consider increasing the dose of erlotinib to 300 mg in patients with NSCLC who are actively smoking, as the metabolism of erlotinib by CYP1A1/1A2 in the liver is induced.
6. In patients who develop a skin rash, topical antibiotics such as clindamycin gel or erythromycin cream/gel or oral clindamycin, oral doxycycline, or oral minocycline may help.
7. Avoid Seville oranges, starfruit, pomelos, grapefruit products, and grapefruit juice while on erlotinib therapy.
8. Avoid the concomitant use of PPIs and H2-blockers as they can reduce the oral bioavailability of erlotinib. If an H2-blocker must be used, erlotinib should be taken 10 hours after the H2-blocker and at least 2 hours before the next H2-blocker.
9. Pregnancy category D. Breastfeeding should be avoided.

TOXICITY 1
Pruritus, dry skin with mainly a pustular, acneiform skin rash occurring most often on face and upper trunk. Nail changes, paronychia, painful fissures or cracking of the skin on hands and feet, and hair growth abnormalities, including alopecia, thinning hair with increased fragility (trichorrhexis), darkening and increased thickness of eyelashes and eyebrows (trichomegaly), and hirsutism.

TOXICITY 2
Diarrhea is most common GI toxicity. Mild nausea/vomiting and mucositis.

TOXICITY 3
Pulmonary toxicity in the form of ILD manifested by increased cough, dyspnea, fever, and pulmonary infiltrates. Occurs rarely and observed in less than 1% of patients and more frequent in patients with underlying pulmonary disease.

TOXICITY 4
Mild-to-moderate elevations in serum transaminases. Usually transient and clinically asymptomatic.

TOXICITY 5
Anorexia.

TOXICITY 6
Conjunctivitis and keratitis. Rare cases of corneal perforation and ulceration.

TOXICITY 7
Rare episodes of GI hemorrhage.

TOXICITY 8
Radiation-recall skin reactions.

Estramustine

TRADE NAMES	Estracyte, Emcyt	**CLASSIFICATION**	Antimicrotubule agent
CATEGORY	Chemotherapy drug	**DRUG MANUFACTURER**	Pfizer

MECHANISM OF ACTION
- Conjugate of nornitrogen mustard and estradiol phosphate.
- Cell cycle–specific agent with activity in the mitosis (M) phase.
- Initially designed to target cancer cells expressing estrogen receptors. However, active against estrogen receptor-negative tumor cells.
- Although this compound was initially designed as an alkylating agent, it has no alkylating activity.
- Inhibits microtubule structure and function and the process of microtubule assembly by binding to microtubule-associated proteins (MAPs).

MECHANISM OF RESISTANCE
- Mechanisms of cellular resistance are different from those identified for other antimicrotubule agents.
- Estramustine-resistant cells do not express increased levels of P170 glycoprotein and are not cross-resistant to other antimicrotubule agents and/or natural products.
- Estramustine-resistant cells display increased efflux of drug with decreased drug accumulation. The underlying mechanism(s) remains ill-defined.

ABSORPTION
Highly bioavailable via the oral route with 70%–75% of an oral dose absorbed.

METABOLISM
Estramustine is supplied as the estramustine phosphate form, which renders it more water-soluble. Rapidly dephosphorylated in the GI tract so that the dephosphorylated form predominates about 4 hours after ingestion. Metabolized primarily in the liver. About 15%–20% of the drug is excreted in urine. Only small amounts of unmetabolized drug are found. Biliary and fecal

excretion of alkylating and estrogenic metabolites has also been demonstrated. Prolonged half-life of 20–24 hours.

INDICATIONS
Hormone-refractory, metastatic prostate cancer.

DOSAGE RANGE
1. Single agent: 14 mg/kg/day PO in 3–4 divided doses.
2. Combination: 600 mg/m^2/day PO days 1–42 every 8 weeks, as part of the estramustine/vinblastine regimen.

DRUG INTERACTIONS
None well characterized.

SPECIAL CONSIDERATIONS
1. Contraindicated in patients with active thrombophlebitis or thromboembolic disorders. Closely monitor patients with history of heart disease and/or stroke.
2. Contraindicated in patients with known hypersensitivity to estradiol or nitrogen mustard.
3. Contraindicated in patients with peptic ulcer disease, severe liver disease, or cardiac disease.
4. Instruct patients to take estramustine with water 1 hour before meals or 2 hours after meals to decrease the risk of GI upset.
5. Administer prophylactic antiemetics to avoid nausea and vomiting.
6. Instruct patients that milk, milk products, and calcium-rich foods may impair absorption of drug.

TOXICITY 1
Nausea and vomiting. Occur within 2 hours of ingestion. Usually mild and respond to antiemetic therapy. However, intractable vomiting may occur after prolonged therapy (6–8 weeks).

TOXICITY 2
Gynecomastia is reported in up to 50% of patients. Can be prevented by prophylactic breast irradiation.

TOXICITY 3
Diarrhea occurs in about 15%–25% of patients.

TOXICITY 4
Cardiovascular complications are rare and include congestive heart failure, cardiac ischemia, and thromboembolism.

TOXICITY 5
Myelosuppression is rare.

TOXICITY 6
Skin rash.

Etoposide

TRADE NAMES	VePesid, VP-16	CLASSIFICATION	Epipodophyllotoxin, topoisomerase II inhibitor
CATEGORY	Chemotherapy drug	DRUG MANUFACTURER	Bristol-Myers Squibb

MECHANISM OF ACTION
- Plant alkaloid extracted from the *Podophyllum peltatum* mandrake plant.
- Cell cycle–specific agent with activity in the late S-and G2-phase.
- Inhibits topoisomerase II by stabilizing the topoisomerase II-DNA complex and preventing the unwinding of DNA.

MECHANISM OF RESISTANCE
- Multidrug-resistant phenotype with increased expression of P170 glycoprotein. Results in enhanced drug efflux and decreased intracellular accumulation of drug. Cross-resistant to vinca alkaloids, anthracyclines, taxanes, and other natural products.
- Decreased expression of topoisomerase II.
- Mutations in topoisomerase II with decreased binding affinity to drug.
- Enhanced activity of DNA repair enzymes.

ABSORPTION
Bioavailability of oral capsules is approximately 50%, requiring an oral dose to be twice that of an IV dose. However, oral bioavailability is non-linear and decreases with higher doses of drug (>200 mg). Presence of food and/or other anticancer agents does not alter drug absorption.

DISTRIBUTION

Rapidly distributed into all body fluids and tissues. Large fraction of etoposide (90%–95%) is protein-bound, mainly to albumin. Decreased albumin levels result in a higher fraction of free drug and a potentially higher incidence of host toxicity.

METABOLISM

Metabolized primarily by the liver via glucuronidation to hydroxyacid metabolites, which are less active than the parent compound. About 30%–50% of etoposide is excreted in urine, and only 2%–6% is excreted in stool via biliary excretion. The elimination half-life ranges from 3 to 10 hours.

INDICATIONS

1. Germ cell tumors.
2. SCLC.
3. NSCLC.
4. Non-Hodgkin's lymphoma.
5. Hodgkin's lymphoma.
6. Gastric cancer.
7. High-dose therapy in transplant setting for various malignancies, including breast cancer, lymphoma, and ovarian cancer.

DOSAGE RANGE

1. IV: Testicular cancer—As part of the PEB regimen, 100 mg/m^2 IV on days 1–5 with cycles repeated every 3 weeks.
2. IV: SCLC—As part of cisplatin/VP-16 regimen, 100–120 mg/m^2 IV on days 1–3 with cycles repeated every 3 weeks.
3. SCLC—50 mg/m^2/day PO for 21 days.

DRUG INTERACTIONS

Warfarin—Etoposide may alter the anticoagulant effect of warfarin by prolonging the PT and INR. Coagulation parameters (PT and INR) need to be closely monitored and dose of warfarin may require adjustment.

SPECIAL CONSIDERATIONS

1. Use with caution in patients with abnormal renal function. Dose reduction is recommended in patients with renal dysfunction. Baseline CrCl should be obtained, and renal status should be carefully monitored during therapy.
2. Use with caution in patients with abnormal liver function. Dose reduction is recommended in this setting.
3. Administer drug over a period of at least 30–60 minutes to avoid the risk of hypotension. Should the blood pressure drop, immediately discontinue the drug and administer IV fluids. Rate of administration must be reduced upon restarting therapy.
4. Carefully monitor for anaphylactic reactions. More commonly observed during the initial infusion of therapy and probably related to the

polysorbate 80 vehicle in which the drug is formulated. In rare instances, such an allergic reaction can be fatal. The drug should be immediately stopped and treatment with antihistamines, steroids, H2-blockers such as cimetidine, and pressor agents should be administered.

5. Closely monitor injection site for signs of phlebitis and avoid extravasation.

6. Pregnancy category D. Breastfeeding should be avoided.

TOXICITY 1
Myelosuppression. Dose-limiting toxicity with leukopenia more common than thrombocytopenia. Nadir usually occurs 10–14 days after therapy with recovery by day 21.

TOXICITY 2
Nausea and vomiting. Occurs in about 30%–40% of patients and generally mild to moderate. More commonly observed with oral administration.

TOXICITY 3
Anorexia.

TOXICITY 4
Alopecia observed in nearly two-thirds of patients.

TOXICITY 5
Mucositis and diarrhea are unusual with standard doses but more often observed with high doses in transplant setting.

TOXICITY 6
Hypersensitivity reaction with chills, fever, bronchospasm, dyspnea, tachycardia, facial and tongue swelling, and hypotension. Occurs in less than 2% of patients.

TOXICITY 7
Metallic taste during infusion of drug.

TOXICITY 8
Local inflammatory reaction at injection site.

TOXICITY 9
Radiation-recall skin changes.

TOXICITY 10
Increased risk of secondary malignancies, especially acute myelogenous leukemia. Associated with 11:23 translocation. Usually develops within 5–8 years of treatment and in the absence of preceding myelodysplastic syndrome.

Etoposide phosphate

TRADE NAME	Etopophos	CLASSIFICATION	Epipodophyllotoxin, topoisomerase II inhibitor
CATEGORY	Chemotherapy drug	DRUG MANUFACTURER	Bristol-Myers Squibb

MECHANISM OF ACTION
- Water-soluble prodrug form of etoposide.
- Cell cycle–specific agent with activity in late S- and G2 phases.
- Must first be dephosphorylated for etoposide to be active.
- Once activated, it inhibits topoisomerase II by stabilizing the topoisomerase II-DNA complex and preventing the unwinding of DNA.

MECHANISM OF RESISTANCE
- Multidrug-resistant phenotype with increased expression of P170 glycoprotein. Results in enhanced drug efflux and decreased intracellular accumulation of drug.
- Decreased expression of topoisomerase II.
- Mutations in topoisomerase II with decreased binding affinity to drug.
- Enhanced activity of DNA repair enzymes.

ABSORPTION
Only administered via the IV route.

DISTRIBUTION
Rapidly distributed into all body fluids and tissues. Large fraction of drug (90%–95%) is protein-bound, mainly to albumin. Decreased albumin levels result in a higher fraction of free drug and a potentially higher incidence of host toxicity.

METABOLISM

Etoposide phosphate is rapidly and completely converted to etoposide in plasma, which is then metabolized primarily by the liver to hydroxyacid metabolites. These metabolites are less active than the parent compound. The elimination half-life of the drug ranges from 3 to 10 hours. About 15%–20% of the drug is excreted in urine and about 2%–6% is excreted in stool within 72 hours after IV administration.

INDICATIONS

1. Germ cell tumors.
2. SCLC.
3. NSCLC.

DOSAGE RANGE

1. Testicular cancer: 100 mg/m^2 IV on days 1–5 with cycles repeated every 3 weeks.
2. SCLC: 100 mg/m^2 IV on days 1–3 with cycles repeated every 3 weeks.

DRUG INTERACTIONS

Warfarin—Etoposide may alter the anticoagulant effect of warfarin by prolonging the PT and INR. Coagulation parameters need to be closely monitored and dose of warfarin may require adjustment.

SPECIAL CONSIDERATIONS

1. Use with caution in patients with abnormal renal function. Dose reduction is recommended in this setting. Baseline CrCl should be obtained and renal status should be closely monitored during therapy.
2. Use with caution in patients with abnormal liver function. Dose reduction is recommended in this setting.
3. Administer drug over a period of at least 30–60 minutes to avoid the risk of hypotension. Should the blood pressure drop, immediately discontinue the drug and administer IV fluids. The rate of administration must be reduced upon restarting therapy.
4. Carefully monitor for anaphylactic reactions. Occur more frequently during the initial infusion of therapy. In rare instances, such an allergic reaction can be fatal. The drug should be immediately stopped and treatment with antihistamines, steroids, H2-blockers such as cimetidine, and pressor agents should be administered.
5. Closely monitor injection site for signs of phlebitis. Carefully avoid extravasation.
6. Pregnancy category D. Breastfeeding should be avoided.

TOXICITY 1

Myelosuppression is dose-limiting with leukopenia more common than thrombocytopenia. Nadir usually occurs 10–14 days after therapy with recovery by day 21.

TOXICITY 2

Nausea and vomiting. Occurs in about 30%–40% of patients and generally mild to moderate.

TOXICITY 3
Anorexia.

TOXICITY 4
Alopecia.

TOXICITY 5
Mucositis and diarrhea are only occasionally seen.

TOXICITY 6
Hypersensitivity reaction with chills, fever, bronchospasm, dyspnea, tachycardia, facial and tongue swelling, and hypotension.

TOXICITY 7
Metallic taste during infusion of drug.

TOXICITY 8
Local inflammatory reaction at the injection site.

TOXICITY 9
Radiation-recall skin changes.

TOXICITY 10
Increased risk of secondary malignancies, especially acute myelogenous leukemia. Associated with 11:23 translocation. Typically develops within 5–8 years of treatment and in the absence of preceding myelodysplastic syndrome.

Everolimus

TRADE NAMES	Afinitor, RAD001	**CLASSIFICATION**	Signal transduction inhibitor
CATEGORY	Chemotherapy drug	**DRUG MANUFACTURER**	Novartis

MECHANISM OF ACTION
- Potent inhibitor of the mammalian target of rapamycin (mTOR), a serine-threonine kinase that is a key component of cellular signaling pathways involved in the growth and proliferation of tumor cells.
- Inhibitor of hypoxia-inducible factor (HIF-1), which leads to reduced expression of VEGF.
- Inhibition of mTOR signaling results in cell cycle arrest, induction of apoptosis, and inhibition of angiogenesis.

MECHANISM OF RESISTANCE
None well characterized to date.

ABSORPTION
Peak drug levels are achieved 1–2 hours after oral administration. Food with a high fat content reduces oral bioavailability by up to 20%.

DISTRIBUTION
Steady-state drug concentrations are reached within 2 weeks after once-daily dosing. Significant binding (up to 75%) to plasma proteins.

METABOLISM
Metabolism in the liver primarily by CYP3A4 microsomal enzymes. Six main metabolites have been identified, including three monohydroxylated metabolites, two hydrolytic ring-opened products, and a phosphatidylcholine conjugate of everolimus. In general, these metabolites are significantly less active than the parent compound. Elimination is mainly hepatic with excretion in feces, and renal elimination of parent drug and its metabolites accounts for only 5% of an administered dose. The terminal half-life of the parent drug is 30 hours.

INDICATIONS
1. FDA-approved for the treatment of advanced renal cell cancer after failure on sunitinib or sorafenib.
2. FDA-approved for the treatment of advanced pancreatic neuroendocrine tumors (PNET) and for progressive, well-differentiated, non-functional neuroendocrine tumors (NET) of GI or lung origin that are unresectable, locally advanced, or metastatic. This agent is not indicated for the treatment of functional carcinoid tumors.
3. FDA-approved for the treatment of renal angiomyolipoma and tuberous sclerosis complex (TSC) patients not requiring surgery.
4. FDA-approved for the treatment of subependymal giant cell astrocytoma associated with TSC patients who require treatment but are not candidates for curative surgery.

5. FDA-approved in combination with exemestane for the treatment of postmenopausal women with advanced hormone receptor (HR)-positive, HER2-negative breast cancer with recurrent or progressive disease after failure of treatment with either letrozole or anastrozole.

DOSAGE RANGE
Recommended dose for advanced breast cancer, NET, and renal cell cancer is 10 mg PO once daily.

DRUG INTERACTION 1
Phenytoin and other drugs that induce liver microsomal CYP3A4 enzymes, including carbamazepine, rifampin, phenobarbital, dexamethasone, and St. John's wort—These drugs may increase the rate of metabolism of everolimus, resulting in its inactivation.

DRUG INTERACTION 2
Drugs that inhibit liver microsomal CYP3A4 enzymes, including ketoconazole, itraconazole, fluconazole, verapamil or diltiazem, erythromycin, and clarithromycin—These drugs may decrease the rate of metabolism of everolimus, resulting in increased drug levels and potentially increased toxicity.

SPECIAL CONSIDERATIONS
1. Everolimus should be taken once daily at the same time with or without food. The tablets should be swallowed whole with a glass of water and never chewed or crushed.
2. Use with caution in patients with moderate liver impairment (Child Pugh Class B), and dose should be reduced to 5 mg daily. Should not be used in patients with severe liver impairment (Child-Pugh Class C).
3. Consider increasing dose in 5 mg increments up to a maximum of 20 mg once daily if used in combination with drugs that are strong inducers of CYP3A4.
4. Closely monitor patients for new or progressive pulmonary symptoms, including cough, dyspnea, and fever. Non-infectious pneumonitis is a class effect of rapamycin analogs, and everolimus therapy should be interrupted pending further diagnostic evaluation.
5. Patients are at increased risk for developing opportunistic infections, such as pneumonia, other bacterial infections, and invasive fungal infections, while on everolimus.
6. Closely monitor serum glucose levels in all patients, especially those with diabetes mellitus.
7. Closely monitor serum triglyceride and cholesterol levels while on therapy.
8. Avoid alcohol or mouthwashes containing peroxide in the setting of oral ulcerations, as they may worsen the condition.
9. Avoid grapefruit products while on everolimus, as they can result in a significant increase in drug levels.
10. Avoid the use of live vaccines and/or close contact with those who have received live vaccines while on everolimus.
11. Pregnancy category D. Breastfeeding should be avoided.

TOXICITY 1

Asthenia and fatigue.

TOXICITY 2

Mucositis, oral ulcerations, and diarrhea.

TOXICITY 3

Nausea/vomiting and anorexia.

TOXICITY 4

Increased risk of opportunistic infections, such as pneumonia, other bacterial infections, and invasive fungal infections.

TOXICITY 5

Pulmonary toxicity in the form of increased cough, dyspnea, fever, and pulmonary infiltrates.

TOXICITY 6

Skin rash.

TOXICITY 7

Myelosuppression with anemia, thrombocytopenia, and neutropenia.

TOXICITY 8

Hyperlipidemia with increased serum triglycerides and/or cholesterol in up to 70%–75% of patients.

TOXICITY 9

Hyperglycemia in up to 50% of patients.

TOXICITY 10

Mild liver toxicity with elevation in serum transaminases and alkaline phosphatase.

Exemestane

TRADE NAME	Aromasin	CLASSIFICATION	Steroidal aromatase inactivator
CATEGORY	Hormonal agent	DRUG MANUFACTURER	Pfizer

MECHANISM OF ACTION
- Permanently binds to and irreversibly inactivates aromatase.
- Inhibits the synthesis of estrogens by inhibiting the conversion of adrenal androgens (androstenedione and testosterone) to estrogens (estrone, estrone sulfate, and estradiol).
- No inhibitory effect on adrenal corticosteroid or aldosterone biosynthesis.

MECHANISM OF RESISTANCE
- There is some degree of cross-resistance between exemestane and nonsteroidal aromatase inhibitors.

ABSORPTION
Excellent bioavailability via the oral route with 85% of a dose absorbed within 2 hours of ingestion. Absorption is not affected by food.

DISTRIBUTION
Widely distributed throughout the body. About 90% of drug is bound to plasma proteins.

METABOLISM
Extensively metabolized in the liver by CYP3A4 enzymes (up to 85%) to inactive forms. Half-life of drug is about 24 hours. Steady-state levels of drug are achieved after 7 days of a once-daily administration. The major route of elimination is hepatobiliary with excretion in feces, with renal excretion accounting for only 10% of drug clearance.

INDICATIONS
Treatment of advanced breast cancer in postmenopausal women whose disease has progressed following tamoxifen therapy.

DOSAGE RANGE
Usual dose is 25 mg PO once daily after a meal.

DRUG INTERACTION 1
Phenytoin and other drugs that stimulate the liver microsomal CYP3A4 enzymes, including carbamazepine, rifampin, phenobarbital, and St. John's wort—These drugs may increase the metabolism of exemestane, resulting in its inactivation.

DRUG INTERACTION 2
Drugs that inhibit the liver microsomal CYP3A4 enzymes, including ketoconazole, itraconazole, erythromycin, and clarithromycin—These drugs may

decrease the metabolism of exemestane, resulting in increased drug levels and potentially increased toxicity.

SPECIAL CONSIDERATIONS
1. No dose adjustments are required for patients with either hepatic or renal dysfunction.
2. Should not be administered to premenopausal women.
3. Should not be administered with estrogen-containing agents, as they may interfere with antitumor activity.
4. Caution patients about the risk of hot flashes.
5. No need for glucocorticoid and/or mineralocorticoid replacement.
6. Pregnancy category D. Breastfeeding should be avoided.

TOXICITY 1
Hot flashes.

TOXICITY 2
Mild nausea.

TOXICITY 3
Fatigue.

TOXICITY 4
Headache.

Floxuridine

TRADE NAMES	5-Fluoro-2'-deoxyuridine, FUDR	CLASSIFICATION	Antimetabolite
CATEGORY	Chemotherapy drug	DRUG MANUFACTURER	Roche

MECHANISM OF ACTION

- Fluoropyrimidine deoxynucleoside analog.
- Cell cycle specific with activity in the S-phase.
- Requires activation to cytotoxic metabolite forms. Metabolized to 5-FU metabolite FdUMP, which inhibits thymidylate synthase (TS). This results in inhibition of DNA synthesis, function, and repair.
- Incorporation of 5-FU metabolite FUTP into RNA resulting in alterations in RNA processing and/or mRNA translation.
- Incorporation of 5-FU metabolite FdUTP into DNA resulting in inhibition of DNA synthesis and function.
- Inhibition of TS leads to accumulation of dUMP, which becomes misincorporated into DNA in the form of dUTP, resulting in inhibition of DNA synthesis and function.

MECHANISM OF RESISTANCE

- Increased expression of thymidylate synthase.
- Decreased levels of reduced folate substrate 5, 10-methylenetetrahydrofolate.
- Decreased incorporation of 5-FU into RNA.
- Decreased incorporation of 5-FU into DNA.
- Increased activity of DNA repair enzymes, uracil glycosylase and dUTPase.
- Increased salvage of physiologic nucleosides including thymidine.
- Increased expression of dihydropyrimidine dehydrogenase.
- Decreased expression of mismatch repair enzymes (hMLH1, hMSH2).
- Alterations in TS with decreased binding affinity of enzyme for FdUMP.

ABSORPTION

Administered only by the IV and IA routes, as it is poorly absorbed by the GI tract.

DISTRIBUTION

After IV administration, floxuridine is rapidly extracted by the liver via first-pass metabolism. After hepatic intra-arterial (IA) administration, greater than 90% of drug is extracted by hepatocytes. Binding to plasma proteins has not been well characterized.

METABOLISM

Undergoes extensive enzymatic metabolism to 5-FU and 5-FU metabolites. Catabolism accounts for >85% of drug metabolism. Dihydropyrimidine dehydrogenase is the main enzyme responsible for 5-FU catabolism, and it is present in liver and extrahepatic tissues, including GI mucosa, WBCs, and the kidneys. About 30% of an administered dose of drug is cleared in urine, mainly as inactive metabolites. The terminal elimination half-life is 20 hours.

INDICATIONS

1. Metastatic colorectal cancer—Intrahepatic arterial treatment of colorectal cancer metastatic to the liver.
2. Metastatic GI adenocarcinoma—Patients with metastatic disease confined to the liver.

DOSAGE RANGE

Recommended dose is 0.1–0.6 mg/kg/day IA for 7–14 days via hepatic artery.

DRUG INTERACTION 1

Leucovorin—Leucovorin enhances the toxicity and antitumor activity of floxuridine. Stabilizes the TS-FdUMP-reduced folate ternary complex, resulting in maximal inhibition of TS.

DRUG INTERACTION 2

Thymidine—Rescues against the toxic effects of floxuridine.

DRUG INTERACTION 3

Vistonuridine (PN401)—Rescues against the toxic effects of floxuridine.

SPECIAL CONSIDERATIONS

1. Contraindicated in patients with poor nutritional status, depressed bone marrow function, or potentially serious infection.
2. No dose adjustments are necessary in patients with mild-to-moderate liver dysfunction or abnormal renal function. However, patients should be closely monitored as they may be at increased risk of toxicity.
3. Patients should be placed on an H2-blocker, such as ranitidine 150 mg PO bid, to prevent the onset of peptic ulcer disease while on therapy. Onset of ulcer-like pain is an indication to stop therapy, as hemorrhage and/or perforation may occur.
4. Patients who experience unexpected, severe grade 3 or 4 host toxicities with initiation of therapy may have an underlying deficiency in dihydropyrimidine dehydrogenase. Therapy must be discontinued immediately. Further testing to identify the presence of this pharmacogenetic syndrome should be considered.
5. Pregnancy category D. Breastfeeding should be avoided.

TOXICITY 1

Hepatotoxicity is dose-limiting. Presents as abdominal pain, elevated alkaline phosphatase, liver transaminases, and bilirubin. Sclerosing cholangitis is a rare event. Other GI toxicities include duodenitis, duodenal ulcer, and gastritis.

TOXICITY 2
Nausea and vomiting are mild. Mucositis and diarrhea also observed.

TOXICITY 3
Hand-foot syndrome (palmar-plantar erythrodysesthesia). Characterized by tingling, numbness, pain, erythema, dryness, rash, swelling, increased pigmentation, and/or pruritus of the hands and feet.

TOXICITY 4
Myelosuppression. Nadir occurs at 7–10 days with full recovery by 14–17 days.

TOXICITY 5
Neurologic toxicity manifested by somnolence, confusion, seizures, cerebellar ataxia, and rarely encephalopathy.

TOXICITY 6
Cardiac symptoms of chest pain, ECG changes, and serum enzyme elevation. Rare event but increased risk in patients with prior history of ischemic heart disease.

TOXICITY 7
Blepharitis, tear-duct stenosis, acute and chronic conjunctivitis.

TOXICITY 8
Catheter-related complications include leakage, catheter occlusion, perforation, dislodgement, infection, bleeding at catheter site, and thrombosis and/or embolism of hepatic artery.

Fludarabine

TRADE NAMES	2-Fluoro-ara-AMP, Fludara	**CLASSIFICATION**	Antimetabolite
CATEGORY	Chemotherapy drug	**DRUG MANUFACTURER**	Sagent Pharmaceuticals and Antisoma (oral form)

MECHANISM OF ACTION
- 5'-monophosphate analog of arabinofuranosyladenosine (F-ara-A) with high specificity for lymphoid cells. Presence of the 2-fluoro group on adenine ring renders fludarabine resistant to breakdown by adenosine deaminase.
- Considered a prodrug. Following administration, it is rapidly dephosphorylated to 2-fluoro-ara-adenosine (F-ara-A). F-ara-A enters cells and is then rephosphorylated first to its monophosphate form and eventually to the active 5-triphosphate metabolite (F-ara-ATP).
- Antitumor activity against both dividing and resting cells.
- Triphosphate metabolite incorporates into DNA resulting in inhibition of DNA chain extension.
- Inhibition of ribonucleotide reductase by the triphosphate metabolite.
- Inhibition of DNA polymerase-α and DNA polymerase-β by the triphosphate metabolite, resulting in inhibition of DNA synthesis and DNA repair.
- Induction of apoptosis (programmed cell death).

MECHANISM OF RESISTANCE
- Decreased expression of the activating enzyme, deoxycytidine kinase.
- Decreased nucleoside transport of drug.

ABSORPTION
Fludarabine is orally bioavailable, in the range of 50%–65%, and an oral tablet form is available. Absorption is not affected by food.

DISTRIBUTION
Widely distributed throughout the body. Concentrates in high levels in liver, kidney, and spleen. Binding to plasma proteins has not been well characterized.

METABOLISM
Rapidly converted to 2-fluoro-ara-A, which enters cells via the nucleoside transport system and is rephosphorylated by deoxycytidine kinase to fludarabine monophosphate. This metabolite undergoes two subsequent phosphorylation steps to yield fludarabine triphosphate, the active species. Major route of elimination is via the kidneys, and approximately 25% of 2-fluoro-ara-A is excreted unchanged in urine. The terminal half-life is on the order of 10–20 hours.

INDICATIONS
1. Chronic lymphocytic leukemia (CLL).
2. Non-Hodgkin's lymphoma (low-grade).
3. Cutaneous T-cell lymphoma.

DOSAGE RANGE
Usual dose is 25 mg/m^2 IV on days 1–5 every 28 days. For oral usage, the recommended dose is 40 mg/m^2 PO on days 1–5 every 28 days.

DRUG INTERACTION 1
Cytarabine—Fludarabine may enhance the antitumor activity of cytarabine by inducing the expression of deoxycytidine kinase.

DRUG INTERACTION 2
Cyclophosphamide, cisplatin, mitoxantrone—Fludarabine may enhance the antitumor activity of cyclophosphamide, cisplatin, and mitoxantrone by inhibiting nucleotide excision repair mechanisms.

SPECIAL CONSIDERATIONS
1. Use with caution in patients with abnormal renal function. Dose should be reduced in proportion to the creatinine clearance.
2. Use with caution in elderly patients and in those with bone marrow impairment as they are at increased risk of toxicity.
3. Monitor for signs of infection. Patients are at increased risk for opportunistic infections, including herpes, fungi, and *Pneumocystis jiroveci*. Patients should be empirically placed on trimethoprim/sulfamethoxazole prophylaxis, 1 DS tablet PO bid three times/week.
4. Monitor for signs of tumor lysis syndrome, especially in patients with a high tumor cell burden. May occur as early as within the first week of treatment.
5. Allopurinol may be given prior to initiation of fludarabine therapy to prevent hyperuricemia.
6. Use irradiated blood products in patients requiring transfusions as transfusion-associated graft-versus-host disease can occur rarely after transfusion of nonirradiated products in patients treated with fludarabine.
7. Pregnancy category D. Breastfeeding should be avoided.

TOXICITY 1
Myelosuppression is dose-limiting. Leukocyte nadir occurs in 10–13 days, with recovery by day 14–21. Autoimmune hemolytic anemia and drug-induced aplastic anemia also occur.

TOXICITY 2
Immunosuppression. Decrease in CD4 and CD8 T cells occurs in most patients. Increased risk of opportunistic infections, including fungus, herpes, and *Pneumocystis jiroveci*. Recovery of CD4 count is slow and may take over a year to return to normal.

TOXICITY 3
Nausea and vomiting are usually mild.

TOXICITY 4
Fever occurs in 20%–30% of patients. Most likely due to release of pyrogens and/or cytokines from tumor cells. Associated with fatigue, malaise, myalgias, arthralgias, and chills.

TOXICITY 5
Hypersensitivity reaction with maculopapular skin rash, erythema, and pruritus.

TOXICITY 6
Tumor lysis syndrome. Rarely seen (in less than 1%–2% of patients), and most often in the setting of high tumor-cell burden. However, it can be fatal upon presentation.

TOXICITY 7
Transient elevation in serum transaminases. Clinically asymptomatic.

5-Fluorouracil

TRADE NAMES	5-FU, Efudex	CLASSIFICATION	Antimetabolite
CATEGORY	Chemotherapy drug	DRUG MANUFACTURER	Roche

MECHANISM OF ACTION
- Fluoropyrimidine analog.
- Cell cycle–specific with activity in the S-phase.
- Requires activation to cytotoxic metabolite forms.
- Inhibition of the target enzyme thymidylate synthase (TS) by the 5-FU metabolite, FdUMP.
- Incorporation of the 5-FU metabolite FUTP into RNA resulting in alterations in RNA processing and/or mRNA translation.
- Incorporation of the 5-FU metabolite FdUTP into DNA, resulting in inhibition of DNA synthesis and function.
- Inhibition of TS leads to accumulation of dUMP, which then gets misincorporated into DNA in the form of dUTP, resulting in inhibition of DNA synthesis and function.

MECHANISM OF RESISTANCE
- Increased expression of thymidylate synthase.
- Decreased levels of reduced folate substrate 5, 10-methylenetetrahydrofolate for TS reaction.
- Decreased incorporation of 5-FU into RNA.
- Decreased incorporation of 5-FU into DNA.
- Increased activity of DNA repair enzymes, uracil glycosylase and dUTPase.
- Increased salvage of physiologic nucleosides including thymidine.
- Increased expression of dihydropyrimidine dehydrogenase.
- Decreased expression of mismatch repair enzymes (hMLH1, hMSH2).
- Alterations in TS with decreased binding affinity of enzyme for FdUMP.

ABSORPTION
Oral absorption is variable and erratic with a bioavailability that ranges from 40% to 70%.

DISTRIBUTION
After IV administration, 5-FU is widely distributed to tissues with highest concentration in GI mucosa, bone marrow, and liver. Penetrates into third-space fluid collections such as ascites and pleural effusions. Crosses the blood-brain barrier and distributes into CSF and brain tissue. Binding to plasma proteins has not been well characterized.

METABOLISM
Undergoes extensive enzymatic metabolism intracellularly to cytotoxic metabolites. Catabolism accounts for >85% of drug metabolism. Dihydropyrimidine dehydrogenase is the main enzyme responsible for 5-FU catabolism, and it is highly expressed in liver and extrahepatic tissues such as GI mucosa, WBCs, and kidney. Greater than 90% of an administered dose of drug is cleared in urine and lungs. The terminal elimination half-life is short, ranging from 10 to 20 min.

INDICATIONS
1. Colorectal cancer—Adjuvant setting and advanced disease.
2. Breast cancer—Adjuvant setting and advanced disease.
3. GI malignancies, including anal, esophageal, gastric, and pancreatic cancer.
4. Head and neck cancer.
5. Hepatoma.
6. Ovarian cancer.
7. Topical use in basal cell cancer of skin and actinic keratoses.

DOSAGE RANGE
1. Bolus monthly schedule: 425–450 mg/m^2 IV on days 1–5 every 28 days.
2. Bolus weekly schedule: 500–600 mg/m^2 IV every week for 6 weeks every 8 weeks.
3. 24-hour infusion: 2400–2600 mg/m^2 IV every week.

4. 96-hour infusion: 800–1000 mg/m^2/day IV.
5. 120-hour infusion: 1000 mg/m^2/day IV on days 1–5 every 21–28 days.
6. Protracted continuous infusion: 200–400 mg/m^2/day IV.

DRUG INTERACTION 1
Leucovorin—Leucovorin enhances the antitumor activity and toxicity of 5-FU. Stabilizes the TS-FdUMP-reduced folate ternary complex resulting in maximal inhibition of TS.

DRUG INTERACTION 2
Methotrexate, trimetrexate—Antifolate analogs increase the formation of 5-FU nucleotide metabolites when given 24 hours before 5-FU.

DRUG INTERACTION 3
Thymidine—Rescues against the TS- and DNA-mediated toxic effects of 5-FU.

DRUG INTERACTION 4
Vistonuridine (uridine triacetate)—Rescues against the toxic effects of 5-FU.

SPECIAL CONSIDERATIONS
1. No dose adjustments are necessary in patients with mild-to-moderate liver or renal dysfunction. However, patients should be closely monitored as they may be at increased risk for toxicity.
2. Contraindicated in patients with bone marrow depression, poor nutritional status, infection, active ischemic heart disease, or history of myocardial infarction within previous 6 months.
3. Patients should be monitored closely for mucositis and/or diarrhea as there is increased potential for dehydration, fluid imbalance, and infection. Elderly patients are at especially high risk for GI toxicity.
4. Patients who experience unexpected, severe grade 3 or 4 myelosuppression, GI toxicity, and/or neurologic toxicity with initiation of therapy may have an underlying deficiency in dihydropyrimidine dehydrogenase. Therapy must be discontinued immediately. Further testing to identify the presence of this pharmacogenetic syndrome should be considered.
5. Vistonuridine, at a dose of 10 g PO every 6 hours, may be used in patients overdosed with 5-FU or in those who experience severe toxicity. For further information, contact Wellstat Therapeutics.
6. Vitamin B6 (pyridoxine 50 mg PO bid) may be used to prevent and/or reduce the incidence and severity of hand-foot syndrome.
7. Use of ice chips in mouth 10–15 minutes pre- and 10–15 minutes post-IV bolus injections of 5-FU may reduce the incidence and severity of mucositis.
8. Pregnancy category D. Breastfeeding should be avoided.

TOXICITY 1
Myelosuppression. Dose-limiting for the qd × 5 or weekly schedules, less frequently observed with infusional therapy. Neutropenia and thrombocytopenia more common than anemia.

TOXICITY 2
Mucositis and/or diarrhea. May be severe and dose-limiting for infusional schedules. Nausea and vomiting are mild and rare.

TOXICITY 3
Hand-foot syndrome (palmar-plantar erythrodysesthesia). Characterized by tingling, numbness, pain, erythema, dryness, rash, swelling, increased pigmentation, nail changes, pruritus of the hands and feet, and/or desquamation. Most often observed with infusional therapy and can be dose-limiting.

TOXICITY 4
Neurologic toxicity manifested by somnolence, confusion, seizures, cerebellar ataxia, and rarely encephalopathy.

TOXICITY 5
Cardiac symptoms of chest pain, ECG changes, and serum enzyme elevation. Rare event but increased risk in patients with prior history of ischemic heart disease.

TOXICITY 6
Blepharitis, tear-duct stenosis, acute and chronic conjunctivitis.

TOXICITY 7
Dry skin, photosensitivity, and pigmentation of the infused vein are common.

TOXICITY 8
Metallic taste in mouth during IV bolus injection.

Flutamide

TRADE NAME	Eulexin	CLASSIFICATION	Antiandrogen
CATEGORY	Hormonal agent	DRUG MANUFACTURER	Schering, Taj Pharmaceuticals

MECHANISM OF ACTION
Nonsteroidal, antiandrogen agent binds to androgen receptor and inhibits androgen uptake as well as inhibiting androgen binding in nucleus in androgen-sensitive prostate cancer cells.

MECHANISM OF RESISTANCE
- Decreased expression of androgen receptor.
- Mutation in androgen receptor leading to decreased binding affinity to flutamide.

ABSORPTION
Rapidly and completely absorbed by the GI tract. Peak plasma levels observed 1–2 hours after oral administration.

DISTRIBUTION
Distribution is not well characterized. Flutamide and its metabolites are extensively bound to plasma proteins (92%–96%).

METABOLISM
Extensive metabolism by the liver cytochrome P450 system to both active and inactive metabolites. The main metabolite, α-hydroxyflutamide, is biologically active. Flutamide and its metabolites are cleared primarily in urine, and only 4% of drug is eliminated in feces. The elimination half-life of flutamide is about 8 hours, whereas the half-life of the hydroxyflutamide metabolite is 8–10 hours.

INDICATIONS
1. Locally confined stage B2–C prostate cancer.
2. Stage D2 metastatic prostate cancer.

DOSAGE RANGE
Recommended dose is 250 mg PO tid at 8-hour intervals.

DRUG INTERACTIONS
Warfarin—Flutamide can inhibit metabolism of warfarin by the liver P450 system leading to increased anticoagulant effect. Coagulation parameters (PT and INR) must be followed closely when warfarin and flutamide are taken concurrently, and dose adjustments may be needed.

SPECIAL CONSIDERATIONS
1. Monitor LFTs at baseline and during therapy. In the presence of elevated serum transaminases to 2–3 times the upper limit of normal (ULN), therapy should be terminated.
2. Caution patients about the risk of diarrhea and, if severe, flutamide may need to be stopped.
3. Caution patients about the potential for hot flashes. Consider the use of clonidine 0.1–0.2 mg PO daily, megestrol acetate 20 mg PO bid, or soy tablets 1 tablet PO tid for prevention and/or treatment.
4. Instruct patients on the potential risk of altered sexual function and impotence.
5. Pregnancy category D. Breastfeeding should be avoided.

TOXICITY 1
Hot flashes occur in 60% of patients, decreased libido (35%), impotence (30%), gynecomastia (10%), nipple pain, and galactorrhea.

TOXICITY 2
Nausea, vomiting, and diarrhea.

TOXICITY 3
Transient elevations in serum transaminases are rare but may necessitate discontinuation of therapy.

TOXICITY 4
Amber-green discoloration of urine secondary to flutamide and/or its metabolites.

Fulvestrant

TRADE NAME	Faslodex	CLASSIFICATION	Estrogen receptor antagonist
CATEGORY	Hormonal agent	DRUG MANUFACTURER	AstraZeneca

MECHANISM OF ACTION
- Potent and selective antagonist of the estrogen receptor (ER) with no known agonist effects. Affinity to the ER is comparable to that of estradiol.
- Downregulates the expression of the ER, presumably through enhanced degradation.

MECHANISM OF RESISTANCE
- Decreased expression of ER.
- Decreased expression of G protein-coupled estrogen receptor 1 (GPER).
- Increased expression of cell division protein kinase 6 (CDK6).
- Overexpression of growth factor receptors, such as EGFR and HER2/neu.

ABSORPTION
Not absorbed orally. After IM injection, peak plasma levels are achieved in approximately 7 days and are maintained for at least 1 month.

DISTRIBUTION
Rapidly and widely distributed throughout the body. Approximately 99% of drug is bound to plasma proteins, and VLDL, LDL, and HDL are the main binding proteins.

METABOLISM
Extensively metabolized in the liver by microsomal CYP3A4 enzymes to both active and inactive forms. Steady-state levels of drug are achieved after 7 days of a once-monthly administration and are maintained for at least up to 1 month. The major route of elimination is fecal (approximately 90%), with renal excretion accounting for only 1% of drug clearance.

INDICATIONS
1. Metastatic breast cancer—Treatment of hormone receptor (HR)-positive metastatic breast cancer in postmenopausal women with disease progression following anti-estrogen therapy.
2. Metastatic breast cancer—Treatment of HR-positive, HER2-negative advanced or metastatic breast cancer in combination with palbociclib in women with disease progression following endocrine therapy.

DOSAGE RANGE
Recommended dose is 500 mg IM on days 1, 15, 29, and once monthly thereafter.

DRUG INTERACTIONS
None well characterized.

SPECIAL CONSIDERATIONS
1. No dose adjustments are required for patients with renal dysfunction.
2. No dose adjustments required for patients with mild liver dysfunction. In patients with moderate liver dysfunction (Child-Pugh Class B), a dose of 250 mg is recommended. The safety and efficacy have not been carefully studied in patients with severe hepatic impairment.
3. Use with caution in patients with bleeding diatheses, thrombocytopenia, and/or in those receiving anticoagulation therapy.
4. Pregnancy category D. Breastfeeding should be avoided as it is not known whether fulvestrant is excreted in human milk.

TOXICITY 1
Asthenia occurs in up to 25% of patients.

TOXICITY 2
Mild nausea and vomiting. Constipation and/or diarrhea can also occur.

TOXICITY 3
Hot flashes seen in 20% of patients.

TOXICITY 4
Mild headache.

TOXICITY 5
Injection site reactions with mild pain and inflammation that are usually transient in nature.

TOXICITY 6
Back pain and arthralgias. Flu-like syndrome in the form of fever, malaise, and myalgias. Occurs in 10% of patients.

TOXICITY 8
Dry, scaling skin rash.

Gefitinib

TRADE NAMES	Iressa, ZD1839	CLASSIFICATION	Signal transduction inhibitor
CATEGORY	Chemotherapy drug	DRUG MANUFACTURER	AstraZeneca

MECHANISM OF ACTION
- Potent and selective small-molecule inhibitor of the EGFR tyrosine kinase, resulting in inhibition of EGFR autophosphorylation and inhibition of EGFR signaling.
- Inhibition of the EGFR tyrosine kinase results in inhibition of critical mitogenic and antiapoptotic signals involved in proliferation, growth, metastasis, angiogenesis, and response to chemotherapy and/or radiation therapy.

MECHANISM OF RESISTANCE
- Mutations in the EGFR tyrosine kinase leading to decreased binding affinity to gefitinib.
- Presence of KRAS mutations.
- Activation/induction of alternative cellular signaling pathways, such as PI3K/Akt and IGF-1R.

ABSORPTION
Oral absorption is relatively slow, and the oral bioavailability is approximately 60%. Food does not affect drug absorption.

DISTRIBUTION
Extensive binding (90%) to plasma proteins, including albumin and α1-acid glycoprotein, and extensive tissue distribution. Steady-state drug concentrations are reached in 7–10 days.

METABOLISM
Metabolism in the liver primarily by CYP3A4 microsomal enzymes. Other cytochrome P450 enzymes play a minor role in its metabolism. The main metabolite is the O-desmethyl piperazine derivative, and this metabolite is significantly less potent than the parent drug. Elimination is mainly hepatic

with excretion in the feces, and renal elimination of the parent drug and its metabolites accounts for less than 4% of an administered dose. The terminal half-life of the parent drug is 48 hours.

INDICATIONS
FDA-approved for the first-line treatment of patients with metastatic NSCLC whose tumors have EGFR exon 19 deletions or exon 21 (L858R) substitution mutations as detected by an FDA-approved test.

DOSAGE RANGE
Recommended dose is 250 mg/day PO.

DRUG INTERACTION 1
Dilantin and other drugs that stimulate the liver microsomal CYP3A4 enzyme, including carbamazepine, rifampin, phenobarbital, and St. John's wort—These drugs increase the rate of metabolism of gefitinib, resulting in its inactivation.

DRUG INTERACTION 2
Drugs that inhibit the liver microsomal CYP3A4 enzyme, including ketoconazole, itraconazole, erythromycin, and clarithromycin—These drugs decrease the rate of metabolism of gefitinib, resulting in increased drug levels and potentially increased toxicity.

DRUG INTERACTION 3
Warfarin—Patients receiving coumarin-derived anticoagulants should be closely monitored for alterations in their clotting parameters (PT and INR) and/ or bleeding as gefitinib inhibits the metabolism of warfarin by the liver P450 system. Dose of warfarin may require careful adjustment in the presence of gefitinib therapy.

SPECIAL CONSIDERATIONS
1. Clinical responses may be observed within the first week of initiation of therapy.
2. Patients with bronchoalveolar NSCLC may be more sensitive to gefitinib therapy than other histologic subtypes. Females and nonsmokers also show increased sensitivity to gefitinib therapy.
3. Closely monitor patients with central lesions, as they may be at increased risk for complications of hemoptysis.
4. Dose of gefitinib may need to be increased when used in patients with seizure disorders who are receiving phenytoin, as the metabolism of gefitinib by the liver P450 system is enhanced in the presence of phenytoin.
5. Coagulation parameters (PT/INR) should be closely monitored when patients are receiving both gefitinib and warfarin, as gefitinib inhibits the metabolism of warfarin by the liver P450 system.
6. In patients who develop a skin rash, topical antibiotics such as clindamycin gel or either oral clindamycin and/or oral minocycline may help.
7. Avoid Seville oranges, starfruit, pomelos, grapefruit, and grapefruit juice while on gefinitib.
8. Pregnancy category D. Breastfeeding should be avoided.

TOXICITY 1
Elevations in blood pressure, especially in those with underlying hypertension.

TOXICITY 2
Pruritus, dry skin with mainly a pustular, acneiform skin rash.

TOXICITY 3
Mild-to-moderate elevations in serum transaminases. Usually transient and clinically asymptomatic.

TOXICITY 4
Asthenia and anorexia.

TOXICITY 5
Mild nausea/vomiting and mucositis.

TOXICITY 6
Conjunctivitis, blepharitis, and corneal erosions. Abnormal eyelash growth may occur in some patients.

TOXICITY 7
Rare episodes of hemoptysis and GI hemorrhage.

Gemcitabine

TRADE NAME	Gemzar	CLASSIFICATION	Antimetabolite
CATEGORY	Chemotherapy drug	DRUG MANUFACTURER	Eli Lilly

MECHANISM OF ACTION
- Fluorine-substituted deoxycytidine analog.
- Cell cycle–specific with activity in the S-phase.
- Requires intracellular activation by deoxycytidine kinase to the monophosphate form with eventual metabolism to the cytotoxic triphosphate nucleotide metabolite (dFdCTP). Antitumor activity of gemcitabine is determined by a balance between intracellular activation and degradation and the formation of cytotoxic triphosphate metabolites.
- Incorporation of dFdCTP triphosphate metabolite into DNA, resulting in chain termination and inhibition of DNA synthesis and function.

- Triphosphate metabolite inhibits DNA polymerases α, β, and γ, which, in turn, interferes with DNA synthesis, DNA repair, and DNA chain elongation.
- Difluorodeoxycytidine diphosphate (dFdCDP) metabolite inhibits the enzyme ribonucleotide reductase, resulting in decreased levels of essential deoxyribonucleotides for DNA synthesis and function.
- Incorporation into RNA, resulting in alterations in RNA processing and mRNA translation.

MECHANISM OF RESISTANCE
- Decreased activation of drug through decreased expression of the anabolic enzyme deoxycytidine kinase.
- Increased breakdown of drug by the catabolic enzymes cytidine deaminase and dCMP deaminase.
- Decreased nucleoside transport of drug into cells.
- Increased concentration of the competing physiologic nucleotide dCTP, through increased expression of CTP synthetase.

ABSORPTION
Poor oral bioavailability as a result of extensive deamination within the GI tract. Administered by the IV route.

DISTRIBUTION
With infusions <70 minutes, drug is not extensively distributed. In contrast, with longer infusions, drug is slowly and widely distributed into body tissues. Does not cross the blood-brain barrier. Binding to plasma proteins is negligible.

METABOLISM
Undergoes extensive metabolism by deamination to the difluorouridine (dFdU) metabolite with approximately >90% of drug being recovered in urine in this form. Deamination occurs in liver, plasma, and peripheral tissues. The principal enzyme involved in drug catabolism is cytidine deaminase. The terminal elimination half-life is dependent on the infusion time. With short infusions <70 minutes, the half-life ranges from 30 to 90 minutes, while for infusions >70 minutes, the half-life is 4–10 hours. Plasma clearance is also dependent on gender and age. Clearance is 30% lower in women and in elderly patients.

INDICATIONS
1. Pancreatic cancer—FDA-approved as monotherapy or in combination with erlotinib for first-line treatment of locally advanced or metastatic disease.
2. Pancreatic cancer—FDA-approved in combination with abraxane for first-line treatment of metastatic disease.
3. NSCLC—FDA-approved in combination with cisplatin for treatment of inoperable, locally advanced, or metastatic disease.
4. Breast cancer—FDA-approved in combination with paclitaxel for first-line treatment of metastatic breast cancer after failure of prior anthracycline-containing adjuvant chemotherapy.
5. Ovarian cancer—FDA-approved in combination with carboplatin for patients with advanced ovarian cancer that has relapsed at least 6 months after completion of platinum-based therapy.
6. Bladder cancer.

7. Soft tissue sarcoma.
8. Hodgkin's lymphoma.
9. Non-Hodgkin's lymphoma.

DOSAGE RANGE

1. Pancreatic cancer: 1000 mg/m^2 IV every week for 7 weeks with 1-week rest. Treatment then continues weekly for 3 weeks followed by 1-week rest.
2. Pancreatic cancer: 1000 mg/m^2 IV on days 1, 8, and 15 in combination with abraxane 125 mg/m^2 IV on days 1, 8, and 15 with cycles repeated every 28 days.
3. Bladder cancer: 1000 mg/m^2 IV on days 1, 8, and 15 every 28 days.
4. NSCLC: 1200 mg/m^2 IV on days 1, 8, and 15 every 28 days.

DRUG INTERACTION 1

Cisplatin—Gemcitabine enhances the cytotoxicity of cisplatin by increasing the formation of cytotoxic platinum-DNA adducts.

DRUG INTERACTION 2

Radiation therapy—Gemcitabine is a potent radiosensitizer.

SPECIAL CONSIDERATIONS

1. Monitor CBCs on a regular basis during therapy. Dose reduction is recommended based on the degree of hematologic toxicity.
2. Use with caution in patients with abnormal liver and/or renal function. Dose modification should be considered in this setting as there is an increased risk for toxicity.
3. Use with caution in women and in elderly patients as gemcitabine clearance is decreased.
4. Pregnancy category D. Breastfeeding should be avoided.

TOXICITY 1

Myelosuppression is dose-limiting. Neutropenia more common than thrombocytopenia. Nadir occurs by days 10–14, with recovery by day 21.

TOXICITY 2

Nausea and vomiting. Usually mild to moderate, occur in 70% of patients. Diarrhea and/or mucositis observed in 15%–20% of patients.

TOXICITY 3

Flu-like syndrome manifested by fever, malaise, chills, headache, and myalgias. Seen in 20% of patients. Fever, in the absence of infection, develops in 40% of patients within the first 6–12 hours after treatment but generally is mild.

TOXICITY 4

Transient hepatic dysfunction with elevation of serum transaminases and bilirubin.

TOXICITY 5

Pulmonary toxicity in the form of mild dyspnea and drug-induced pneumonitis. ARDS has been reported rarely.

TOXICITY 6

Infusion reaction presents as flushing, facial swelling, headache, dyspnea, and/or hypotension. Usually related to the rate of infusion and resolves with slowing or discontinuation of infusion.

TOXICITY 7

Mild proteinuria and hematuria. In rare cases, renal microangiopathy syndromes, including hemolytic-uremic syndrome (HUS) and thrombotic thrombocytopenic purpura (TTP), have been reported.

TOXICITY 8

Maculopapular skin rash generally involving the trunk and extremities with pruritus. Peripheral edema involving the lower extremities, which can be asymptomatic, or in some cases, painful and tender. Radiation-recall dermatitis may occur. Alopecia is rarely observed.

Goserelin

TRADE NAME	Zoladex	CLASSIFICATION	LHRH agonist
CATEGORY	Hormonal agent	DRUG MANUFACTURER	AstraZeneca

MECHANISM OF ACTION

- Administration leads to initial release of follicle-stimulating hormone (FSH) and luteinizing hormone (LH) followed by suppression of gonadotropin secretion as a result of desensitization of the pituitary to gonadotropin-releasing hormone. This results in decreased secretion of LH and FSH from the pituitary.

ABSORPTION

Not orally absorbed because of extensive proteolysis in the GI tract. Bioavailability of subcutaneously administered drug is 75%–90%.

DISTRIBUTION

Distribution is not well characterized. Slowly released over a 28-day period. Peak serum concentrations are achieved 10–15 days after drug administration. About 30% of goserelin is bound to plasma proteins.

METABOLISM

Metabolism of goserelin occurs mainly via hydrolysis of the C-terminal amino acids. Goserelin is nearly completely eliminated in urine. The elimination half-life is normally 4–5 hours but is prolonged in patients with impaired renal function (12 hours).

INDICATIONS

Advanced prostate cancer.

DOSAGE RANGE
Administer 3.6 mg SC every 28 days or 10.8 mg SC every 90 days.

DRUG INTERACTIONS
None known.

SPECIAL CONSIDERATIONS
1. Initiation of treatment with goserelin may induce a transient tumor flare. Goserelin should not be given in patients with impending ureteral obstruction and/or spinal cord compression or in those with painful bone metastases.
2. Serum testosterone levels decrease to castrate levels within 2–4 weeks after initiation of therapy.
3. Use with caution in patients with abnormal renal function.
4. Caution patients about the potential for hot flashes. Consider the use of soy tablets, 1 tablet PO tid for prevention and/or treatment.

TOXICITY 1
Hot flashes occur in 50% of patients, decreased libido (10%), impotence (10%), and gynecomastia (10%).

TOXICITY 2
Tumor flare. Occurs in up to 20% of patients, usually within the first 2 weeks of starting therapy, and presents as increased bone pain, urinary retention, or back pain with spinal cord compression. Usually prevented by pretreating with an antiandrogen agent such as flutamide, bicalutamide, or nilutamide.

TOXICITY 3
Local discomfort at the site of injection.

TOXICITY 4
Elevated serum cholesterol levels.

TOXICITY 5
Hypersensitivity reaction.

TOXICITY 6
Nausea and vomiting. Rarely observed.

TOXICITY 7
Myelosuppression. Rarely observed.

Hydroxyurea

$$H_2N-\overset{\overset{\displaystyle O}{\|}}{C}-\overset{\overset{\displaystyle H}{|}}{N}-OH$$

TRADE NAME	Hydrea	CLASSIFICATION	Antimetabolite
CATEGORY	Chemotherapy drug	DRUG MANUFACTURER	MGI Pharma

MECHANISM OF ACTION
- Cell cycle–specific analog of urea with activity in the S-phase.
- Inhibits the enzyme ribonucleotide reductase (RR), a key enzyme that converts ribonucleotides to deoxyribonucleotides, which are critical precursors for de novo DNA biosynthesis and DNA repair.

MECHANISM OF RESISTANCE
Increased expression of ribonucleotide reductase due to gene amplification, increased transcription, and post-transcriptional mechanisms.

ABSORPTION
Oral absorption is rapid and nearly complete with a bioavailability ranging between 80% and 100%. Peak plasma concentrations are achieved in 1–1.5 hours.

DISTRIBUTION
Widely distributed in all tissues. High concentrations are found in third-space collections, including pleural effusions and ascites. Crosses the blood-brain barrier and enters the CSF. Excreted in significant levels in human breast milk.

METABOLISM
Approximately 50% of drug is metabolized in the liver. About 50% of drug is excreted unchanged in urine. The carbon dioxide that results from drug metabolism is released through the lungs. Plasma half-life on the order of 3 to 4.5 hours.

INDICATIONS
1. Chronic myelogenous leukemia.
2. Essential thrombocytosis.
3. Polycythemia vera.
4. Acute myelogenous leukemia, blast crisis.
5. Head and neck cancer (in combination with radiation therapy).
6. Refractory ovarian cancer.

DOSAGE RANGE
1. Continuous therapy: 20–30 mg/kg PO daily.
2. Intermittent therapy: 80 mg/kg PO every third day.

3. Combination therapy with irradiation of head and neck cancer: 80 mg/kg PO every third day. In this setting, hydroxyurea is used as a radiation sensitizer and initiated at least 7 days before radiation therapy.

DRUG INTERACTION 1
5-FU—Hydroxyurea may enhance the risk of 5-FU toxicity.

DRUG INTERACTION 2
Antiretroviral agents—Hydroxyurea may enhance the anti-HIV activity of azidothymidine (AZT), dideoxycytidine (ddC), and dideoxyinosine (ddl).

SPECIAL CONSIDERATIONS
1. Contraindicated in patients with bone marrow suppression presenting as WBC <2500/mm^3 or platelet count <100,000/mm^3.
2. Monitor CBC on a weekly basis during therapy. Treatment should be stopped if the WBC count falls to less than 2500/mm^3 or the platelet count drops to less than 100,000/mm^3 and held until the counts rise above these values.
3. Use with caution in patients previously treated with chemotherapy and/or radiation therapy as there is an increased risk of myelosuppression.
4. Use with caution in patients with abnormal renal function. Doses should be reduced in the setting of renal dysfunction.
5. Pregnancy category D. Breastfeeding should be avoided as the drug is excreted in human breast milk.

TOXICITY 1
Myelosuppression with neutropenia is dose-limiting. Median onset 7–10 days with recovery of WBC counts 7–10 days after stopping the drug. Median onset of thrombocytopenia and anemia usually by day 10. Effect on bone marrow may be more severe in patients previously treated with chemotherapy and/or radiation therapy.

TOXICITY 2
Nausea and vomiting. Generally mild. Incidence can be reduced by dividing the daily dose into two or three doses. Stomatitis also occurs.

TOXICITY 3
Maculopapular rash, facial and acral erythema, hyperpigmentation, dry skin with atrophy, and pruritus.

TOXICITY 4
Radiation-recall skin reaction.

TOXICITY 5
Headache, drowsiness, and confusion.

TOXICITY 6
Transient elevations of serum transaminases and bilirubin.

TOXICITY 7
Teratogenic. Carcinogenic potential is not known.

Ibritumomab

TRADE NAMES	Zevalin, IDEC-Y2B8	CLASSIFICATION	Monoclonal antibody
CATEGORY	Biologic response modifier agent	DRUG MANUFACTURER	Spectrum

MECHANISM OF ACTION

- Immunoconjugate consisting of a stable thiourea covalent bond between the monoclonal antibody ibritumomab and the linker-chelator tiuxetan. This linker-chelator provides a high-affinity, conformationally-restricted site for indium-111 and/or yttrium-90.
- The antibody moiety is ibritumomab, which targets the CD20 antigen, a 35 kDa cell-surface non-glycosylated phosphoprotein expressed during early pre–B-cell development until the plasma cell stage. Binding of antibodies to CD20 induces a transmembrane signal that blocks cell activation and cell cycle progression,
- CD20 is expressed on more than 90% of all B-cell non-Hodgkin's lymphomas and leukemias. CD20 is not expressed on early pre–B cells, plasma cells, normal bone marrow stem cells, antigen-presenting dendritic reticulum cells, or other normal tissues.
- The beta emission from yttrium-90 induces cellular damage by the formation of free radicals in the target and neighboring cells.

ABSORPTION

Ibritumomab is given only by the IV route.

DISTRIBUTION

Peak and trough levels of rituximab correlate inversely with the number of circulating CD20-positive B cells. When In-111-ibritumomab is administered without unlabeled ibritumomab, only 18% of known sites of disease are imaged. In contrast, when In-111-ibritumomab administration is preceded by unlabeled ibritumomab, up to 90% of known sites of disease can be imaged.

METABOLISM

The mean effective half-life of yttrium-90 in blood is 30 hours, and the mean area under the fraction of injected activity (FIA) versus time curve in blood is 39 hours. Over a period of 7 days, a median of 7.2% of the injected activity is excreted in urine.

INDICATIONS

1. FDA-approved for relapsed and/or refractory low-grade, follicular, or transformed B-cell non-Hodgkin's lymphoma (NHL), including patients refractory to rituximab therapy.
2. FDA-approved for patients with previously untreated follicular NHL who achieve either a PR or CR to first-line chemotherapy.

DOSAGE RANGE

The regimen consists of the following: On day 1, an IV infusion of 250 mg/m^2 of rituximab; on day 7 and day 8 or 9, an IV infusion of 250 mg/m^2 of rituximab; and within 4 hours of each rituximab infusion, a therapeutic dose of 0.4 mCi/kg for patients with platelet counts greater than 150,000 or 0.3 mCi/kg for patients with platelet counts between 100,000 and 149,000. In either case, the maximum allowable dose of ibritumomab is 32 mCi, and patients should not be treated with a platelet count <100,000.

DRUG INTERACTIONS

None well characterized to date.

SPECIAL CONSIDERATIONS

1. Contraindicated in patients with known type I hypersensitivity, anaphylactic reactions to murine proteins, or sensitivity to any component of the product, including rituximab, yttrium chloride, and indium chloride.
2. Should not be administered to patients with an altered biodistribution of In-111 ibritumomab.
3. The prescribed and administered dose of yttrium-90 should not exceed the absolute maximum allowable dose of 32 mCi.
4. This therapy should be used only by physicians and healthcare professionals who are qualified and experienced in the safe use and handling of radioisotopes.
5. Patients should be premedicated with acetaminophen and diphenhydramine before each infusion of rituximab to reduce the incidence of infusion-related reactions.
6. Rituximab infusion should be started at an initial rate of 50 mg/hour. If no toxicity is observed during the first hour, the infusion rate can be escalated by increments of 50 mg/hour every 30 minutes to a maximum of 400 mg/hour. If the first treatment is well tolerated, the starting infusion rate for the second infusion can be administered at 100 mg/hour with 100 mg/hour increments at 30-minute intervals up to 400 mg/hour. Rituximab should **NOT** be given by IV push.
7. Monitor for infusion-related events resulting from rituximab infusion, which usually occur 30–120 minutes after the start of the first infusion. Infusion should be immediately stopped if signs or symptoms of an allergic reaction are observed. Immediate institution of diphenhydramine, acetaminophen, corticosteroids, IV fluids, and/or vasopressors may be necessary. In most instances, the infusion can be restarted at a reduced rate (50%) once symptoms have completely resolved. Resuscitation equipment should be readily available at bedside.
8. Infusion-related deaths within 24 hours of rituximab infusions have been reported.
9. Ibritumomab therapy should not be given to patients with >25% involvement of the bone marrow by lymphoma and/or impaired bone marrow reserve.
10. Ibritumomab therapy should not be given to patients with platelet counts below 100,000.

11. CBCs and platelet counts should be monitored weekly following ibritumomab therapy and should continue until levels recover.
12. The ibritumomab regimen should be given only as a single-course treatment.
13. The ibritumomab regimen may have direct toxic effects on the male and female reproductive organs, and effective contraception should be used during therapy and for up to 12 months following the completion of therapy.
14. Pregnancy category D. Breastfeeding should be avoided, as it is not known whether ibritumomab is excreted in human milk.

TOXICITY 1
Infusion-related symptoms, including fever, chills, urticaria, flushing, fatigue, headache, bronchospasm, rhinitis, dyspnea, angioedema, nausea, and/or hypotension. Severe symptoms include pulmonary infiltrates, acute respiratory distress syndrome, myocardial infarction, ventricular fibrillation, and/or cardiogenic shock. Usually occur within 30 minutes to 2 hours after the start of the first infusion. Usually resolve upon slowing or interrupting the infusion and with supportive care.

TOXICITY 2
Myelosuppression is the most common side effect. Thrombocytopenia is observed more frequently than neutropenia. The median duration of cytopenias ranges from 22 to 35 days, and the median time to nadir is 7–9 weeks. In <5% of patients, severe cytopenias remained beyond 12 weeks after therapy.

TOXICITY 3
Mild asthenia occurs in up to 40% of patients.

TOXICITY 4
Infections develop in nearly 30% of patients during the first 3 months after therapy.

TOXICITY 5
Mild nausea and vomiting.

TOXICITY 6
Cough, rhinitis, dyspnea, and sinusitis are observed in up to 35% of patients.

TOXICITY 7
Secondary malignancies occur in about 2% of patients. Acute myelogenous leukemia and myelodysplastic syndrome have been reported at a range of 8–34 months following therapy.

TOXICITY 8
Development of human anti-mouse (HAMA) and human antichimeric antibodies (HACA). Rare event in less than 1%–2% of patients.

Ibrutinib

TRADE NAME	Imbruvica	**CLASSIFICATION**	Signal transduction inhibitor
CATEGORY	Chemotherapy drug	**DRUG MANUFACTURER**	Pharmacyclics/ Janssen Biotech

MECHANISM OF ACTION
- Irreversible small-molecule inhibitor of Bruton's tyrosine kinase (BTK).
- BKT is a key signaling molecule of the B-cell antigen receptor (BCR) and cytokine receptor pathways.

MECHANISM OF RESISTANCE
- None well-characterized to date.

ABSORPTION
The absolute oral bioavailability has not been well characterized to date. Peak plasma drug levels are achieved in 1-2 hours after ingestion.

DISTRIBUTION
Extensive binding (97%) to plasma proteins. Steady-state drug levels are reached in approximately 8 days.

METABOLISM
Metabolism in the liver primarily by CYP3A4 and to a minor extent by CYP2D6 with formation of several metabolites. PCI-45227 is a dihydrodiol metabolite with inhibitory activity against BTK, although significantly less than parent drug. Elimination is mainly hepatic (80%) with excretion in the feces. Renal elimination of parent drug and its metabolites account for only <10% of an administered dose. The terminal half-life of the parent drug is 7–8 hours.

INDICATIONS
1. FDA-approved for patients with mantle cell lymphoma (MCL) who have received at least one prior therapy.
2. FDA-approved for patients with CLL/small lymphocytic lymphoma who have received at least one prior therapy.
3. FDA-approved for patients with CLL/small lymphocytic lymphoma and 17p deletion.
4. FDA-approved for patients with Waldenstrom's macroglobulinemia.

DOSAGE RANGE
1. MCL: Recommended dose is 560 mg PO daily
2. CLL, small lymphocytic lymphoma, Waldenstrom's macroglobulinemia: Recommended dose Is 420 mg PO daily

DRUG INTERACTION 1
Phenytoin and other drugs that stimulate the liver microsomal CYP3A4 enzymes, including carbamazepine, rifampin, phenobarbital, and St. John's Wort—These drugs may increase the metabolism of ibrutinib, resulting in its inactivation.

DRUG INTERACTION 2
Drugs that inhibit the liver microsomal CYP3A4 enzymes, including ketoconazole, itraconazole, erythromycin, and clarithromycin—These drugs may decrease the metabolism of ibrutinib, resulting in increased drug levels and potentially increased toxicity.

DRUG INTERACTION 3
Warfarin—Patients receiving coumarin-derived anticoagulants should be closely monitored for alterations in their clotting parameters (PT and INR) and/or bleeding, as ibrutinib may inhibit the metabolism of warfarin by the liver P450 system. Dose of warfarin may require careful adjustment in the presence of ibrutinib therapy.

SPECIAL CONSIDERATIONS
1. Ibrutinib capsules should be swallowed whole with water.
2. Closely monitor CBCs on a monthly basis.
3. Ibrutinib may increase the risk of bleeding in patients on antiplatelet or anticoagulant therapies.
4. Patients should be advised to maintain their hydration status.
5. Closely monitor renal function.
6. Closely monitor patients for fever and signs of infection.
7. Pregnancy category D. Breastfeeding should be avoided.

TOXICITY 1
Bleeding in the form of ecchymoses, GI bleeding, and hematuria.

TOXICITY 2
Infections.

TOXICITY 3
Myelosuppression with neutropenia, thrombocytopenia, and anemia.

y
TOXICITY 4
Renal toxicity with increases in serum creatinine. Serious and even fatal cases of renal failure have occurred.

TOXICITY 5
Second primary cancers with skin cancer and other solid tumors.

TOXICITY 6
Fatigue.

Idarubicin

TRADE NAMES	Idamycin, 4-Deme thoxydaunorubicin	CLASSIFICATION	Antitumor antibiotic
CATEGORY	Chemotherapy drug	DRUG MANUFACTURER	Pfizer

MECHANISM OF ACTION
- Semisynthetic anthracycline glycoside analog of daunorubicin.
- Intercalates into DNA, which results in inhibition of DNA synthesis and function.
- Inhibits topoisomerase II by forming a cleavable complex with topoisomerase II and DNA.
- In the presence of iron, drug forms oxygen free radicals, which cause single- and double-stranded DNA breaks.
- Specificity, in part, for the late S- and G2-phases of the cell cycle.

MECHANISM OF RESISTANCE
- Increased expression of the multidrug-resistant gene with enhanced drug efflux. This results in decreased intracellular drug accumulation.
- Decreased expression of topoisomerase II.
- Mutation in topoisomerase II with decreased binding affinity to drug.
- Increased expression of sulfhydryl proteins, including glutathione and glutathione-associated enzymes.

ABSORPTION
Administered only by the IV route.

DISTRIBUTION
Rapid and extensive tissue distribution. Peak concentrations in nucleated blood and bone marrow cells are achieved within minutes of administration and are 100-fold greater than those in plasma. Drug and its major metabolite, idarubicinol, are extensively bound (>90%) to plasma proteins.

METABOLISM
Significant metabolism in liver and in extrahepatic tissues. Metabolism by the liver microsomal system yields the active metabolite, idarubicinol, which may be responsible for the cardiotoxic effects. Idarubicin is eliminated mainly by biliary excretion into feces, with renal clearance accounting for only about 15% of drug elimination. The half-life of the parent drug is on the order of 20 hours, while the half-life of drug metabolites may exceed 45 hours.

INDICATIONS
1. Acute myelogenous leukemia.
2. Acute lymphoblastic leukemia.
3. Chronic myelogenous leukemia in blast crisis.
4. Myelodysplastic syndromes.

DOSAGE RANGE
Acute myelogenous leukemia, induction therapy—12 mg/m^2 IV on days 1–3 in combination with cytarabine, 100 mg/m^2/day IV continuous infusion for 7 days.

DRUG INTERACTION 1
Probenecid and sulfinpyrazone—Avoid concomitant use of probenecid and sulfinpyrazone, as these are uricosuric agents and may lead to uric acid nephropathy.

DRUG INTERACTION 2
Heparin—Idarubicin is incompatible with heparin as it forms a precipitate.

SPECIAL CONSIDERATIONS
1. Use with caution in patients with abnormal liver function. Dose modification should be considered in patients with liver dysfunction. Dose reduction by 50% is recommended for serum bilirubin in the range of 2.6–5.0 mg/dL. Absolutely contraindicated in patients with bilirubin >5.0 mg/dL.
2. Careful administration of drug, usually through a central venous catheter, is necessary as it is a strong vesicant. If peripheral venous access is used, careful monitoring of drug administration is necessary to avoid extravasation. If extravasation is suspected, stop infusion immediately, withdraw fluid, elevate arm, and apply ice to site. In severe cases, consult a plastic surgeon.
3. Alkalinization of the urine, allopurinol, and vigorous IV hydration are recommended to prevent tumor lysis syndrome in patients with acute myelogenous leukemia.

4. Monitor cardiac function before (baseline) and periodically during therapy with either MUGA radionuclide scan or echocardiogram to assess LVEF. Risk of cardiotoxicity is higher in elderly patients >70 years of age, in patients with prior history of hypertension or pre-existing heart disease, in patients previously treated with anthracyclines, or in patients with prior radiation therapy to the chest. While maximum dose of idarubicin that may be administered safely is not known, cumulative doses of >150 mg/m^2 have been associated with decreased LVEF.
5. Caution patients against sun exposure and to wear sun protection when outside.
6. Caution patients about the potential for red discoloration of urine for 1–2 days after drug administration.
7. Pregnancy category D. Breastfeeding should be avoided.

TOXICITY 1
Myelosuppression is dose-limiting with neutropenia and thrombocytopenia. Nadir typically occurs at 10–14 days after treatment, with recovery of counts by day 21. Risk of myelosuppression is greater in elderly patients and in those previously treated with chemotherapy and/or radiation therapy.

TOXICITY 2
Nausea and vomiting. Usually mild and occurs in up to 80%–90% of patients.

TOXICITY 3
Cardiotoxicity. Cardiac effects are similar to but less severe than those of doxorubicin. Acute toxicity presents as atrial arrhythmias, chest pain, and myopericarditis syndrome that typically occur within the first 24–48 hours of drug administration. Dilated cardiomyopathy with congestive heart failure can occur, usually with higher cumulative doses above 150 mg/m^2.

TOXICITY 4
Alopecia is nearly universal but reversible.

TOXICITY 5
Generalized skin rash, increased sensitivity to sunlight, hyperpigmentation of nails and at the injection site. Rarely, radiation-recall skin reaction.

TOXICITY 6
Strong vesicant. Extravasation can lead to extensive tissue damage.

TOXICITY 7
Mucositis and diarrhea. Common but usually not severe.

TOXICITY 8
Reversible effects on liver enzymes, including SGOT and SGPT.

TOXICITY 9
Red discoloration of urine. Usually within the first 1–2 days after drug administration.

Idelalisib

TRADE NAME	Zydelig	CLASSIFICATION	Signal transduction inhibitor
CATEGORY	Chemotherapy drug	DRUG MANUFACTURER	Gilead

MECHANISM OF ACTION
- Small-molecule inhibitor of PI3Kδ kinase, which is expressed in normal and malignant B-cells.
- Inhibits several key cell signaling pathways, including B-cell receptor signaling and CXCR4 and CXCR5 signaling.

MECHANISM OF RESISTANCE
- None well characterized to date.

ABSORPTION
The absolute oral bioavailability has not been well characterized to date. Peak plasma drug levels are achieved in about 1.5 hours after ingestion. Ingestion of a high-fat meal may slightly increase the idelalisib AUC.

DISTRIBUTION
Significant binding (>84%) to plasma proteins. Steady-state drug levels are reached in approximately 8 days.

METABOLISM
Metabolism in the liver primarily by CYP3A4 and to a minor extent by UGT1A4. GS-563117 is the major metabolite, and it is inactive against the phosphoinositide 3-kinase (PI3K) target. Elimination is mainly hepatic (approximately 80%) with excretion in the feces. Renal elimination of parent drug and its metabolites account for only about 14% of an administered dose. The terminal half-life of the parent drug is approximately 8 hours.

INDICATIONS

1. FDA-approved for relapsed CLL in combination with rituximab, and in patients for whom rituximab alone would be considered appropriate therapy due to other comorbidities.
2. FDA-approved for relapsed follicular non-Hodgkin's lymphoma after at least 2 prior systemic therapies.
3. FDA-approved for relapsed small lymphocytic lymphoma (SLL) after at least 2 prior systemic therapies.

DOSAGE RANGE

Recommended dose is 150 mg PO bid.

DRUG INTERACTION 1

Phenytoin and other drugs that stimulate the liver microsomal CYP3A4 enzymes, including carbamazepine, rifampin, phenobarbital, and St. John's Wort—These drugs may increase the metabolism of idelalisib, resulting in its inactivation.

DRUG INTERACTION 2

Drugs that inhibit the liver microsomal CYP3A4 enzymes, including ketoconazole, itraconazole, erythromycin, and clarithromycin—These drugs may decrease the metabolism of idelalisib, resulting in increased drug levels and potentially increased toxicity.

DRUG INTERACTION 3

Warfarin—Patients receiving coumarin-derived anticoagulants should be closely monitored for alterations in their clotting parameters (PT and INR) and/or bleeding, as idelalisib may inhibit the metabolism of warfarin by the liver P450 system. Dose of warfarin may require careful adjustment in the presence of idelalisib therapy.

SPECIAL CONSIDERATIONS

1. Idelalisib tablets should be swallowed whole and can be taken with or without food.
2. Closely monitor liver function during treatment. Fatal and/or serious hepatoxicity occurs in 14% of patients, and this represents a black-box warning.
3. Closely monitor patients for severe diarrhea and/or colitis. Severe diarrhea and/or colitis occurs in 14% of patients, and this represents a black-box warning.
4. Closely monitor patients for pulmonary symptoms and bilateral interstitial infiltrates. Fatal and/or serious pneumonitis represents a black-box warning.
5. Idelalisib treatment can result in the development of intestinal perforations, which in some cases has resulted in death. These GI perforations represent a black-box warning.
6. Closely monitor CBCs every 2 weeks for the first 3 months of therapy.
7. Closely monitor patients for serious allergic reactions at anaphylaxis has been reported. Idelalisib therapy should be discontinued permanently, and appropriate supportive measures need to be instituted.
8. Pregnancy category D. Breastfeeding should be avoided.

TOXICITY 1
Hepatotoxicity with elevations in LFTs and serum bilirubin.

TOXICITY 2
Diarrhea and/or colitis.

TOXICITY 3
Myelosuppression with neutropenia.

TOXICITY 4
GI perforations, which present as abdominal pain, diarrhea, fever, chills, and nausea/vomiting.

TOXICITY 5
Allergic reactions, including anaphylaxis.

TOXICITY 6
Skin toxicity, including erythema, pruritus, maculopapular rash, generalized skin rash.

Ifosfamide

TRADE NAMES	Ifex, Isophosphamide	CLASSIFICATION	Alkylating agent
CATEGORY	Chemotherapy drug	DRUG MANUFACTURER	Teva

MECHANISM OF ACTION
- Inactive in its parent form.
- Activated by the liver cytochrome P450 microsomal system to various cytotoxic metabolites, including ifosfamide mustard and acrolein.
- Cytotoxic metabolites form cross-links with DNA resulting in inhibition of DNA synthesis and function.
- Cell cycle–nonspecific agent, active in all phases of the cell cycle.

MECHANISM OF RESISTANCE
- Decreased cellular uptake of drug.
- Decreased expression of liver P450 activating enzymes.

- Increased expression of sulfhydryl proteins, including glutathione and glutathione-associated enzymes.
- Increased expression of aldehyde dehydrogenase, resulting in enhanced inactivation of drug.
- Enhanced activity of DNA repair enzymes.

ABSORPTION

Well absorbed by the GI tract with a bioavailability of nearly 100%. However, only IV form is available commercially because oral form is highly neurotoxic.

DISTRIBUTION

Widely distributed into body tissues. About 20% of drug is bound to plasma proteins.

METABOLISM

Extensively metabolized in the liver by the cytochrome P450 system. Activated at a four-fold slower rate than cyclophosphamide because of lower affinity to the liver P450 system. For this reason, about four-fold more drug is required to produce equitoxic antitumor effects with cyclophosphamide. The half-life of the drug is 3–10 hours for standard therapy and up to 14 hours for high-dose therapy. Approximately 50%–70% of the drug and its metabolites are excreted in urine.

INDICATIONS

1. Recurrent germ cell tumors.
2. Soft tissue sarcoma, osteogenic sarcoma.
3. Non-Hodgkin's lymphoma.
4. Hodgkin's lymphoma.
5. SCLC and NSCLC.
6. Bladder cancer.
7. Head and neck cancer.
8. Cervical cancer.
9. Ewing's sarcoma.

DOSAGE RANGE

1. Testicular cancer: 1200 mg/m^2 IV on days 1–5 every 21 days, as part of the VeIP salvage regimen.
2. Soft tissue sarcoma: 2000 mg/m^2 IV continuous infusion on days 1–3 every 21 days, as part of the MAID regimen.
3. Non-Hodgkin's lymphoma: 1000 mg/m^2 on days 1 and 2 every 28 days, as part of the ICE regimen.
4. Head and neck cancer: 1000 mg/m^2 on days 1–3 every 21–28 days, as part of the TIC regimen.

DRUG INTERACTION 1

Phenobarbital, phenytoin, and other drugs that stimulate the liver P450 system—Increase the rate of metabolic activation of ifosfamide to its toxic metabolites resulting in enhanced toxicity.

DRUG INTERACTION 2

Cimetidine and allopurinol—Increase the formation of ifosfamide metabolites resulting in increased toxicity.

DRUG INTERACTION 3

Cisplatin—Increases ifosfamide-associated renal toxicity.

DRUG INTERACTION 4

Warfarin—Ifosfamide may enhance the anticoagulant effects of warfarin. Need to closely monitor coagulation parameters, PT and INR.

SPECIAL CONSIDERATIONS

1. Administer prophylactic antiemetics to avoid nausea and vomiting.
2. Use with caution in patients with abnormal renal function. Dose reduction is necessary in this setting. Baseline CrCl must be obtained, and renal function should be monitored during therapy.
3. Uroprotection with mesna and hydration must be used to prevent bladder toxicity. Pre- and post-hydration (1500–2000 mL/day) or continuous bladder irrigations are recommended to prevent hemorrhagic cystitis. Important to monitor urine for presence of gross and/or microscopic hematuria before each cycle of therapy
4. Monitor coagulation parameters, including PT and INR, when ifosfamide is used concurrently with warfarin, as ifosfamide may enhance its anticoagulant effects.
5. Contraindicated in patients with peptic ulcer disease, severe liver disease, and/or cardiac disease.
6. Pregnancy category D. Breastfeeding should be avoided.

TOXICITY 1

Myelosuppression is dose-limiting. Mainly leukopenia and to a lesser extent thrombocytopenia. Nadir occurs at 10–14 days with recovery in 21 days.

TOXICITY 2

Bladder toxicity can be dose-limiting and manifested by hemorrhagic cystitis, dysuria, and increased urinary frequency. Chronic fibrosis of bladder leads to an increased risk of secondary bladder cancer. Uroprotection with mesna and hydration must be used to prevent bladder toxicity.

TOXICITY 3

Nausea and vomiting. Usually occurs within 3–6 hours of therapy and may last up to 3 days. Anorexia is fairly common.

TOXICITY 4

Neurotoxicity in the form of lethargy, confusion, seizure, cerebellar ataxia, weakness, hallucinations, cranial nerve dysfunction, and rarely stupor and coma. Incidence may be higher in patients receiving high-dose therapy and in those with impaired renal function.

TOXICITY 5
Alopecia is common (>80%). Skin rash, hyperpigmentation, and nail changes are occasionally seen.

TOXICITY 6
Syndrome of inappropriate antidiuretic hormone secretion (SIADH).

TOXICITY 7
Amenorrhea, oligospermia, and infertility.

TOXICITY 8
Mutagenic, teratogenic, and carcinogenic.

Imatinib

TRADE NAMES	STI571, Gleevec	CLASSIFICATION	Signal transduction inhibitor
CATEGORY	Chemotherapy drug	DRUG MANUFACTURER	Novartis

MECHANISM OF ACTION
- Phenylaminopyrimidine methanesulfonate compound that occupies the ATP binding site of the Bcr-Abl protein and a very limited number of other tyrosine kinases. Binding in this ATP pocket results in subsequent inhibition of substrate phosphorylation.
- Potent and selective inhibitor of the P210 Bcr-Abl tyrosine kinase resulting in inhibition of clonogenicity and tumorigenicity of Bcr-Abl and Ph+ cells.
- Induces apoptosis in Bcr-Abl positive cells without causing cell differentiation.
- Inhibits other activated Abl tyrosine kinases, including P185 Bcr-Abl, and inhibits other receptor tyrosine kinases for platelet-derived growth factor receptor (PDGFR) and c-Kit.

MECHANISM OF RESISTANCE

- Increased expression of Bcr-Abl tyrosine kinase through amplification of the Bcr-Abl gene.
- Mutations in the Bcr-Abl tyrosine kinase resulting in altered binding affinity to the drug.
- Increased expression of P170 glycoprotein resulting in enhanced drug efflux and decreased intracellular drug accumulation.
- Increased degradation and/or metabolism of the drug through as yet undefined mechanisms.
- Increased expression of c-Kit through amplification of the c-Kit gene.
- Mutations in the c-Kit tyrosine kinase resulting in altered binding affinity to the drug.

ABSORPTION
Oral bioavailability is nearly 100%.

DISTRIBUTION
Extensive binding (95%) to plasma proteins, including albumin and α1-acid glycoprotein. Steady-state drug concentrations are reached in 2–3 days.

METABOLISM
Metabolism in the liver primarily by CYP3A4 microsomal enzymes. Other cytochrome P450 enzymes play a minor role in its metabolism. The main metabolite is the N-desmethylated piperazine derivative, and this metabolite shows in vitro potency similar to that of the parent drug. Elimination is mainly in the feces, predominantly as metabolites. The terminal half-life of the parent drug is 18 hours, while that of its main metabolite, the N-desmethyl derivative, is on the order of 40 hours.

INDICATIONS
1. Chronic phase of CML—FDA-approved first-line therapy in adult patients.
2. Chronic phase of CML after failure on interferon-α therapy—FDA-approved.
3. CML in accelerated phase and/or in blast crisis—FDA-approved.
4. Newly diagnosed pediatric patients with Ph+ acute lymphocytic leukemia (Ph+ ALL)—FDA-approved.
5. Chronic phase Ph+ CML in pediatric patients whose disease has recurred after stem cell transplant or is resistant to interferon-α.
6. Myelodysplastic/myeloproliferative diseases (MDS/MPD) associated with PDGFR gene rearrangements.
7. Hypereosinophilic syndrome/chronic eosinophilic leukemia (HES/CEL).
8. Relapsed/refractory adult Ph+ ALL.
9. Gastrointestinal stromal tumors (GIST) expressing c-Kit (CD117)—Unresectable and/or metastatic disease.
10. GIST expressing c-Kit (CD117)—Adjuvant therapy following resection of localized disease.

DOSAGE RANGE

1. Recommended starting dose is 400 mg/day for patients in chronic phase CML and 600 mg/day for patients in accelerated phase or blast crisis. Dose increases from 400 mg to 600 mg or 800 mg in patients with chronic phase disease, or from 600 mg to a maximum of 800 mg (given as 400 mg twice daily) in patients with accelerated phase or blast crisis may be considered in the absence of severe adverse drug reaction and severe non–leukemia-related neutropenia or thrombocytopenia in the following circumstances: disease progression (at any time); failure to achieve a satisfactory hematologic response after at least 3 months of treatment; failure to achieve a cytogenetic response after 12 months of treatment; or loss of a previously achieved hematologic and/or cytogenetic response. Patients should be monitored closely following dose escalation given the potential for an increased incidence of adverse reactions at higher dosages.
2. Recommended starting dose is 400 mg/day for patients with unresectable and/or metastatic GIST. Limited data exist on the effect of dose increases from 400 mg to 600 mg or 800 mg in patients progressing at the lower dose.
3. Recommended dose is 400 mg/day for 3 years of adjuvant therapy of patients with early-stage GIST.
4. Recommended starting dose is 400 mg/day for patients with MDS/MPD.
5. Recommended starting dose is 400 mg/day for patients with HES/CEL.
6. Recommended starting dose is 600 mg/day for patients with Ph+ ALL.

DRUG INTERACTION 1

Phenytoin and other drugs that stimulate the liver microsomal CYP3A4 enzymes, including carbamazepine, rifampin, phenobarbital, and St. John's wort—These drugs increase the rate of metabolism of imatinib resulting in its inactivation.

DRUG INTERACTION 2

Drugs that inhibit the liver microsomal CYP3A4 enzymes, including ketoconazole, itraconazole, erythromycin, and clarithromycin—These drugs decrease the rate of metabolism of imatinib resulting in increased drug levels and potentially increased toxicity.

DRUG INTERACTION 3

Warfarin—Patients on coumarin-derived anticoagulants should be closely monitored for alterations in their clotting parameters (PT and INR) and/or bleeding as imatinib inhibits the metabolism of warfarin by the liver P450 system. Dose of warfarin may require careful adjustment in the presence of imatinib therapy.

SPECIAL CONSIDERATIONS

1. Patients should be weighed and monitored regularly for signs and symptoms of fluid retention. The risk of fluid retention and edema is increased with higher drug doses and in patients whose age >65 years.
2. Use with caution in patients with underlying hepatic impairment. Dose adjustment is not required in patients with mild to moderate hepatic impairment. Patients with severe hepatic impairment should have a 25% reduction in the recommended dose.

3. Use with caution in patients with underlying renal impairment. For patients with moderate renal impairment (CrCL 20–39 mL/min), doses greater than 400 mg are not recommended, and patients should have a 50% reduction in the recommended starting dose. For patients with mild renal impairment (CrCL 40–59 mL/min), doses greater than 600 mg are not recommended.

4. Monitor CBC on a weekly basis for the first month, biweekly for the second month, and periodically thereafter.

5. Imatinib should be taken with food and a large glass of water to decrease the risk of GI irritation. Imatinib tablets can be dissolved in water or apple juice for patients who have difficulty swallowing.

6. Hematologic responses typically occur within 2 weeks after initiation of therapy while complete hematologic responses are observed within 4 weeks after starting therapy.

7. Cytogenetic responses are observed as early as 2 months and up to 10 months after starting therapy. The median time to best cytogenetic response is about 5 months.

8. Carefully monitor dose of drug when used in patients with seizure disorders on phenytoin. Dose of drug may need to be increased as the metabolism of imatinib by the CYP3A4 enzyme is enhanced in the presence of phenytoin.

9. Patients who require anticoagulation should receive low-molecular weight or standard heparin, as imatinib inhibits the metabolism of warfarin.

10. Monitor cardiac function before (baseline) and periodically during therapy with either MUGA radionuclide scan or echocardiogram to assess LVEF. The diagnosis of CHF should be considered in patients who experience edema while on imatinib.

11. Avoid Seville oranges, starfruit, pomelos, grapefruit juice, and grapefruit products while on imatinib therapy.

12. Patients should be closely monitored for depressive symptoms and suicidal ideation while on therapy.

13. Musculoskeletal pain may be a sign of potential withdrawal syndrome in patients who had stopped imatinib therapy after having been on treatment for more than 3 years. Pain sites include shoulder and hip regions, extremities, and hands and feet along with muscle tenderness.

14. Screen all patient for hepatitis B (HBV) infection before initiation of imatinib therapy. Closely monitor HBV carriers for signs of active HBV infection during imatinib therapy. Imatinib therapy can increase the risk of HBV reactivation, and imatinib therapy should be permanently discontinued in the event of HBV reactivation.

15. Pregnancy category D. Breastfeeding should be avoided.

TOXICITY 1
Nausea and vomiting occur in 40%–50% of patients. Usually related to the swallowing of capsules and relieved when the drug is taken with food.

TOXICITY 2
Transient ankle and periorbital edema. Usually mild to moderate in nature.

TOXICITY 3
Occasional myalgias.

TOXICITY 4
Fluid retention with pleural effusion, ascites, pulmonary edema, and weight gain. Usually dose-related and more common in elderly patients and in those in blast crisis and the accelerated phase of CML. CHF is a rare but serious adverse event.

TOXICITY 5
Diarrhea is observed in 25%–30% of patients.

TOXICITY 6
Myelosuppression with neutropenia and thrombocytopenia.

TOXICITY 7
Mild, transient elevation in serum transaminases. Clinically asymptomatic in most cases.

TOXICITY 8
Skin toxicity in the form of bullous reactions, including erythema multiforme and Stevens-Johnson syndrome.

TOXICITY 9
Insomnia, depression, and suicidal ideation.

Interferon-α

TRADE NAMES	α-interferon, IFN-α, Interferon-α2a, Roferon Interferon-α2b, Intron A, Sylatron (Peginterferon-α2b)	CLASSIFICATION	Immunotherapy
CATEGORY	Biologic response modifier agent	DRUG MANUFACTURER	Roche (Roferon), Merck (Intron A), Merck (Sylatron)

MECHANISM OF ACTION
- Precise mechanism of antitumor action remains unknown.
- Direct antiproliferative effects on tumor cell mediated by: induction of 2', 5'-oligoadenylate synthetase and protein kinase leading to decreased translation and inhibition of tumor cell protein synthesis; induction of differentiation; prolongation of the cell cycle; modulation of oncogene expression.
- Indirect induction of host antitumor mechanisms mediated by: induced activity of at least four immune effector cells, including cytotoxic T cells, helper T cells, NK cells, and macrophages; enhancement of tumor

surface expression of critical antigens that are recognized by the immune system; inhibition of angiogenesis through decreased expression of various angiogenic factors.

MECHANISM OF RESISTANCE
- Development of neutralizing antibodies to interferon-α.
- Decreased expression of cell surface receptors to interferon-α.

ABSORPTION
Not available for oral use and is administered only via the parenteral route. Approximately 80%–90% of interferon-α is absorbed into the systemic circulation after IM or SC injection. Peak plasma levels are achieved in 4 hours after intramuscular injection and 7 hours after subcutaneous administration.

DISTRIBUTION
Does not cross the blood-brain barrier. Binding to plasma proteins has not been well characterized.

METABOLISM
Interferon-α is catabolized by renal tubule cells to various breakdown products. The major route of elimination is through the kidneys by both glomerular filtration and tubular secretion. Hepatic metabolism and biliary excretion play only a minor role in drug clearance. The elimination half-life is approximately 2–7 hours and depends on the specific route of drug administration.

INDICATIONS
1. Malignant melanoma—Adjuvant therapy.
2. Chronic myelogenous leukemia—Chronic phase.
3. Hairy cell leukemia.
4. AIDS-related Kaposi's sarcoma.
5. Cutaneous T-cell lymphoma.
6. Multiple myeloma.
7. Low-grade, non-Hodgkin's lymphoma.
8. Renal cell cancer.
9. Hemangioma.

DOSAGE RANGE
1. Chronic myelogenous leukemia: 9 million IU SC or IM daily.
2. Hairy cell leukemia: 3 million IU SC or IM daily for 16–24 weeks.
3. Malignant melanoma: 20 million IU/m^2 IV, 5 times weekly for 4 weeks, then 10 million IU/m^2 SC, three times weekly for 48 weeks.
4. Malignant melanoma (Peginterferon-α2b): 6 mg/kg/week SC for 8 doses followed by 3 mg/kg/week SC for up to 5 years.
5. Kaposi's sarcoma: 36 million IU SC or IM daily for 12 weeks.

DRUG INTERACTION 1
Phenytoin, phenobarbital—Effects of phenytoin and phenobarbital may be increased as interferon-α inhibits the liver P450 system. Drug levels should be monitored closely and dose adjustments made accordingly.

DRUG INTERACTION 2

Live vaccines—Vaccination with live vaccines is contraindicated during and for at least 3 months after completion of interferon-α therapy.

SPECIAL CONSIDERATIONS

1. Use with caution in patients with pre-existing cardiac, pulmonary, CNS, hepatic, and/or renal impairment, as they are at increased risk for developing serious and sometimes fatal reactions.
2. Contraindicated in patients with history of autoimmune disease, autoimmune hepatitis, or in those who have received immunosuppressive therapy for organ transplants.
3. Contraindicated in patients with a known allergy to benzyl alcohol as the injectable solution form contains benzyl alcohol.
4. Use with caution in patients with myelosuppression or those who are receiving concurrent agents known to cause myelosuppression.
5. Use with caution in patients with a history of depression and/or other neuropsychiatric disorders. Routine neuropsychiatric monitoring of all patients on interferon-α is recommended. Therapy should be permanently discontinued in patients with persistently severe or worsening signs or symptoms of depression, psychosis, or encephalopathy.
6. Use with caution in older patients (>65 years of age) as they are at increased risk for developing fatigue and neurologic toxicities secondary to interferon-α.
7. Premedicate patient with acetaminophen to reduce the risk and/or severity of flu-like symptoms, including fever and chills. In the event that acetaminophen is unsuccessful, indomethacin can be used.
8. Pregnancy category C. Breastfeeding should be avoided.

TOXICITY 1

Flu-like symptoms with fever, chills, headache, myalgias, and arthralgias. Occur in 80%–90% of patients, usually beginning a few hours after the first injection and lasting for up to 8–9 hours. Incidence decreases with subsequent injections. Can be controlled with acetaminophen and/or indomethacin.

TOXICITY 2

Fatigue and anorexia are dose-limiting with chronic administration.

TOXICITY 3

Somnolence, confusion, or depression. Patients >65 years of age are more susceptible to the neurologic sequelae of interferon-α.

TOXICITY 4

Myelosuppression with mild leukopenia and thrombocytopenia. Reversible upon discontinuation of therapy.

TOXICITY 5

Mild, transient elevations in serum transaminases. Dose-dependent toxicity observed more frequently in the presence of pre-existing liver abnormalities.

TOXICITY 6
Renal toxicity is uncommon and is manifested by mild proteinuria and hypocalcemia. Acute renal failure and nephrotic syndrome have been reported in rare instances.

TOXICITY 7
Alopecia, skin rash, pruritus with dry skin, and irritation at the injection site.

TOXICITY 8
Cardiotoxicity in the form of chest pain, arrhythmias, and congestive heart failure. Uncommon and almost always reversible.

TOXICITY 9
Impotence, decreased libido, menstrual irregularities, and an increased incidence of spontaneous abortions.

TOXICITY 10
Rare cases of autoimmune disorders, including thrombocytopenia, vasculitis, Raynaud's disease, lupus, rheumatoid arthritis, and rhabdomyolysis

TOXICITY 11
Retinopathy with macular edema, retinal artery or vein thrombosis, optic neuritis, retinal detachment, cotton-wool spots, and small hemorrhages.

Ipilimumab

TRADE NAME	Yervoy	CLASSIFICATION	Monoclonal antibody
CATEGORY	Biologic response modifier agent	DRUG MANUFACTURER	Bristol-Myers Squibb

MECHANISM OF ACTION
- Ipilimumab binds to cytotoxic T-lymphocyte-associated antigen 4 (CTLA-4), which is expressed on the surface of activated CD4 and CD8 T lymphocytes, resulting in inhibition of the interaction between CTLA-4 and its target ligands CD80/CD86.
- Blockade of CTLA-4 enhances T-cell immune responses, including T-cell activation and proliferation.

MECHANISM OF RESISTANCE
None well characterized to date.

ABSORPTION
Administered only by the IV route.

DISTRIBUTION
Distribution is not well characterized. Steady-state concentrations are generally reached by the third dose.

METABOLISM
Metabolism of ipilimumab has not been extensively characterized. The terminal half-life is on the order of 385–400 hours.

INDICATIONS
1. FDA-approved for the treatment of unresectable or metastatic malignant melanoma.
2. FDA-approved for the adjuvant treatment of cutaneous melanoma with pathologic involvement of regional lymph nodes of more than 1 mm who have undergone complete resection, including total lymphadenectomy.

DOSAGE RANGE
1. Metastatic melanoma: Recommended dose is 3 mg/kg IV over 90 minutes every 3 weeks for a total of 4 doses.
2. Adjuvant melanoma: Recommended dose is 10 mg/kg every 3 weeks for 4 doses, followed by 10 mg/kg every 12 weeks for up to 3 years.

DRUG INTERACTIONS
None characterized to date.

SPECIAL CONSIDERATIONS
1. Ipilimumab can result in severe and fatal immune-mediated adverse reactions due to T-cell activation and proliferation. These immune-mediated reactions may involve any organ system, with the most common reactions being enterocolitis, hepatitis, dermatitis, neuropathy, and endocrinopathy. They typically occur during treatment, although some of these reactions may occur weeks to months after completion of therapy. These reactions represent a black-box warning.
2. Ipilumumab should be permanently discontinued for any of the following:
   - Persistent moderate adverse reactions or inability to reduce daily steroid dose to 7.5 mg prednisone
   - Failure to complete the full treatment course within 16 weeks from administration of first dose
   - Colitis with abdominal pain, fever, ileus, or peritoneal signs; increase in stool frequency with 7 or more over baseline; stool incontinence; need for IV hydration for more than 24 hours; GI hemorrhage; and GI perforation
   - SGOT/SGPT >5×ULN or total bilirubin >3×ULN
   - Stevens-Johnson syndrome, toxic epidermal necrolysis, or rash complicated by full thickness dermal ulceration, or necrotic, bullous, or hemorrhagic manifestations

- Severe motor or sensory neuropathy, Guillain-Barré syndrome, or myasthenia gravis
- Severe immune-mediated reactions involving any organ system
- Immune-mediated ocular disease that is unresponsive to topical immunosuppressive therapy

3. Ipilumumab should be withheld for any moderate immune-mediated adverse reaction or for symptomatic endocrinopathy. For patients with partial or complete resolution of symptoms (grade 0–1) and who are receiving less than 7.5 mg prednisone, ipilumumab may be resumed at a dose of 3 mg/kg every 3 weeks until administration of all four planned doses or 16 weeks from first dose, whichever occurs earlier.

4. Closely monitor for signs and symptoms of enterocolitis, such as diarrhea and abdominal pain. Patients with inflammatory bowel disease may not be appropriate candidates for ipilimumab.

5. In patients with moderate enterocolitis, withhold ipilumumab therapy and administer antidiarrheal treatment. If symptoms persist for more than 1 week, administer prednisone at 0.5 mg/kg. In patients with severe enterocolitis, permanently discontinue ipilumumab and administer prednisone at 1–2 mg/kg/day.

6. Administer steroid eye drops to patients who develop uveitis, iritis, or episcleritis. Permanently discontinue ipilumumab for immune-mediated ocular disease that is unresponsive to local immunosuppressive therapy. In this setting, administer prednisone at 1–2 mg/ kg/day.

7. FDA-approved Risk Evaluation and Mitigation Strategy (REMS) program has been developed to inform healthcare providers about the risk of serious immune-mediated adverse reactions caused by ipilimumab.

8. Monitor thyroid function tests at the start of treatment and before each dose.

9. Pregnancy category C. Breastfeeding should be avoided.

TOXICITY 1
Fatigue and anorexia.

TOXICITY 2
Immune-mediated entercolitis presenting as diarrhea, abdominal pain, fever, and ileus.

TOXICITY 3
Immune-mediated hepatitis that can range from moderate to severe life-threatening hepatotoxicity.

TOXICITY 4
Immune-mediated dermatitis with rash and pruritis. Severe, life-threatening dermatitis in the form of Stevens-Johnson syndrome, toxic epidermal necrolysis, full thickness dermal ulceration, or necrotic, bullous, or hemorrhagic skin lesions occur rarely.

TOXICITY 5
Immune-mediated endocrinopathies with hypophysitis, adrenal insufficiency, hypopituitarism, hypogonadism, and hyperthyroidism or hypothyroidism.

TOXICITY 6

Immune-mediated neuropathies with motor weakness, sensory alterations, or paresthesias with severe neuropathies such as myasthenia gravis and Guillain-Barré–like syndromes.

TOXICITY 7

Ocular toxicities in the form of uveitis, iritis, conjunctivitis, blepharitis, or episcleritis.

TOXICITY 8

Other immune-mediated adverse reactions, including myocarditis, temporal arteritis, polymyalgia rheumatica, vasculitis, arthritis, and autoimmune thyroiditis.

Irinotecan

TRADE NAMES	Camptosar, CPT-11	CLASSIFICATION	Topoisomerase I inhibitor
CATEGORY	Chemotherapy drug	DRUG MANUFACTURER	Pfizer

MECHANISM OF ACTION

- Semisynthetic derivative of camptothecin, an alkaloid extract from the *Camptotheca acuminata* tree.
- Inactive in its parent form. Converted by the carboxylesterase enzyme to its active metabolite, SN-38.
- SN-38 binds to and stabilizes the topoisomerase I-DNA complex and prevents the religation of DNA after it has been cleaved by topoisomerase I. The collision between this stable, cleavable complex and the advancing replication fork results in double-strand DNA breaks and cellular death.
- Antitumor activity of drug requires the presence of ongoing DNA synthesis.
- Cell cycle-nonspecific agent with activity in all phases of the cell cycle.
- Colorectal tumors express higher levels of topoisomerase I than normal colonic mucosa, making this an attractive target for chemotherapy.

MECHANISM OF RESISTANCE

- Decreased expression of topoisomerase I.
- Mutations in topoisomerase I enzyme with decreased affinity for the drug.
- Increased expression of the multidrug-resistant phenotype with over-expression of P170 glycoprotein. Results in enhanced efflux of drug and decreased intracellular accumulation of drug.
- Decreased formation of the cytotoxic metabolite SN-38 through decreased activity and/or expression of the carboxylesterase enzyme.
- Decreased accumulation of drug into cells by mechanisms not well identified.

ABSORPTION

Irinotecan is administered only by the IV route.

DISTRIBUTION

Widely distributed in body tissues. Irinotecan exhibits moderate binding to plasma proteins (30%–60%). In contrast, SN-38 shows extensive plasma protein binding (95%). Peak levels of SN-38 are achieved within 1 hour after drug administration.

METABOLISM

The conversion of irinotecan to the active metabolite SN-38 occurs primarily in the liver. However, this conversion can also take place in plasma and in intestinal mucosa. SN-38 subsequently undergoes conjugation in the liver to the glucuronide metabolite, which is essentially inactive. In aqueous solution, the lactone ring undergoes rapid hydrolysis to the carboxylate form. Only about 34%–44% of CPT-11 and 45%–64% of the active metabolite SN-38 are present in the active lactone form at 1 hour after drug administration. The major route of elimination of both irinotecan and SN-38 is in bile and feces, accounting for 50%–70% of drug clearance. Only 10%–14% of CPT-11 and <1% of SN-38 is cleared in urine. The half-lives of irinotecan and SN-38 are 6–12 and 10–20 hours, respectively.

INDICATIONS
1. Colorectal cancer—FDA-approved in combination with 5-FU and leucovorin (5-FU/LV) as first-line treatment of patients with metastatic colorectal cancer.
2. Colorectal cancer—FDA-approved as a single agent for second-line treatment of patients with metastatic colorectal cancer after failure of 5-FU–based chemotherapy.
3. NSCLC.
4. SCLC.

DOSAGE RANGE
1. Irinotecan can be administered at 180 mg/m^2 IV as monotherapy or in combination with infusional 5-FU/LV on an every-2-week schedule.
2. An alternative regimen is 300–350 mg/m^2 IV on an every-3-week schedule.

DRUG INTERACTION 1
Phenytoin and other drugs that stimulate the liver microsomal CYP3A4 enzyme, including carbamazepine, rifampin, phenobarbital, and St. John's wort—These drugs increase the rate of metabolism of irinotecan and SN-38, resulting in its inactivation.

DRUG INTERACTION 2
Drugs that inhibit the liver microsomal CYP3A4 enzymes, including ketoconazole, itraconazole, erythromycin, and clarithromycin—These drugs decrease the rate of metabolism of irinotecan and SN-38, resulting in increased drug levels and potentially increased toxicity.

SPECIAL CONSIDERATIONS
1. Irinotecan is an emetogenic drug (level 4). Patients should routinely receive antiemetic prophylaxis with a 5-HT3 antagonist, such as ondansetron or granisetron, in combination with dexamethasone.
2. Treatment with irinotecan is complicated by a syndrome of "early diarrhea," which consists of diarrhea, diaphoresis, and abdominal cramping during the infusion or within 24 hours of drug administration. This complication is thought to be due to a cholinergic effect. The recommended treatment is atropine (0.25–1.0 mg) administered IV unless clinically contraindicated. The routine use of atropine for prophylaxis is not recommended. However, atropine prophylaxis should be administered if a cholinergic event has been experienced.
3. Instruct patients about the possibility of late diarrhea (starting after 24 hours of drug administration), which can lead to serious dehydration

and/or electrolyte imbalances if not managed promptly. This side effect is thought to be due to a direct irritation of the gastrointestinal mucosa by SN-38, although other as yet unidentified mechanisms may be involved. Loperamide should be taken immediately after the first loose bowel movement. The recommended dose is 4 mg PO as a loading dose, followed by 2 mg every 2 hours around the clock (4 mg every 4 hours during the night). Loperamide can be discontinued once the patient is diarrhea-free for 12 hours. If diarrhea should continue without improvement in the first 24 hours, an oral fluoroquinolone should be added. Hospitalization with IV antibiotics and IV hydration should be considered with continued diarrhea.

4. Irinotecan should be held for grade 3 (7–9 stools/day, incontinence, or severe cramping) and/or grade 4 (<10 stools/day, grossly bloody stool, or need for parenteral support) diarrhea. Dose of drug must be reduced upon recovery by the patient.

5. Patients should be warned against taking laxatives while on therapy.

6. Carefully monitor administration of drug, as it is a moderate vesicant. The site of infusion should be carefully inspected for extravasation, in which case flushing with sterile water, elevation of the extremity, and local application of ice are recommended.

7. Use with caution in patients >65 years of age, in patients with poor performance status, and in those previously treated with pelvic and/or abdominal irradiation as they are at increased risk for myelosuppression and diarrhea.

8. Careful monitoring of patients on a weekly basis, especially during the first treatment cycle. Monitor complete blood cell count and platelet count on a weekly basis.

9. Patients with the UGT1A1 7/7 genotype may be at increased risk for developing GI toxicity and myelosuppression. Approximately 10% of the North American population is homozygous for this genotype. Dose reduction should be considered in this setting.

10. Patients should be warned to be off St. John's wort for at least 2 weeks before starting irinotecan therapy and should remain off until after the completion of irinotecan therapy. St. John's wort has been shown to reduce the efficacy of irinotecan chemotherapy by inhibiting metabolism of irinotecan to the active SN-38 metabolite.

11. Pregnancy category D. Breastfeeding should be avoided.

TOXICITY 1

Myelosuppression. Dose-limiting with neutropenia being most commonly observed. Patients with prior history of abdominal/pelvic irradiation are particularly prone to developing myelosuppression after treatment with irinotecan. Typical nadir occurs at days 7–10 with full recovery by days 21–28.

TOXICITY 2

Diarrhea. Dose-limiting with two different forms: early and late. Early form occurs within 24 hours of drug treatment and is thought to be a cholinergic event. Characterized by flushing, diaphoresis, abdominal pain, and diarrhea. Late-form diarrhea occurs after 24 hours, typically at 3–10 days after treatment, can be severe and prolonged, and can lead to dehydration and electrolyte imbalance. Up to 80%–90% of patients may experience some aspect of late diarrhea, although only 10%–20% of patients will experience grade 3 or 4 diarrhea. Anorexia, nausea, and vomiting are usually mild and dose-related.

TOXICITY 3
Mild alopecia.

TOXICITY 4
Transient elevation in serum transaminases, alkaline phosphatase, and bilirubin.

TOXICITY 5
Asthenia and fever.

Irinotecan liposome

TRADE NAMES	Onivyde	**CLASSIFICATION**	Topoisomerase I inhibitor
CATEGORY	Chemotherapy drug	**DRUG MANUFACTURER**	Merrimack

MECHANISM OF ACTION
- Semisynthetic derivative of camptothecin, an alkaloid extract from the *Camptotheca acuminata* tree that is encapsulated in a liposome.
- Inactive in its parent form. Converted by a carboxylesterase enzyme to its active metabolite, SN-38.
- SN-38 binds to and stabilizes the topoisomerase I-DNA complex and prevents the religation of DNA after it has been cleaved by topoisomerase I. The collision between this stable, cleavable complex and the advancing replication fork results in double-strand DNA breaks and cellular death.

- Antitumor activity of drug requires the presence of ongoing DNA synthesis.
- Cell cycle–nonspecific agent with activity in all phases of the cell cycle.

MECHANISM OF RESISTANCE
- Decreased expression of topoisomerase I.
- Mutations in topoisomerase I enzyme with decreased affinity for the drug.
- Increased expression of the multidrug-resistant phenotype with over-expression of P170 glycoprotein. Results in enhanced efflux of drug and decreased intracellular accumulation of drug.
- Decreased formation of the cytotoxic metabolite SN-38 through decreased activity and/or expression of the carboxylesterase enzyme.

ABSORPTION
Administered only by the IV route.

DISTRIBUTION
Approximately 95% of irinotecan remains liposome-encapsulated. Plasma protein binding is <0.44% of the total irinotecan in the liposome preparation.

METABOLISM
The metabolism of irinotecan liposome has not been well characterized. Conversion of irinotecan to the active metabolite SN-38 occurs primarily in the liver. However, this conversion can also take place in plasma and in intestinal mucosa. SN-38 subsequently undergoes conjugation in the liver to form the inactive glucuronide metabolite. The metabolic clearance of irinotecan liposome has not been well characterized. The major route of elimination of both irinotecan and SN-38 is in bile and feces, accounting for 50%–70% of drug clearance. Only 11%–20% of CPT-11 and <1% of SN-38 is cleared in urine. The half-lives of irinotecan and SN-38 are about 26 and 68 hours, respectively.

INDICATIONS
FDA-approved in combination with 5-FU and leucovorin (5-FU/LV) for the treatment of patients with metastatic pancreatic cancer after disease progression following gemcitabine-based therapy.

DOSAGE RANGE
1. Recommended dose is 70 mg/m^2 IV in combination with 5-FU/LV every 2 weeks.
2. A lower dose of 50 mg/m^2 IV is recommended every 2 weeks for patients found to be homozygous for UGT1A1*28.

DRUG INTERACTION 1
Phenytoin and other drugs that stimulate the liver microsomal CYP3A4 enzyme, including carbamazepine, rifampin, phenobarbital, and St. John's wort—These drugs increase the rate of metabolism of irinotecan and SN-38, resulting in its inactivation.

DRUG INTERACTION 2

Drugs that inhibit the liver microsomal CYP3A4 enzymes, including ketoconazole, itraconazole, erythromycin, and clarithromycin—These drugs decrease the rate of metabolism of irinotecan and SN-38, resulting in increased drug levels and potentially increased toxicity.

DRUG INTERACTION 3

Drugs that inhibit UGT1A1, including atazanavir, gemfibrozil, and indinavir—These drugs may increase the systemic exposure to irinotecan and SN-38, resulting in increased drug levels and potentially increased toxicity.

SPECIAL CONSIDERATIONS

1. Irinotecan is an emetogenic drug. Patients should routinely receive antiemetic prophylaxis with a 5-HT3 antagonist, such as ondansetron or granisetron, in combination with dexamethasone.
2. Treatment with irinotecan is complicated by an acute cholinergic effect, which consists of diarrhea, diaphoresis, and abdominal cramping during the infusion or within 24 hours of drug administration. The recommended treatment is atropine (0.25–1.0 mg) administered IV unless clinically contraindicated. The routine use of atropine for prophylaxis is not recommended. However, atropine prophylaxis should be administered if a cholinergic event has been experienced.
3. Instruct patients about the possibility of late diarrhea (starting after 24 hours of drug administration), which can lead to serious dehydration and/or electrolyte imbalances if not managed promptly. This represents a black-box warning. This side effect is thought to be due to a direct irritation of the gastrointestinal mucosa by SN-38, although other as yet unidentified mechanisms may be involved. Loperamide should be taken immediately after the first loose bowel movement. The recommended dose is 4 mg PO as a loading dose, followed by 2 mg every 2 hours around the clock (4 mg every 4 hours during the night). Loperamide can be discontinued once the patient is diarrhea-free for 12 hours. If diarrhea should continue without improvement in the first 24 hours, an oral fluoroquinolone should be added. Hospitalization with IV antibiotics and IV hydration should be considered with continued diarrhea.
4. Irinotecan liposome should not be given to patients with bowel obstruction.
5. Patients should be warned against taking laxatives while on therapy.
6. Closely monitor CBCs on days 1 and 8 of every cycle as irinotecan liposome can cause severe life-threatening neutropenia and neutropenic sepsis. This represents a black-box warning.
7. Irinotecan liposome should be withheld for ANC < 1500/mm^3 or neutropenic fever.
8. Patients with the UGT1A1 7/7 genotype are at increased risk for developing GI toxicity and myelosuppression. Approximately 10% of the North American population is homozygous for this genotype. Dose reduction to 50 mg/m^2 is recommended in this setting.

9. Patients should be warned to be off St. John's wort for at least 2 weeks before starting irinotecan therapy and should remain off until after the completion of irinotecan therapy. St. John's wort has been shown to reduce the efficacy of irinotecan chemotherapy by inhibiting metabolism of irinotecan to the active SN-38 metabolite.
10. Pregnancy category D. Breastfeeding should be avoided.

TOXICITY 1
Myelosuppression. Dose-limiting with neutropenia being most commonly observed. Severe neutropenia occurs in 20% of patients and neutropenic fever or sepsis occurs in 3% of patients.

TOXICITY 2
Diarrhea with two different forms: early and late. Early form occurs within 24 hours of drug treatment and this is a cholinergic event. Characterized by flushing, diaphoresis, abdominal pain, and diarrhea. Late-form diarrhea occurs after 24 hours, typically at 3–10 days after treatment, can be severe and prolonged, and can lead to dehydration and electrolyte imbalance. Severe late diarrhea occurs in 13% of patients.

TOXICITY 3
Interstitial lung disease with dyspnea, cough, and fever.

TOXICITY 4
Hypersensitivity reactions.

TOXICITY 5
Fatigue, decreased appetite, and anorexia.

Ixabepilone

TRADE NAMES	Ixempra, BMS-247550	**CLASSIFICATION**	Epothilone, antimicrotubule agent
CATEGORY	Chemotherapy drug	**DRUG MANUFACTURER**	Bristol-Myers Squibb

MECHANISM OF ACTION
- Semisynthetic analog of epothilone B.
- Cell cycle–specific, active in the mitosis (M) phase of the cell cycle.
- Binds directly to β-tubulin subunits on microtubules, leading to inhibition of normal microtubule dynamics.
- Exhibits activity in drug-resistant tumors that overexpress P-glycoprotein, MRP-1, βIII tubulin isoforms, and tubulin mutations.

MECHANISM OF RESISTANCE
None well characterized to date.

ABSORPTION
Not orally bioavailable. Administered only by the IV route.

DISTRIBUTION
Distributes widely to all body tissues. Moderate binding (60%–70%) to plasma proteins.

METABOLISM
Metabolized extensively by the hepatic P450 microsomal system via oxidation by CYP3A4. About 85% of drug is excreted via fecal elimination. Less than 10% is eliminated as the parent form with the majority being eliminated as metabolites. Renal clearance is relatively minor with less than 10% of drug cleared via the kidneys. The terminal elimination half-life is on the order of 52 hours. Gender, race, and age do not impact drug pharmacokinetics.

INDICATIONS
1. FDA-approved in combination with capecitabine for metastatic or locally advanced breast cancer resistant to treatment with an anthracycline and a taxane, or in patients whose cancer is taxane-resistant and for whom further anthracycline therapy is contraindicated.
2. FDA-approved as monotherapy for metastatic or locally advanced breast cancer in patients whose tumors are resistant or refractory to anthracyclines, taxanes, and capecitabine.

DOSAGE RANGE
Recommended dose is 40 mg/m^2 IV every 3 weeks.

DRUG INTERACTION 1
Drugs such as ketoconazole, fluconazole, itraconazole, erythromycin, clarithromycin, and verapamil may decrease the rate of metabolism of

ixabepilone, resulting in increased drug levels and potentially increased toxicity.

DRUG INTERACTION 2
Drugs such as rifampin, phenytoin, phenobarbital, and carbamazepine may increase the rate of metabolism of ixabepilone, resulting in its inactivation.

DRUG INTERACTION 3
St. John's Wort may alter the metabolism of ixabepilone and should be avoided while on therapy.

DRUG INTERACTION 4
Ixabepilone does not appear to affect the metabolism of drugs that are substrates of liver CYP enzymes.

SPECIAL CONSIDERATIONS
1. Contraindicated in patients with history of severe hypersensitivity reaction to paclitaxel or to other drugs formulated in Cremophor EL.
2. Use with caution in patients with abnormal liver function. When used as monotherapy, dose reduction is required in the setting of mild-to-moderate hepatic impairment. Contraindicated when used in combination with capecitabine in patients with SGOT or SGPT >2.5×ULN or bilirubin >1×ULN.
3. Contraindicated in patients with a neutrophil count <1500 cells/mm^3 or a platelet count <100,000 cells/mm^3.
4. Use with caution in patients with prior history of diabetes mellitus and chronic alcoholism or prior therapy with known neurotoxic agents such as cisplatin.
5. Patients should receive premedication prior to treatment to prevent the incidence of hypersensitivity reactions. Give an H1-antagonist (diphenhydramine 50 mg PO) and an H2-antagonist (cimetidine 300 mg) 1 hour prior to drug administration. Patients experiencing a hypersensitivity reaction require premedication with dexamethasone 20 mg IV 30 minutes before drug treatment, along with diphenhydramine 50 mg IV and cimetidine 300 mg IV.
6. Medical personnel should be available at the time of drug administration. Emergency equipment, including Ambu bag, ECG machine, IV fluids, pressors, and other drugs for resuscitation, must be at bedside before initiation of treatment.
7. Pregnancy category D. Breastfeeding should be avoided.

TOXICITY 1
Myelosuppression with neutropenia and thrombocytopenia. Neutropenia typically occurs on days 10–14 with recovery by day 21.

TOXICITY 2
Hypersensitivity reaction characterized by generalized skin rash, flushing, erythema, hypotension, dyspnea, and/or bronchospasm. Premedication

regimen, as outlined in Special Considerations, has significantly decreased incidence.

TOXICITY 3
Neurotoxicity mainly in the form of peripheral sensory neuropathy with numbness and paresthesias. Occurs in up to 20% of patients.

TOXICITY 4
Fatigue and asthenia.

TOXICITY 5
GI toxicity in the form of nausea/vomiting, mucositis, and/or diarrhea.

TOXICITY 6
Myalgias, arthralgias, and musculoskeletal pain.

Ixazomib

TRADE NAME	Ninlaro	CLASSIFICATION	Proteasome inhibitor
CATEGORY	Chemotherapy drug	DRUG MANUFACTURER	Millennium and Takeda Oncology

MECHANISM OF ACTION:
- Ixazomib is a reversible proteasome inhibitor. It preferentially binds and inhibits the chymotrypsin-like activity of the $\beta 5$ subunit of the 20S proteasome, which then results in activation of signaling cascades, cell-cycle arrest, and apoptosis.
- Ixazomib has in vitro cytotoxicity against myeloma-derived cell lines from patients who had progressed on previous therapies, including bortezomib, lenalidomide, and dexamethasone.

- The combination of ixazomib and lenalidomide has synergistic cytotoxicity in multiple myeloma cell lines in vitro and in vivo antitumor activity in myeloma tumor xenograft models.

MECHANISM OF RESISTANCE:

None well characterized to date.

ABSORPTION:

The absolute oral bioavailability is 58%, and the median T_{max} is 1 hour. Food with a high fat content reduces AUC by 28% and C_{max} by 69%, respectively.

DISTRIBUTION:

Ixazomib is highly bound to plasma proteins (99%). The steady-state volume of distribution is 543 liters.

METABOLISM

Metabolized primarily in the liver by multiple liver microsomal CYP enzymes, with CYP3A4 being the major metabolizing enzyme. Non-CYP proteins are also involved in ixazomib metabolism. After drug administration, approximately 60% is excreted in urine with <3.5% as unchanged drug and 22% is excreted in feces. The terminal half-life is 9.5 days.

INDICATIONS

FDA-approved in combination with lenalidomide and dexamethasone for the treatment of patients with multiple myeloma who have received at least one prior therapy.

DOSAGE RANGE

Recommended dose is 4 mg PO on days 1, 8, and 15 of a 28-day cycle.
To be used in combination with lenalidomide 25 mg/day PO on days 1 through 21 and dexamethasone 40 mg PO on days 1, 8, 15, and 22.

DRUG INTERACTION 1

Phenytoin and other drugs that stimulate the liver microsomal CYP3A4 enzymes, including carbamazepine, rifampin, phenobarbital, and St. John's wort—These drugs may increase the metabolism of ixazomib, resulting in reduced effective drug levels in the blood.

SPECIAL CONSIDERATIONS:

1. Closely monitor CBCs on a periodic basis with more frequent monitoring during the first three cycles.
2. Thrombocytopenia is an especially important issue with platelet nadirs usually occurring between days 14–21 of each 28-day cycle with recovery to baseline by the start of the next cycle. Thrombocytopenia should be managed with dose modification as per the package insert as well as with platelet transfusion.
3. No dose adjustment is needed for mild hepatic dysfunction. The dose of ixazomib should be reduced to 3 mg in patients with moderate (total

bilirubin >1.5-3 × ULN) or severe (total bilirubin >3 × ULN) hepatic dysfunction.

4. No dose reduction is needed for mild or moderate renal dysfunction. The dose of ixazomib should be reduced to 3 mg in patients with severe renal dysfunction (CrCl<30 mL/min) or in those with end-stage renal disease. Ixazomib is not dialyzable, and as such, it may be administered without regard to the timing of dialysis.

5. LFTs should be closely monitored with dose adjustments for grade 3 or 4 liver toxicity.

6. Patients should be closely followed for the development of skin rash and other cutaneous reactions with dose adjustments as needed.

TOXICITY 1:
Myelosuppression with thrombocytopenia and neutropenia.

TOXICITY 2
Neurologic toxicity with peripheral neuropathy most commonly reported and rare cases of peripheral motor neuropathy.

TOXICITY 3
GI toxicity with diarrhea, constipation, nausea/vomiting.

TOXICITY 4
Dermatologic toxicity with maculopapular and macular skin rash.

TOXICITY 5
Hepatotoxicity with drug-induced liver injury, hepatic steatosis, and cholestatic hepatitis.

TOXICITY 6
Peripheral edema.

TOXICITY 7
Fatigue.

Lapatinib

TRADE NAMES	Tykerb, GW572016	CLASSIFICATION	Signal transduction inhibitor
CATEGORY	Chemotherapy drug	DRUG MANUFACTURER	GlaxoSmithKline

MECHANISM OF ACTION
- Potent small-molecule inhibitor of the tyrosine kinases associated with epidermal growth factor receptor (ErbB1; EGFR) and HER2 (ErbB2), resulting in inhibition of phosphorylation and downstream signaling.
- Inhibition of the EGFR and HER2 tyrosine kinases results in inhibition of critical mitogenic and antiapoptotic signals involved in proliferation, growth, invasion/metastasis, angiogenesis, and response to chemotherapy and/or radiation therapy.

MECHANISM OF RESISTANCE
- Mutations in the EGFR and HER2/neu growth factor receptors leading to decreased binding affinity to lapatinib.
- Increased expression of HER3.
- Increased ERα transcription and ER signaling.
- Increased expression of c-Met.
- Increased expression of RON.
- Increased expression and activation of AXL.
- Activation/induction of alternative cellular signaling pathways, such as PI3K, as a result of activating PIK3CA mutations or loss of PTEN.

ABSORPTION
Oral absorption is incomplete and variable and is increased when administered with food.

DISTRIBUTION
Extensive binding (99%) to plasma proteins, including albumin and α1-acid glycoprotein, and extensive tissue distribution. Peak plasma levels are achieved 4 hours after ingestion. Steady-state drug concentrations are reached in 6 to 7 days.

METABOLISM
Metabolism in the liver primarily by the CYP3A4 and CYP3A5 microsomal enzymes and by CYP2C19 and CYP2C8 to a lesser extent. Elimination is mainly hepatic with excretion in the feces, and renal elimination of parent drug and its metabolites accounts for less than 2% of an administered dose. The terminal half-life of the parent drug is 14 hours, and with repeat dosing, the effective half-life is 24 hours.

INDICATIONS
FDA-approved in combination with capecitabine for the treatment of patients with advanced or metastatic breast cancer whose tumors overexpress HER2 and who have received prior therapy, including an anthracycline, a taxane, and trastuzumab.

DOSAGE RANGE
Recommended dose is 1250 mg PO daily on days 1–21 continuously in combination with capecitabine 1000 mg/m^2 PO bid on days 1–14, with each cycle repeated every 21 days.

DRUG INTERACTION 1
Phenytoin and other drugs that stimulate the liver microsomal CYP3A4 enzymes, including carbamazepine, rifampin, phenobarbital, and St. John's wort. These drugs may increase the rate of metabolism of lapatinib, resulting in its inactivation.

DRUG INTERACTION 2
Drugs that inhibit the liver microsomal CYP3A4 enzymes, including ketoconazole, itraconazole, erythromycin, and clarithromycin. These drugs may decrease the rate of metabolism of lapatinib, resulting in increased drug levels and potentially increased toxicity.

DRUG INTERACTION 3
Warfarin—Patients receiving coumarin-derived anticoagulants should be closely monitored for alterations in their clotting parameters (PT and INR) and/or bleeding, as lapatinib may inhibit the metabolism of warfarin by the liver P450 system. The dose of warfarin may require careful adjustment in the presence of lapatinib therapy.

SPECIAL CONSIDERATIONS
1. Use with caution in patients with hepatic impairment, and dose reduction and/or interruption should be considered.
2. Monitor cardiac function at baseline and periodically during therapy with either MUGA or echocardiogram to assess LVEF. The majority of LVEF decreases occur within the first 9 weeks of therapy. Use with caution in patients with pre-existing conditions that could impair LVEF.

3. Monitor ECG with QT measurement at baseline and periodically during therapy, as QT prolongation has been observed. Use with caution in patients at risk of developing QT prolongation, including hypokalemia, hypomagnesemia, congenital long QT syndrome, patients taking antiarrhythmic medications or any other products that may cause QT prolongation, and cumulative high-dose anthracycline therapy.
4. Lapatinib should be taken 1 hour before or after a meal, and the daily dose should not be divided. When capecitabine is co-administered, capecitabine should be taken with a glass of water within 30 minutes after a meal.
5. Avoid Seville oranges, starfruit, pomelos, and grapefruit products while on therapy.
6. Closely monitor patients for diarrhea, as severe diarrhea may develop while on therapy. Aggressive management with antidiarrheal agents as well as replacement of fluids. Electrolyte status should be closely followed.
7. Pregnancy category D. Breastfeeding should be avoided.

TOXICITY 1
Diarrhea is the most common dose-limiting toxicity and occurs in 65% of patients. Mild nausea/vomiting may also occur.

TOXICITY 2
Cardiac toxicity with reduction in LVEF. QT prolongation observed rarely.

TOXICITY 3
Myelosuppression with anemia more common than thrombocytopenia or neutropenia.

TOXICITY 4
Fatigue and anorexia.

TOXICITY 5
Mild-to-moderate elevation of serum transaminases and serum bilirubin.

TOXICITY 6
Hand-foot syndrome (palmar-plantar erythrodysesthesia) and skin rash.

Lenalidomide

TRADE NAMES	Revlimid, CC-5013	CLASSIFICATION	Immunomodulatory analog of thalidomide, antiangiogenic agent
CATEGORY	Unclassified therapeutic agent, biologic response modifier agent	DRUG MANUFACTURER	Celgene

MECHANISM OF ACTION

- Mechanism of action is not fully characterized.
- Immunomodulatory drug that stimulates T-cell proliferation as well as IL-2 and IFN-γ production.
- Inhibition of TNF-α and IL-6 synthesis and downmodulation of cell surface adhesion molecules similar to thalidomide.
- May exert antiangiogenic effect by inhibition of basic fibroblast growth factor (bFGF) and vascular endothelial growth factor (VEGF) through as yet undefined mechanisms.
- Overcomes cellular drug resistance to thalidomide.

MECHANISM OF RESISTANCE

None characterized to date.

ABSORPTION

Lenalidomide is rapidly absorbed following oral administration with peak plasma concentrations at 60–90 minutes post ingestion. Co-administration with food does not alter the extent of absorption (AUC) but does reduce maximal plasma concentration (C_{max}) by 36%.

DISTRIBUTION

Not well characterized.

METABOLISM

Lenalidomide does not appear to be metabolized or induced by the cytochrome P450 pathway. Approximately 66% of an administered dose is excreted unchanged in the urine. The elimination half-life of the drug is approximately 3 hours.

INDICATIONS

1. FDA-approved for the treatment of low- or intermediate-1-risk myelodysplastic syndromes (MDS) associated with the deletion 5q (del 5q) cytogenetic abnormality with or without additional cytogenetic abnormalities.
2. FDA-approved for the treatment of multiple myeloma in combination with dexamethasone for patients who have received at least one prior therapy.
3. FDA-approved for the treatment of mantle cell lymphoma in patients whose disease has relapsed or progressed after two prior therapies, one of which included bortezomib.

DOSAGE RANGE
1. Myelodysplastic syndrome: 10 mg PO daily.
2. Multiple myeloma: 25 mg PO daily on days 1–21 and 40 mg dexamethasone PO on days 1–4, 9–12, and 17–20 of a 28-day cycle. An alternative regimen is to use 40 mg dexamethasone PO on days 1, 8, 15, and 22 of a 28-day cycle.
3. Mantle cell lymphoma: 25 mg PO daily on days 1–21 of a 28-day cycle.

DRUG INTERACTIONS
None well characterized to date.

SPECIAL CONSIDERATIONS
1. Pregnancy category X. Lenalidomide is a thalidomide analog, a known human teratogen that causes severe or life-threatening birth defects. As such, women who are pregnant or who wish to become pregnant should not take lenalidomide. Severe fetal malformations can occur if even one capsule is taken by a pregnant woman. All women should have a baseline β-human chorionic gonadotropin (β-HCG) before starting lenalidomide therapy. Women of reproductive age must have two negative pregnancy tests before starting therapy: one should be 10 to 14 days before therapy is begun, and the second should be 24 hours before therapy.
2. All women of childbearing potential should practice two forms of birth control throughout therapy with lenalidomide: one highly effective form (intrauterine device, hormonal contraception [patch, implant, pill, injection], partner's vasectomy, or tubal ligation) and one additional barrier method (latex condom, diaphragm, or cervical cap). It is strongly recommended that these precautionary measures be taken 1 month before initiation of therapy, continued while on therapy, and continued at least 1 month after therapy is discontinued.
3. Lenalidomide is only available under a special restricted distribution program called "RevAssist®." Only prescribers and pharmacists registered with the RevAssist® program are able to prescribe and dispense the drug. Lenalidomide should only be dispensed to those patients who are registered and meet all the conditions of the RevAssist® program.
4. Breastfeeding while on therapy should be avoided, as it remains unknown if lenalidomide is excreted in breast milk.
5. Men taking lenalidomide must use latex condoms for every sexual encounter with a woman of childbearing potential, as the drug may be present in semen.
6. Patients taking lenalidomide should not donate blood or semen while receiving treatment, and for at least 1 month after stopping this drug.
7. Monitor complete blood counts while on therapy as lenalidomide has hematologic toxicity, especially in patients with del 5q MDS.
8. Use with caution in patients with impaired renal function, as the risk of toxicity may be greater.
9. There is a significantly increased risk of thromboembolic complications, including deep venous thrombosis (DVT) and pulmonary embolism

(PE), especially in myeloma patients treated with lenalidomide and dexamethasone. Prophylaxis with low-molecular weight heparin or aspirin (325 mg PO qd) can help prevent and/or reduce this risk.

TOXICITY 1
Potentially severe or fatal teratogenic effects.

TOXICITY 2
Myelosuppression with neutropenia and thrombocytopenia that is usually reversible.

TOXICITY 3
Increased risk of thromboembolic complications, such as DVT and PE.

TOXICITY 4
Nausea/vomiting, diarrhea, and constipation are most common GI side effects.

TOXICITY 5
Neurotoxic side effects are rare with almost no sedation.

TOXICITY 6
Increased risk for second primary tumors, including acute myeloid leukemia, solid tumors, and myelodysplastic syndrome.

Lenvatinib

TRADE NAMES	Lenvima, E7080	**CLASSIFICATION**	Signal transduction inhibitor
CATEGORY	Chemotherapy drug	**DRUG MANUFACTURER**	Eisai

MECHANISM OF ACTION
- Small-molecule, multitargeted receptor tyrosine kinase inhibitor (TKI) that inhibits the kinase activities of vascular endothelial growth factor receptor 1 (VEGFR-1), VEGFR-2, and VEGFR-3.

- Inhibits other tyrosine kinase inhibitors, including fibroblast growth factor receptor 1 (FGFR-1), FGFR-2, FGFR-3, FGFR-4, platelet-derived growth factor receptor-α (PDGFR-α), Kit, and RET, which are involved in tumor angiogenesis, tumor growth, and cancer progression.

MECHANISM OF RESISTANCE

- Increased expression of the target receptor tyrosine kinases (RTKs), such as VEGFR.
- Alterations in binding affinity of the drug to the RTKs resulting from mutations in the tyrosine kinase domain.
- Activation of the hepatocyte growth factor pathway through its cognate receptor c-Met.
- Activation/induction of alternative cellular signaling pathways, such as IGF-1R.

ABSORPTION

Oral absorption is relatively fast with peak plasma concentrations achieved within 1 to 4 hours after ingestion. Food does not affect the extent of absorption but decreases the rate of absorption and delays the median T_{max} from 2 to 4 hours.

DISTRIBUTION

Extensive binding of lenvatinib to human plasma proteins (98% to 99%).

METABOLISM

Metabolized to a large extent by the liver CYP3A enzymes and aldehyde oxidase as well as by non-enzymatic processes. Approximately 64% and 25% of drug is eliminated in feces and urine, respectively. The terminal elimination half-life of lenvatinib is approximately 28 hours.

INDICATIONS

1. FDA-approved for the treatment of locally recurrent or metastatic, progressive, radioactive iodine-refractory differentiated thyroid cancer.
2. FDA-approved in combination with everolimus for the treatment of advanced renal cell cancer following one prior anti-angiogenic therapy.

DOSAGE RANGE

1. Thyroid cancer: Recommended dose is 24 mg PO once daily with or without food.
2. Renal cell cancer: Recommended dose is 18 mg of lenvatinib PO once daily in combination with everolimus 5 mg PO once daily.

DRUG INTERACTION 1

Drugs that stimulate liver microsomal CYP3A4 enzymes, including phenytoin, carbamazepine, rifampin, phenobarbital, and St. John's Wort—These drugs may increase the metabolism of lenvatinib, resulting in lower drug levels and potentially reduced clinical activity.

DRUG INTERACTION 2

Drugs that inhibit liver microsomal CYP3A4 enzymes, including ketoconazole, itraconazole, erythromycin, and clarithromycin—These drugs may reduce the metabolism of lenvatinib, resulting in increased drug levels and potentially increased toxicity.

SPECIAL CONSIDERATIONS

1. Dose modification is not required in patients with mild and moderate hepatic impairment. However, dose reduction is recommended in the setting of severe hepatic impairment (Child-Pugh C), and the recommended dose is 14 mg PO daily for thyroid cancer and 10 mg PO daily for renal cell cancer.
2. Dose modification is not required in patients with mild and moderate renal impairment. However, dose reduction is recommended in the setting of severe renal impairment (CrCl< 30 mL/min), and the recommended dose is 14 mg PO daily for thyroid cancer and 10 mg PO daily for renal cancer.
3. Closely monitor blood pressure while on therapy and treat as needed with standard oral antihypertensive medication. Should be discontinued in patients who develop hypertensive crisis.
4. Baseline and periodic evaluation of LVEF should be performed while on lenvatinib therapy. Lenvatinib should be withheld if grade 3 cardiac dysfunction occurs, until improved to grade 0 or 1 or baseline. Either resume at a reduced dose or discontinue depending on the severity and persistence of cardiac dysfunction. Lenvatinib should be discontinued for grade 4 cardiac dysfunction.
5. Patients should be warned of the risk of arterial thromboembolic events, and the drug should be discontinued following an arterial thrombotic event.
6. Monitor liver function tests prior to initiation of therapy and every 2 weeks thereafter for the first 2 months, and then at least monthly during treatment. Lenvatinib should be withheld for the development of grade 3 or greater liver impairment until resolved to grade 0 to 1 or baseline. Lenvatinib should be discontinued in the setting of liver failure.
7. Monitor renal function while on therapy as renal impairment has been observed in up to 14% of patients treated with lenvatinib therapy.
8. Monitor urine for protein at baseline and periodically throughout treatment. If urine dipstick proteinuria is greater than or equal to 2+, a 24-hour urine collection for protein needs to be obtained. Lenvatinib should be withheld for ⩾2 g of proteinuria/24 hours and resumed at a reduced dose when proteinuria is < 2 g/24 hours. Lenvatinib should be terminated in patients who develop the nephrotic syndrome.
9. Monitor ECG with QTc measurement at baseline and periodically during therapy as QTc prolongation has been observed in nearly 10% of patients. Use with caution in patients at increased risk of developing QT prolongation, including hypokalemia, hypomagnesemia, congenital QT syndrome, and in patients on antiarrhythmic medications or any other products that may cause QT prolongation.
10. Lenvatinib treatment can result in RPLS, as manifested by headache, seizure, lethargy, confusion, blindness and other visual side effects, as

well as other neurologic disturbances. Magnetic resonance imaging is helpful in confirming the diagnosis. Once confirmed by MRI, the drug should be withheld until RPLS is fully resolved. Upon resolution, resume at a reduced dose or discontinue depending on the severity and persistence of neurologic symptoms.

11. Monitor electrolyte status and especially serum calcium levels on at least a monthly basis.
12. Monitor TSH levels on a monthly basis, and adjust thyroid replacement medication as needed.
13. Pregnancy category D.

TOXICITY 1
Hypertension.

TOXICITY 2
Nausea/vomiting, anorexia, diarrhea, and mucositis.

TOXICITY 3
Mild to moderate bleeding complications with epistaxis being most commonly observed.

TOXICITY 4
Increased risk of arterial thromboembolic events, including MI, angina, stroke, and transient ischemic attack (TIA).

TOXICITY 5
Hepatotoxicity.

TOXICITY 6
Impairment of renal function and proteinuria.

TOXICITY 7
Cardiac toxicity in the form of cardiac dysfunction and/or cardiac failure. QTc prolongation may also occur.

TOXICITY 8
Hypocalcemia.

TOXICITY 9
GI perforation, fistula formation, and wound-healing complications.

TOXICITY 10
Impairment of thyroid stimulating hormone suppression.

TOXICITY 11
RPLS with seizures, headache, visual disturbances, confusion, or altered mental function.

Letrozole

TRADE NAME	Femara	CLASSIFICATION	Aromatase inhibitor
CATEGORY	Hormonal agent	DRUG MANUFACTURER	Novartis

MECHANISM OF ACTION
- Nonsteroidal, competitive inhibitor of aromatase. Nearly 200-fold more potent than aminoglutethimide.
- Inhibits synthesis of estrogens by inhibiting the conversion of adrenal androgens (androstenedione and testosterone) to estrogens (estrone, estrone sulfate, and estradiol). Serum estradiol levels are suppressed by 90% within 14 days, and nearly completely suppressed after 6 weeks of therapy.
- No inhibitory effect on adrenal corticosteroid biosynthesis.

MECHANISM OF RESISTANCE
- Decreased expression of ER.
- Mutations in the ER leading to decreased binding affinity to letrozole.
- Overexpression of growth factor receptors, such as EGFR, HER2/ neu, IGF-1R, or TGF-β that counteract the inhibitory effects of letrozole.
- Presence of ESR1 mutations.

ABSORPTION
Rapidly and completely absorbed after oral administration. Food does not interfere with oral absorption.

DISTRIBUTION
Significant uptake in peripheral tissues and in breast cancer cells.

METABOLISM
Metabolism occurs in the liver by the cytochrome P450 system. Process of glucuronidation leads to inactive metabolites. Parent drug and metabolites are excreted via the kidneys with over 75%–90% cleared in urine.

INDICATIONS
1. First-line treatment of postmenopausal women with hormone-receptor positive or hormone-receptor unknown locally advanced or metastatic breast cancer.

2. Second-line treatment of postmenopausal women with advanced breast cancer after progression on antiestrogen therapy.
3. Adjuvant treatment of postmenopausal women with hormone-receptor positive early-stage breast cancer.
4. Extended adjuvant treatment of early-stage breast cancer in postmenopausal women who have received 5 years of adjuvant tamoxifen therapy.

DOSAGE RANGE
1. Metastatic disease: 2.5 mg PO qd until disease progression.
2. Adjuvant setting: 2.5 mg PO qd until disease relapse.

DRUG INTERACTION 1
Phenytoin and other drugs that stimulate the liver microsomal CYP3A4 enzymes, including carbamazepine, rifampin, phenobarbital, and St. John's Wort. These drugs may increase the rate of metabolism of letrozole, resulting in its inactivation.

DRUG INTERACTION 2
Drugs that inhibit the liver microsomal CYP3A4 enzymes, including ketoconazole, itraconazole, erythromycin, and clarithromycin. These drugs may decrease the rate of metabolism of letrozole, resulting in increased drug levels and potentially increased toxicity.

DRUG INTERACTION 3
Warfarin—Patients receiving coumarin-derived anticoagulants should be closely monitored for alterations in their clotting parameters (PT and INR) and/or bleeding, as letrozole may inhibit the metabolism of warfarin by the liver P450 system. The dose of warfarin may require careful adjustment in the presence of letrozole therapy.

DRUG INTERACTION 4
Clopidogrel (Plavix)—Letrozole therapy may reduce the clinical efficacy of clopidrogel, as it is an inhibitor of CYP2C19, which is required for activation of clopidrogel.

SPECIAL CONSIDERATIONS
1. Letrozole is indicated only for postmenopausal women. Efficacy in premenopausal women has not been established, and there may be an increased risk of benign ovarian tumors and cystic ovarian disease in this population.
2. Use with caution in patients with abnormal liver function. Monitor liver function at baseline and periodically during therapy. The dose should be reduced by 50% in patients with cirrhosis and severe hepatic dysfunction. In this setting, the recommended dose is 2.5 mg PO every other day.
3. No need for glucocorticoid and/or mineralocorticoid replacement.
4. Closely monitor women with osteoporosis or at risk of osteoporosis by performing bone densitometry at the start of therapy and at regular

intervals. Treatment or prophylaxis for osteoporosis should be initiated when appropriate.

5. Letrozole can be taken with or without food.
6. Pregnancy category D. Breastfeeding should be avoided.

TOXICITY 1
Mild musculoskeletal pains and arthralgias are the most common adverse events.

TOXICITY 2
Headache and fatigue.

TOXICITY 3
Mild nausea with less frequent vomiting and anorexia. Thromboembolic events are rare, and less common than with megestrol acetate.

TOXICITY 4
Hot flashes occur in less than 10% of patients.

TOXICITY 5
Mild elevation in serum transaminases and serum bilirubin. Most often seen in patients with established metastatic disease in the liver.

TOXICITY 6
Thromboembolic events are rarely observed.

Leuprolide

TRADE NAME	Lupron	**CLASSIFICATION**	LHRH agonist
CATEGORY	Hormonal agent	**DRUG MANUFACTURER**	TAP Pharmaceuticals

MECHANISM OF ACTION
Administration of this LHRH agonist leads to initial release of FSH and LH followed by suppression of gonadotropin secretion as a result of desensitization of the pituitary to gonadotropin-releasing hormone. This eventually leads to decreased secretion of LH and FSH from the pituitary, resulting in castration levels of testosterone. Plasma levels of testosterone fall to castrate levels after 2–4 weeks of therapy.

ABSORPTION
Leuprolide is not orally absorbed. After SC injection, approximately 90% of a dose is absorbed into the systemic circulation.

DISTRIBUTION

Distribution is not well characterized. Leuprolide is slowly released over a 28-day period. Peak serum concentrations are achieved 10–15 days after drug administration. About 45%–50% of drug is bound to plasma proteins.

METABOLISM

Metabolism of leuprolide occurs mainly via hydrolysis of the C-terminal amino acids. Leuprolide is nearly completely eliminated in its parent form in urine (>90%) with an elimination half-life of 3–4 hours. Half-life is prolonged in patients with impaired renal function.

INDICATIONS

1. Advanced prostate cancer.
2. Neoadjuvant therapy of early-stage prostate cancer.

DOSAGE RANGE

Administer 22.5 mg SC every 3 months. Can also be given as 30 mg SC every 4 months.

DRUG INTERACTIONS

None known.

SPECIAL CONSIDERATIONS

1. Initiation of treatment with leuprolide may induce a transient tumor flare due to the initial release of LH and FSH. Patients with impending ureteral obstruction and/or spinal cord compression or those with painful bone metastases are at especially high risk. To prevent tumor flare, patients should be started on antiandrogen therapy at least 2 weeks before starting leuprolide.
2. Serum testosterone levels decrease to castrate levels within 2–4 weeks after initiation of therapy.
3. Use with caution in patients with abnormal renal function.
4. Caution patients about the possibility of hot flashes. Consider the use of clonidine 0.1–0.2 mg PO daily, megestrol acetate 20 mg PO bid, or soy tablets 1 tablet PO tid for prevention and/or treatment.

TOXICITY 1

Hot flashes, impotence, and gynecomastia. Decreased libido occurs less commonly.

TOXICITY 2

Tumor flare. May occur in up to 20% of patients, usually within the first 2 weeks of starting therapy. May observe increased bone pain, urinary retention, or back pain with spinal cord compression. May be prevented by pretreating with an antiandrogen agent such as flutamide, bicalutamide, or nilutamide.

TOXICITY 3

Local discomfort at the site of injection.

TOXICITY 4
Elevated serum cholesterol levels.

TOXICITY 5
Nausea and vomiting. Rarely observed.

TOXICITY 6
Hypersensitivity reaction.

TOXICITY 7
Myelosuppression. Rarely observed.

TOXICITY 8
Peripheral edema. Results from sodium retention.

TOXICITY 9
Asthenia.

Lomustine

TRADE NAME	CCNU	CLASSIFICATION	Alkylating agent
CATEGORY	Chemotherapy drug	DRUG MANUFACTURER	Bristol-Myers Squibb

MECHANISM OF ACTION
- Cell cycle–nonspecific nitrosourea analog.
- Alkylation and carbamoylation by lomustine metabolites interfere with the synthesis and function of DNA, RNA, and proteins.
- Antitumor activity appears to correlate best with formation of intrastrand cross-linking of DNA.

MECHANISM OF RESISTANCE
- Decreased cellular uptake of drug.
- Increased intracellular thiol content due to glutathione and/or glutathione-related enzymes.
- Enhanced activity of DNA repair enzymes.

ABSORPTION
Readily and completely absorbed orally. Peak plasma concentrations are observed within 3 hours after oral administration.

DISTRIBUTION
Lipid-soluble drug with broad tissue distribution. Well-absorbed after oral administration and crosses the blood-brain barrier. CNS levels approach 15%–30% of plasma levels.

METABOLISM
Metabolized by the liver microsomal P450 system to active metabolites. The elimination half-life of the drug is about 72 hours, and excretion mainly occurs via the kidneys. Approximately 50% of a dose is excreted in urine within the first 12–24 hours, while 60% of a dose is excreted after 48 hours.

INDICATIONS
1. Brain tumors—Early-stage or metastatic.
2. Hodgkin's lymphoma.
3. Non-Hodgkin's lymphoma.

DOSAGE RANGE
Recommended dose as a single agent in previously untreated patients is 130 mg/m^2 PO every 6 weeks. In patients with compromised bone marrow function, the dose should be reduced to 100 mg/m^2 PO every 6 weeks.

DRUG INTERACTION 1
Cimetidine—Cimetidine enhances the toxicity of lomustine.

DRUG INTERACTION 2
Alcohol—Ingestion of alcohol should be avoided for at least 1 hour before and after administration of lomustine.

SPECIAL CONSIDERATIONS
1. Monitor CBC while on therapy. Subsequent cycles should not be given before 6 weeks, given the delayed and potentially cumulative effects of the drug. Platelet and leukocyte counts must return to normal before starting the next course of therapy.
2. PFTs should be obtained at baseline and monitored periodically during therapy. There is an increased risk of pulmonary toxicity in patients with a prior history of lung disease and a baseline FVC or DLCO below 70% of predicted.
3. Administer drug on an empty stomach as food may inhibit absorption.
4. Pregnancy category D. Breastfeeding should be avoided.

TOXICITY 1
Myelosuppression is dose-limiting. In contrast to most other anticancer agents, myelosuppression involving all elements is delayed and cumulative. Nadirs typically occur 4–6 weeks after therapy and may persist for 1–3 weeks.

TOXICITY 2

Nausea and vomiting may occur within 2–6 hours after a dose of drug and can last for up to 24 hours.

TOXICITY 3

Anorexia may be present but short-lived. Mucositis is unusual.

TOXICITY 4

Impotence, male sterility, amenorrhea, ovarian suppression, menopause, and infertility. Gynecomastia is occasionally observed.

TOXICITY 5

Pulmonary toxicity is uncommon at doses lower than 1100 mg/m^2.

TOXICITY 6

ILD and pulmonary fibrosis in the form of an insidious cough, dyspnea, pulmonary infiltrates, and/or respiratory failure may be observed.

TOXICITY 7

Renal toxicity is uncommon at total cumulative doses of lower than 1000 mg/m^2. Usually manifested by progressive azotemia and decrease in kidney size, which can progress to renal failure.

TOXICITY 8

Neurotoxicity in the form of confusion, lethargy, dysarthria, and ataxia.

TOXICITY 9

Increased risk of secondary malignancies with long-term use, especially acute myelogenous leukemia and myelodysplasia.

TOXICITY 10

Alopecia is rarely seen.

Mechlorethamine

$$CICH_2CH_2 - \overset{\overset{\displaystyle CH_3}{\underset{\displaystyle |}{|}}}{\underset{\overset{\displaystyle |}{\displaystyle H}}{\overset{\oplus}{N}}} - CH_2CH_2CI$$

TRADE NAMES	Mustargen, Nitrogen mustard	CLASSIFICATION	Alkylating agent
CATEGORY	Chemotherapy drug	DRUG MANUFACTURER	Merck

MECHANISM OF ACTION
- Analog of mustard gas.
- Classic alkylating agent that forms interstrand and intrastrand crosslinks with DNA resulting in inhibition of DNA synthesis and function.
- Cell cycle–nonspecific with activity in all phases of the cell cycle.

MECHANISM OF RESISTANCE
- Decreased cellular uptake of drug.
- Increased inactivation of cytotoxic species through increased expression of sulfhydryl proteins, including glutathione and glutathione-associated enzymes.
- Enhanced activity of DNA repair enzymes.

ABSORPTION
Not orally bioavailable.

DISTRIBUTION
Distribution of drug is not well characterized.

METABOLISM
Undergoes rapid hydrolysis in plasma to reactive metabolites. Extremely short plasma half-life on the order of 15–20 minutes. No significant organ metabolism. Greater than 50% of inactive drug metabolites are excreted in urine within 24 hours.

INDICATIONS
1. Hodgkin's lymphoma.
2. Non-Hodgkin's lymphoma.
3. Cutaneous T-cell lymphoma (topical use).
4. Intrapleural, intrapericardial, and intraperitoneal treatment of metastatic disease resulting in pleural effusion.

DOSAGE RANGE

1. Hodgkin's lymphoma: Administer 6 mg/m^2 IV on days 1 and 8 every 28 days, as part of the MOPP regimen.
2. Cutaneous T-cell lymphoma: Dilute 10 mg in 60 mL sterile water and apply topically to skin lesions.
3. Intracavitary use: Administer 0.2–0.4 mg/kg into the pleural and/or peritoneal cavity.

DRUG INTERACTIONS

Sodium thiosulfate—Sodium thiosulfate inactivates the activity of mechlorethamine.

SPECIAL CONSIDERATIONS

1. Mechlorethamine is a potent vesicant, and caution should be exercised in preparing and administering the drug.
2. Administer drug into either a new IV site or one that is less than 24 hours old to decrease the risk of extravasation.
3. In the event of drug extravasation, inflammation and necrosis may be prevented by the immediate instillation of 2.6% sodium thiosulfate solution into the area to neutralize the active drug. Elevate arm and apply ice packs for 6–12 hours. May need to consult a plastic surgeon for further evaluation.
4. Pregnancy category D. Breastfeeding should be avoided.

TOXICITY 1

Myelosuppression is dose-limiting with leukopenia and thrombocytopenia. Nadirs occur at day 7–10 and recover by day 21.

TOXICITY 2

Nausea and vomiting. Usually occur within the first 3 hours after drug administration, lasting for 4–8 hours and up to 24 hours, and often severe. Can be dose-limiting in some patients.

TOXICITY 3

Potent vesicant. Pain, inflammation, erythema, induration, and necrosis can be observed at the injection site.

TOXICITY 4

Alopecia.

TOXICITY 5

Amenorrhea and azoospermia.

TOXICITY 6

Hyperuricemia.

TOXICITY 7

CNS toxicities, including weakness, sleepiness, and headache, are rare.

TOXICITY 8
Hypersensitivity reactions. Rarely observed.

TOXICITY 9
Increased risk of secondary malignancies, including acute myelogenous leukemia with IV administration and basal cell and squamous cell cancers of the skin with topical application.

Megestrol acetate

TRADE NAME	Megace	CLASSIFICATION	Progestational agent
CATEGORY	Hormonal agent	DRUG MANUFACTURER	Bristol-Myers Squibb

MECHANISM OF ACTION
- Synthetic derivative of the naturally occurring steroid hormone progesterone.
- Possesses antiestrogenic effects. Induces the activity of 17-hydroxysteroid dehydrogenase, which then oxidizes estradiol to the less-active metabolite estrone. Also activates estrogen sulfatransferase, which metabolizes estrogen to less potent metabolites.
- Inhibits release of luteinizing hormone receptors, resulting in a decrease in estrogen levels.
- Inhibits stability, availability, and turnover of estrogen receptors.

MECHANISM OF RESISTANCE
None known.

ABSORPTION
Rapidly and completely absorbed after an oral dose. Peak plasma concentration is reached within 1–3 hours after oral administration.

DISTRIBUTION
Large fraction of megestrol is distributed into body fat.

METABOLISM

About 70% of drug is metabolized in the liver to inactive steroid metabolites. The drug is primarily eliminated in urine in the form of parent drug and metabolites, and 60%–80% of the drug is renally excreted within 10 days after administration. Elimination half-life is quite variable and ranges from 15 to 105 hours with a mean of 34 hours.

INDICATIONS

1. Breast cancer.
2. Endometrial cancer.
3. Renal cell cancer.
4. Appetite stimulant in cancer and HIV patients.

DOSAGE RANGE

1. Breast cancer: 40 mg PO qid.
2. Endometrial cancer: 40 mg PO qid.
3. Appetite stimulant: 80–200 mg PO qid.

DRUG INTERACTIONS

Aminoglutethimide—Aminoglutethimide enhances the hepatic metabolism of megestrol, resulting in decreased serum levels.

SPECIAL CONSIDERATIONS

1. Use with caution in patients with either a history of thromboembolic or hypercoagulable disorders, as megestrol acetate has been associated with an increased incidence of thromboembolic events.
2. Use with caution in patients with diabetes mellitus, as megestrol may exacerbate this condition.
3. Use with caution in patients with abnormal liver function. Dose reduction is recommended in this setting.
4. Caution patients on the risk of weight gain and fluid retention. Patients should be advised to go on a low-salt diet.
5. Pregnancy category D. Breastfeeding should be avoided.

TOXICITY 1

Weight gain results from a combination of fluid retention and increased appetite.

TOXICITY 2

Thromboembolic events are rarely observed.

TOXICITY 3

Nausea and vomiting.

TOXICITY 4

Breakthrough menstrual bleeding.

TOXICITY 5

Tumor flare.

TOXICITY 6
Hyperglycemia.

TOXICITY 7
Hot flashes, sweating, and mood changes.

Melphalan

TRADE NAMES	Alkeran, Phenylalanine mustard, L-PAM	CLASSIFICATION	Alkylating agent
CATEGORY	Chemotherapy drug	DRUG MANUFACTURER	GlaxoSmithKline

MECHANISM OF ACTION
- Analog of nitrogen mustard.
- Classic bifunctional alkylating agent that forms interstrand and intrastrand cross-links with DNA, resulting in inhibition of DNA synthesis and function.
- Cell cycle–nonspecific as it acts at all stages of the cell cycle.

MECHANISM OF RESISTANCE
- Decreased cellular uptake of drug.
- Increased inactivation of cytotoxic species through increased expression of sulfhydryl proteins, including glutathione and glutathione-associated enzymes.
- Enhanced activity of DNA repair enzymes.

ABSORPTION
Oral absorption is poor and incomplete. Oral bioavailability ranges between 25% and 90% with a mean of 60%, and oral absorption is decreased when taken with food.

DISTRIBUTION
Widely distributed in all tissues. Approximately 80%–90% of drug is bound to plasma proteins.

METABOLISM
Undergoes rapid hydrolysis in plasma to reactive metabolites. Short plasma half-life on the order of 60–90 minutes. No significant organ metabolism. About 25%–30% of drug is excreted in urine within 24 hours after administration, with the majority of the drug being excreted in feces (up to 50%) over 6 days.

INDICATIONS
1. Multiple myeloma.
2. Breast cancer.
3. Ovarian cancer.
4. High-dose chemotherapy and transplant setting.
5. Polycythemia vera.

DOSAGE RANGE
1. Multiple myeloma: 9 mg/m^2 IV on days 1–4 every 4 weeks as part of the melphalan-prednisone regimen.
2. Transplant setting: 140 mg/m^2 as a single agent in bone marrow/stem cell transplant setting.

DRUG INTERACTION 1
Cimetidine—Cimetidine decreases the oral bioavailability of melphalan by up to 30%.

DRUG INTERACTION 2
Steroids—Steroids enhance the antitumor effects of melphalan.

DRUG INTERACTION 3
Cyclosporine—Cyclosporine enhances the risk of renal toxicity secondary to melphalan.

SPECIAL CONSIDERATIONS
1. Use with caution in patients with abnormal renal function. Although the drug has been used in high doses in the transplant setting in the face of renal dysfunction without increased toxicity, dose reduction should be considered in the setting of renal dysfunction.
2. When administered orally, drug should be taken on an empty stomach to maximize absorption.
3. IV administration may cause hypersensitivity reaction.
4. Monitor complete blood cell count as melphalan therapy is associated with delayed and prolonged nadir.
5. Monitor injection site for erythema, pain, and/or burning.
6. Pregnancy category D. Breastfeeding should be avoided.

TOXICITY 1

Myelosuppression is dose-limiting with leukopenia and thrombocytopenia equally affected. Effect may be prolonged and cumulative with a nadir 4–6 weeks after therapy.

TOXICITY 2

Nausea and vomiting, mucositis, and diarrhea. Generally mild with conventional doses, but severe with high-dose therapy.

TOXICITY 3

Hypersensitivity reactions are rare with oral form. Observed in about 10% of patients treated with IV form of drug, and manifested as diaphoresis, urticaria, skin rashes, bronchospasm, dyspnea, tachycardia, and hypotension.

TOXICITY 4

Alopecia is uncommon.

TOXICITY 5

Skin ulcerations and other skin reactions at the injection site are uncommon.

TOXICITY 6

Increased risk of secondary malignancies including acute myelogenous leukemia and myelodysplasia with prolonged use. Mutagenic and teratogenic.

Mercaptopurine

TRADE NAMES	6-MP, Purinethol	CLASSIFICATION	Antimetabolite
CATEGORY	Chemotherapy drug	DRUG MANUFACTURER	GlaxoSmithKline

MECHANISM OF ACTION
- Cell cycle–specific purine analog with activity in the S-phase.
- Parent drug is inactive. Requires intracellular phosphorylation by the enzyme hypoxanthine-guanine phosphoribosyltransferase (HGPRT) to the cytotoxic monophosphate form, which is then metabolized to the eventual triphosphate metabolite.
- Inhibits de novo purine synthesis by inhibiting 5-phosphoribosyl-1 pyrophosphate (PRPP) amidotransferase.
- Incorporation of thiopurine triphosphate nucleotides into DNA, resulting in inhibition of DNA synthesis and function.
- Incorporation of thiopurine triphosphate nucleotides into RNA, resulting in alterations in RNA processing and/or mRNA translation.

MECHANISM OF RESISTANCE
- Decreased expression of the activating enzyme HGPRT.
- Increased expression of the catabolic enzyme alkaline phosphatase or the conjugating enzyme thiopurine methyltransferase (TPMT).
- Decreased transmembrane transport of drug.
- Decreased expression of mismatch repair enzymes (e.g., hMLH1, hMSH2).
- Cross-resistance observed between mercaptopurine and thioguanine.

ABSORPTION
Oral absorption is erratic and incomplete. Only 50% of an oral dose is absorbed. A new oral suspension has been recently approved by the FDA as it has greater oral bioavailability than tablets.

DISTRIBUTION
Widely distributed in total body water. Does not cross the blood-brain barrier. About 20%–30% of drug is bound to plasma proteins.

METABOLISM
Metabolized in the liver by methylation to inactive metabolites and via oxidation by xanthine oxidase to inactive metabolites. About 50% of parent drug and metabolites are eliminated in urine within the first 24 hours. Plasma half-life after oral administration is 1.5 hours in contrast to the plasma half-life after IV administration, which ranges between 20 and 50 minutes.

INDICATIONS
Acute lymphoblastic leukemia.

DOSAGE RANGE
1. Induction therapy: 2.5 mg/kg PO daily.
2. Maintenance therapy: 1.5–2.5 mg/kg PO daily.

DRUG INTERACTION 1
Warfarin—Anticoagulant effects of warfarin are inhibited by 6-MP through an unknown mechanism. Monitor coagulation parameters (PT/ INR), and adjust dose accordingly.

DRUG INTERACTION 2
Allopurinol—Allopurinol inhibits xanthine oxidase and the catabolic breakdown of 6-MP, resulting in enhanced toxicity. Dose of mercaptopurine must be reduced by 50%–75% when given concurrently with allopurinol.

DRUG INTERACTION 3
Trimethoprim/sulfamethoxazole (Bactrim DS) may enhance the myelosuppressive effects of 6-MP when given concurrently.

SPECIAL CONSIDERATIONS
1. Dose reduction of 50%–75% is required when 6-MP is given concurrently with allopurinol. This is because allopurinol inhibits the catabolic breakdown of 6-MP by xanthine oxidase.
2. Use with caution in patients with abnormal liver and/or renal function. Dose reduction should be considered in this setting.
3. Use with caution in the presence of other hepatotoxic drugs as risk of 6-MP-associated hepatic toxicity is increased.
4. Patients with a deficiency in the metabolizing enzyme thiopurine methyltransferase (TPMT) are at increased risk for developing severe toxicities with myelosuppression and GI toxicity. This enzyme deficiency is a pharmacogenetic syndrome.
5. Administer on an empty stomach to facilitate oral absorption. Advise patient to take 6-MP at bedtime.
6. Pregnancy category D. Breastfeeding should be avoided.

TOXICITY 1
Myelosuppression. Mild to moderate with leukopenia more common than thrombocytopenia. Leukopenia nadir at days 10–14 with recovery by day 21.

TOXICITY 2
Mucositis and/or diarrhea. Usually seen with higher doses.

TOXICITY 3
Hepatotoxicity in the form of elevated serum bilirubin and transaminases, presenting as jaundice. Usually occurs 2–3 months after therapy.

TOXICITY 4
Mild nausea and vomiting.

TOXICITY 5
Dry skin, urticaria, and photosensitivity.

TOXICITY 6
Immunosuppression with increased risk of bacterial, fungal, and parasitic infections.

TOXICITY 7
Mutagenic, teratogenic, and carcinogenic.

Methotrexate

TRADE NAMES	MTX, Amethopterin	**CLASSIFICATION**	Antimetabolite
CATEGORY	Chemotherapy drug	**DRUG MANUFACTURER**	Lederle Laboratories and Immunex

MECHANISM OF ACTION

- Cell cycle–specific antifolate analog, active in S-phase of the cell cycle.
- Enters cells through specific transport systems mediated by the reduced folate carrier and the folate receptor protein.
- Requires polyglutamation by the enzyme folylpolyglutamate synthase (FPGS) for its cytotoxic activity.
- Inhibition of dihydrofolate reductase (DHFR), resulting in depletion of critical reduced folates.
- Inhibition of de novo thymidylate synthesis.
- Inhibition of de novo purine synthesis.
- Incorporation of dUTP into DNA, resulting in inhibition of DNA synthesis and function.

MECHANISM OF RESISTANCE

- Increased expression of the target enzyme DHFR through either gene amplification or increased transcription, translation, and/or post-translational events.
- Alterations in the binding affinity of DHFR for methotrexate.
- Decreased carrier-mediated transport of drug into cell through decreased expression and/or activity of reduced folate carrier (RFC) or folate-receptor protein (FRP).
- Decreased formation of cytotoxic methotrexate polyglutamates through either decreased expression of FPGS or increased expression of γ-glutamyl hydrolase (GGH).
- Decreased expression of mismatch repair enzymes may contribute to drug resistance.

ABSORPTION

Oral bioavailability is saturable and erratic at doses greater than 25 mg/m². Peak serum levels are achieved within 1–2 hours of oral administration. Methotrexate is completely absorbed from parenteral routes of administration, and peak serum concentrations are reached in 30–60 minutes after IM injection.

DISTRIBUTION

Widely distributed throughout the body. At conventional doses, CSF levels are only about 5%–10% of those in plasma. High-dose methotrexate yields therapeutic concentrations in the CSF. Distributes into third-space fluid collections such as pleural effusion and ascites. Only about 50% of drug bound to plasma proteins, mainly to albumin.

METABOLISM

Extensive metabolism in liver and in cells by FPGS to higher polyglutamate forms. About 10%–20% of parent drug and the 7-hydroxymetabolite are eliminated in bile and then reabsorbed via enterohepatic circulation. Renal excretion is the main route of elimination and is mediated by glomerular filtration and tubular secretion. About 80%–90% of an administered dose is eliminated unchanged in urine within 24 hours. Terminal half-life of drug is on the order of 8–10 hours.

INDICATIONS

1. Breast cancer.
2. Head and neck cancer.
3. Osteogenic sarcoma.
4. Acute lymphoblastic leukemia.
5. Non-Hodgkin's lymphoma.
6. Primary CNS lymphoma.
7. Meningeal leukemia and carcinomatous meningitis.
8. Bladder cancer.
9. Gestational trophoblastic cancer.

DOSAGE RANGE

1. Low dose: 10–50 mg/m^2 IV every 3–4 weeks.
2. Low dose weekly: 25 mg/m^2 IV weekly.
3. Moderate dose: 100–500 mg/m^2 IV every 2–3 weeks.
4. High dose: 1–12 g/m^2 IV over a 3- to 24-hour period every 1–3 weeks.
5. Intrathecal: 10–15 mg IT two times weekly until CSF is clear, then weekly dose for 2–6 weeks, followed by monthly dose.
6. Intramuscular: 25 mg/m^2 IM every 3 weeks.

DRUG INTERACTION 1

Aspirin, penicillins, probenecid, NSAIDs, and cephalosporins—These drugs inhibit the renal excretion of methotrexate, leading to enhanced drug effect and toxicity.

DRUG INTERACTION 2

Warfarin—Methotrexate may enhance the anticoagulant effect of warfarin through competitive displacement from plasma proteins.

DRUG INTERACTION 3

5-FU—Methotrexate enhances the antitumor activity of 5-FU when given 24 hours before fluoropyrimidine treatment.

DRUG INTERACTION 4
Leucovorin—Leucovorin rescues the toxic effects of methotrexate and may also impair the antitumor activity. The active form of leucovorin is the L-isomer.

DRUG INTERACTION 5
Thymidine—Thymidine rescues the toxic effects of methotrexate and may also impair the antitumor activity.

DRUG INTERACTION 6
Folic acid supplements—These supplements may counteract the antitumor effects of methotrexate and should be discontinued while on therapy.

DRUG INTERACTION 7
Proton pump inhibitors—Proton pump inhibitors may reduce the elimination of methotrexate, which can then result in increased serum methotrexate levels, leading to increased toxicity. This is an especially important issue for patients receiving high-dose methotrexate.

DRUG INTERACTION 8
L-Asparaginase—L-Asparaginase antagonizes the antitumor activity of methotrexate.

SPECIAL CONSIDERATIONS
1. Use with caution in patients with abnormal renal function. Dose should be reduced in proportion to the creatinine clearance. Important to obtain baseline creatinine clearance and to monitor renal status during therapy.
2. Instruct patients to stop folic acid supplements during therapy as they may counteract the effects of methotrexate.
3. Monitor CBCs on a weekly basis and more frequently with high-dose therapy.
4. Use with caution in patients with third-space fluid collections such as pleural effusion and ascites, as the half-life of methotrexate is prolonged, leading to enhanced clinical toxicity. Fluid collections should be drained before methotrexate therapy.
5. Use with caution in patients with bladder cancer status post cystectomy and ileal conduit diversion, as they are at increased risk for delayed elimination of methotrexate and subsequent toxicity.
6. With high-dose therapy, methotrexate doses >1 g/m^2, important to vigorously hydrate the patient with 2.5–3.5 liters/m^2/day of IV 0.9% sodium chloride starting 12 hours before and for 24–48 hours after methotrexate infusion. Sodium bicarbonate (1–2 amps/L solution) should be included in the IV fluid to ensure that the urine pH is greater than 7.0 at the time of drug infusion and ideally for up to 48–72 hours after drug is given.
7. Methotrexate blood levels should be monitored in patients receiving high-dose therapy, patients with renal dysfunction (CrCl <60 mL/min) regardless of dose, and patients who have experienced excessive toxicity with prior treatment with methotrexate.
8. With high-dose therapy, methotrexate blood levels should be monitored every 24 hours starting at 24 hours after methotrexate infusion. Rescue

with leucovorin or L-leucovorin, the active isomer of leucovorin, should begin at 24 hours after drug infusion and should continue until the methotrexate drug level is <50 nM.

9. Glucarpidase is indicated for the treatment of toxic plasma methotrexate concentrations (>1 mM) in patients with delayed drug clearance due to impaired renal function.

10. Patients should be instructed to lie on their side for at least 1 hour after intrathecal administration of methotrexate. This will ensure adequate delivery of drug throughout the CSF.

11. Intrathecal administration of methotrexate may lead to myelosuppression and/or mucositis as therapeutic blood levels can be achieved.

12. Methotrexate overdose can be treated with leucovorin, L-leucovorin, and/ or thymidine.

13. Instruct patients to avoid sun exposure for at least 1 month after therapy.

14. Caution patients about drinking carbonated beverages as they can increase the acidity of urine, resulting in impaired drug elimination.

15. Pregnancy category D. Breastfeeding should be avoided.

TOXICITY 1
Myelosuppression is dose-limiting toxicity with leukocyte nadir at days 4–7 and recovery usually by day 14.

TOXICITY 2
Mucositis can be dose-limiting. Typical onset is 3–7 days after methotrexate therapy and precedes the decrease in leukocyte and platelet count. Nausea and vomiting are dose-dependent.

TOXICITY 3
Acute renal failure, azotemia, urinary retention, and uric acid nephropathy. Renal toxicity results from the intratubular precipitation of methotrexate and its metabolites. Methotrexate itself may exert a direct toxic effect on the renal tubules.

TOXICITY 4
Transient elevation in serum transaminases and bilirubin are often observed with high-dose therapy. May occur within the first 12–24 hours after start of infusion and returns to normal within 10 days.

TOXICITY 5
Poorly defined pneumonitis characterized by fever, cough, and interstitial pulmonary infiltrates.

TOXICITY 6
Acute chemical arachnoiditis with headaches, nuchal rigidity, seizures, vomiting, fever, and an inflammatory cell infiltrate in the CSF observed immediately after intrathecal administration. Chronic, demyelinating encephalopathy observed in children months to years after intrathecal methotrexate and presents as dementia, limb spasticity, and in advanced cases, coma.

TOXICITY 7

Acute cerebral dysfunction with paresis, aphasia, behavioral abnormalities, and seizures observed in 5%–15% of patients receiving high-dose methotrexate. Usually occurs within 6 days of treatment and resolves within 48–72 hours. A chronic form of neurotoxicity manifested as an encephalopathy with dementia and motor paresis can develop 2–4 months after treatment.

TOXICITY 8

Erythematous skin rash, pruritus, urticaria, photosensitivity, and hyperpigmentation. Radiation-recall skin reaction is also observed.

TOXICITY 9

Menstrual irregularities, abortion, and fetal deaths in women. Reversible oligospermia with testicular failure reported in men with high-dose therapy.

Mitomycin-C

TRADE NAMES	Mutamycin, Mitomycin	CLASSIFICATION	Antitumor antibiotic
CATEGORY	Chemotherapy drug	DRUG MANUFACTURER	Bristol-Myers Squibb

MECHANISM OF ACTION

- Isolated from the broth of *Streptomyces caespitosus* species.
- Acts as an alkylating agent to cross-link DNA, resulting in inhibition of DNA synthesis and function.
- Inhibits transcription by targeting DNA-dependent RNA polymerase.
- Bioreductive activation by NADPH cytochrome P450 reductase, NADH cytochrome B450 reductase, and DT-diaphorase to oxygen free radical forms, semiquinone or hydroquinone species, which target DNA and inhibit DNA synthesis and function.
- Preferential activation of mitomycin-C in hypoxic tumor cells.

MECHANISM OF RESISTANCE

- Increased expression of the multidrug-resistant gene with elevated P170 protein levels. This leads to increased drug efflux and decreased intracellular drug accumulation. Cross-resistance to anthracyclines, vinca alkaloids, and other natural products.

- Decreased bioactivation through decreased expression of DT-diaphorase.
- Increased activity of DNA excision repair enzymes.
- Increased expression of glutathione and glutathione-dependent detoxifying enzymes.

ABSORPTION

Not available for oral use and is administered only by the IV route.

DISTRIBUTION

Rapidly cleared from plasma after IV administration and widely distributed to tissues. Does not cross the blood-brain barrier.

METABOLISM

Metabolism in the liver with formation of both active and inactive metabolites. Mediated by the liver cytochrome P450 system and DT-diaphorase. Bioactivation can also occur in spleen, kidney, and heart. Parent compound and its metabolites are excreted mainly through the hepatobiliary system into feces. Renal clearance accounts for only 8%–10% of drug elimination. Elimination half-life of about 50 minutes.

INDICATIONS

1. Gastric cancer.
2. Pancreatic cancer.
3. Breast cancer.
4. NSCLC
5. Cervical cancer.
6. Head and neck cancer (in combination with radiation therapy).
7. Superficial bladder cancer.

DOSAGE RANGE

1. Gastric cancer: 10 mg/m^2 IV every 8 weeks, as part of the FAM regimen.
2. Breast cancer: Usual dose in various combination regimens is 10 mg/m^2 IV every 8 weeks.
3. Intravesicular therapy: Usual dose for intravesicular instillation is 40 mg administered in 20 mL of water.

DRUG INTERACTIONS

None well characterized.

SPECIAL CONSIDERATIONS

1. Use with caution in patients with abnormal liver function. Dose reduction is required in the setting of liver dysfunction.
2. Because mitomycin-C is a potent vesicant, administer slowly over 30–60 minutes with a rapidly flowing IV. Administer drug carefully, usually through a central venous catheter. Careful monitoring is necessary to avoid extravasation. If extravasation is suspected, immediately stop infusion, withdraw fluid, elevate extremity, and apply ice to involved site. May administer topical DMSO. In severe cases, consult a plastic surgeon.

3. Monitor complete blood cell counts on a weekly basis. Mitomyin-C therapy results in delayed and cumulative myelosuppression.
4. Monitor patients for acute dyspnea and severe bronchospasm following drug administration. Bronchodilators, steroids, and/or oxygen may help to relieve symptoms. Risk of pulmonary toxicity increased with cumulative doses of mitomycin-C >50 mg/m^2.
5. FIO$_2$ concentrations in the perioperative period should be maintained below 50% as patients receiving mitomycin-C concurrently with other anticancer agents are at increased risk for developing ARDS. Careful attention to fluid status is important.
6. Monitor for signs of hemolytic-uremic syndrome (anemia with fragmented cells on peripheral blood smear, thrombocytopenia, and renal dysfunction), especially when total cumulative doses of mitomycin-C are >50 mg/m^2.
7. Monitor when used in combination with other myelosuppressive anticancer agents.
8. Pregnancy category D. Breastfeeding should be avoided.

TOXICITY 1
Myelosuppression is dose-limiting and cumulative toxicity with leukopenia more common than thrombocytopenia. Nadir counts are delayed at about 4–6 weeks.

TOXICITY 2
Nausea and vomiting. Usually mild and occurs within 1–2 hours of treatment, lasting for up to 3 days.

TOXICITY 3
Mucositis is common but not dose-limiting. Observed within the first week of treatment.

TOXICITY 4
Potent vesicant. Extravasation can lead to tissue necrosis and chemical thrombophlebitis at the site of injection.

TOXICITY 5
Anorexia and fatigue are common.

TOXICITY 6
Hemolytic-uremic syndrome. Consists of microangiopathic hemolytic anemia (hematocrit <25%), thrombocytopenia (<100,000/mm^3), and renal failure (serum creatinine >1.6 mg/dL). Other complications include pulmonary edema, neurologic abnormalities, and hypertension. Rare event, seen in <2% of patients treated. Can occur at any time during treatment but usually occurs at total doses >50 mg/m^2. In rare cases, syndrome can be fatal.

TOXICITY 7
Interstitial pneumonitis. Presents with dyspnea, nonproductive cough, and interstitial infiltrates on chest X-ray. Occurs more frequently with total cumulative doses >50 mg/m^2.

TOXICITY 8

Hepatic veno-occlusive disease. Presents with abdominal pain, hepatomegaly, and liver failure. Occurs only with high-dose therapy in transplant setting.

TOXICITY 9

Chemical cystitis and bladder contraction. Observed only in setting of intravesicular therapy.

Mitotane

TRADE NAME	Lysodren	CLASSIFICATION	Adrenolytic agent
CATEGORY	Chemotherapy drug	DRUG MANUFACTURER	Bristol-Myers Squibb

MECHANISM OF ACTION

- Dichloro derivative of the insecticide DDD.
- Direct toxic effect on mitochondria of adrenal cortical cells resulting in inhibition of adrenal steroid production.
- Alters the peripheral metabolism of steroids, resulting in decreased levels of 17-OH corticosteroid.

ABSORPTION

About 35%–45% of an oral dose is absorbed. Peak plasma levels are achieved in 3–5 hours.

DISTRIBUTION

Widely distributed to tissues. Highly fat-soluble with large amounts of drug distributed in adipose tissues. Mitotane is slowly released with drug levels being detectable for up to 10 weeks. Does not cross the blood-brain barrier.

METABOLISM

Metabolism in the liver with formation of both active and inactive metabolites. Parent compound and its metabolites are excreted mainly through the hepatobiliary system into feces (60%). Renal clearance accounts for only 10%–25% of drug elimination. Variable elimination half-life of up to 160 hours due to storage of drug in adipose tissue.

INDICATIONS
Adrenocortical cancer.

DOSAGE RANGE
Usual dose is 2–10 g/day PO in three or four divided doses.

DRUG INTERACTION 1
Warfarin—Mitotane alters the metabolism of warfarin, leading to an increased requirement for warfarin. Coagulation parameters, including PT and INR, should be monitored closely, and dose adjustments made accordingly.

DRUG INTERACTION 2
Barbiturates, phenytoin, cyclophosphamide—Mitotane alters the metabolism of various drugs that are metabolized by the liver microsomal P450 system, including barbiturates, phenytoin, and cyclophosphamide.

DRUG INTERACTION 3
Steroids—Mitotane interferes with steroid metabolism. If steroid replacement is required, doses higher than those for physiologic replacement may be needed.

SPECIAL CONSIDERATIONS
1. Use with caution in patients with abnormal liver function. Dose reduction is required in the setting of liver dysfunction.
2. Adrenal insufficiency may develop, and adrenal steroid replacement with glucocorticoid and/or mineralocorticoid therapy is indicated.
3. Stress-dose IV steroids are required in the event of infection, stress, trauma, and/or shock.
4. Patients should be cautioned about driving, operating complicated machinery, and/or other activities that require increased mental alertness, as mitotane causes lethargy and somnolence.
5. Concurrent use of mitotane and warfarin requires careful monitoring of coagulation parameters, including PT and INR, as mitotane can alter warfarin metabolism.
6. Pregnancy category C. Breastfeeding should be avoided.

TOXICITY 1
Mild nausea and vomiting. Dose-limiting, occurs in 80% of patients.

TOXICITY 2
Lethargy, somnolence, vertigo, and dizziness. CNS side effects occur in 40% of patients.

TOXICITY 3
Mucositis is common but not dose-limiting. Observed within the first week of treatment.

TOXICITY 4
Transient skin rash and hyperpigmentation.

TOXICITY 5

Adrenal insufficiency. Rarely occurs with steroid replacement therapy.

Mitoxantrone

TRADE NAME	Novantrone	**CLASSIFICATION**	Antitumor antibiotic
CATEGORY	Chemotherapy drug	**DRUG MANUFACTURER**	OSI

MECHANISM OF ACTION
- Synthetic planar anthracenedione analog.
- Intercalates into DNA, resulting in inhibition of DNA synthesis and function.
- Inhibits topoisomerase II by forming a cleavable complex with topoisomerase II and DNA.

MECHANISM OF RESISTANCE
- Increased expression of the multidrug-resistant gene with enhanced drug efflux, resulting in decreased intracellular drug accumulation.
- Decreased expression of topoisomerase II.
- Mutation in topoisomerase II with decreased binding affinity to drug.
- Increased expression of sulfhydryl proteins, including glutathione and glutathione-associated enzymes.

ABSORPTION
Administered only by the IV route, as it is not orally bioavailable.

DISTRIBUTION
Rapid and extensive distribution to formed blood elements and to body tissues. Distributes in high concentrations in liver, bone marrow, heart, lung, and kidney. Does not cross the blood-brain barrier. Extensively bound (about 80%) to plasma proteins. Peak plasma levels are achieved immediately after IV injection.

METABOLISM
Metabolism by the liver microsomal P450 system. Elimination is mainly through the hepatobiliary route, with 25% of the drug excreted in feces. Renal clearance

accounts for only 6%–10% of drug elimination, mainly as unchanged drug. The elimination half-life ranges from 23 to 215 hours with a median of 75 hours.

INDICATIONS
1. Advanced, hormone-refractory prostate cancer—Used in combination with prednisone as initial chemotherapy.
2. Acute myelogenous leukemia.
3. Breast cancer.
4. Non-Hodgkin's lymphoma.

DOSAGE RANGE
1. Acute myelogenous leukemia, induction therapy: 12 mg/m^2 IV on days 1–3, given in combination with ara-C, 100 mg/m^2/day IV continuous infusion for 5–7 days.
2. Prostate cancer: 12 mg/m^2 IV on day 1 every 21 days, given in combination with prednisone 5 mg PO bid.
3. Non-Hodgkin's lymphoma: 10 mg/m^2 IV on day 1 every 21 days, given as part of the CNOP or FND regimens.

DRUG INTERACTIONS
Heparin—Mitoxantrone is incompatible with heparin, as a precipitate will form.

SPECIAL CONSIDERATIONS
1. Use with caution in patients with abnormal liver function. Dose modification should be considered in patients with liver dysfunction.
2. Carefully monitor the IV injection site as mitoxantrone is a vesicant. Skin may turn blue at site of injection. Avoid extravasation, but ulceration and tissue injury are rare when drug is properly diluted.
3. Alkalinization of the urine, allopurinol, and vigorous IV hydration are recommended to prevent tumor lysis syndrome in patients with acute myelogenous leukemia.
4. Monitor cardiac function prior to (baseline) and periodically during therapy with either MUGA radionuclide scan or echocardiogram to assess LVEF. Risk of cardiac toxicity is higher in elderly patients >70 years of age, in patients with prior history of hypertension or pre-existing heart disease, in patients previously treated with anthracyclines, or in patients with prior radiation therapy to the chest. Cumulative doses of 140 mg/m^2 in patients with no prior history of anthracycline therapy and 120 mg/m^2 in patients with prior anthracycline therapy are associated with increased risk for cardiotoxicity. A decrease in LVEF by 15%–20% is an indication to discontinue treatment.
5. Monitor CBCs while on therapy.
6. Patients may experience blue-green urine for up to 24 hours after drug administration.
7. Pregnancy category D. Breastfeeding should be avoided.

TOXICITY 1

Myelosuppression is dose-limiting with neutropenia more common than thrombocytopenia. Nadir typically occurs at 10–14 days after treatment but may occur earlier in acute leukemia, with recovery of counts by day 21. Risk of myelosuppression is greater in elderly patients and in those previously treated with chemotherapy and/or radiation therapy.

TOXICITY 2

Nausea and vomiting are observed in 70% of patients. Usually mild, occurs less frequently than with doxorubicin.

TOXICITY 3

Mucositis and diarrhea. Common but usually not severe.

TOXICITY 4

Cardiotoxicity. Cardiac effects are similar to but less severe than those of doxorubicin. Acute toxicity presents as atrial arrhythmias, chest pain, and myopericarditis syndrome that typically occurs within the first 24–48 hours of drug administration. Transient and mostly asymptomatic.

Chronic toxicity is manifested in the form of a dilated cardiomyopathy with congestive heart failure. Cumulative doses of 140 mg/m^2 in patients with no prior history of anthracycline therapy and 120 mg/m^2 in patients with prior anthracycline therapy are associated with increased risk for developing congestive cardiomyopathy.

TOXICITY 5

Alopecia. Observed in 40% of patients but less severe than with doxorubicin.

TOXICITY 6

Transient and reversible effects on liver enzymes including SGOT and SGPT.

TOXICITY 7

Blue discoloration of fingernails, sclera, and urine for 1–2 days after treatment.

TOXICITY 8

Secondary acute myelogenous leukemia.

Necitumumab

TRADE NAME	Portrazza	CLASSIFICATION	Monoclonal antibody, anti-EGFR antibody
CATEGORY	Biologic response modifier agent	DRUG MANUFACTURER	Eli Lilly

MECHANISM OF ACTION
- Recombinant human IgG1 monoclonal antibody directed against the epidermal growth factor receptor (EGFR). EGFR is overexpressed in a broad range of human solid tumors, including colorectal cancer, head and neck cancer, NSCLC, pancreatic cancer, and breast cancer.
- Binds with higher affinity to EGFR than normal ligands EGF and TGF-α, which then results in inhibition of EGFR. Prevents both homodimerization and heterodimerization of the EGFR, leading to inhibition of autophosphorylation and inhibition of EGFR signaling.
- Inhibition of the EGFR signaling pathway results in inhibition of critical mitogenic and antiapoptotic signals involved in proliferation, growth, invasion/metastasis, and angiogenesis.
- Inhibition of the EGFR pathway enhances the response to chemotherapy and/or radiation therapy.
- Immunologic mechanisms may also be involved in antitumor activity, and they include recruitment of ADCC and/or complement-mediated cell lysis.

MECHANISM OF RESISTANCE
- Mutations in EGFR leading to decreased binding affinity to necitumumab.
- Decreased expression of EGFR.
- Increased expression of TGF-α ligand.
- Presence of KRAS mutations.
- Presence of BRAF mutations.
- Presence of NRAS mutations.
- Increased expression of HER2 through gene amplification.
- Increased HER3 expression.
- Activation/induction of alternative cellular signaling pathways, such as PI3K/Akt and IGF-1R.

DISTRIBUTION
Distribution in the body is not well characterized. The time to reach steady-state is 100 days.

METABOLISM
Metabolism of necitumumab has not been extensively characterized. Half-life is on the order of 14 days.

INDICATIONS

FDA-approved in combination with gemcitabine and cisplatin for the first-line treatment of metastatic squamous NSCLC. Necitumumab is not recommended for the treatment of non-squamous NSCLC.

DOSAGE RANGE

The recommended dose is 800 mg IV on days 1 and 8 on an every 21-day cycle.

DRUG INTERACTIONS

None well characterized to date.

SPECIAL CONSIDERATIONS

1. The level of EGFR expression does not accurately predict for necitumumab clinical activity. As such, EGFR testing should not be required for the clinical use of necitumumab.
2. Electrolyte status should be closely monitored prior to each infusion, especially serum magnesium, calcium, and potassium levels, as hypomagnesemia has been observed with necitumumab treatment. This represents a black-box warning. Electrolyte status should continue to be monitored for at least 8 weeks following the completion of therapy.
3. There is an increased risk of cardiopulmonary arrest or sudden death in patients treated with necitumumab plus gemcitabine and cisplatin. This represents a black-box warning. Caution should be used in patients with significant coronary artery disease, MI within the previous 6 months, history of CHF, and/or arrhythmias.
4. In patients who develop a skin rash, topical antibiotics such as clindamycin gel or erythromycin cream or either oral clindamycin, oral doxycycline, or oral minocycline may help. Patients should be warned to avoid sunlight exposure.
5. Most infusion reactions occur after the first or second infusion. For patients who have experienced a prior grade 1 or 2 infusion reaction, patients should be premedicated with diphenhydramine prior to all subsequent infusions. For patients who have experienced a second grade 1 or 2 infusion reaction, need to be more aggressive with premedication regimen and treat with diphenhydramine, acetaminophen, and dexamethasone prior to each infusion.
6. Necitumumab should not be used in the setting of non-squamous NSCLC as it results in increased toxicity and increased mortality.
7. Pregnancy category D. Breastfeeding should be avoided.

TOXICITY 1

Infusion-related symptoms with fever, chills, urticaria, flushing, fatigue, headache, bronchospasm, dyspnea, angioedema, and hypotension. Usually mild-to-moderate in severity and observed most commonly after the first or second infusion.

TOXICITY 2

Pruritus, dry skin with mainly a pustular, acneiform skin rash. Presents mainly on the face, neck region, and upper trunk. Improves with continued treatment and resolves upon cessation of therapy. Nailbed changes may also be observed with prolonged use.

TOXICITY 3

Cardiopulmonary arrest and/or sudden death. Occurs in about 3% of patients.

TOXICITY 4

Hypomagnesemia occurs in approximately 80% of patients with severe cases observed in 20% of patients.

TOXICITY 5

Increased risk of venous and arterial thrombo-embolic events.

Nelarabine

TRADE NAMES	Arranon, 2-amino-9-β-D-arabinofuranosyl-6-methoxy-9H-purine	**CLASSIFICATION**	Antimetabolite
CATEGORY	Chemotherapy drug	**DRUG MANUFACTURER**	GlaxoSmithKline

MECHANISM OF ACTION
- Prodrug of 9-β-D-arabinofuranosylguanine (ara-G).
- Cell cycle–specific with activity in the S-phase.
- Requires intracellular activation to the nucleotide metabolite ara-GTP.
- Incorporation of ara-GTP into DNA, resulting in chain termination and inhibition of DNA synthesis and function.

MECHANISM OF RESISTANCE
- Decreased activation of drug through decreased expression of the anabolic enzyme deoxycytidine kinase.
- Decreased transport of drug into cells.

ABSORPTION
Poor oral bioavailability. Administered only by the IV route.

DISTRIBUTION
Extensively distributed in the body. Binding to plasma proteins has not been well characterized.

METABOLISM
Undergoes metabolism by adenosine deaminase to form ara-G, which is subsequently phosphorylated to the active ara-GTP form. A minor route of nelarabine metabolism is via hydrolysis to form methylguanine, which is then demethylated to form guanine. Nelarabine and ara-G are rapidly eliminated from plasma with a half-life in adults of approximately 30 minutes and 3 hours, respectively. Nelarabine (5%–10%) and ara-G (20%–30%) are eliminated, to a minor extent, by the kidneys. The mean clearance of nelarabine is approximately 30% higher in pediatric patients than adult patients, while the clearance of ara-G is similar in the two patient populations. Age and gender have no effects on nelarabine or ara-G pharmacokinetics.

INDICATIONS
1. FDA-approved for T-cell acute lymphoblastic leukemia (T-ALL) that has not responded to or has relapsed following treatment with at least two chemotherapy regimens.
2. FDA-approved for T-cell lymphoblastic lymphoma (T-LBL) that has not responded to or has relapsed following treatment with at least two chemotherapy regimens.

DOSAGE RANGE
1. Pediatric patients: 650 mg/m^2/day IV over 1 hour on days 1–5 every 21 days.
2. Adult patients: 1500 mg/m^2/day IV over 2 hours on days 1, 3, and 5 every 28 days.

DRUG INTERACTIONS
None well characterized to date.

SPECIAL CONSIDERATIONS
1. Monitor CBCs on a regular basis during therapy.
2. Closely monitor for neurologic events, as this represents a black-box warning.
3. Patients treated previously or concurrently with intrathecal chemotherapy and/or previously with craniospinal radiation therapy may be at increased risk for developing neurotoxicity.
4. Patients should be advised against performing activities that require mental alertness, including operating hazardous machinery and driving.

5. Alkalinization of the urine (pH >7.0), allopurinol, and vigorous IV hydration are recommended to prevent tumor lysis syndrome.
6. Pregnancy category D. Breastfeeding should be avoided.

TOXICITY 1
Myelosuppression is the most common toxicity with neutropenia, thrombocytopenia, and anemia.

TOXICITY 2
Nausea and vomiting. Mild-to-moderate emetogenic agent.

TOXICITY 3
Neurotoxicity is dose-limiting with headache, altered mental status, seizures, and peripheral neuropathy with numbness, paresthesias, motor weakness, and paralysis. Rare events of demyelination and ascending peripheral neuropathies similar to Guillain-Barré syndrome have been reported.

TOXICITY 4
Mild hepatic dysfunction with elevation of serum transaminases and bilirubin.

TOXICITY 5
Fatigue and asthenia.

Nilotinib

TRADE NAMES	Tasigna, AMN107	CLASSIFICATION	Signal transduction inhibitor
CATEGORY	Chemotherapy drug	DRUG MANUFACTURER	Novartis

MECHANISM OF ACTION
- Second-generation phenylaminopyrimidine inhibitor of the Bcr-Abl, c-Kit, and PDGFR-β tyrosine kinases.
- Higher binding affinity (up to 20- to 50-fold) and selectivity for Abl kinase domain when compared to imatinib and overcomes imatinib resistance resulting from Bcr-Abl mutations.

MECHANISM OF RESISTANCE
Single-point mutation within the ATP-binding pocket of the Abl tyrosine kinase (T3151).

ABSORPTION
Nilotinib has good oral bioavailability. Rapidly absorbed following oral administration. Peak plasma concentrations are observed within 3 hours of oral ingestion.

DISTRIBUTION
Extensive binding of parent drug to plasma proteins in the range of 95%–98%.

METABOLISM
Metabolized in the liver primarily by CYP3A4 microsomal enzymes. Other liver P450 enzymes, such as UGT, play a relatively minor role in metabolism. None of the metabolites are biologically active. Approximately 90% of an administered dose is eliminated in feces within 7 days. The terminal half-life of the parent drug is in the order of 15–17 hours.

INDICATIONS
1. FDA-approved for the treatment of adults with chronic phase (CP) and accelerated phase (AP) Ph+ CML with resistance or intolerance to prior therapy that included imatinib.
2. FDA-approved for the front-line treatment of patients with newly diagnosed CP Ph+ CML.

DOSAGE RANGE
Recommended dose is 400 mg PO bid.

DRUG INTERACTION 1
Nilotinib is an inhibitor of CYP3A4 and may decrease the metabolic clearance of drugs that are metabolized by CYP3A4.

DRUG INTERACTION 2
Drugs such as ketoconazole, itraconazole, erythromycin, and clarithromycin may decrease the rate of metabolism of nilotinib, resulting in increased drug levels and potentially increased toxicity.

DRUG INTERACTION 3
Drugs such as rifampin, phenytoin, phenobarbital, carbamazepine, and St. John's wort may increase the rate of metabolism of nilotinib, resulting in its inactivation.

DRUG INTERACTION 4
Nilotinib is a substrate of the P-glycoprotein transporter. Caution should be used in patients on drugs that inhibit P-glycoprotein (e.g., verapamil) as this may lead to increased concentrations of nilotinib.

SPECIAL CONSIDERATIONS
1. Nilotinib tablets should not be taken with food for at least 2 hours before a dose is taken and for at least 1 hour after a dose is taken.
2. Important to review patient's list of medications, as nilotinib has several potential drug–drug interactions.
3. Monitor CBC every 2 weeks for the first 2 months, and monthly thereafter.
4. Use with caution in patients with a prior history of pancreatitis. Serum lipase levels should be checked periodically.
5. Nilotinib should not be used in patients with hypokalemia, hypomagnesemia, or long QT syndrome. Electrolyte abnormalities must be corrected prior to initiation of therapy, and electrolyte status should be monitored periodically during therapy.
6. ECGs should be performed at baseline, 7 days after initiation of therapy, and periodically thereafter.
7. Patients should be warned about not taking St. John's wort while on nilotinib therapy.
8. Avoid Seville oranges, starfruit, pomelos, grapefruit juice, and grapefruit products while on therapy.
9. Pregnancy category D. Breastfeeding should be avoided.

TOXICITY 1
Myelosuppression with thrombocytopenia, neutropenia, and anemia.

TOXICITY 2
Prolongation of QT interval, which on rare occasions, may lead to sudden death.

TOXICITY 3
Elevations in serum lipase.

TOXICITY 4
Electrolyte abnormalities with hypophosphatemia, hypokalemia, hypocalcemia, and hyponatremia.

TOXICITY 5
Fatigue, asthenia, and anorexia.

TOXICITY 6
Elevations in serum transaminases and/or bilirubin (usually indirect bilirubin).

N

Nilutamide

TRADE NAME	Nilandron	CLASSIFICATION	Antiandrogen
CATEGORY	Hormonal agent	DRUG MANUFACTURER	Sanofi-Aventis

MECHANISM OF ACTION
Nonsteroidal, antiandrogen agent that binds to androgen receptor and inhibits androgen uptake. Also inhibits androgen binding in the nucleus of androgen-sensitive prostate cancer cells.

MECHANISM OF RESISTANCE
- Decreased expression of androgen receptor.
- Mutation in androgen receptor, leading to decreased binding affinity to nilutamide.

ABSORPTION
Rapidly and completely absorbed by the GI tract. Absorption is not affected by food.

DISTRIBUTION
Distribution is not well characterized. Moderate binding of nilutamide to plasma proteins.

METABOLISM
Extensive metabolism occurs in the liver to both active and inactive metabolites. About 60% of the drug is excreted in urine, mainly in metabolite form, and only minimal clearance in feces. The elimination half-life is approximately 41–49 hours.

INDICATIONS
Stage D2 metastatic prostate cancer in combination with surgical castration.

DOSAGE RANGE
Recommended dose is 300 mg PO daily for 30 days, then 150 mg PO daily.

DRUG INTERACTION 1
Warfarin—Nilutamide can inhibit metabolism of warfarin by the liver P450 system leading to increased anticoagulant effect. Coagulation parameters, PT and INR, must be followed routinely, and dose adjustments may be needed.

DRUG INTERACTION 2
Drugs metabolized by the liver P450 system—Nilutamide inhibits the activity of liver cytochrome P450 enzymes and may therefore reduce the metabolism of various compounds, including phenytoin and theophylline. Enhanced toxicity of these agents may be observed, requiring dose adjustment.

DRUG INTERACTION 3
Alcohol—Increased risk of alcohol intolerance following treatment with nilutamide.

SPECIAL CONSIDERATIONS
1. Should be given on the same day or on the day after surgical castration to achieve maximal benefit.
2. Nilutamide can be taken with or without food.
3. Should be used with caution in patients with abnormal liver function and is contraindicated in patients with severe liver impairment. Monitor LFTs at baseline and during therapy.
4. Contraindicated in patients with severe respiratory insufficiency. Baseline PFTs and chest X-ray should be obtained in all patients and periodically during therapy. If findings of interstitial pneumonitis appear on chest X-ray or there is a significant decrease by 20%–25% in DLCO and FVC on PFTs, treatment with nilutamide should be terminated.
5. Caution patients about the potential for hot flashes. Consider the use of clonidine 0.1–0.2 mg PO daily, megestrol acetate 20 mg PO bid, or soy tablets 1 tablet PO tid for prevention and/or treatment.
6. Instruct patients on the potential risk of altered sexual function and impotence.
7. Patients should be advised to abstain from alcohol while on nilutamide as there is an increased risk of intolerance (facial flushes, malaise, hypotension) to alcohol.
8. Pregnancy category C. Breastfeeding should be avoided.

TOXICITY 1
Hot flashes, decreased libido, impotence, gynecomastia, nipple pain, and galactorrhea.

TOXICITY 2
Visual disturbances in the form of impaired adaptation to dark, abnormal vision, and alterations in color vision. Occurs in up to 60% of patients and results in treatment discontinuation in 1%–2% of patients.

TOXICITY 3
Anorexia, nausea, and constipation. Transient elevations in serum transaminases are uncommon.

TOXICITY 4
Cough, dyspnea, and interstitial pneumonitis occur rarely in about 2% of patients. Usually observed within the first 3 months of treatment. Incidence may be higher in patients of Asian descent.

Nivolumab

TRADE NAMES	Opdivo, MDX-1106, BMS-936558	CLASSIFICATION	Monoclonal antibody
CATEGORY	Immune checkpoint inhibitor	DRUG MANUFACTURER	Bristol-Myers Squibb

MECHANISM OF ACTION
- Fully human IgG4 monoclonal antibody that binds to the programmed death (PD)-1 receptor, which is expressed on T cells, and inhibits the interaction between the PD-L1 and PD-L2 ligands and the PD-1 receptor.
- Blockade of the PD-1 pathway-mediated immune checkpoint enhances T-cell immune response, leading to T-cell activation and proliferation.

MECHANISM OF RESISTANCE
None well characterized to date.

DISTRIBUTION
The mean volume of distribution is 9.5 mL/hr. Steady-state concentrations are achieved by 12 weeks.

METABOLISM
Metabolism of nivolumab has not been extensively characterized. The mean elimination half-life is on the order of 26.7 days.

INDICATIONS
1. FDA-approved for unresectable or metastatic melanoma and disease progression following ipilumumab therapy, and if BRAF V600 mutation positive, a BRAF inhibitor.
2. FDA-approved for metastatic squamous NSCLC with progression on or after platinum-based chemotherapy.
3. FDA-approved for BRAF V600 mutation-positive unresectable or metastatic melanoma in combination with ipilumumab.
4. FDA-approved for metastatic squamous NSCLC with progression on or after platinum-based chemotherapy. Patients with EGFR or ALK mutations should have disease progression on FDA-approved targeted therapy prior to receiving nivolumab.
5. FDA-approved for advanced renal cell cancer following prior anti-angiogenic therapy.
6. FDA-approved for Hodgkin's lymphoma that has relapsed or progressed after autologous stem cell transplantation and post-transplantation brentuximab therapy.

DOSAGE RANGE

1. Unresectable or metastatic melanoma: Recommended dose as a single agent is 240 mg IV every 2 weeks.
2. Unresectable or metastatic melanoma: Recommended dose in combination with ipilumumab is 1 mg/kg IV every 3 weeks for 4 doses, then 240 mg IV every 2 weeks as a single agent.
3. NSCLC: Recommended dose is 240 mg IV every 2 weeks.
4. Renal cell cancer: Recommended dose is 240 mg IV every 2 weeks.
5. Hodgkin's lymphoma: Recommended dose is 3 mg/kg IV every 2 weeks.

DRUG INTERACTIONS

None well characterized to date.

SPECIAL CONSIDERATIONS

1. Nivolumab can result in significant immune-mediated adverse reactions due to T-cell activation and proliferation. These immune-mediated reactions may involve any organ system, with the most common reactions being pneumonitis, enterocolitis, hepatitis, dermatitis, hypophysitis, nephritis, and thyroid dysfunction.
2. Nivolumab should be withheld for any of the following:
   - Grade 2 pneumonitis
   - Grade 2 or 3 colitis
   - SGOT/SGPT >3×ULN and up to 5×ULN or total bilirubin >1.5×ULN and up to 3×ULN
   - Serum creatinine >1.5×ULN and up to 6×ULN or >1.5×baseline
   - Any other severe or grade 3 treament-related toxicity
3. Nivolumab should be permanently discontinued for any of the following:
   - Any life-threatening or grade 4 toxicity
   - Grade 3 or 4 pneumonitis
   - Grade 4 colitis
   - SGOT/SGPT >5×ULN or total bilirubin >3×ULN
   - Serum creatinine >6×ULN
   - Any severe or grade 3 toxicity that recurs
   - Inability to reduce steroid dose to 10 mg or less of prednisone or equivalent per day within 12 weeks
   - Persistent grade 2 or 3 toxicity that does not recover to grade 1 or resolve within 12 weeks after the last dose of drug
4. Monitor thyroid function prior to and during therapy.
5. Immune-mediated reactions may occur even after discontinuation of therapy.
6. Pregnancy category D.

TOXICITY 1

Colitis with diarrhea and abdominal pain.

TOXICITY 2

Pneumonitis with dyspnea and cough.

TOXICITY 3
GI side effects with nausea/vomiting; dry mouth; hepatitis with elevations in SGOT/SGPT, alkaline phosphatase, and serum bilirubin; and pancreatitis.

TOXICITY 4
Fatigue, anorexia, and asthenia.

TOXICITY 5
Nephritis.

TOXICITY 6
Myalgias and arthralgias.

TOXICITY 7
Maculopapular skin rash, erythema, dermatitis, and pruritus.

TOXICITY 8
Hypothyroidism.

Obinutuzumab

TRADE NAME	Gazyva	**CLASSIFICATION**	Monoclonal antibody
CATEGORY	Biologic response modifier agent	**DRUG MANUFACTURER**	Genentech/Roche

MECHANISM OF ACTION
- Novel glycoengineered type II anti-CD20 monoclonal antibody with a higher affinity for the CD20 epitope than rituximab. Binds to CD20 in a different orientation than type I anti-CD20 antibodies.
- More potent anti-CD20 antibody when compared to rituximab.
- CD20 is expressed on more than 90% of all B-cell, non-Hodgkin's lymphomas and leukemias.
- CD20 is not expressed on early pre–B cells, plasma cells, normal bone marrow stem cells, antigen-presenting dendritic reticulum cells, or other normal tissues.
- More effectively mediates antibody-dependent cellular cytotoxicity (ADCC) and direct cell death when compared to rituximab.

ABSORPTION
Administered only by the IV route.

DISTRIBUTION
The volume of distribution at steady-state is approximately 3.8 L.

METABOLISM
Obinutuzumab is eliminated through both a linear clearance mechanism and a time-dependent, non-linear clearance mechanism. The mean terminal half-life of obinutuzumab is approximately 28.4 days.

INDICATIONS
1. FDA-approved in combination with chlorambucil for previously untreated CLL.
2. FDA-approved in combination with bendamustine followed by obinutuzumab monotherapy for patients with follicular lymphoma (NHL) who relapsed after or are refractory to a rituximab-containing regimen.

DOSAGE RANGE
Recommended dose for 6 cycles (28-day cycles) is as follows:
CLL:
- 100 mg on cycle 1, day 1
- 900 mg on cycle 1, day 2
- 1000 mg on cycle 1, days 8 and 15
- 1000 mg on cycles 2–6, day 1

NHL:

- 1000 mg on cycle 1, day 1, 8, and 15
- 1000 mg on cycles 2-6, day 1
- and then 1000 mg on day 1 every 2 months for 2 years

DRUG INTERACTIONS
None wellcharacterized to date.

SPECIAL CONSIDERATIONS

1. Closely monitor patients for infusion reactions. Usually occur during the infusion, but infusion reactions have been observed within 24 hours of receiving obinutuzumab. Patients should be premedicated 30 min to 2 hours with oral acetaminophen (1000 mg), oral or IV diphenhydramine, and IV corticosteroid (prednisolone 100 mg) to prevent the incidence of infusion-related reactions.
2. Monitor for infusion-related events, especially during the first two infusions. Infusions should be immediately stopped if signs or symptoms of an allergic reaction are observed. Immediate institution of diphenhydramine, corticosteroids, albuterol, IV fluids, and/or vasopressors may be necessary. For grade 1/2 reactions, the infusion rate can be reduced or the infusion interrupted and the symptoms treated; if the patient's symptoms have resolved, the infusion rate escalation may resume at the increments and intervals as appropriate for the treatment cycle dose. For grade 3 reactions, the infusion should be interrupted and if the reaction symptoms resolves, the infusion can be resumed at a rate no more than half the previous rate; if no further infusion reactions are experienced, the infusion rate escalation may resume at the increments and intervals as appropriate for the treatment cycle dose. For grade 4 reactions, the infusion should be stopped immediately and permanently discontinued.
3. Consider holding off on antihypertensive treatments for 12 hours prior to and throughout each obinutuzumab infusion given the potential risk of hypotension.
4. Monitor for tumor lysis syndrome, especially in patients with high numbers of peripheral circulating cells (>25,000/mm^3). In this setting, patients should be premedicated with allopurinol starting 12–24 hours prior to the start of therapy as well as be adequately hydrated.
5. Monitor CBCs at regular intervals during therapy.
6. Consider the diagnosis of progressive multifocal leukoencephalopathy (PML) in patients who present with new onset or changes in pre-existing neurological signs or symptoms.
7. Obinutuzumab should not be given to patients with active infection, as serious bacterial, fungal, and new or reactivated viral infections can occur during and following treatment.
8. Screen all patients for hepatitis B (HBV) infection before initiation of obinutuzumab therapy. Closely monitor hepatitis B carriers for signs of active HBV infection during treatment with obinutuzumab and for 6–12 months following the last infusion. Obinutuzumab therapy should be permanently discontinued in the event of HBV reactivation.
9. Pregnancy category C. Breastfeeding should be avoided.

TOXICITY 1
Infusion-related symptoms occur especially during the first cycle of therapy, and present as nausea/vomiting, flushing, headache, fever, and chills. More serious symptoms include bronchospasm, dyspnea, laryngeal edema, and pulmonary edema.

TOXICITY 2
Myelosuppression with neutropenia and thrombocytopenia.

TOXICITY 3
Progressive multifocal leukoencephalopathy (PML).

TOXICITY 4
Hepatitis B reactivation.

TOXICITY 5
Increased risk of bacterial, viral, and fungal infections.

TOXICITY 6
Mild nausea.

TOXICITY 7
Headache.

TOXICITY 8
Musculoskeletal disorders, including pain.

Ofatumumab

TRADE NAMES	Arzerra, HuMax-CD20	CLASSIFICATION	Monoclonal antibody
CATEGORY	Biologic response modifier agent	DRUG MANUFACTURER	GlaxoSmithKline and Genman A/S

MECHANISM OF ACTION
- Fully human IgG1-κ immunoglobulin monoclonal antibody that binds specifically to both the small and large extracellular loops of the CD20 antigen on B cells.
- Targets a different CD20 epitope and binds CD20 with a reduced off-rate when compared to rituximab, resulting in prolonged antitumor activity.
- Maintains activity in rituximab-resistant tumors, which express low levels of CD20 and/or high levels of complement-regulatory proteins.
- CD20 is expressed on more than 90% of all B-cell, non-Hodgkin's lymphomas and leukemias.

- CD20 is not expressed on early pre–B cells, plasma cells, normal bone marrow stem cells, antigen-presenting dendritic reticulum cells, or other normal tissues.
- Mediates antibody-dependent cellular cytotoxicity (ADCC) and stronger complement-dependent cellular cytotoxicity (CDCC) when compared to rituximab.

ABSORPTION
Administered only by the IV route.

DISTRIBUTION
Mean volume of distribution at steady-state ranges from 1.7 to 5.1 L. The volume of distribution increases with body weight and male gender, but dose adjustment is not required based on body weight or gender.

METABOLISM
Ofatumumab is eliminated through both a B cell–mediated and a target-independent route. Due to the depletion of B cells, the clearance of ofatumumab is reduced significantly after subsequent infusions compared to the first infusion. The mean half-life of ofatumumab between the 4th and 12th infusions is approximately 14 days.

INDICATIONS
1. Refractory CLL—FDA-approved for CLL that is refractory to fludarabine and alemtuzumab.
2. FDA-approved for previously untreated CLL where fludarabine-based therapy is considered not appropriate.
3. FDA-approved for extended treatment of patients who are in complete or partial response after at least two lines of therapy for recurrent or progressive CLL.
4. FDA-approved in combination with fludarabine and cyclophosphamide for relapsed CLL.
5. Relapsed and/or refractory follicular, CD20+, B-cell non-Hodgkin's lymphoma.
6. Intermediate- and/or high-grade, CD20+, B-cell non-Hodgkin's lymphoma.

DOSAGE RANGE
Previously untreated CLL:
- 300 mg on day 1 followed by 1000 mg on day 8 (cycle 1)
- 1000 mg on day 1 of subsequent 28-day cycles for a minimum of 3 cycles until best response or a maximum of 12 cycles

Extended treatment of CLL:
- 300 mg on day 1 followed by
- 1000 mg one week later on day 8, followed by
- 1000 mg 7 weeks later and every 8 weeks thereafter for up to a maximum of 2 years

Refractory CLL:
- 300 mg initial dose on day 1 followed one week later by
- 2000 mg weekly for 7 doses, followed 4 weeks later by
- 2000 mg every 4 weeks for 4 doses

DRUG INTERACTIONS
None characterized to date.

SPECIAL CONSIDERATIONS

1. Patients should be premedicated 30 minutes to 2 hours with oral acetaminophen (1000 mg), oral or IV diphenhydramine, and IV corticosteroid (prednisolone 100 mg) to prevent the incidence of infusion-related reactions. The steroid dose for doses 1, 2, and 9 should not be reduced. If grade 3 or greater infusion reaction did not occur with the preceding dose, the steroid dose may be gradually reduced for doses 3 through 8.

2. Infusion should be started at an initial rate of 3.6 mg/hr (12 mL/hr). If no toxicity observed, rate may be escalated in 2-fold increments at 30-minute intervals to a maximum of 200 mL/hr. Second dose infusion should be started at an initial rate of 24 mg/hr (12 mL/hr). If no toxicity is observed, rate may be escalated in 2-fold increments at 30-minute intervals to a maximum of 200 mL/hr. For doses 3 through 12, infusion should be started at an initial rate of 50 mg/hr (25 mL/hr). If infusion is well tolerated, rate may be escalated in 2-fold increments at 30-minute intervals to a maximum of 400 mL/hr. Ofatumumab should NOT be given by IV push.

3. Monitor for infusion-related events, especially during the first two infusions. Infusions should be immediately stopped if signs or symptoms of an allergic reaction are observed. Immediate institution of diphenhydramine, corticosteroids, albuterol, IV fluids, and/or vasopressors may be necessary. For grade 1/2 reactions, the infusion can be restarted at a reduced rate (50%) once symptoms have completely resolved. For grade 3 reactions, interrupt infusion and if reaction resolves or remains less than or equal to grade 2, resume infusion at a rate of 12 mL/hr; resume infusion at normal escalation as tolerated. For grade 4 reactions, the infusion should be discontinued.

4. Use with caution in patients with moderate-to-severe chronic obstructive pulmonary disease.

5. Do not administer live viral vaccines to patients who have recently received ofatumumab. The ability to generate an immune response to any vaccine following administration of ofatumumab has not been studied.

6. Monitor CBCs at regular intervals during therapy.

7. Consider the diagnosis of progressive multifocal leukoencephalopathy (PML) in patients who present with new onset or changes in pre-existing neurological signs or symptoms.

8. Use with caution in patients with renal or hepatic impairment, as no formal studies of ofatumumab have been conducted in these patient populations.

9. Screen patients at high risk of hepatitis B infection before initiation of ofatumumab therapy. Closely monitor hepatitis B carriers for signs of active HBV infection during treatment with ofatumumab and for 6–12 months following the last infusion.

10. Pregnancy category C. Breastfeeding should be avoided.

TOXICITY 1
Infusion-related symptoms occur especially during the first two infusions, and present as bronchospasm, dyspnea, laryngeal edema, pulmonary edema, angioedema, syncope, back pain, abdominal pain, rash, and cardiac ischemia/infarction.

TOXICITY 2
Myelosuppression with neutropenia and thrombocytopenia.

TOXICITY 3
Progressive multifocal leukoencephalopathy (PML), with rare cases resulting in death.

TOXICITY 4
Hepatitis B reactivation.

TOXICITY 5
Small intestine obstruction.

TOXICITY 6
Increased risk of bacterial, viral, and fungal infections. Nasopharyngitis and upper respiratory infections are most commonly observed.

TOXICITY 7
Skin reactions, including macular and vesicular rash with or without urticaria.

TOXICITY 8
Mild nausea and diarrhea.

TOXICITY 9
Cough and dyspnea.

TOXICITY 10
Fatigue.

Olaparib

TRADE NAME	Lynparza	CLASSIFICATION	Signal transduction inhibitor
CATEGORY	Chemotherapy drug	DRUG MANUFACTURER	AstraZeneca

MECHANISM OF ACTION
- Small-molecule inhibitor of poly (ADP-ribose) polymerase (PARP) enzymes, including PARP1, PARP2, and PARP3.
- Inhibition of PARP enzymatic activity with increased formation of PARP-DNA complexes, results in cell death.
- Enhanced antitumor activity in tumors that are *BRCA*-deficient.

MECHANISM OF RESISTANCE
- Increased expression of the P-glycoprotein drug efflux transporter protein
- Reduced expression of p53-binding protein 1 (53BP1), which is a critical component of DNA double-strand break (DSB) signaling and repair in mammalian cells.
- Secondary mutations in *BRCA1* or *BRCA2* that result in restoration of BRCA function.
- Loss of REV7 expression and function leads to restoration of homologous recombination, resulting in PARP resistance.

ABSORPTION
Oral absorption is rapid, with peak plasma concentrations achieved between 1 and 3 hours after administration. Food with high fat content can slow the rate of absorption but does not alter systemic drug exposure.

DISTRIBUTION
Fairly extensive binding of olaparib to plasma proteins (82%). With daily dosing, steady-state blood levels are achieved in about 3–4 days.

METABOLISM
Metabolized in the liver primarily by CYP3A4 microsomal enzymes. A large fraction of an administered dose of drug is metabolized by oxidation reactions with several of the metabolites undergoing subsequent glucuronide or sulfate conjugation. Nearly 90% of drug is recovered with 42% in feces and 44% in urine, with the majority of drug being in metabolite form. The terminal half-life is on the order of 12 hours.

INDICATIONS
FDA-approved for the treatment of *BRCA*-mutated advanced ovarian cancer

DOSAGE RANGE
Recommended dose is 400 mg PO bid. Olaparib may be taken with or without food.

DRUG INTERACTION 1
Drugs that stimulate liver microsomal CYP3A4 enzymes, including phenytoin, carbamazepine, rifampin, phenobarbital, and St. John's wort—These drugs

may increase the metabolism of olaparib, resulting in lower drug levels, and potentially reduced clinically activity.

DRUG INTERACTION 2
Drugs that inhibit liver microsomal CYP3A4 enzymes, including ketoconazole, itraconazole, erythromycin, and clarithromycin—These drugs may reduce the metabolism of olaparib, resulting in increased drug levels, and potentially increased toxicity.

SPECIAL CONSIDERATIONS
1. Olaparib has not been studied in patients with liver impairment, and there are no formal recommendations for dosing in this setting.
2. No dose modification is needed in patients with mild renal impairment (CrCl 50–80 mL/min). Olaparib has not been studied in patients with moderate to severe renal impairment, and there are no formal recommendations for dosing in this setting.
3. Olaparib capsules should be swallowed whole and should not be chewed, dissolved, or crushed.
4. Closely monitor for new onset of pulmonary symptoms, and if pneumonitis is confirmed, olaparib therapy should be stopped.
5. Closely monitor blood counts at monthly intervals. For prolonged hematologic toxicities, interrupt therapy, and monitor CBCs on a weekly basis until recovery. If blood counts have not recovered within 4 weeks, bone marrow analysis and peripheral blood for cytogenetics should be performed to rule out the possibility of MDS/AML.
6. Pregnancy category D.

TOXICITY 1
Fatigue, anorexia, and asthenia.

TOXICITY 2
Increased risk of infections with nasopharyngitis, pharyngitis, and URI.

TOXICITY 3
Pneumonitis with dyspnea, fever, cough, and wheezing.

TOXICITY 4
GI side effects in the form of nausea/vomiting, abdominal pain, diarrhea, and constipation.

TOXICITY 5
Arthralgias and myalgias.

TOXICITY 6
Myelosuppression with anemia, thrombocytopenia, and neutropenia.

TOXICITY 7
MDS/AML.

O

Omacetaxine mepesuccinate

TRADE NAME	Synribo	**CLASSIFICATION**	Protein synthesis inhibitor
CATEGORY	Chemotherapy drug	**DRUG MANUFACTURER**	Cephalon/Teva

MECHANISM OF ACTION
- Precise mechanism of action not fully characterized but is independent of direct binding to Bcr-Abl.
- Inhibits protein translation by preventing the initial elongation step. It does so by interacting with the ribosomal A-site and prevents the correct positioning of amino acid side chains of incoming aminoacyl-tRNAs.
- Reduces protein expression of Bcr-Abl and Mcl-1 independent of direct Bcr-Abl binding.
- Induces apoptosis through mitochondrial disruption and cytochrome c release leading to caspase-9 and caspase-3 activation.
- Has preclinical in vivo activity against wild-type and T315I-mutated Bcr-Abl CML.

MECHANISM OF RESISTANCE
Not well characterized to date.

ABSORPTION
Following SC administration, maximum drug concentrations are achieved within 30 minutes. The absolute SC bioavailability has not yet been determined.

DISTRIBUTION
Binding to plasma proteins is <50%.

METABOLISM
Omacetaxine mepesuccinate is primarily hydrolyzed to 4′-DMHHT by plasma esterases with minimal hepatic microsomal oxidative and/or esterase-mediated metabolism. The major route of drug elimination is unknown at this time. Less than 15% of an administered dose of drug is excreted unchanged in the urine. The mean half-life is approximately 6 hours.

INDICATIONS

FDA-approved for adult patients with chronic or accelerated phase chronic myeloid leukemia (CML) with resistance and/or intolerance to two or more tyrosine kinase inhibitors.

DOSAGE RANGE

1. Recommended induction dose is 1.25 mg/m^2 SC bid for 14 consecutive days every 28 days until patients achieve a hematologic response.
2. Maintenance schedule is 1.25 mg/m^2 SC bid for 7 consecutive days every 28 days.
3. Continue treatment as long as patients are clinically benefiting.

DRUG INTERACTIONS

None well characterized to date.

SPECIAL CONSIDERATIONS

1. Patients should be weighed and monitored regularly for symptoms and signs of fluid retention, especially when using higher drug doses and in patients age >65 years.
2. Monitor CBC on a weekly basis during induction and early maintenance cycles and every 2 weeks during later maintenance cycles.
3. Patients should be warned of the risk of increased bleeding.
4. Patients should avoid anticoagulants, aspirin, and NSAIDs while on therapy.
5. Monitor blood glucose levels frequently in patients with diabetes or in patients with risk factors for diabetes. Omacetaxine mepesuccinate should be avoided in patients with poorly controlled diabetes until good glycemic control has been established.
6. Pregnancy Category D. Breastfeeding should be avoided.

TOXICITY 1

Myelosuppression with thrombocytopenia, neutropenia, and anemia. Febrile neutropenia observed in 20% of patients.

TOXICITY 2

Impaired glucose tolerance with severe hyperglycemia in up to 10% of patients.

TOXICITY 3

Increased risk of bleeding complications in the setting of thrombocytopenia. Severe, nonfatal, GI bleeding occurs rarely (2%) as well as cerebral bleeding leading to death (2%).

TOXICITY 4

Gastrointestinal toxicity with diarrhea, nausea/vomiting, abdominal pain, and anorexia.

TOXICITY 5

Mild-to-moderate headaches occur in nearly 20%.

TOXICITY 6
Fatigue and asthenia.

TOXICITY 7
Injection site reactions.

Osimertinib

TRADE NAME	Tagrisso	**CLASSIFICATION**	Signal transduction inhibitor
CATEGORY	Chemotherapy drug	**DRUG MANUFACTURER**	AstraZeneca

MECHANISM OF ACTION
- Potent and selective small-molecule inhibitor of the EGFR, which binds irreversibly to specific mutant forms of EGFR, including T790M, L858R, and exon 19 deletion.
- Inhibition of these EGFR mutants results in inhibition of critical mitogenic and antiapoptotic signals involved in proliferation, growth, invasion/metastasis, angiogenesis, and response to chemotherapy and/or radiation therapy.

MECHANISM OF RESISTANCE
- Amplification of the c-Met gene with increased gene copy number.
- Presence of BRAF mutations.
- Activation/induction of alternative cellular signaling pathways such as PI3K/Akt.

ABSORPTION
Oral bioavailability is on the order of 92%. C_{max} and AUC of osimertinib are increased by 14% and 19%, respectively following a high-fat, high-calorie meal compared to fasting state. Peak plasma drug levels are achieved in 2-5 hours after ingestion.

DISTRIBUTION
Extensive binding to plasma proteins. Steady-state drug levels are reached in approximately 15 days.

METABOLISM

Metabolism in the liver primarily by CYP3A4 microsomal enzymes with formation of two active metabolites AZ7550 and AZ5104. Elimination is mainly hepatic (approximately 70%) with excretion in the feces. The mean exposure of each of these metabolites was approximately 10% of the exposure of parent drug at steady-state. Renal elimination of parent drug and its metabolites account for only about 14% of an administered dose. The terminal half-life of the parent drug is 48 hours.

INDICATIONS

FDA-approved for treatment of metastatic NSCLC with EGFR T790M mutation as detected by an FDA-approved test who have progressed on or after TKI therapy.

DOSAGE RANGE

Recommended dose is 80 mg/day PO.

DRUG INTERACTION 1

Phenytoin and other drugs that stimulate the liver microsomal CYP3A4 enzymes, including carbamazepine, rifampin, phenobarbital, and St. John's wort—These drugs may increase the metabolism of osimertinib, resulting in its inactivation.

DRUG INTERACTION 2

Drugs that inhibit the liver microsomal CYP3A4 enzymes, including ketoconazole, itraconazole, erythromycin, and clarithromycin—These drugs may decrease the metabolism of osimertinib, resulting in increased drug levels and potentially increased toxicity.

DRUG INTERACTION 3

Warfarin—Patients receiving coumarin-derived anticoagulants should be closely monitored for alterations in their clotting parameters (PT and INR) and/or bleeding, as osimertinib may inhibit the metabolism of warfarin by the liver P450 system. Dose of warfarin may require careful adjustment in the presence of osimertinib therapy.

SPECIAL CONSIDERATIONS

1. Dose reduction is not recommended in patients with mild hepatic dysfunction. However, osimertinib has not been studied in patients with moderate or severe hepatic dysfunction, and caution should be used in this setting.
2. Dose reduction is not recommended in patients with mild or moderate renal dysfunction. However, osimertinib has not been studied in patients with severe renal dysfunction and caution should be used in this setting.
3. Closely monitor patients for new or progressive pulmonary symptoms, including cough, dyspnea, and fever. Osimertinib therapy should be interrupted pending further diagnostic evaluation.
4. Baseline and periodic evaluations of ECG and electrolyte status should be performed while on therapy. If the QTc >500 msec, therapy should be interrupted. Use with caution in patients at risk of developing QT

prolongation, including hypokalemia, hypomagnesemia, congenital long QT syndrome, and in patients taking antiarrhythmic medications or any other drugs that may cause QT prolongation.

5. Baseline and periodic evaluations of LVEF should be performed while on therapy. If there is an absolute decrease in LVEF of 10% from baseline and below 50%, therapy should be interrupted for up to 4 weeks. If the LVEF improves to baseline, therapy can resume. However, if the LVEF does not return to baseline, therapy should be terminated. In the setting of symptomatic CHF, therapy should be permanently discontinued.

6. Patients should be warned to avoid sunlight exposure.

7. Avoid Seville oranges, starfruit, pomelos, grapefruit, and grapefruit juice while on osimertinib therapy.

8. Pregnancy category D. Breastfeeding should be avoided.

TOXICITY 1
Skin toxicity in the form of rash, dry skin, pruritus, and nail bed changes.

TOXICITY 2
Diarrhea is most common GI toxicity. Mild nausea/vomiting, mucositis, and constipation are also observed.

TOXICITY 3
Pulmonary toxicity in the form of ILD manifested by increased cough, dyspnea, fever, and pulmonary infiltrates. Observed in approximately 3% of patients.

TOXICITY 4
QTc prolongation.

TOXICITY 5
Fatigue, anorexia, and reduced appetite.

TOXICITY 6
Cardiomyopathy and CHF.

Oxaliplatin

TRADE NAMES	Eloxatin, Diaminocyclohexane platinum	CLASSIFICATION	Platinum analog
CATEGORY	Chemotherapy drug	DRUG MANUFACTURER	Sanofi-Aventis

MECHANISM OF ACTION

- Third-generation platinum compound.
- Cell cycle–nonspecific with activity in all phases of the cell cycle.
- Covalently binds to DNA with preferential binding to the N-7 position of guanine and adenine.
- Reacts with two different sites on DNA to produce cross-links, either intrastrand (<90%) or interstrand (<5%). Formation of DNA adducts results in inhibition of DNA synthesis and function as well as inhibition of transcription.
- DNA mismatch repair enzymes are unable to recognize oxaliplatin-DNA adducts in contrast with other platinum-DNA adducts as a result of their bulkier size.
- Binding to nuclear and cytoplasmic proteins may result in additional cytotoxic effects.

MECHANISM OF RESISTANCE

- Decreased drug accumulation due to alterations in cellular transport.
- Increased inactivation by thiol-containing proteins such as glutathione and glutathione-related enzymes.
- Increased DNA repair enzyme activity (e.g., ERCC-1).
- Non–cross-resistant to cisplatin and carboplatin in tumor cells that are deficient in MMR enzymes (e.g., hMHL1, hMSH2).

ABSORPTION

Not orally bioavailable.

DISTRIBUTION

Widely distributed to all tissues with a 50-fold higher volume of distribution than cisplatin. About 40% of drug is sequestered in red blood cells within 2–5 hours of infusion. Extensively binds to plasma proteins in time-dependent manner (up to 98%).

METABOLISM

Oxaliplatin undergoes extensive non-enzymatic conversion to its active cytotoxic species. As observed with cisplatin, oxaliplatin undergoes aquation reaction in the presence of low concentrations of chloride. The major species are monochloro-DACH, dichloro-DACH, and mono-diaquo-DACH platinum. Renal excretion accounts for >50% of oxaliplatin clearance. More than 20 different metabolites have been identified in the urine. Only 2% of drug is excreted in feces. Prolonged terminal half-life of up to 240 hours.

INDICATIONS

1. Metastatic colorectal cancer—FDA-approved in combination with infusional 5-FU/LV in patients with advanced, metastatic disease.
2. Early-stage colon cancer—FDA-approved as adjuvant therapy in combination with infusional 5-FU/LV in patients with stage III colon cancer and also effective in patients with high-risk stage II disease.
3. Metastatic pancreatic cancer.
4. Metastatic gastric cancer and gastroesophageal cancer.

DOSAGE RANGE

Recommended dose is 85 mg/m^2 IV over 2 hours, on an every 2-week schedule. Can also administer 100–130 mg/m^2 IV on an every 3-week schedule.

DRUG INTERACTIONS

None known.

SPECIAL CONSIDERATIONS

1. Use with caution in patients with abnormal renal function, especially when CrCl <20 mL/min. Baseline creatinine clearance should be obtained, and renal status should be closely monitored during treatment.
2. Oxaliplatin should not be administered with basic solutions (e.g., solutions containing 5-FU), as it may be partially degraded.
3. Careful neurologic evaluation should be performed before starting therapy and at the beginning of each cycle as the dose-limiting toxicity of oxaliplatin is neurotoxicity.
4. Caution patients to avoid exposure to cold following drug administration, which can trigger and/or worsen acute neurotoxicity.
5. Calcium/magnesium infusions (1 g calcium gluconate/1 g magnesium sulfate) prior to and at the completion of the oxaliplatin infusion can be used to reduce the incidence of acute neurotoxicity. There is no evidence that these infusions impair the clinical activity of oxaliplatin.
6. May lengthen oxaliplatin infusion from 2 to up to 4 hours to reduce the incidence of acute neurotoxicity.
7. Anaphylactic reactions to oxaliplatin have been reported and may occur within minutes of drug administration. This adverse event represents a black-box warning.
8. Pregnancy category D. Breastfeeding should be avoided.

TOXICITY 1

Neurotoxicity with acute and chronic forms. Acute toxicity is seen in up to 80%–85% of patients and is characterized by a peripheral sensory neuropathy with distal paresthesia and visual and voice changes, often triggered or exacerbated by cold. Dysesthesias in the upper extremities and laryngopharyngeal region with episodes of difficulty breathing or swallowing are also observed usually within hours or 1–3 days after therapy. Risk increases upon exposure to cold and usually is spontaneously reversible. Chronic toxicity is dose-dependent with a 15% and >50% risk of impairment in proprioception and neurosensory function at cumulative doses of 850 and 1200 mg/m^2, respectively.

In contrast to cisplatin-induced neurotoxicity, oxaliplatin-induced neuropathy is more readily reversible, and returns to normal usually within 3–4 months of discontinuation of oxaliplatin. Gait abnormalities and cognitive dysfunction can also occur.

TOXICITY 2
Nausea/vomiting. Occurs in 65% of patients treated with single-agent oxaliplatin and in 90% of patients treated with the combination of 5-FU/LV and oxaliplatin. Usually well-controlled with antiemetic therapy.

TOXICITY 3
Diarrhea.

TOXICITY 4
Myelosuppression. Relatively mild with thrombocytopenia and anemia more common than neutropenia. Autoimmune thrombocytopenia, autoimmune hemolytic anemia, and TTP have also been observed, albeit rarely.

TOXICITY 5
Allergic reactions with facial flushing, rash, urticaria, and less frequently, bronchospasm and hypotension. In rare cases, anaphylactic-like reactions can occur.

TOXICITY 6
Hepatotoxicity with sinusoidal injury resulting in portal hypertension, ascites, splenomegaly, thrombocytopenia, and varices.

TOXICITY 7
RPLS has been observed with headache, lethargy, seizures, visual disturbances, and encephalopathy.

TOXICITY 8
Rare cases of bronchiolitis obliterans organizing pneumonia (BOOP), acute ILD, and pulmonary fibrosis.

P

Paclitaxel

TRADE NAME	Taxol	CLASSIFICATION	Taxane, antimicrotubule agent
CATEGORY	Chemotherapy drug	DRUG MANUFACTURER	Bristol-Myers Squibb

MECHANISM OF ACTION
- Isolated from the bark of the Pacific yew tree, *Taxus brevifolia*.
- Cell cycle–specific, active in the mitosis (M) phase of the cell cycle.
- High-affinity binding to microtubules enhances tubulin polymerization. Normal dynamic process of microtubule network is inhibited, leading to inhibition of mitosis and cell division.

MECHANISM OF RESISTANCE
- Alterations in tubulin with decreased binding affinity for drug.
- Multidrug-resistant phenotype with increased expression of P170 glycoprotein. Results in enhanced drug efflux with decreased intracellular accumulation of drug. Cross-resistant to other natural products, including vinca alkaloids, anthracyclines, taxanes, and etoposide.

ABSORPTION
Poorly soluble and not orally bioavailable.

DISTRIBUTION
Distributes widely to all body tissues, including third-space fluid collections such as ascites. Negligible penetration into the CNS. Extensive binding (>90%) to plasma and cellular proteins.

METABOLISM
Metabolized extensively by the hepatic P450 microsomal system. About 70%–80% of drug is excreted via fecal elimination. Less than 10% is eliminated as the parent form with the majority being eliminated as metabolites. Renal clearance

is relatively minor with less than 10% of drug cleared via the kidneys. Terminal elimination half-life ranges from 9 to 50 hours depending on the schedule of administration.

INDICATIONS
1. Ovarian cancer.
2. Breast cancer.
3. SCLC and NSCLC.
4. Head and neck cancer.
5. Esophageal cancer.
6. Prostate cancer.
7. Bladder cancer.
8. AIDS-related Kaposi's sarcoma.

DOSAGE RANGE
1. Ovarian cancer: 135–175 mg/m^2 IV as a 3-hour infusion every 3 weeks.
2. Breast cancer: 175 mg/m^2 IV as a 3-hour infusion every 3 weeks.
3. Bladder cancer, head and neck cancer: 250 mg/m^2 IV as a 24-hour infusion every 3 weeks.
4. Weekly schedule: 80–100 mg/m^2 IV each week for 3 weeks with 1-week rest.
5. Infusional schedule: 140 mg/m^2 as a 96-hour infusion.

DRUG INTERACTION 1
Radiation therapy—Paclitaxel is a radiosensitizing agent.

DRUG INTERACTION 2
Concomitant use of inhibitors and/or activators of the liver P450 CYP3A4 enzyme system may affect paclitaxel metabolism and its subsequent antitumor and toxic effects.

DRUG INTERACTION 3
Phenytoin, phenobarbital—Accelerate the metabolism of paclitaxel resulting in lower plasma levels of drug.

DRUG INTERACTION 4
Cisplatin, carboplatin—Myelosuppression is greater when platinum compound is administered before paclitaxel. Platinum compounds inhibit plasma clearance of paclitaxel. When a platinum analog is used in combination, paclitaxel must be given first.

DRUG INTERACTION 5
Cyclophosphamide—Myelosuppression is greater when cyclophosphamide is administered before paclitaxel.

DRUG INTERACTION 6
Doxorubicin—Paclitaxel reduces the plasma clearance of doxorubicin by about 30%, resulting in increased severity of myelosuppression.

SPECIAL CONSIDERATIONS

1. Contraindicated in patients with history of severe hypersensitivity reaction to paclitaxel or to other drugs formulated in Cremophor EL, including cyclosporine, etoposide, or teniposide.
2. Use with caution in patients with abnormal liver function. Dose reduction is required in this setting. Patients with abnormal liver function are at significantly higher risk for toxicity. Contraindicated in patients with severe hepatic dysfunction.
3. Use with caution in patients with prior history of diabetes mellitus and chronic alcoholism or prior therapy with known neurotoxic agents such as cisplatin.
4. Use with caution in patients with previous history of ischemic heart disease, with MI within the preceding 6 months, conduction system abnormalities, or on medications known to alter cardiac conduction (beta blockers, calcium channel blockers, and digoxin).
5. Patients should receive premedication to prevent the incidence of hypersensitivity reactions. Give dexamethasone 20 mg PO at 12 and 6 hours before drug administration, diphenhydramine 50 mg IV, and cimetidine 300 mg IV at 30 minutes before drug administration. Patients experiencing major hypersensitivity reaction may be rechallenged after receiving multiple high doses of steroids, dexamethasone 20 mg IV every 6 hr for 4 doses. Patients should also be treated with diphenhydramine 50 mg IV and cimetidine 300 mg IV 30 minutes before the rechallenge.
6. Medical personnel should be readily available at the time of drug administration. Emergency equipment, including Ambu bag, ECG machine, IV fluids, pressors, and other drugs for resuscitation, must be at bedside before initiation of treatment.
7. Monitor patient's vital signs every 15 minutes during the first hour of drug administration. Hypersensitivity reaction usually occurs within 2–3 minutes of start of infusion and almost always within the first 10 minutes.
8. Patients who have received >6 courses of weekly paclitaxel should be advised to avoid sun exposure of their skin as well as their fingernails and toenails, as they are at increased risk for developing onycholysis. This side effect is not observed with the every-3-week schedule.
9. Pregnancy category D. Breastfeeding should be avoided.

TOXICITY 1

Myelosuppression. Dose-limiting neutropenia with nadir at day 8–10 and recovery by day 15–21. Decreased incidence of neutropenia with 3-hour schedule when compared to 24-hour schedule.

TOXICITY 2

Infusion reactions. Occurs in up to 20%–40% of patients. Characterized by generalized skin rash, flushing, erythema, hypotension, dyspnea, and/or bronchospasm. Usually occurs within the first 2–3 minutes of an infusion and almost always within the first 10 minutes. Incidence of hypersensitivity reaction is the same with 3- and 24-hour schedules. Premedication regimen, as outlined in Special Considerations, has significantly decreased incidence.

TOXICITY 3

Neurotoxicity mainly in the form of sensory neuropathy with numbness and paresthesias. Dose-dependent effect. Other risk factors include prior exposure to known neurotoxic agents (e.g., cisplatin) and pre-existing medical disorders such as diabetes mellitus and chronic alcoholism. More frequent with longer infusions and at doses >175 mg/m^2. Motor and autonomic neuropathy observed at high doses. Optic nerve disturbances with scintillating scotomata observed rarely.

TOXICITY 4

Transient asymptomatic sinus bradycardia is most commonly observed cardiotoxicity. Occurs in 30% of patients. Other rhythm disturbances are seen, including Mobitz type I, Mobitz type II, and third-degree heart block, as well as ventricular arrhythmias.

TOXICITY 5

Alopecia. Occurs in nearly all patients, with loss of total body hair.

TOXICITY 6

Mucositis and/or diarrhea seen in 30%–40% of patients. Mucositis is more common with the 24-hour schedule. Mild-to-moderate nausea and vomiting, usually of brief duration.

TOXICITY 7

Transient elevations in serum transaminases, bilirubin, and alkaline phosphatase.

TOXICITY 8

Onycholysis. Mainly observed in those receiving >6 courses on the weekly schedule. Not seen with the every-3-week schedule.

Palbociclib

TRADE NAMES	Ibrance, PD 0332991	CLASSIFICATION	Signal transduction inhibitor
CATEGORY	Chemotherapy drug	DRUG MANUFACTURER	Pfizer

MECHANISM OF ACTION
- Inhibitor of cyclin-dependent kinase (CDK) 4 and 6.
- Inhibition of CDK 4/6 leads to inhibition of cell proliferation and growth by blocking progression of cells from G1 to the S-phase of the cell cycle.
- Decreased retinoblastoma (Rb) protein phosphorylation resulting in reduced E2F expression and signaling.
- Induces cell senescence.

MECHANISM OF RESISTANCE
None well characterized to date.

ABSORPTION
Oral bioavailability is on the order of 46%. Food intake appears to reduce the interpatient variability of drug exposure.

DISTRIBUTION
Significant binding (85%) to plasma proteins and extensive tissue distribution. Steady-state drug levels are achieved within 8 days following repeat daily dosing.

METABOLISM
Extensively metabolized in the liver primarily by CYP3A4 microsomal enzymes with oxidation and sulfonation reactions being most important. Acylation and glucuronidation play only minor roles in drug metabolism. Nearly 92% of drug is recovered with 74% in feces and 17.5% in urine, with the majority of drug being in metabolite form. The elimination half-life of the drug is 26 hours.

INDICATIONS
1. FDA-approved in combination with letrozole for patients with hormone receptor (HR)-positive, HER2-negative advanced or metastatic breast cancer as initial endocrine-based therapy in post-menopausal women.
2. FDA-approved in combination with fulvestrant for patients with hormone receptor (HR)-positive, HER2-negative advanced or metastatic breast cancer in women with disease progression following endocrine therapy.

DOSAGE RANGE
Recommended dose is 125 mg PO daily for 21 days followed by 7 days off.

DRUG INTERACTION 1
Drugs that stimulate liver microsomal CYP3A4 enzymes, including phenytoin, carbamazepine, rifampin, phenobarbital, and St. John's wort—These drugs may increase the metabolism of palbociclib, resulting in lower drug levels, and potentially reduced clinically activity.

DRUG INTERACTION 2
Drugs that inhibit liver microsomal CYP3A4 enzymes, including ketoconazole, itraconazole, erythromycin, and clarithromycin—These drugs may reduce the metabolism of palbociclib, resulting in increased drug levels and potentially increased toxicity.

SPECIAL CONSIDERATIONS
1. Dose reduction is not required in the setting of mild hepatic impairment. Use with caution in patients with moderate or severe hepatic impairment, although no specific dose recommendations have been provided.
2. Dose reduction is not required in the setting of mild and moderate renal impairment. Use with caution in patients with severe renal impairment as palbociclib has not been studied in this setting.
3. Closely monitor CBC and platelet count every 2 weeks during the first 2 months of therapy and at monthly intervals thereafter.
4. Monitor for signs and symptoms of infection.
5. Monitor for signs and symptoms of pulmonary embolism.
6. Pregnancy category D.

TOXICITY 1
Myelosuppression with neutropenia, anemia, and thrombocytopenia.

TOXICITY 2
Fatigue and anorexia.

TOXICITY 3
Increased risk of infections with URI being most common.

TOXICITY 4
Nausea/vomiting, abdominal pain, and diarrhea.

TOXICITY 5
Increased risk of pulmonary emboli.

TOXICITY 6
Alopecia.

Panitumumab

TRADE NAME	Vectibix	CLASSIFICATION	Monoclonal antibody, anti-EGFR antibody
CATEGORY	Biologic response modifier agent	DRUG MANUFACTURER	Amgen

MECHANISM OF ACTION
- Fully human IgG2 monoclonal antibody directed against the EGFR.
- Precise mechanism(s) of action remains unknown.
- Binds with nearly 40-fold higher affinity to EGFR than normal ligands EGF and TGF-α, which results in inhibition of EGFR. Prevents both

homodimerization and heterodimerization of the EGFR, which leads to inhibition of autophosphorylation and inhibition of EGFR signaling.
- Inhibition of the EGFR signaling pathway results in inhibition of critical mitogenic and antiapoptotic signals involved in proliferation, growth, invasion/metastasis, and angiogenesis.
- Inhibition of the EGFR pathway enhances the response to chemotherapy and/or radiation therapy.

MECHANISM OF RESISTANCE
- Mutations in the EGFR leading to decreased binding affinity to panitumumab.
- Decreased expression of EGFR.
- KRAS mutations, which mainly occur in codons 12 and 13.
- BRAF mutations.
- NRAS mutations.
- Increased expression of HER2 through gene amplification.
- Increased expression of HER3.
- Activation/induction of alternative cellular signaling pathways, such as PI3K/Akt and IGF-1R.

DISTRIBUTION
Distribution in the body is not well characterized.

METABOLISM
Metabolism of panitumumab has not been extensively characterized. Pharmacokinetic studies showed clearance of antibody was saturated at a weekly dose of 2 mg/kg. Half-life is on the order of 6–7 days.

INDICATIONS
1. FDA-approved as monotherapy for the treatment of advanced colorectal cancer following fluoropyrimidine-, oxaliplatin-, and irinotecan-containing regimens. Use of panitumumab is not recommended in mutant KRAS mCRC.
2. Approved in Europe as monotherapy for advanced, refractory disease in wild-type KRAS CRC.
3. FDA-approved for the first-line treatment of wild-type KRAS (exon 2 in codons 12 or 13) mCRC in combination with FOLFOX chemotherapy.

DOSAGE RANGE
1. Recommended dose for the treatment of mCRC is 6 mg/kg IV on an every 2-week schedule.
2. An alternative schedule is 2.5 mg/kg IV every week.

DRUG INTERACTIONS
No formal drug interactions have been characterized to date.

SPECIAL CONSIDERATIONS
1. The incidence of infusion reactions is lower when compared with cetuximab, as panitumumab is a fully human antibody. Reduce infusion

rate by 50% in patients who experience grade 1/2 infusion reaction for the duration of that infusion. The infusion should be terminated in patients who experience a severe infusion reaction.

2. The level of EGFR expression does not correlate with clinical activity, and as such, EGFR testing should not be required for clinical use.

3. Extended RAS testing should be performed in all patients to determine KRAS and NRAS status. Only patients whose tumors express wild-type KRAS and NRAS should receive panitumumab therapy.

4. Development of skin toxicity appears to be a surrogate marker for panitumumab clinical activity. Refer to the prescribing information for dose modifications in the setting of skin toxicity.

5. Use with caution in patients with underlying ILD as these patients are at increased risk for developing worsening of their ILD.

6. In patients who develop a skin rash, topical antibiotics such as clindamycin gel or erythromycin cream/gel either oral clindamycin, oral doxycycline, or oral minocycline may help. Patients should be warned to avoid sunlight exposure.

7. Electrolyte status (magnesium and calcium) should be closely monitored during therapy and for up to 8 weeks after completion of therapy.

8. Pregnancy category C. Breastfeeding should be avoided.

TOXICITY 1
Pruritus, dry skin with mainly a pustular, acneiform skin rash. Presents mainly on the face and upper trunk. Improves with continued treatment and resolves upon cessation of therapy. Skin toxicity occurs in up to 90% of patients with grade 3/4 toxicity occurring in 15% of patients.

TOXICITY 2
Infusion-related symptoms with fever, chills, urticaria, flushing, and headache. Usually minor in severity and observed most commonly with administration of the first infusion.

TOXICITY 3
Pulmonary toxicity in the form of ILD manifested by increased cough, dyspnea, and pulmonary infiltrates. Observed rarely in less than 1% of patients and more frequent in patients with underlying pulmonary disease.

TOXICITY 4
Hypomagnesemia.

TOXICITY 5
Diarrhea.

TOXICITY 6
Asthenia and generalized malaise observed in up to 10%–15%.

TOXICITY 7
Paronychial inflammation with swelling of the lateral nail folds of the toes and fingers. Usually occurs with prolonged use of panitumumab.

Panobinostat

TRADE NAMES	Farydak, LBH 589	**CLASSIFICATION**	Histone deacetylase (HDAC) inhibitor
CATEGORY	Chemotherapy drug	**DRUG MANUFACTURER**	Novartis

MECHANISM OF ACTION
- Potent pan-inhibitor of histone deacetylase (HDAC) enzymes.
- Inhibition of HDAC activity leads to accumulation of acetyl groups on the histone lysine residues, resulting in open chromatin structure and transcriptional activation.
- HDAC inhibition activates differentiation, inhibits the cell cycle, and induces cell cycle arrest and apoptosis.
- Increased expression of HDAC in human tumors, including multiple myeloma.

MECHANISM OF RESISTANCE
None well characterized to date.

DISTRIBUTION
Approximately 90% of drug is bound to plasma proteins. Oral bioavailability is on the order of 21%, and peak plasma levels are achieved within 2 hours after ingestion.

METABOLISM
Extensively metabolized in the liver by microsomal enzymes, with CYP3A4 accounting for about 40% of drug metabolism. Only 2% of parent drug is recovered in urine. The drug is a P-glycoprotein substrate and a CYP2D6 inhibitor. Approximately equal amounts of an administered dose of drug is excreted in feces and in urine, and only less than 2% of parent drug is recovered in urine. The elimination half-life is on the order of 30 hours.

INDICATIONS
FDA-approved for the treatment of patients with multiple myeloma who have received at least 2 prior regimens, including bortezomib and an immunomodulatory agent.

DOSAGE RANGE

Recommended dose is 20 mg PO on days 1, 3, 5, 8, 10, and 12 of weeks 1 and 2 with cycles repeated every 21 days for 8 cycles.

DRUG INTERACTION 1

Drugs that stimulate liver microsomal CYP3A4 enzymes, including phenytoin, carbamazepine, rifampin, phenobarbital, and St. John's wort—These drugs may increase the metabolism of panobinostat, resulting in lower drug levels, and potentially reduced clinically activity.

DRUG INTERACTION 2

Drugs that inhibit liver microsomal CYP3A4 enzymes, including ketoconazole, itraconazole, erythromycin, and clarithromycin—These drugs may reduce the metabolism of panobinostat, resulting in increased drug levels, and potentially increased toxicity.

DRUG INTERACTION 3

Drugs that serve as substrates of CYP2D6, including perphenazine, atomoxetine, desipramine, dextromethorphan, metoprolol, nebivolol, tolterodine, and venlafaxine—Panobinostat is a CYP2D6 inhibitor, and co-administration with CYP2D6 substrates may result in higher drug levels and potentially increased toxicity.

SPECIAL CONSIDERATIONS

1. Use with caution in patients with hepatic impairment. Dose modification is recommended in the setting of mild and moderate hepatic impairment. Panobinostat should not be administered to patients with severe hepatic impairment as the drug has not been used in this setting.
2. Panobinostat can be used safely in patients with mild, moderate, and severe renal dysfunction. However, it has not been tested in patients with end-stage renal disease or in those undergoing dialysis.
3. Closely monitor patients for diarrhea, which can occur at any time. Important to monitor the hydration status of the patient and closely follow serum electrolytes, including potassium, magnesium, and phosphate. Anti-diarrheal medication should be started at the onset of diarrhea, and panobinostat should be interrupted with the onset of moderate diarrhea. This represents a black-box warning.
4. Closely monitor for cardiac toxicities, which include ECG changes, arrhythmias, and cardiac ischemic events. Panobinostat should not be given to patients with history of recent MI or unstable angina. This represents a black-box warning.
5. Monitor CBC and platelet count on a weekly basis during treatment.
6. Monitor liver function tests before treatment and before the start of each cycle. Interrupt and/or adjust dosage until recovery, or permanently discontinue based on the severity of the hepatic toxicity.
7. Monitor ECG with QTc measurement at baseline and periodically during therapy as QTc prolongation has been observed.

8. Monitor patients for infections, as pneumonia, bacterial infections, fungal infections, and viral infections have been observed. Panobinostat should be interrupted and/or terminated with the development of active infections.
9. Pregnancy category D.

TOXICITY 1

Diarrhea and nausea/vomiting are the most common GI side effects.

TOXICITY 2

Myelosuppression with thrombocytopenia and neutropenia more common than anemia.

TOXICITY 3

Cardiac toxicity with ECG changes, arrhythmias, and cardiac ischemic events. QTc prolongation has been observed.

TOXICITY 4

Hepatotoxicity.

TOXICITY 5

Increased risk of infections with pneumonia, bacterial infections, fungal infections, and viral infections.

TOXICITY 6

Electrolyte abnormalities with hypokalemia, hypomagnesemia, and hypophosphatemia.

TOXICITY 7

Peripheral neuropathy.

Pazopanib

TRADE NAME	Votrient	CLASSIFICATION	Signal transduction inhibitor
CATEGORY	Chemotherapy drug	DRUG MANUFACTURER	GlaxoSmithKline

MECHANISM OF ACTION
- Oral multikinase inhibitor of angiogenesis.
- Inhibits VEGFR-1, VEGFR-2, VEGFR-3, platelet-derived growth factor receptor (PDGFR)-α and PDGFR–β, fibroblast growth factor receptor (FGFR)-1 and FGFR-3, c-Kit, interleukin-2 receptor inducible T-cell kinase (Itk), leukocyte-specific protein tyrosine kinase (Lck), and transmembrane glycoprotein receptor tyrosine kinase (c-Fms).

MECHANISM OF RESISTANCE
- Mechanisms of resistance have not been well characterized.
- Increased expression of VEGFR-1, VEGFR-2, VEGFR-3, PDGFR, FGFR, and c-Kit.
- Mutations in target receptors resulting in alterations in drug-binding affinity.
- Increased degradation and/or metabolism of the drug.

ABSORPTION
Pazopanib is absorbed orally with median time to peak concentrations of 2–4 hours. Systemic exposure to pazopanib is increased when administered with food. The bioavailability and the rate of pazopanib oral absorption are also increased after administration of the crushed tablet relative to administration of the whole tablet.

DISTRIBUTION
Extensive binding (>99%) of pazopanib to plasma proteins.

METABOLISM
Pazopanib undergoes oxidative metabolism primarily by CYP3A4 microsomal enzymes and to a lesser extent by CYP1A2 and CYP2C8 isoenzymes. Pazopanib is a weak inhibitor of CYP2C8 and CYP2D6, as well as UGT1A1 and OATP1B1, and it is a substrate for P-glycoprotein. Elimination is primarily via feces, with renal elimination accounting for less than 4% of the administered dose. In patients with moderate hepatic impairment, clearance is decreased by 50%. A plateau in steady-state drug exposure is observed at doses of $\geqslant$ 800 mg once daily, and the half-life is 31 hours.

INDICATIONS
1. FDA-approved for the treatment of advanced renal cell carcinoma.
2. FDA-approved for the treatment of advanced soft tissue sarcoma (STS) following treatment with prior chemotherapy. The efficacy of pazaponib has not been docmented in adipocytic STS or GIST.

DOSAGE RANGE

Recommended dose is 800 mg PO once daily without food at least 1 hour before or 2 hours after a meal.

DRUG INTERACTION 1

Concomitant administration of CYP3A4 inhibitors such as ketoconazole, itraconazole, clarithromycin, atazanavir, indinavir, nefazodone, nelfinavir, ritonavir, saquinavir, telithromycin, and voriconazole decrease the rate of pazopanib metabolism, resulting in increased drug levels and potentially increased toxicity.

DRUG INTERACTION 2

Concomitant administration of CYP3A4 inducers such as phenytoin, carbamazepine, rifampin, phenobarbital, and St. John's wort increase the rate of metabolism of pazopanib, resulting in its inactivation and reduced drug levels.

SPECIAL CONSIDERATIONS

1. Baseline and periodic evaluation of liver function tests (at weeks 3, 5, 7, and 9 and at month 3 and 4) should be performed while on pazopanib therapy. Patients with isolated SGOT elevations between 3 × ULN and 8 × ULN may be continued on therapy with weekly monitoring of LFTs until they return to grade 1 or baseline. In this setting, the dose of pazopanib should be reduced to 200 mg PO once daily. Patients with isolated SGOT elevations of more than 8 × ULN should have pazopanib therapy interrupted.
2. Use with caution in patients with moderate hepatic impairment, as drug clearance is reduced by at least 50% in this setting. No data is presently available in patients with mild or severe hepatic impairment.
3. Closely monitor ECG with QT measurement at baseline and periodically during therapy, as QT prolongation has been observed. Use with caution in patients at risk of developing QT prolongation, including hypokalemia, hypomagnesemia, congenital long QT syndrome, patients taking antiarrhythmic medications or any other products that may cause QT prolongation, and in those with pre-existing cardiac disease.
4. Avoid use in patients with a prior history of hemoptysis and cerebral or clinically significant GI hemorrhage within 6 months of initiation of pazopanib.
5. Use with caution in patients with cardiovascular and cerebrovascular disease, especially those with prior MI, angina, stroke, and TIA.
6. Closely monitor blood pressure while on therapy.
7. Blood pressure should be well controlled prior to initiation of pazopanib.
8. Closely monitor thyroid function tests, as pazopanib therapy results in hypothyroidism.
9. Baseline and periodic urinalysis during treatment is recommended, and pazopanib should be discontinued in the setting of grade 4 proteinuria.
10. Avoid Seville oranges, starfruit, pomelos, grapefruit, and grapefruit products while on pazopanib therapy, as they can inhibit CYP3A4 activity, resulting in increased drug levels.
11. Pregnancy category D. Breastfeeding should be avoided.

TOXICITY 1
Hypertension occurs in nearly 50% of patients. Usually occurs within the first 18 weeks of therapy and is well controlled with oral antihypertensive medications.

TOXICITY 2
Diarrhea, nausea/vomiting, and abdominal pain are the most common GI side effects. Elevations in serum lipase have been observed in up to 30% of patients. Increased risk of GI fistulas and/or perforations.

TOXICITY 3
Fatigue, asthenia, and anorexia may be significant in some patients.

TOXICITY 4
Hair color changes with depigmentation.

TOXICITY 5
Bleeding complications with hematuria, epistaxis, and hemoptysis.

TOXICITY 6
Increased risk of arterial thrombolic events, including MI, angina, TIA, and stroke.

TOXICITY 7
Proteinuria develops in 8% of patients.

TOXICITY 8
Myelosuppression with neutropenia and thrombocytopenia. Usually mild to moderate in severity.

TOXICITY 9
Hypothyroidism.

TOXICITY 10
Elevations in serum transaminases usually observed within the first 18 weeks of therapy. Indirect hyperbilirubinemia may occur in patients with underlying Gilbert's syndrome.

TOXICITY 11
Cardiac toxicity with QT prolongation ($\geq$ 500 msec) and torsades de pointes.

TOXICITY 12
Electrolyte abnormalities with hyperglycemia, hypophosphatemia, hyponatremia, hypomagnesemia, and hypoglycemia.

Pembrolizumab

TRADE NAMES	Keytruda, MK-3475	CLASSIFICATION	Monoclonal antibody
CATEGORY	Immune checkpoint inhibitor	DRUG MANUFACTURER	Merck

MECHANISM OF ACTION
- Humanized IgG4 antibody that binds to the PD-1 receptor, which is expressed on T cells, and inhibits the interaction between the PD-L1 and PD-L2 ligands and the PD-1 receptor.
- Blockade of the PD-1 pathway-mediated immune checkpoint enhances T-cell immune response, leading to T-cell activation and proliferation.

MECHANISM OF RESISTANCE
None well characterized to date.

DISTRIBUTION
Distribution in body is not well characterized. Steady-state levels are achieved by 18 weeks.

METABOLISM
Metabolism of pembrolizumab has not been extensively characterized. The terminal half-life is on the order of 26 days.

INDICATIONS
1. FDA-approved for unresectable or metastatic melanoma.
2. FDA-approved for patients with metastatic NSCLC whose tumors express PD-L1 as determined by an FDA-approved test and who have disease progression on or after platinum-based chemotherapy. Patients with EGFR or ALK genomic alterations should have disease progression on FDA-approved targeted therapy prior to receiving pembrolizumab.
3. FDA-approved for recurrent or metastatic head and neck cancer with disease progression on or after platinum-based chemotherapy.

DOSAGE RANGE
1. Melanoma: Recommended dose is 2 mg/kg IV every 3 weeks.
2. NSCLC: Recommended dose is 200 mg IV every 3 weeks.
3. Head and neck cancer: Recommended dose is 200 mg IV every 3 weeks.

DRUG INTERACTIONS
None well characterized to date

SPECIAL CONSIDERATIONS
1. Pembrolizumab can result in significant immune-mediated adverse reactions due to T-cell activation and proliferation. These

immune-mediated reactions may involve any organ system, with the most common reactions being pneumonitis, colitis, hepatitis, hypophysitis, nephritis, and thyroid dysfunction.

2. Pembrolizumab should be withheld for any of the following:
   - Grade 2 pneumonitis
   - Grade 2 or 3 colitis
   - SGOT/SGPT >3×ULN and up to 5×ULN or total bilirubin >1.5×ULN and up to 3×ULN
   - Grade 2 nephritis
   - Symptomatic hypophysitis
   - Grade 3 hyperthyroidism
   - Any other severe or grade 3 treatment-related toxicity

3. Pembrolizumab should be permanently discontinued for any of the following:
   - Any life-threatening toxicity
   - Grade 3 or 4 pneumonitis
   - SGOT/SGPT >5×ULN or total bilirubin >3×ULN
   - Grade 3 or 4 infusion-related reactions
   - Grade 3 or 4 nephritis
   - Any severe or grade 3 toxicity that recurs
   - Inability to reduce steroid dose to 10 mg or less of prednisone or equivalent per day within 12 weeks

4. Monitor thyroid function prior to and during therapy.
5. Dose modification is not needed for patients with renal dysfunction.
6. Dose modification is not needed for patients with mild hepatic dysfunction. Pembrolizumab has not been studied in patients with moderate to severe hepatic dysfunction.
7. Pregnancy category D.

TOXICITY 1
Colitis with diarrhea and abdominal pain.

TOXICITY 2
Pneumonitis with dyspnea and cough.

TOXICITY 3
GI side effects with nausea/vomiting; dry mouth; hepatitis with elevations in SGOT/SGPT, alkaline phosphatase, and serum bilirubin seen in up to 20%–30% of patients; and pancreatitis.

TOXICITY 4
Fatigue, anorexia, and asthenia.

TOXICITY 5
Nephritis.

TOXICITY 6
Myalgias and arthralgias.

TOXICITY 7

Maculopapular skin rash, erythema, dermatitis, and pruritus.

TOXICITY 8

Hypothyroidism.

Pemetrexed

TRADE NAMES	Alimta, LY231514	CLASSIFICATION	Antimetabolite
CATEGORY	Chemotherapy drug	DRUG MANUFACTURER	Eli Lilly

MECHANISM OF ACTION

- Pyrrolopyrimidine antifolate analog with activity in the S-phase of the cell cycle.
- Transported into the cell primarily via the RFC and to a smaller extent by the folate-receptor protein (FRP).
- Metabolized intracellularly to higher polyglutamate forms by the enzyme folylpolyglutamate synthase (FPGS). The pentaglutamate form is the predominant intracellular species. Pemetrexed polyglutamates are approximately 60-fold more potent than the parent monoglutamate compound, and they exhibit prolonged cellular retention.
- Inhibition of the folate-dependent enzyme thymidylate synthase (TS) resulting in inhibition of de novo thymidylate and DNA synthesis. This represents the main site of action of the drug.
- Inhibition of TS leads to accumulation of dUMP and subsequent incorporation of dUTP into DNA, resulting in inhibition of DNA synthesis and function.
- Inhibition of dihydrofolate reductase, resulting in depletion of reduced folates and of critical one-carbon carriers for cellular metabolism.
- Inhibition of de novo purine biosynthesis through inhibition of glycinamide ribonucleotide formyltransferase (GART) and aminoimidazole carboxamide ribonucleotide formyltransferase (AICART).

MECHANISM OF RESISTANCE

- Increased expression of the target enzyme TS.
- Alterations in the binding affinity of TS for pemetrexed.

- Decreased transport of drug into cells through decreased expression of the RFC and/or FRP.
- Decreased polyglutamation of drug, resulting in decreased formation of cytotoxic metabolites.

ABSORPTION
Pemetrexed is given only by the IV route.

DISTRIBUTION
Peak plasma levels are reached in less than 30 minutes. Widely distributed throughout the body. Tissue concentrations highest in liver, kidneys, small intestine, and colon.

METABOLISM
Significant intracellular metabolism of drug to the polyglutamated species. Metabolism in the liver through as yet undefined mechanisms. Principally cleared by renal excretion, with as much as 90% of the drug in the urine unchanged during the first 24 hours after administration. Short distribution half-life in plasma with a mean of 3 hours. However, relatively prolonged terminal half-life of about 20 hours and a prolonged intracellular half-life as a result of pemetrexed polyglutamates.

INDICATIONS
1. Mesothelioma—FDA-approved in combination with cisplatin for treatment of locally advanced or metastatic nonsquamous NSCLC.
2. NSCLC—FDA-approved in combination with cisplatin for the initial treatment of locally advanced or metastatic nonsquamous NSCLC.
3. NSCLC—FDA-approved as second-line monotherapy for locally advanced or metastatic nonsquamous NSCLC.
4. NSCLC—FDA-approved as maintenance treatment of locally advanced or metastatic nonsquamous NSCLC whose disease has not progressed after four cycles of platinum-based first-line chemotherapy.
5. Pemetrexed should not be used in patients with squamous cell NSCLC.

DOSAGE RANGE
1. Recommended dose as a single agent is 500 mg/m^2 IV every 3 weeks.
2. When used in combination with cisplatin, recommended dose is 500 mg/m^2 IV every 3 weeks.

DRUG INTERACTION 1
Thymidine—Thymidine rescues against the host toxic effects of pemetrexed.

DRUG INTERACTION 2
5-FU—Pemetrexed may enhance the antitumor activity of 5-FU. Precise mechanism of interaction remains unknown.

DRUG INTERACTION 3
Leucovorin—Administration of leucovorin may decrease the antitumor activity of pemetrexed.

DRUG INTERACTION 4
NSAIDs and aspirin—Concomitant administration of NSAIDs and aspirin may inhibit the renal excretion of pemetrexed, resulting in enhanced drug toxicity.

SPECIAL CONSIDERATIONS
1. Use with caution in patients with abnormal renal function. Important to obtain baseline CrCl and to monitor renal function before each cycle of therapy. Should not be given if CrCl <45 mL/ min.
2. Dose reduction is not necessary in patients with mild-to-moderate liver impairment.
3. Monitor CBCs on a periodic basis.
4. Use with caution in patients with third-space fluid collections such as pleural effusion and ascites, as the half-life of pemetrexed may be prolonged, leading to enhanced toxicity. Should consider draining of fluid collections prior to initiation of therapy.
5. Dietary folate status of patient may be an important factor in determining risk for clinical toxicity. Patients with insufficient folate intake may be at increased risk for host toxicity. Evaluation of serum homocysteine and folate levels at baseline and during therapy may be helpful. A baseline serum homocysteine level >10 is a good predictor for the development of grade 3/4 toxicities.
6. All patients should receive vitamin supplementation with 350 μg/day of folic acid PO and 1000 μg of vitamin B12 IM every three cycles to reduce the risk and incidence of toxicity while on drug therapy. Folic acid supplementation should begin 7 days prior to initiation of pemetrexed treatment, and the first vitamin B12 injection should be administered at least 1 week prior to the start of pemetrexed. No evidence has been found to suggest that vitamin supplementation reduces clinical efficacy.
7. Prophylactic use of steroids may ameliorate and/or completely eliminate the development of skin rash. Dexamethasone can be given at a dose of 4 mg PO bid for 3 days beginning the day before therapy.
8. NSAIDs and aspirin should be discontinued for at least 2 days before therapy with pemetrexed and should not be restarted for at least 2 days after a drug dose. These agents may inhibit the renal clearance of pemetrexed, resulting in enhanced toxicity.
9. Pregnancy category D. Breastfeeding should be avoided.

TOXICITY 1
Myelosuppression. Dose-limiting, dose-related toxicity with neutropenia and thrombocytopenia being most commonly observed.

TOXICITY 2
Skin rash, usually in the form of the hand-foot syndrome.

TOXICITY 3
Mucositis, diarrhea, and nausea and vomiting.

TOXICITY 4
Transient elevation in serum transaminases and bilirubin. Occurs in 10%–15% of patients. Clinically asymptomatic in most cases.

TOXICITY 5
Fatigue.

Pertuzumab

TRADE NAMES	Perjeta, Anti-HER2-antibody	CLASSIFICATION	Monoclonal antibody
CATEGORY	Biologic response modifier agent	DRUG MANUFACTURER	Genentech/ Roche

MECHANISM OF ACTION
- Recombinant humanized IgG1 monoclonal antibody directed against the extracellular dimerization domain (subdomain II) of the HER2/neu growth factor receptor.
- Binding of pertuzumab to HER2 leads to inhibition of heterodimerization of HER2 with other HER family members, including EGFR, HER3, and HER4.
- Inhibition of these heterodimerization processes leads to the inhibition of downstream signaling pathways, which includes mitogen-activated protein (MAP) kinase, phosphoinositide 3-kinase (PI3K), and initiation of cell apoptosis.
- Immunologic mechanisms may also be involved in antitumor activity, including ADCC.
- Pertuzumab binds to a different HER2 epitope than trastuzumab.

MECHANISM OF RESISTANCE
- Mutations in HER2/neu receptor leading to decreased binding affinity to pertuzumab.
- Activation/induction of alternative cellular signaling pathways, such as IGF-1R, c-MET, PIK3CA/Akt, Ras/Raf MEK/ERK.
- Loss of PTEN.

ABSORPTION
Pertuzumab is only given intravenously.

DISTRIBUTION
Steady-state drug levels are generally achieved after the first maintenance dose.

METABOLISM

Metabolism of pertuzumab has not been extensively evaluated. The terminal half-life is approximately 18 days using an every–3-week infusion schedule.

INDICATIONS

1. FDA-approved in combination with trastuzumab and docetaxel for patients with HER2-positive metastatic breast cancer who have not received prior anti-HER2 therapy or chemotherapy for metastatic disease.
2. Patients must express HER2/neu protein to be treated with this monoclonal antibody.

DOSAGE RANGE

Recommended initial dose is 840 mg IV administered over 60 minutes, followed by a maintenance dose of 420 mg over 30–60 minutes every 3 weeks.

DRUG INTERACTIONS

No drug–drug interactions were observed between pertuzumab and trastuzumab or between pertuzumab and docetaxel. No other drug interactions have been formally investigated to date.

SPECIAL CONSIDERATIONS

1. Pertuzumab has been associated with decreased LVEF. Patients with prior exposure to anthracyclines or radiotherapy to the chest may be at increased risk of developing a decline in LVEF. Caution should be exercised in treating patients with pre-existing cardiac disease such as congestive heart failure, ischemic heart disease, myocardial infarction, valvular heart disease, or arrhythmias.
2. Careful baseline assessment of cardiac function (LVEF) before treatment and frequent monitoring (every 3 months) of cardiac function while on therapy. Pertuzumab should be held for at least 3 weeks if there is a drop in LVEF <45% or an LVEF of 45%–49% with a 10% or greater absolute decline from baseline. If cardiac function does not improve after 3 weeks of withholding therapy, consider permanently discontinuing therapy.
3. Carefully monitor for infusion-related and hypersensitivity reactions. Monitor patients 60 minutes after the first infusion and for 30 minutes after subsequent infusions for infusion reactions or cytokine release syndrome. If an infusion reaction occurs, slow and/or interrupt treatment. Immediate institution of diphenhydramine, acetaminophen, corticosteroids, IV fluids, and/or vasopressors may be necessary. Resuscitation equipment should be readily available at bedside.
4. The pregnancy status of a female patient must be verified prior to the start of pertuzumab therapy. Patients should be advised of the risks of embryo-fetal deaths and birth defects, and the need for contraception during and after treatment.
5. Pregnancy category D. Breastfeeding should be avoided.

TOXICITY 1
Embryo-fetal deaths and/or severe birth defects.

TOXICITY 2
Cardiotoxicity with a reduced LVEF.

TOXICITY 3
Infusion-related symptoms with fever, chills, urticaria, flushing, fatigue, headache, hypersensitivity, and myalgia. Occurs in up to 13% of patients. Most commonly observed with administration of first infusion.

TOXICITY 4
Fatigue.

TOXICITY 5
Diarrhea and nausea/vomiting.

Pomalidomide

TRADE NAME	Pomalyst	CLASSIFICATION	Immunomodulatory analog of thalidomide, antiangiogenic agent
CATEGORY	Unclassified therapeutic agent, biologic response modifier agent	DRUG MANUFACTURER	Celgene

MECHANISM OF ACTION
- Mechanism of action is not fully characterized.
- More potent antiproliferative immunomodulating agent than thalidomide and lenalidomide.
- Immunomodulatory drug that stimulates T-cell proliferation as well as IL-2 and IFN-γ production.
- Inhibition of TNF-α and IL-6 synthesis and down-modulation of cell surface adhesion molecules similar to thalidomide.

- May exert antiangiogenic effect by inhibition of basic fibroblast growth factor (bFGF) and vascular endothelial growth factor (VEGF) and through as yet undefined mechanisms.
- Overcomes cellular drug resistance to thalidomide and lenalidomide.

MECHANISM OF RESISTANCE
None characterized to date.

ABSORPTION
Well-absorbed following oral administration, with peak plasma concentrations at 2–3 hours post ingestion.

DISTRIBUTION
Binding to plasma proteins ranges from 12%–44%. Distributed in male semen at concentrations of approximately 67% of plasma levels after 4 days of treatment.

METABOLISM
Pomalidomide is mainly metabolized in the liver by CYP1A2 and CYP3A4 with minor effects by CYP2C19 and CYP2D6. Approximately 75% of an administered dose is excreted in urine, primarily in the form of drug metabolites, while 15% of an administered dose is eliminated in feces. The elimination half-life of the drug is approximately 7.5 hours.

INDICATIONS
FDA-approved for the treatment of patients with multiple myeloma who have received at least two prior therapies, including lenalidomide and bortezomib, and who have disease progression on or within 60 days of completion of the previous therapy.

DOSAGE RANGE
1. Recommended dose is 4 mg PO daily on days 1–21 of a 28-day cycle.
2. May be given in combination with Decadron 40 mg PO daily on days 1, 8, 15, and 22 of a 28-day cycle.

DRUG INTERACTIONS
None well characterized to date.

SPECIAL CONSIDERATIONS
1. Pregnancy category X. Pomalidomide is a thalidomide analog, a known human teratogen that causes severe or life-threatening birth defects. As such, women who are pregnant or who wish to become pregnant should not take pomalidomide. Severe fetal malformations can occur if even one capsule is taken by a pregnant woman. All women should have a baseline β-human chorionic gonadotropin (β-HCG) before starting pomalidomide therapy. Women of reproductive age must have two negative pregnancy tests before starting therapy: one should be 10 to 14 days before therapy is begun, and the second should be 24 hours before therapy. This is a black-box warning.

2. All women of childbearing potential should practice two forms of birth control throughout therapy with pomalidomide: one highly effective form (intrauterine device, hormonal contraception [patch, implant, pill, injection], partner's vasectomy, or tubal ligation) and one additional barrier method (latex condom, diaphragm, or cervical cap). It is strongly recommended that these precautionary measures be taken 1 month before initiation of therapy, continue while on therapy, and continue at least 1 month after therapy is discontinued.

3. Pomalidomide is only available under a special restricted distribution program called "POMALYST REMS." Only prescribers and pharmacists registered with this program are able to prescribe and dispense the drug. Pomalidomide should only be dispensed to those patients who are registered and meet all the conditions of this program.

4. Breastfeeding while on therapy should be avoided, as it remains unknown if pomalidomide is excreted in breast milk.

5. Men taking pomalidomide must use latex condoms for every sexual encounter with a woman of childbearing potential, as the drug may be present in semen.

6. Patients taking pomalidomide should not donate blood or semen while receiving treatment, and for at least 1 month after stopping this drug.

7. Monitor CBCs while on therapy, as pomalidomide has hematologic toxicity.

8. Use with caution in patients with impaired renal function, as pomalidomide and its metabolites are mainly excreted by the kidneys. Although no formal renal dysfunction studies have been performed, the use of pomalidomide should be avoided in patients with a serum creatinine >3 mg/dL.

9. There is a significantly increased risk of thromboembolic complications, including DVT and PE. This represents a black-box warning. Prophylaxis with low-molecular weight heparin or aspirin (325 mg PO qd) is recommended to prevent and/or reduce this risk.

10. Smoking should be avoided while on therapy, as cigarette smoking may reduce pomalidomide exposure secondary to CYP1A2 induction.

TOXICITY 1
Potentially severe or fatal teratogenic effects.

TOXICITY 2
Myelosuppression with neutropenia and thrombocytopenia that is usually reversible.

TOXICITY 3
Increased risk of thromboembolic complications, such as DVT and PE.

TOXICITY 4
Nausea/vomiting, diarrhea, and constipation are most common GI side effects.

TOXICITY 5
Dizziness and confusion are the two most common neurologic side

TOXICITY 6
Hypersensitivity reactions. More likely to occur in patients with a prior history of hypersensitivity reactions to thalidomide or lenalidomide.

TOXICITY 7
Neuropathy observed in nearly 20% of patients, with approximately 10% in the form of peripheral neuropathy. Usually mild with no grade 3 or higher neuropathy reported.

Ponatinib

TRADE NAMES	Iclusig, AP24534	CLASSIFICATION	Signal transduction inhibitor
CATEGORY	Chemotherapy drug	DRUG MANUFACTURER	ARIAD Pharmaceuticals

MECHANISM OF ACTION
1. Potent inhibitor of the non-mutant Bcr-Abl tyrosine kinase. In contrast to other Bcr-Abl inhibitors, ponatinib demonstrates inhibitory effects against all known Bcr-Abl mutations, including the T315I mutation. Ponatinib was specifically designed to bind and inhibit these mutant forms.
2. Inhibits other tyrosine kinases, some of which are involved in tumor growth and tumor angiogenesis, including VEGFR, PDGFR, FGFR, Flt3, Tie-2, Src family kinases, Kit, RET, and EPH.

MECHANISM OF RESISTANCE
None well characterized to date.

ABSORPTION
Absorbed following oral administration at varying levels of bioavailability based on pH levels, with higher gastric pH levels leading to lower oral bioavailability. Peak plasma concentrations are achieved at 6 hours, and steady-state drug levels are achieved at 28 days.

DISTRIBUTION
Extensive plasma proteins binding of >99%.

METABOLISM
Metabolized in the liver primarily by the CYP3A4 microsomal enzymes. CYP2C8, CYP2D6, and CYP3A5 liver microsomal enzymes are also involved. Phase II metabolism occurs via esterases and/or amidases. The mean terminal elimination half-life is 24 hours. Approximately 87% and 5% of an administered dose is eliminated in feces and urine, respectively.

INDICATIONS
1. FDA-approved for the treatment of adult patients with chronic-, accelerated-, or blast-phase CML that is resistant or intolerant to prior tyrosine kinase inhibitor therapy.
2. FDA-approved for the treatment of Ph+ ALL that is resistant or intolerant to prior tyrosine kinase inhibitor therapy.

DOSAGE RANGE
1. Recommended dose is 45 mg PO once daily with or without food.
2. Recommended dose is 30 mg PO once daily if given concurrently with strong CYP3A inhibitors.

DRUG INTERACTION 1
Phenytoin and other drugs that stimulate liver microsomal CYP3A4 enzymes, including carbamazepine, rifampin, phenobarbital, and St. John's wort—These drugs increase the rate of metabolism of ponatinib resulting in its inactivation and reduced drug levels.

DRUG INTERACTION 2
Drugs that inhibit liver microsomal CYP3A4 enzymes, including ketoconazole, voriconazole, posaconazole, itraconazole, erythromycin, and clarithromycin—These drugs decrease the rate of metabolism of ponatinib resulting in increased drug levels and potentially increased toxicity.

DRUG INTERACTION 3
Warfarin—Patients on coumarin-derived anticoagulants should be closely monitored for alterations in their clotting parameters (PT and INR) and/or bleeding as ponatinib inhibits the metabolism of warfarin by the liver P450 system. Dose of warfarin may require careful adjustment in the presence of ponatinib therapy.

DRUG INTERACTION 4
Proton pump inhibitors and H2-blockers can reduce the plasma drug concentrations of ponatinib.

SPECIAL CONSIDERATIONS
1. Patients should be closely monitored for an increased risk of arterial thromboembolic events, such as cardiovascular, cerebrovascular, and peripheral vascular thrombosis, including fatal myocardial infarction and stroke. This represents a black-box warning.

2. Closely monitor hepatic function prior to and at least monthly thereafter, as hepatotoxicity, liver failure, and death have been reported in patients treated with ponatinib. This represents a black-box warning.
3. Severe bleeding can occur, and caution should be taken in patients with thrombocytopenia or in those on anticoagulation.
4. Ponatinib therapy should be interrupted in patients undergoing major surgical procedures.
5. Ponatinib therapy can result in the development of gastrointestinal perforation and fistula formation.
6. Monitor CBC every 2 weeks during the first 3 months then monthly thereafter.
7. Closely monitor blood pressure, especially in patients with underlying hypertension as ponatinib can worsen hypertension.
8. Tumor lysis syndrome has been reported. Monitor uric acid levels and consider allopurinol and adequate hydration.
9. Monitor patients for fluid retention that can manifest as peripheral edema, pericardial effusion, pleural effusion, pulmonary edema, or ascites.
10. Avoid grapefruit, grapefruit juice, starfruit, pomelos, and St. John's wort while on therapy.
11. Avoid PPIs and H2-blockers, as they can reduce the oral bioavailability and subsequent efficacy of ponatinib.
12. Pregnancy category D. Breastfeeding should be avoided.

TOXICITY 1
Arterial thromboembolic events, such as myocardial infarction and stroke. Serious arterial thrombosis occurs in up to 10% of patients.

TOXICITY 2
Hepatotoxicity with elevation in SGOT/SGPT in 60% of patients with liver failure and death patients.

TOXICITY 3
Pancreatitis occurs in 6% of patients.

TOXICITY 4
Hypertension.

TOXICITY 5
Cardiac arrhythmias in the form of complete heart block, sick sinus syndrome, atrial fibrillation, and sinus bradycardia.

TOXICITY 6
Fluid retention manifesting as peripheral edema, pericardial effusion, pleural effusion, pulmonary edema, or ascites.

TOXICITY 7
Bleeding complications usually associated with severe thrombocytopenia.

TOXICITY 8
Myelosuppression with neutropenia, thrombocytopenia, and anemia.

TOXICITY 9
Tumor lysis syndrome occurs rarely in less than 1%.

TOXICITY 10
Gastrointestinal perforation, fistula formation, and wound-healing complications.

TOXICITY 11
Skin toxicity including skin rash and dry skin.

Pralatrexate

and epimer at C*

TRADE NAME	Folotyn	CLASSIFICATION	Antimetabolite
CATEGORY	Chemotherapy drug	DRUG MANUFACTURER	Allos Therapeutics

MECHANISM OF ACTION
- 10-deazaaminopterin antifolate analog with activity in the S-phase of the cell cycle.
- Transported selectively into the cell by the reduced folate carrier type 1 (RFC-1) and was rationally designed to have greater affinity to this transport protein.
- Requires polyglutamation by the enzyme folylpolyglutamate synthase (FPGS) for its cytotoxic activity.
- Inhibition of dihydrofolate reductase (DHFR), resulting in depletion of critical reduced folates.
- Inhibition of de novo thymidylate synthesis.
- Inhibition of de novo purine synthesis.
- Incorporation of dUTP into DNA, resulting in inhibition of DNA synthesis and function.

MECHANISM OF RESISTANCE
- Increased expression of the target enzyme DHFR through either gene amplification or increased transcription, translation, and/or post-translational events.
- Alterations in the binding affinity of DHFR.
- Decreased carrier-mediated transport of drug into cell through decreased expression and/or activity of RFC-1.
- Decreased formation of cytotoxic pralatrexate polyglutamates through either decreased expression of FPGS or increased expression of γ-glutamyl hydrolase (GGH).

ABSORPTION
Administered only by the IV route.

DISTRIBUTION
Approximately 67% of drug is bound to plasma proteins.

METABOLISM
Significant intracellular metabolism of drug to the polyglutamated species. Metabolism in the liver through as yet undefined mechanisms. Principally cleared by renal excretion with approximately 34% of an administered dose of drug excreted unchanged in urine. Age-related decline in renal function may lead to a reduction in pralatrexate clearance and an increase in plasma exposure. The terminal half-life of pralatrexate is 12–18 hours with a prolonged intracellular half-life as a result of pralatrexate polyglutamates.

INDICATIONS
FDA-approved for the treatment of patients with relapsed or refractory peripheral T-cell lymphoma (PTCL).

DOSAGE RANGE
Recommended dose is 30 mg/m^2 IV weekly for 6 weeks in 7-week cycles.

DRUG INTERACTION 1
Aspirin, NSAIDs, penicillins, probenecid, cephalosporins, and trimethroprim/sulfamethoxazole—These drugs inhibit the renal excretion of pralatrexate leading to enhanced drug effect and toxicity.

DRUG INTERACTION 2
Leucovorin—Leucovorin rescues the toxic effects of pralatrexate and may also impair the antitumor activity. The active form of leucovorin is the L-isomer.

DRUG INTERACTION 3
Thymidine—Thymidine rescues the toxic effects of pralatrexate and may also impair the antitumor activity.

SPECIAL CONSIDERATIONS

1. Closely monitor CBCs on a periodic basis.
2. Use with caution in patients with abnormal renal function. Dose should be reduced in proportion to the creatinine clearance. Important to obtain baseline CrCl and to monitor renal function before each cycle of therapy.
3. Closely monitor liver function while on treatment. Patients who develop evidence of hepatic impairment or hepatic disease may require dose modification.
4. Dietary folate status of the patient may be an important factor in determining risk for toxicity. Patients with insufficient folate intake may be at increased risk for toxicity. Evaluation of serum homocysteine and methylmalonic acid may be helpful.
5. All patients should receive supplementation with folic acid and vitamin B12 to reduce the incidence and severity of adverse reactions. Folic acid 1–1.25 mg PO daily should begin 10 days prior to the first dose of pralatrexate and continue during the full course of therapy, until 30 days after the last dose of pralatrexate. Vitamin B12 1000 μg IM should begin no more than 10 weeks prior to the first dose of pralatrexate and should be repeated every 8–10 weeks during therapy. Subsequent vitamin B12 injections may be given on the same day as pralatrexate.
6. Pregnancy category D. Breastfeeding should be avoided.

TOXICITY 1
Myelosuppression with thrombocytopenia, neutropenia, and anemia.

TOXICITY 2
Mucositis, nausea/vomiting, diarrhea, and abdominal pain.

TOXICITY 3
Transient elevations in serum transaminases reported in 10%–15% of patients. Clinically asymptomatic in most cases.

TOXICITY 4
Fatigue and asthenia.

TOXICITY 5
Skin rash.

Procarbazine

TRADE NAMES	Matulane, N-Methylhydrazine	CLASSIFICATION	Nonclassic alkylating agent
CATEGORY	Chemotherapy drug	DRUG MANUFACTURER	Roche

MECHANISM OF ACTION

1. Hydrazine analog that acts as an alkylating agent. Weak monoamine oxidase (MAO) inhibitor and a relative of the MAO inhibitor 1-methyl-2-benzylhydrazine.
2. Requires metabolic activation for cytotoxicity. Occurs spontaneously through a non-enzymatic process and/or by an enzymatic reaction mediated by the liver cytochrome P450 system.
3. While the precise mechanism of cytotoxicity is unclear, this drug inhibits DNA, RNA, and protein synthesis.
4. Cell cycle–nonspecific drug.

MECHANISM OF RESISTANCE

1. Enhanced DNA repair secondary to increased expression of AGAT.
2. Enhanced DNA repair secondary to AGAT-independent mechanisms.

ABSORPTION

Rapid and complete absorption from the GI tract, reaching peak plasma levels within 1 hour.

DISTRIBUTION

Rapidly and extensively metabolized by the liver cytochrome P450 microsomal system. Procarbazine metabolites cross the blood-brain barrier, and peak CSF levels of drug occur within 30–90 minutes after drug administration.

METABOLISM

Metabolized to active and inactive metabolites by two main pathways, chemical breakdown in aqueous solution and liver microsomal P450 system. Possible formation of free radical intermediates. About 70% of procarbazine is excreted in urine within 24 hours. Less than 5%–10% of the drug is eliminated in an unchanged form. The elimination half-life is short, being less than 1 hour after oral administration.

INDICATIONS

1. Hodgkin's lymphoma.
2. Non-Hodgkin's lymphoma.
3. Brain tumors adjuvant and/or advanced disease.
4. Cutaneous T-cell lymphoma (CTCL).

DOSAGE RANGE

1. Hodgkin's lymphoma: 100 mg/m^2 PO daily for 14 days, as part of MOPP regimen.
2. Brain tumors: 60 mg/m^2 PO daily for 14 days, as part of PCV regimen.

DRUG INTERACTION 1
Alcohol- or tyramine-containing foods—Concurrent use with procarbazine can result in nausea, vomiting, increased CNS depression, hypertensive crisis, visual disturbances, and headache.

DRUG INTERACTION 2
Antihistamines, CNS depressants—Concurrent use of procarbazine with antihistamines can result in CNS and/or respiratory depression.

DRUG INTERACTION 3
Levodopa, meperidine—Concurrent use of procarbazine with levodopa or meperidine results in hypertension.

DRUG INTERACTION 4
Tricyclic antidepressants—Concurrent use of procarbazine with sympathomimetics and tricyclic antidepressants may result in CNS excitation, hypertension, tremors, palpitations, and in severe cases, hypertensive crisis and/or angina.

DRUG INTERACTION 5
Antidiabetic agents—Concurrent use of procarbazine with antidiabetic agents such as sulfonylurea compounds and insulin may potentiate hypoglycemic effect.

SPECIAL CONSIDERATIONS
1. Monitor CBC while on therapy.
2. Prophylactic use of antiemetics 30 minutes before drug administration to decrease risk of nausea and vomiting. Incidence and severity of nausea usually decrease with continued therapy.
3. Important to review patient's list of concurrent medications as procarbazine has several potential drug–drug interactions.
4. Instruct patients against ingestion of alcohol while on procarbazine. May result in disulfiram (Antabuse)-like effect.
5. Instruct patients about specific types of food to avoid during drug therapy (e.g., dark beer, wine, cheese, bananas, yogurt, and pickled and smoked foods).
6. Pregnancy category D. Breastfeeding should be avoided.

TOXICITY 1
Myelosuppression is dose-limiting. Thrombocytopenia is most pronounced with nadir in 4 weeks and returns to normal in 4–6 weeks. Neutropenia usually occurs after thrombocytopenia. Patients with G6PD deficiency may present with hemolytic anemia while on procarbazine therapy.

TOXICITY 2
Nausea and vomiting usually develop in the first days of therapy and improve with continued therapy. Diarrhea may also be observed.

TOXICITY 3
Flu-like syndrome in the form of fever, chills, sweating, myalgias, and arthralgias. Usually occurs with initial therapy.

TOXICITY 4
CNS toxicity in the form of paresthesias, neuropathies, ataxia, lethargy, headache, confusion, and/or seizures.

TOXICITY 5
Hypersensitivity reaction with pruritus, urticaria, maculopapular skin rash, flushing, eosinophilia, and pulmonary infiltrates. Skin rash responds to steroid therapy, and drug treatment may be continued. However, procarbazine-induced interstitial pneumonitis usually mandates discontinuation of therapy.

TOXICITY 6
Amenorrhea and azoospermia.

TOXICITY 7
Immunosuppressive activity with increased risk of infections.

TOXICITY 8
Increased risk of secondary malignancies in the form of acute leukemia. The drug is teratogenic, mutagenic, and carcinogenic.

Ramucirumab

TRADE NAMES	Cyramza, IMC-1121B	CLASSIFICATION	Monoclonal antibody
CATEGORY	Anti-VEGFR2 antibody	DRUG MANUFACTURER	Eli Lilly

MECHANISM OF ACTION
- Recombinant fully human IgG1 monoclonal antibody directed against the vascular endothelial growth factor receptor 2 (VEGFR-2) and prevents binding of the VEGF-A, VEGF-C, and VEGF-D ligands to its target VEGFR-2.
- Binds with high affinity to VEGFR-2 (50 pM) and results in inhibition of VEGFR-mediated signaling, which leads to reduced endothelial cell permeability, migration, and proliferation.
- Precise mechanism of action remains unknown.
- Inhibits formation of new blood vessels in primary tumor and metastatic tumors.
- Inhibits tumor blood vessel permeability and reduces interstitial tumoral pressures, and in so doing, may enhance blood flow delivery within tumor.

MECHANISM OF RESISTANCE
- Activation and/or upregulation of alternative pro-angiogenic factor ligands, such as bFGF and HGF.
- Recruitment of bone marrow-derived cells, which circumvents the requirement of VEGF signaling and restores neovascularization and tumor angiogenesis.

DISTRIBUTION
Distribution in the body is not well characterized. The estimated time to reach steady-state levels is approximately 28 days.

METABOLISM
The metabolism of ramucirumab has not been extensively characterized. The mean drug clearance was similar for patients with gastric cancer, NSCLC, and mCRC, and the mean terminal half-life is 14 days.

INDICATIONS
1. Advanced metastatic colorectal cancer—FDA-approved for use in combination with FOLFIRI chemotherapy in patients with disease progression on or after prior therapy with FOLFOX/XELOX plus bevacizumab.
2. Advanced metastatic gastric or gastro-esophageal junction adenocarcinoma—FDA-approved for use as monotherapy or in

combination with paclitaxel in patients with disease progression on or after fluoropyrimidine or platinum-containing chemotherapy.

3. Advanced metastatic NSCLC—FDA-approved for NSCLC in combination with docetaxel in patients with disease progression on or after platinum-based chemotherapy.

DOSAGE RANGE

1. Recommended dose for the treatment of mCRC is 8 mg/kg IV every 2 weeks in combination with FOLFIRI.
2. Recommended dose for the treatment of advanced gastric or gastro-esophageal junction adenocarcinoma is 8 mg/kg IV every 2 weeks as monotherapy or in combination with paclitaxel.
3. Recommended dose for the treatment of NSCLC is 10 mg/kg IV every 3 weeks in combination with docetaxel.

DRUG INTERACTIONS

None well characterized to date.

SPECIAL CONSIDERATIONS

1. Serious, sometimes fatal, arterial thromboembolic events including myocardial infarction, cardiac arrest, cerebrovascular accident, and cerebral ischemia may occur. Permanently discontinue ramucirumab in patients who experience a severe arterial thromboembolic event.
2. Patients should be warned of the potential for increased risk of hemorrhage and gastrointestinal hemorrhage, including severe and sometimes fatal hemorrhagic events. Patients with gastric cancer receiving NSAIDs were excluded from studies. As a result, the risk of gastric hemorrhage in patients with gastric tumors receiving NSAIDs is unknown.
3. Ramucirumab treatment can cause an increased incidence of severe hypertension. Use with caution in patients with uncontrolled hypertension. Closely monitor blood pressure every 2 weeks or more frequently as indicated during treatment. Should be permanently discontinued in patients who develop hypertensive crisis.
4. Carefully monitor for infusion-related symptoms. May need to treat with benadryl and acetaminophen.
5. Potentially fatal gastrointestinal perforation can occur. Ramucirumab should be permanently discontinued in patients who experience a gastrointestinal perforation.
6. Impaired wound healing can occur with antibodies inhibiting the VEGF signaling pathway. Ramucirumab has not been studied in patients with serious or non-healing wounds. However, ramucirumab has the potential to adversely affect wound healing. Ramucirumab should be discontinued in patients with impaired wound healing and withheld prior to surgery. Resume following surgery based on clinical judgment of adequate wound healing. If a patient develops wound-healing complications during therapy, discontinue until the wound is fully healed.
7. Clinical deterioration, as manifested by new-onset or worsening encephalopathy, ascites, or hepatorenal syndrome was reported in

patients with Child-Pugh B or C cirrhosis who received single-agent ramucirumab.

8. Ramucirumab should be used with caution in patients with renal disease. Severe proteinuria including nephrotic syndrome has been reported. Ramucirumab should be withheld for urine protein levels that are >2 g over 24 hours and reinitiated at a reduced dose once the urine protein level returns to <2 g over 24 hours. Permanently discontinue if urine protein levels >3 g over 24 hours or in the setting of nephrotic syndrome.
9. Closely monitor thyroid function.
10. Pregnancy category B.

TOXICITY 1
Hypertension occurs in up to 20%–30% of patients with grade 3 hypertension observed in 8%–15% of patients. Usually well controlled with oral anti-hypertensive medication.

TOXICITY 2
Bleeding complications with epistaxis and GI hemorrhage, including severe and sometimes fatal hemorrhagic events.

TOXICITY 3
Fatigue and headache.

TOXICITY 4
Nausea/vomiting, anorexia, abdominal pain, and diarrhea.

TOXICITY 5
GI perforations and wound-healing complications.

TOXICITY 6
Proteinuria with nephrotic syndrome.

TOXICITY 7
Infusion-related symptoms with fever, chills, urticaria, flushing, fatigue, headache, bronchospasm, dyspnea, angioedema, and hypotension. Relatively uncommon (<5%).

TOXICITY 8
Increased risk of arterial thromboembolic events, including myocardial infarction, angina, and stroke. There is also an increased incidence of venous thromboembolic events.

TOXICITY 9
Hypothyroidism.

TOXICITY 10
RPLS occurs rarely (<0.1%), presenting with headache, seizure, lethargy, confusion, blindness, and other visual disturbances.

Regorafenib

TRADE NAMES	Stivarga, BAY 73-4506	CLASSIFICATION	Signal transduction inhibitor
CATEGORY	Chemotherapy drug	DRUG MANUFACTURER	Bayer, Onyx

MECHANISM OF ACTION
- Regorafenib is a small-molecule inhibitor of multiple membrane-bound and intracellular kinases involved in oncogenesis, tumor angiogenesis, and maintenance of the tumor microenvironment.
- Inhibits vascular endothelial growth factor receptors (VEGFR-1, VEGFR-2, VEGFR-3), platelet-derived growth factor receptors (PDGFR)-α, PDGFR-β, and Tie-2.
- Inhibits oncogenic kinases such as c-Kit, RET, RAF-1, and BRAF.
- Inhibits fibroblast growth factor receptor FGFR-1, FGFR-2, DDR2, Trk2A, Eph2A, SAPK2, PTK5, and Abl.

MECHANISM OF RESISTANCE
- Activation of Akt signaling.
- Activation of Notch-1 signaling.
- Increased expression and activity of the multidrug resistant-associated transporter protein 2 (MRP2).
- Mutations in the *KRAS* gene.
- Defects in PUMA-mediated apoptosis.

ABSORPTION
Rapidly absorbed after an oral dose. Peak plasma levels are reached at a median time of 4 hours. The mean relative bioavailablity of tablets compared to oral solution is 69% to 83%. Food with a high fat content increases oral bioavailability of parent drug by 48%.

DISTRIBUTION
Highly bound (99.5%) to human plasma proteins.

METABOLISM
Metabolized in the liver primarily by CYP3A4 and UGT1A9. The main circulating metabolites are M-2 (N-oxide) and M-5 (N-oxide and N-desmethyl), both of

which have similar biological activity as parent drug. Approximately 71% of an administered drug is excreted in the feces with 47% in parent form and 24% as metabolites, and 19% is eliminated in the urine. The terminal half-life of regorafenib is 28 hours, while the terminal half-lives of the M-2 and M-5 metabolites are approximately 25 and 51 hours, respectively.

INDICATIONS
1. FDA-approved for metastatic colorectal cancer following treatment with fluoropyrimidine-, oxaliplatin-, and irinotecan-based chemotherapy; an anti-VEGF therapy; and an anti-EGFR therapy if KRAS wild-type.
2. FDA-approved for locally advanced, unresectable, or metastatic GIST previously treated with imatinib and sunitinib.

DOSAGE RANGE
Recommended dose is 160 mg PO once daily with a low-fat breakfast for the first 21 days of each 28-day cycle.

DRUG INTERACTION 1
Strong inhibitors of CYP3A4 such as ketoconazole, itraconazole, clarithromycin, nefazodone, telithromycin, and voriconazole decrease the rate of metabolism of regorafenib, resulting in increased drug levels and potentially increased toxicity.

DRUG INTERACTION 2
Drugs such as rifampin, phenytoin, phenobarbital, carbamazepine, and St. John's wort increase the rate of metabolism of regorafenib, resulting in its inactivation.

DRUG INTERACTION 3
Concomitant use of regorafenib, a UGT1A1 inhibitor, and irinotecan, a UGT1A1 substrate, may result in increased exposure of irinotecan and the active metabolite SN-38, potentially leading to increased toxicity.

SPECIAL CONSIDERATIONS
1. Regorafenib should be taken at the same time each day with a low-fat breakfast that contains less than 30% fat.
2. No initial dosage adjustment is needed in patients with pre-existing mild or moderate hepatic disease; however, regorafenib has not been studied in patients with severe hepatic disease, and the use in this population is not recommended. No dose adjustments are necessary in patients with mild-to-moderate renal dysfunction.
3. Regorafenib should be held for > grade 2/3 hand-foot skin reaction, symptomatic grade 2 hypertension, and any NCI CTCAE v3.0 grade 3/4 toxicity.
4. Patients should be warned of the risk of liver toxicity, which represents a black-box warning. LFTs need to be closely monitored while on therapy.
5. Regorafenib should be stopped permanently if a reduced dose of 80 mg is not tolerated, SGOT/SGPT >20×ULN, SGOT/SGPT >3×ULN with serum bilirubin >2×ULN, recurrence of SGOT/SGPT >5×ULN with dose reduction to 120 mg, and for any grade 4 side effects.

6. The dose of regorafenib can be reduced to 120 mg and 80 mg, respectively, based on specific conditions, which are outlined in the full prescribing information.
7. Use with caution when administering with agents that are metabolized and/or eliminated by the UGT1A1 pathway, such as irinotecan, as regorafenib is an inhibitor of UGT1A1.
8. Patients receiving regorafenib along with oral warfarin anticoagulant therapy should have their coagulation parameters (PT and INR) monitored frequently as elevations in INR and bleeding events have been observed.
9. Closely monitor blood pressure while on therapy, especially during the first 6 weeks of therapy, and treat as needed with standard oral antihypertensive medication.
10. Closely monitor LFTs at least every 2 weeks during the first 2 months of therapy and monthly thereafter.
11. Skin toxicities, including rash and hand-foot reaction, should be managed early in the course of therapy with topical treatments for symptomatic relief, temporary interruption, dose reduction, and/or discontinuation. Sun exposure should be avoided, and periodic dermatologic evaluation is recommended.
12. Regorafenib therapy should be interrupted in patients undergoing major surgical procedures.
13. Avoid Seville oranges, starfruit, pomelos, grapefruit, and grapefruit juice while on regorafenib therapy.
14. Pregnancy category D. Breastfeeding should be avoided.

TOXICITY 1
Hypertension occurs in nearly 30% of patients. Usually occurs within 6 weeks of starting therapy and well controlled with oral antihypertensive medications. Hypertensive crisis has been reported rarely.

TOXICITY 2
Skin toxicity in the form of the hand-foot syndrome and skin rash occur in up to 45% and 26%, respectively. Generally appears within the first cycle of drug treatment.

TOXICITY 3
Bleeding complications occur in approximately 20% of patients.

TOXICITY 4
Diarrhea and nausea are the most common GI side effects.

TOXICITY 5
Fatigue and asthenia.

TOXICITY 6
Hepatotoxicity with elevations in SGOT, SGPT, and serum bilirubin. Severe drug-induced liver injury resulting in death has been reported rarely.

TOXICITY 7
GI perforation and GI fistula occur rarely.

TOXICITY 9
Myocardial ischemia and/or infarction occurred in 1.2% of patients.

TOXICITY 10
CNS toxicity in the form of RPLS.

Rituximab

TRADE NAME	Rituxan	**CLASSIFICATION**	Monoclonal antibody
CATEGORY	Biologic response modifier agent	**DRUG MANUFACTURER**	Biogen-IDEC and Genentech

MECHANISM OF ACTION
- Chimeric anti-CD20 antibody consisting of human IgG1-κ constant regions and variable regions from the murine monoclonal anti-CD20 antibody.
- Targets the CD20 antigen, a 35 kDa cell-surface, non-glycosylated phosphoprotein expressed during early pre B cell development until the plasma cell stage. Binding of antibodies to CD20 results in inhibition of CD20-mediated signaling that leads to inhibition of cell activation and cell cycle progression.
- CD20 is expressed on more than 90% of all B-cell non-Hodgkin's lymphomas and leukemias.
- CD20 is not expressed on early pre–B cells, plasma cells, normal bone marrow stem cells, antigen-presenting dendritic reticulum cells, or other normal tissues.
- Chimeric antibody mediates complement-dependent cell lysis (CDC) in the presence of human complement and antibody-dependent cellular cytotoxicity (ADCC) with human effector cells.

ABSORPTION
Rituximab is given only by the IV route.

DISTRIBUTION
Peak and trough levels of rituximab correlate inversely with the number of circulating CD20-positive B cells.

METABOLISM
Antibody can be detected in serum up to 3–6 months after completion of therapy. Elimination pathway has not been well characterized, although antibody-coated cells are reported to undergo elimination via Fc-receptor binding and phagocytosis by the reticuloendothelial system.

INDICATIONS
1. FDA-approved for relapsed and/or refractory low-grade or follicular, CD20+, B-cell non-Hodgkin's lymphoma as a single agent.
2. FDA-approved for previously untreated low-grade or follicular, CD20+, B-cell non-Hodgkin's lymphoma in combination with first-line chemotherapy and, in patients achieving a complete or partial response to rituximab therapy in combination with chemotherapy, as single-agent maintenance therapy.
3. FDA-approved for non-progressing (including stable disease) low-grade CD20-positive, B-cell non-Hodgkin's lymphoma as a single agent after CVP chemotherapy.
4. FDA-approved for previously untreated diffuse large B-cell, CD20+, non-Hodgkin's lymphoma in combination with CHOP or other anthracycline-based chemotherapy regimens.
5. FDA-approved in combination with fludarabine and cyclophosphamide for the treatment of previously untreated and previously treated patients with CD20-positive CLL.

DOSAGE RANGE
1. NHL: Recommended dose for relapsed or refractory low-grade or follicular NHL is 375 mg/m^2 IV on a weekly schedule for 4 or 8 weeks.
2. NHL: Recommended dose for retreatment of relapsed or refractory low-grade or follicular NHL is 375 mg/m^2 IV on a weekly schedule for 4 weeks.
3. NHL: Recommended dose for previously untreated low-grade or follicular NHL is 375 mg/m^2 IV on day 1 of each cycle of chemotherapy for up to 8 doses. For maintenance therapy, rituximab should be started 8 weeks following completion of rituximab plus chemotherapy, and administered as a single agent every 8 weeks for up to 12 doses.
4. NHL: Recommended dose for non-progressing low-grade or follicular NHL after first-line CVP chemotherapy is 375 mg/m^2 IV on a weekly schedule for 4 weeks at 6-month intervals up to a maximum of 16 doses.
5. NHL: Recommended dose for diffuse large B-cell NHL is 375 mg/m^2 IV on day 1 of each cycle of chemotherapy for up to 8 doses.
6. CLL: Recommended dose is 375 mg/m^2 on the day prior to initiation of FC chemotherapy of the first cycle and then 500 mg/m^2 on day 1 of cycles 2-6, with each cycle administered every 28 days.

DRUG INTERACTIONS
None well characterized to date.

SPECIAL CONSIDERATIONS

1. Contraindicated in patients with known type 1 hypersensitivity or anaphylactic reactions to murine proteins or product components.
2. Patients should be premedicated with acetaminophen and diphenhydramine to reduce the incidence of infusion-related reactions.
3. Infusion should be started at an initial rate of 50 mg/hour. If no toxicity is observed during the first hour, the infusion rate can be escalated by increments of 50 mg/hour every 30 minutes to a maximum of 400 mg/hour. If the first treatment is well tolerated, the starting infusion rate for the second and subsequent infusions can be administered at 100 mg/hour with 100 mg/hour increments at 30-minute intervals up to 400 mg/hour. Rituximab should **NOT** be given by IV push.
4. Monitor for infusion-related events, which usually occur 30–120 minutes after the start of the first infusion. Infusion should be immediately stopped if signs or symptoms of an allergic reaction are observed. Immediate institution of diphenhydramine, acetaminophen, corticosteroids, IV fluids, and/or vasopressors may be necessary. In most instances, the infusion can be restarted at a reduced rate (50%) once symptoms have completely resolved. Resuscitation equipment should be readily available at bedside.
5. Infusion-related deaths within 24 hours have been reported. Usually occur with the first infusion. Other risk factors include female gender, patients with pre-existing pulmonary disease, and patients with CLL or mantle cell lymphoma.
6. Monitor for tumor lysis syndrome, especially in patients with high numbers of circulating cells ($>25,000/mm^3$) or high tumor burden. In this case, the first dose of rituximab can be split into two doses with 50% of the total dose to be given on days 1 and 2.
7. Use with caution in patients with pre-existing heart disease, including arrhythmias and angina, as there is an increased risk of cardiotoxicity. The development of cardiac arrhythmias requires cardiac monitoring with subsequent infusion of drug. Patients should be monitored during the infusion and in the immediate post-transfusion period.
8. Monitor for the development of skin reactions. Patients experiencing severe skin reactions should not receive further therapy, and skin biopsies may be required to guide future treatment.
9. Pregnancy category C. Breastfeeding should be avoided.

TOXICITY 1

Infusion-related symptoms, including fever, chills, urticaria, flushing, fatigue, headache, bronchospasm, rhinitis, dyspnea, angioedema, nausea, and/or hypotension. Usually occur within 30 minutes to 2 hours after the start of the first infusion. Usually resolves upon slowing or interrupting the infusion and with supportive care. Incidence decreases with subsequent infusion.

TOXICITY 2

Tumor lysis syndrome. Characterized by hyperkalemia, hyperuricemia, hyperphosphatemia, hypocalcemia, and renal insufficiency. Usually occurs within the first 12–24 hours of treatment. Risk is increased in patients with high numbers of circulating malignant cells (>25,000/mm^3) and/or high tumor burden/bulky lymph nodes.

TOXICITY 3
Skin reactions, including pemphigus, Stevens-Johnson syndrome, lichenoid dermatitis, and toxic epidermal neurolysis. Usual onset ranges from 1 to 13 weeks following drug treatment.

TOXICITY 4
Arrhythmias and chest pain, usually occurring during drug infusion. Increased risk in patients with pre-existing cardiac disease.

TOXICITY 5
Myelosuppression is rarely observed.

TOXICITY 6
Nausea and vomiting. Generally mild.

Romidepsin

TRADE NAMES	Istodax, depsipeptide	CLASSIFICATION	Histone deacetylase (HDAC) inhibitor
CATEGORY	Chemotherapy drug	DRUG MANUFACTURER	Celgene

MECHANISM OF ACTION
- Bicyclic peptide isolated from *Chromobacterium violaceum*.
- Potent inhibitor of histone deacetylases HDAC1 and HDAC2.
- Inhibition of HDAC activity leads to accumulation of acetyl groups on the histone lysine residues, resulting in chromatin remodeling and open chromatin structure. Induction of cell-cycle arrest in G1 and G2/M phases and/or apoptosis may then occur.

- Modulator of transcription of genes and cellular gene expression.
- The precise mechanism(s) by which romidepsin exerts its antitumor activity has not been fully characterized.

MECHANISM OF RESISTANCE
None well characterized to date.

ABSORPTION
Administered only via the IV route.

DISTRIBUTION
Significant binding (90%–95%) to plasma proteins.

METABOLISM
Extensive metabolism by CYP3A4 with minor contribution from CYP3A5, CYP1A1, CYP2B6, and CYP2C19. Elimination is mainly via metabolism. The terminal half-life of the parent drug is approximately 3–3.5 hours.

INDICATIONS
FDA-approved for the treatment of patients with CTCL who have received at least one prior systemic therapy.

DOSAGE RANGE
Recommended dose is 14 mg/m^2 on days 1, 8, and 15 of a 28-day cycle.

DRUG INTERACTIONS
1. Warfarin—Patients receiving coumarin-derived anticoagulants should be closely monitored for alterations in their clotting parameters (PT and INR) and/or bleeding, as prolongation of PT and INR has been observed with concomitant use of romidepsin. The dose of warfarin may require careful adjustment in the presence of romidepsin therapy.
2. Phenytoin and other drugs that stimulate liver microsomal CYP3A4 enzymes, including carbamazepine, rifampin, phenobarbital, and St. John's wort—These drugs may increase the rate of metabolism of romidepsin, resulting in its inactivation.
3. Drugs that inhibit liver microsomal CYP3A4 enzymes, including ketoconazole, itraconazole, voriconazole, atazanavir, indinavir, ritonavir, erythromycin, and clarithromycin—These drugs may decrease the rate of metabolism of romidepsin, resulting in increased drug levels and potentially increased toxicity.
4. P-glycoprotein inhibitors—Romidepsin is a substrate for the efflux transport protein P-glycoprotein. Caution should be used when romidepsin is given concomitantly with drugs that inhibit P-glycoprotein, as increased drug levels of romidepsin may be observed.

SPECIAL CONSIDERATIONS

1. Use with caution in patients with moderate and severe hepatic impairment, although no specific dose recommendations have been provided.
2. Use with caution in patients with end-stage renal disease.
3. Closely monitor CBC and platelet count while on therapy.
4. Monitor ECG with QT measurement at baseline and periodically during therapy, as QTc prolongation has been observed. Use with caution in patients at risk of developing QT prolongation, including hypokalemia, hypomagnesemia, congenital long QT syndrome, and in patients taking antiarrhythmic medications or any other products that may cause QT prolongation.
5. Pregnancy category D. Breastfeeding should be avoided.

TOXICITY 1
Nausea and vomiting are the most common GI toxicities.

TOXICITY 2
Myelosuppression with neutropenia, thrombocytopenia, and anemia.

TOXICITY 3
Fatigue and anorexia.

TOXICITY 4
Infections involving skin, upper respiratory tract, pulmonary, GI, and urinary tract.

TOXICITY 5
ECG changes consisting of T-wave flattening, ST segment depression, and rare cases of QTc prolongation. These ECG changes are usually not associated with functional cardiac toxicity.

Sipuleucel-T

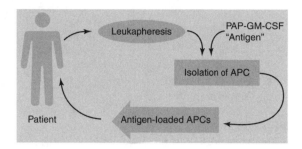

TRADE NAMES	Provenge, APC8015	CLASSIFICATION	Immunotherapy
CATEGORY	Biologic response modifier agent	DRUG MANUFACTURER	Dendreon

MECHANISM OF ACTION

- Sipuleucel-T is an autologous vaccine prepared using a patient's own peripheral blood mononuclear cells.
- Stimulates T-cell immunity to prostatic acid phosphatase (PAP), an antigen expressed in the majority of prostate cancer but not in non-prostate tissue.
- Composed of autologous antigen-presenting cells (APCs) cultured ex vivo with a fusion protein, termed PA2024, which is made up of PAP linked to GM-CSF. PA2024 provides efficient loading and processing of antigen by APCs.
- Activated APCs trigger autologous immune reaction against PAP-expressing prostate cancer cells.

MECHANISM OF RESISTANCE

- Downregulation of the cell surface expression of PAP.
- Increased tumor load rendering vaccine therapy ineffective.
- Activation of the immune checkpoint molecule PD-1, which is expressed on the surface of activated T cells, resulting in inhibition of the immune response.

ABSORPTION

Administered only by the IV route.

INDICATIONS

FDA-approved for the treatment of asymptomatic or minimally symptomatic, metastatic, castrate-resistant (hormone-refractory) prostate cancer.

DOSAGE RANGE

- Sipuleucel-T is for autologous use only.
- Recommended course is three doses infused over 60 minutes at 2-week intervals.
- Each dose contains a minimum of 50 million autologous CD54+ cells activated with PAP-GM-CSF in a sealed, patient-specific infusion bag.

DRUG INTERACTIONS

None well characterized to date.

SPECIAL CONSIDERATIONS

1. Patients should be premedicated 30 minutes prior to administration with acetaminophen 1000 mg PO and diphenhydramine 50 mg PO to reduce the incidence of acute infusion reactions.
2. Monitor for infusion-related events, which typically occur within 1 day of infusion and are more severe following the second infusion.
3. Use with caution in patients with underlying cardiac or pulmonary disease.
4. Universal precautions need to be employed, as sipuleucel-T is not routinely tested for transmissible infectious diseases.
5. The concomitant use of chemotherapy and immunosuppressive medications should be avoided as they have the potential to reduce the efficacy and/or alter the toxicity of sipuleucel-T.
6. No pregnancy category has been assigned.

TOXICITY 1

Acute infusion reactions in the form of chills, fever, fatigue, and headache. In more severe cases, patients present with dyspnea, cough, hypoxia, and bronchospasm.

TOXICITY 2

Arthralgias, myalgias, muscle cramps/spasms, and bone pain.

TOXICITY 3

Mild nausea, vomiting, constipation, diarrhea, and anorexia.

Sonidegib

TRADE NAME	Odomzo, LDE225	CLASSIFICATION	Signal transduction inhibitor
CATEGORY	Chemotherapy drug	DRUG MANUFACTURER	Novartis

MECHANISM OF ACTION
- Small-molecule inhibitor of the Hedgehog pathway.
- Binds to and inhibits smoothened, a transmembrane protein that is involved in Hedgehog signaling.

MECHANISM OF RESISTANCE
- Increased expression of MAPK signaling.
- Activation/induction of alternative cellular signaling pathways, such as c-Met, FGFR, EGFR, and PI3K/Akt.
- Reactivation of Ras/Raf signaling via mutations in KRAS, NRAS, and BRAF.
- Cross-resistance between sonidegib and vismodegib.

ABSORPTION
Oral bioavailability is low at about 10%. The median time to peak drug levels (T_{max}) is 2-4 hours. Food with high fat content can significantly increase AUC drug exposure.

DISTRIBUTION
Extensive binding (97%) of sonidegib to plasma proteins.

METABOLISM
Metabolism occurs mainly in the liver by CYP3A enzymes. The main route of elimination of parent drug and its metabolites is hepatic with excretion in feces (70%), with renal elimination accounting for 30% of an administered dose. The elimination half-life of sonidegib is approximately 28 days. Population pharmacokinetic analyses show that age, body weight, and sex do not impact on systemic exposure to drug.

INDICATIONS
FDA-approved for patients with locally advanced basal cell cancer that has recurred following surgery or radiation therapy, or in those who are not candidates for surgery and/or radiation.

DOSAGE RANGE
Recommended dose is 200 mg PO once daily on an empty stomach, at least 1 hour before or 2 hours after a meal.

DRUG INTERACTION 1
Phenytoin and other drugs that stimulate the liver microsomal CYP3A4 enzymes, including carbamazepine, rifampin, phenobarbital, and St. John's wort—These drugs may increase the metabolism of sonidegib, resulting in its inactivation.

DRUG INTERACTION 2
Drugs that inhibit the liver microsomal CYP3A4 enzymes, including ketoconazole, itraconazole, erythromycin, and clarithromycin—These drugs may decrease the metabolism of sonidegib, resulting in increased drug levels and potentially increased toxicity.

SPECIAL CONSIDERATIONS
1. Sonidegib should be taken on an empty stomach at least 1 hour before or 2 hours after a meal.
2. Dose reduction is not required in patients with mild, moderate, or severe hepatic impairment.
3. Dose reduction is not required in patients with mild or moderate renal impairment. However, the drug has not been well studied in this setting or severe renal impairment.
4. Patients should be advised not to donate blood or blood products while on sonidegib and for at least 20 months after the last drug dose.
5. The pregnancy status of female patients must be verified prior to the start of vismodegib therapy given the risk of embryo-fetal death and/or severe birth defects. This is a black-box warning.
6. Female and male patients of reproductive potential should be counseled on pregnancy prevention and planning. Female patients should be advised on the need for contraception and for at least 20 months after the last dose. Male patients should be advised of the potential risk of drug exposure through semen and to use condoms with a pregnant partner or a female partner of reproductive potential during treatment with sonidegib and for at least 8 months after the last dose. This is a black-box warning.
7. In contrast to vismodegib, proton pump inhibitors can be used while on sonidegib therapy.
8. Closely monitor serum CK and creatinine levels at baseline and periodically while on sonidegib therapy, as musculoskeletal adverse reactions, including rhabdomyolysis, has been reported.
9. Patients should be advised to report any new unexplained muscle pain, tenderness or weakness that occurs during treatment or that persists after sonidgeib therapy has been stopped.
10. Pregnancy category X. Breastfeeding should be avoided.

TOXICITY 1
Embryo-fetal deaths and/or severe birth defects.

TOXICITY 2
Musculoskeletal side effects, which include muscle spasms, musculoskeletal pain, myalgia, muscle tenderness or weakness. Rhabdomyolysis is a rare event.

TOXICITY 3
Elevations in CK.

TOXICITY 4
Decreased appetite, weight loss, fatigue, and asthenia.

TOXICITY 5
Change in taste and/or loss of taste.

TOXICITY 6
Alopecia.

TOXICITY 7
Nausea/vomiting, constipation, and diarrhea.

TOXICITY 8
Hepatotoxicity with elevations in SGOT/SGPT.

TOXICITY 9
Elevations in serum lipase and amylase.

Sorafenib

TRADE NAMES	Nexavar, BAY 43-9006	CLASSIFICATION	Signal transduction inhibitor
CATEGORY	Chemotherapy drug	DRUG MANUFACTURER	Bayer and Onyx

MECHANISM OF ACTION
- Inhibits multiple receptor tyrosine kinases (RTKs), some of which are involved in tumor growth, tumor angiogenesis, and metastasis.
- Potent inhibitor of intracellular kinases, including c-Raf and wild-type and mutant B-Raf.
- Targets vascular endothelial growth factor receptors, VEGF-R2 and VEGF-R3, and platelet-derived growth factor receptor-β (PDGFR-β), and in so doing, inhibits angiogenesis.

MECHANISM OF RESISTANCE
None well characterized to date.

ABSORPTION
Rapidly absorbed after an oral dose with peak plasma levels achieved within 2 to 7 hours. Oral administration should be without food at least 1 hour before or 2 hours after eating, as food with a high fat content reduces oral bioavailability by up to 29%.

DISTRIBUTION
Extensive binding (99%) to plasma proteins. Steady-state drug concentrations are reached in 7 days.

METABOLISM
Metabolized in the liver, primarily by CYP3A4 microsomal enzymes and by glucuronidation mediated by UGT1A9. Parent drug accounts for 70%–85% at steady state, while the pyridine-N-oxide metabolite, which has similar biological activity to sorafenib, accounts for 9%–16%. Elimination is hepatic with excretion in feces (~77%), with renal elimination of the glucuronidated metabolites accounting for 19% of the administered dose. The terminal half-life of sorafenib is approximately 25 to 48 hours.

INDICATIONS
1. FDA-approved for the treatment of advanced renal cell cancer.
2. FDA-approved for the treatment of unresectable hepatocellular cancer (HCC).

DOSAGE RANGE
Recommended dose is 400 mg PO bid. Dose may need to be reduced in Asian patients, as they appear to experience increased toxicity to sorafenib.

DRUG INTERACTION 1
Drugs such as ketoconazole and other CYP3A4 inhibitors, may decrease the rate of metabolism of sorafenib. However, one study with ketoconazole administered at a dose of 400 mg once daily for 7 days did not alter the mean AUC of a single oral dose of sorafenib 50 mg in healthy volunteers.

DRUG INTERACTION 2

Drugs such as rifampin, phenytoin, phenobarbital, carbamazepine, and St. John's wort increase the rate of metabolism of sorafenib, resulting in its inactivation.

SPECIAL CONSIDERATIONS

1. Sorafenib should be taken without food at least 1 hour before or 2 hours after a meal.
2. No dose adjustment is necessary in patients with Child-Pugh A and B liver dysfunction. However, sorafenib has not been studied in patients with Child-Pugh C liver disease, and caution should be used in this setting.
3. No dose adjustments are necessary in patients with mild-to-moderate renal dysfunction. Sorafenib has not been studied in patients undergoing dialysis.
4. Use with caution when administering sorafenib with agents that are metabolized and/or eliminated by the UGT1A1 pathway, such as irinotecan, as sorafenib is an inhibitor of UGT1A1.
5. Patients receiving sorafenib along with oral warfarin anticoagulant therapy should have their coagulation parameters (PT and INR) monitored frequently as elevations in INR and bleeding events have been observed.
6. Closely monitor blood pressure while on therapy, especially during the first 6 weeks of therapy, and treat as needed with standard oral antihypertensive medication.
7. Skin toxicities, including rash and hand-foot reaction, should be managed early in the course of therapy with topical treatments for symptomatic relief, temporary interruption, dose reduction, and/or discontinuation. Sun exposure should be avoided, and periodic dermatologic evaluation is recommended.
8. Sorafenib therapy should be interrupted in patients undergoing major surgical procedures.
9. Avoid Seville oranges, starfruit, pomelos, grapefruit, and grapefruit juice while on sorafenib therapy.
10. Pregnancy category D. Breastfeeding should be avoided.

TOXICITY 1

Hypertension usually occurs within 6 weeks of starting therapy and well-controlled with oral antihypertensive medication.

TOXICITY 2

Skin rash. Hand-foot skin reaction occurs in up to 30%. Rare cases of actinic keratoses and cutaneous squamous cell cancer have been reported.

TOXICITY 3

Bleeding complications with epistaxis most commonly observed.

TOXICITY 4

Wound-healing complications.

TOXICITY 5
Constitutional side effects with fatigue and asthenia.

TOXICITY 6
Diarrhea and nausea are the most common GI side effects.

TOXICITY 7
Hypophosphatemia occurs in up to 45% of patients, but usually clinically asymptomatic.

Streptozocin

TRADE NAMES	Streptozotocin, Zanosar	CLASSIFICATION	Alkylating agent
CATEGORY	Chemotherapy drug	DRUG MANUFACTURER	Teva

MECHANISM OF ACTION
- Cell cycle–nonspecific nitrosourea analog.
- Formation of intrastrand cross-links of DNA resulting in inhibition of DNA synthesis and function.
- Selectively targets pancreatic β cells, possibly due to the presence of a glucose moiety on the compound.
- In contrast with other nitrosourea analogs, no effect on RNA or protein synthesis.

MECHANISM OF RESISTANCE
- Decreased cellular uptake of drug.
- Increased intracellular thiol content due to glutathione and/or glutathione-related enzymes.
- Enhanced activity of DNA repair enzymes.

ABSORPTION
Not absorbed orally.

DISTRIBUTION

Rapidly cleared from plasma with an elimination half-life of 35 minutes. Drug concentrates in the liver and kidney, reaching concentrations equivalent to those in plasma. Drug metabolites cross the blood-brain barrier and enter the CSF. Selectively concentrates in pancreatic β cells presumably due to the glucose moiety on the molecule.

METABOLISM

Metabolized primarily by the liver to active metabolites. The elimination half-life of the drug is short, being less than 1 hour. About 60%–70% of drug is excreted in urine, 20% in unchanged form. Less than 1% of drug is eliminated in stool.

INDICATIONS

1. Pancreatic islet cell cancer.
2. Carcinoid tumors.

DOSAGE RANGE

1. Weekly schedule: 1000–1500 mg/m^2 IV weekly for 6 weeks followed by 4 weeks of observation.
2. Daily schedule: 500 mg/m^2 IV for 5 days every 6 weeks.

DRUG INTERACTION 1

Steroids—Concurrent use of steroids and streptozocin may result in severe hyperglycemia.

DRUG INTERACTION 2

Phenytoin—Phenytoin antagonizes the antitumor effect of streptozocin.

DRUG INTERACTION 3

Nephrotoxic drugs—Avoid concurrent use of streptozocin with nephrotoxic agents, as renal toxicity may be enhanced.

SPECIAL CONSIDERATIONS

1. Use with caution in patients with abnormal renal function. Dose reduction is recommended in this setting as nephrotoxicity is dose-limiting and can be severe and/or fatal. Baseline CrCl is required, as is monitoring of renal function before each cycle of therapy. Hydration with 1–2 liters of fluid is recommended to prevent nephrotoxicity.
2. Monitor CBC while on therapy.
3. Avoid the use of other nephrotoxic agents in combination with streptozocin.
4. Carefully administer drug to minimize and/or avoid burning, pain, and extravasation.
5. Pregnancy category D. Breastfeeding should be avoided.

TOXICITY 1

Renal toxicity is dose-limiting. Seen in 40%–60% of patients and manifested initially by proteinuria and azotemia. Can also present as glucosuria, hypophosphatemia, and nephrogenic diabetes insipidus. Permanent renal damage can occur in rare instances.

TOXICITY 2

Nausea and vomiting occur in 90% of patients. More frequently observed with the daily dosage schedule and can be severe.

TOXICITY 3

Myelosuppression. Usually mild with nadir occurring at 3–4 weeks.

TOXICITY 4

Pain and/or burning at the injection site.

TOXICITY 5

Altered glucose metabolism resulting in either hypoglycemia or hyperglycemia.

TOXICITY 6

Mild and transient increases in SGOT, alkaline phosphatase, and bilirubin. Usual onset is within 2–3 weeks of starting therapy.

Sunitinib

TRADE NAMES	Sutent, SU11248	CLASSIFICATION	Signal transduction inhibitor
CATEGORY	Chemotherapy drug	DRUG MANUFACTURER	Pfizer

MECHANISM OF ACTION

- Inhibits multiple RTKs, some of which are involved in tumor growth, tumor angiogenesis, and metastasis.
- Potent inhibitor of platelet-derived growth factor receptors (PDGFR-α and PDGFR-β), vascular endothelial growth factor receptors (VEGFR-1, VEGFR-2, and VEGFR-3), stem cell factor receptor (Kit), Fms-like tyrosine kinase-3 (Flt3), colony-stimulating factor receptor type 1 (CSF-1R), and the glial cell-line derived neurotrophic factor receptor (RET).

MECHANISM OF RESISTANCE

- Increased expression of PDGFR-α, PDGFR-β, VEGFR-1, VEGFR-2, VEGFR-3, c-Kit, CSF-1R, and RET.
- Alterations in binding affinity of the drug to the RTK resulting from mutations in the RTKs.
- Increased degradation and/or metabolism of the drug through as yet ill-defined mechanisms.

ABSORPTION

Oral bioavailability is nearly 100%. Sunitinib may be taken with or without food, as food does not affect oral bioavailability.

DISTRIBUTION

Extensive binding (90%–95%) of sunitinib and its primary metabolite to plasma proteins. Peak plasma levels are achieved 6 to 12 hours after ingestion. Steady-state drug concentrations of sunitinib and its primary active metabolite are reached in 10 to 14 days.

METABOLISM

Metabolized in the liver primarily by CYP3A4 microsomal enzymes to produce its primary active metabolite, which is further metabolized by CYP3A4. The primary active metabolite comprises 23%–37% of the total exposure. Elimination is hepatic with excretion in feces (~60%), with renal elimination accounting for 16% of the administered dose. The terminal half-lives of sunitinib and its primary active metabolite are approximately 40–60 hours and 80–110 hours, respectively. With repeated daily administration, sunitinib accumulates 3- to 4-fold, while the primary metabolite accumulates 7- to 10-fold.

INDICATIONS

1. FDA-approved for GIST after disease progression on or intolerance to imatinib.
2. FDA-approved for advanced renal cell cancer.
3. FDA-approved for progressive, well-differentiated PNET in patients with unresectable locally advanced or metastatic disease.

DOSAGE RANGE

1. GIST and RCC: Recommended dose is 50 mg/day PO for 4 weeks followed by 2 weeks off.
2. PNET: Recommended dose is 37.5 mg/day PO continuously.

DRUG INTERACTION 1

Drugs such as ketoconazole, itraconazole, erythromycin, clarithromycin, atazanavir, indinavir, nefazodone, nelfinavir, ritonavir, saquinavir, telithromycin, and voriconazole decrease the rate of metabolism of sunitinib, resulting in increased drug levels and potentially increased toxicity.

DRUG INTERACTION 2

Drugs such as rifampin, phenytoin, phenobarbital, carbamazepine, and St. John's wort increase the rate of metabolism of sunitinib, resulting in its inactivation.

SPECIAL CONSIDERATIONS

1. Baseline and periodic evaluations of LVEF should be performed while on sunitinib therapy.
2. Use with caution in patients with underlying cardiac disease, especially those who presented with cardiac events within 12 months prior to initiation of sunitinib, such as MI (including severe/unstable angina), coronary/peripheral artery bypass graft, and CHF.
3. In the presence of clinical manifestations of CHF, discontinuation of sunitinib is recommended. The dose of sunitinib should be interrupted and/or reduced in patients without clinical evidence of CHF but with an ejection fraction <50% and >20% below pretreatment baseline.
4. Closely monitor blood pressure while on therapy and treat as needed with standard oral antihypertensive medication. In cases of severe hypertension, temporary suspension of sunitinib is recommended until hypertension is controlled.
5. Monitor for adrenal insufficiency in patients who experience increased stress such as surgery, trauma, or severe infection.
6. Closely monitor thyroid function tests and TSH at 2- to 3-month intervals, as sunitinib treatment results in hypothyroidism. The incidence of hypothyroidism is increased with prolonged duration of therapy.
7. Avoid Seville oranges, starfruit, pomelos, grapefruit, and grapefruit, products while on sunitinib therapy.
8. Pregnancy category D. Breastfeeding should be avoided.

TOXICITY 1

Hypertension occurs in up to nearly 30% of patients. Usually occurs within 3–4 weeks of starting therapy and well-controlled with oral antihypertensive medication.

TOXICITY 2

Yellowish discoloration of the skin occurs in approximately 30% of patients. Skin rash, dryness, thickness, and/or cracking of skin. Depigmentation of hair and/or skin may also occur.

TOXICITY 3

Bleeding complications with epistaxis most commonly observed.

TOXICITY 4

Constitutional side effects with fatigue and asthenia, which may be significant in some patients.

TOXICITY 5

Diarrhea, stomatitis, altered taste, and abdominal pain are the most common GI side effects. Pancreatitis has been reported rarely with elevations in serum lipase and amylase.

TOXICITY 6

Myelosuppression with neutropenia and thrombocytopenia.

TOXICITY 7

Increased risk of left ventricular dysfunction, which in some cases results in CHF.

TOXICITY 8

Adrenal insufficiency and hypothyroidism.

Talimogene laherparepvec

TRADE NAMES	Imlygic; T-vec	**CLASSIFICATION**	Immunotherapy
CATEGORY	Biologic response modifier agent; Oncolytic virus	**DRUG MANUFACTURER**	Amgen

MECHANISM OF ACTION
- Talimogene laherparepvec (T-vec) is a first-in-class oncolytic virus based on a modified herpes simplex virus (HSV) type 1 that selectively replicates in and lyses tumor cells.
- T-vec is modified through deletion of two non-essential viral genes, which reduces viral pathogenicity and enhances tumor-selective replication.
- T-vec is further modified with insertion and expression of the gene encoding human granulocyte macrophage colony-stimulating factor (GM-CSF). This results in local production of GM-CSF that then recruits and activates antigen-presenting dendritic cells with subsequent induction of tumor-specific T-cell responses.
- A local antitumor immune response is generated through the combined effects of release of tumor-derived antigens and GM-CSF production. There also appears to be generation of a systemic immune response that acts at non-injected sites, a phenomenon known as an abscopal effect.
- Clinical studies have shown an association between clinical response and presence of interferon-γ-producing MART-1-specific CD8+ T cells and reduction in CD4+ FoxP3+ regulatory T cells, which are consistent with induction of host antitumor immunity.

MECHANISM OF RESISTANCE
None well characterized to date.

ABSORPTION
Administered only via the intratumoral route.

DISTRIBUTION
Distribution in the body has not been well-characterized.

METABOLISM
Metabolism of T-vec has not been well-characterized.

INDICATIONS
FDA-approved for the local treatment of unresectable cutaneous, subcutaneous, and nodal lesions in patients with recurrent melanoma following initial surgery.

DOSAGE RANGE
Initial dose: 10^6 PFU per mL solution

Second dose to be administered 3 weeks after initial treatment: 10^8 PFU per mL solution

All subsequent doses: 10^8 PFU per mL solution to be administered 2 weeks after the second treatment

The following guidelines are used to determine the volume of T-vec to be injected (lesion size is based on longest dimension; when lesions are clustered together, they are to be injected as a single lesion):

- If the lesion size is >5 cm, inject up to 4 mL.
- If the lesion size is >2.5 cm to 5 cm, inject up to 2 mL.
- If the lesion size is >1.5 cm to 2.5 cm, inject up to 1 mL.
- If the lesion size is >0.5 cm to 1.5 cm, inject up to 0.5 mL.
- If the lesion size is ≤0.5 cm, inject up to 0.1 mL.

DRUG INTERACTION

Acyclovir or other antiviral agents may reduce clinical efficacy of T-vec.

SPECIAL CONSIDERATIONS:

1. T-vec should be administered by intralesional injection into cutaneous, subcutaneous, and/or nodal lesions that are visible, palpable, or detectable by ultrasound. Please see package insert for complete details regarding how the intralesional injection should be performed.
2. Accidental exposure may lead to transmission of T-vec and herpetic infection. If accidental exposure occurs, exposed individuals should clean the affected areas thoroughly. If signs or symptoms of herpetic infection develop, the exposed individuals must contact their healthcare provide for appropriate treatment.
3. Healthcare providers who are immunocompromised or pregnant should not prepare or administer talimogene laherparepvec and should not come into direct contact with injection sites, dressings, or body fluids of treated patients.
4. T-vec should **NOT** be administered to immunocompromised patients, including those with a history of leukemia, lymphoma, AIDS or other clinical manifestations of infections with human immunodeficiency viruses, and those on immunosuppressive therapy.
5. T-vec should **NOT** be administered to pregnant patients.
6. There are no formal recommendations for dosing in the setting of hepatic or renal impairment as studies have not been conducted in these clinical settings.
7. Pregnancy category D. Breastfeeding should be avoided.

TOXICITY 1

Generalized symptoms including fatigue, low-grade fever, chills, and myalgias are most commonly observed.

TOXICITY 2

Herpetic infections with cold sores and herpetic keratitis. Disseminated herpes infection may occur in immunocompromised patients.

TOXICITY 3
Injection-site complications, including pain, erythema, and pruritus at the injection site; necrosis; tumor tissue ulceration; and cellulitis.

TOXICITY 4
Immune-mediated events, including glomerulonephritis, pneumonitis, vasculitis, vitiligo, and psoriasis.

TOXICITY 5
Influenza-like illness.

TOXICITY 6
GI side effects with nausea/vomiting, diarrhea, and constipation.

Tamoxifen

TRADE NAME	Nolvadex	CLASSIFICATION	Antiestrogen
CATEGORY	Hormonal agent	DRUG MANUFACTURER	AstraZeneca

MECHANISM OF ACTION
- Nonsteroidal antiestrogen with weak estrogen agonist effects.
- Competes with estrogen for binding to ERs. Binding of tamoxifen to ER leads to ER dimerization. The tamoxifen-bound ER dimer is transported to the nucleus, where it binds to DNA sequences referred to as ER elements. This interaction results in inhibition of critical transcriptional processes and signal transduction pathways that are required for cellular growth and proliferation.
- Cell cycle–specific agent that blocks cells in the mid-G1 phase of the cell cycle. Effect may be mediated by cyclin D.
- Stimulates the secretion of transforming growth factor-β (TGF-β), which then acts to inhibit the expression and/or activity of TGF-α and IGF-1, two genes that are involved in cell growth and proliferation.

MECHANISM OF RESISTANCE
- Decreased expression of ER.
- Mutations in the ER leading to decreased binding affinity to tamoxifen.
- Overexpression of growth factor receptors, such as as EGFR, HER2/neu, IGF-1R, or TGF-β that counteract the inhibitory effects of tamoxifen.
- Presence of ESR1 mutations.

ABSORPTION
Rapidly and completely absorbed in the GI tract. Peak plasma levels are achieved within 4–6 hours after oral administration.

DISTRIBUTION
Distributes to most body tissues, especially in those expressing estrogen receptors. Present in very low concentrations in CSF. Nearly all of drug is bound to plasma proteins.

METABOLISM
Extensively metabolized by liver cytochrome P450 enzymes after oral administration. The main metabolite, N-desmethyl tamoxifen, has biologic activity similar to that of the parent drug. Both tamoxifen and its metabolites are excreted primarily (75%) in feces with minimal clearance in urine. The terminal half-lives of tamoxifen and its metabolites are relatively long, approaching 7–14 days.

INDICATIONS
1. Adjuvant therapy in axillary node-negative breast cancer following surgical resection.
2. Adjuvant therapy in axillary node-positive breast cancer in postmenopausal women following surgical resection.
3. Adjuvant therapy in women with ductal carcinoma in situ (DCIS) after surgical resection and radiation therapy.
4. Metastatic breast cancer in women and men.
5. Approved as a chemopreventive agent for women at high risk for breast cancer. "High-risk" women are defined as women >35 years and with a 5-year predicted risk of breast cancer $\geqslant$1.67%, according to the Gail model.
6. Endometrial cancer.

DOSAGE RANGE
Recommended dose for treatment of breast cancer patients is 20 mg PO every day.

DRUG INTERACTION 1
Warfarin—Tamoxifen can inhibit metabolism of warfarin by the liver P450 system leading to increased anticoagulant effect. Coagulation parameters, including PT and INR, must be closely monitored, and dose adjustments may be required.

DRUG INTERACTION 2

Drugs activated by liver P450 system—Tamoxifen and its metabolites are potent inhibitors of hepatic P450 enzymes and may inhibit the metabolic activation of drugs utilizing this pathway, including cyclophosphamide.

DRUG INTERACTION 3

Drugs metabolized by liver P450 system—Tamoxifen and its metabolites are potent inhibitors of hepatic P450 enzymes and may inhibit the metabolism of various drugs, including erythromycin, calcium channel blockers, and cyclosporine.

DRUG INTERACTION 4

Antidepressants that act as selective serotonin reuptake inhibitors (SSRIs) or selective noradrenergic reuptake inhibitors (SNRIs)—Drugs such as paroxetine, fluoxetine, bupropion, duloxetine, and sertraline are inhibitors of CYP2D6, which can then interfere and inhibit tamoxifen metabolism, resulting in lower blood levels of the active tamoxifen metabolites.

DRUG INTERACTION 5

Antipsychotics—Drugs such as thioridazine, perphenazine, and pimozide are inhibitors of CYP2D6, which can then interfere and inhibit tamoxifen metabolism, resulting in lower blood levels of the active tamoxifen metabolites.

DRUG INTERACTION 6

Drugs such as cimetidine, quinidine, ticlopidine, and terfenadine are inhibitors of CYP2D6, which can then interfere and inhibit tamoxifen metabolism, resulting in lower blood levels of the active tamoxifen metabolites.

SPECIAL CONSIDERATIONS

1. Instruct patients to notify physician about menstrual irregularities, abnormal vaginal bleeding, and pelvic pain and/or discomfort while on therapy.
2. Patients should have routine follow-up with a gynecologist, as tamoxifen therapy is associated with an increased risk of endometrial hyperplasia, polyps, and endometrial cancer.
3. Use with caution in patients with abnormal liver function as there may be an increased risk of drug accumulation resulting in toxicity.
4. Use with caution in patients with either personal history or family history of thromboembolic disease or hypercoagulable states, as tamoxifen is associated with an increased risk of thromboembolic events. Tamoxifen therapy is associated with antithrombin III deficiency.
5. Initiation of treatment with tamoxifen may induce a transient tumor flare. Tamoxifen should not be given in patients with impending ureteral obstruction, spinal cord compression, or in those with extensive painful bone metastases.
6. Premenopausal patients should be warned about the possibility of developing menopausal symptoms with tamoxifen therapy.

7. Monitor CBC during therapy with tamoxifen as myelosuppression can occur, albeit rarely.
8. Testing for CYP2D6 is recommended prior to initiation of tamoxifen therapy. Up to 10% of patients are poor metabolizers of tamoxifen based on CYP2D6 alleles, which might result in reduced clinical efficacy.
9. Consider using citalopram, escitalopram, fluvoxamine, mirtazapine, and venlafaxine if an antidepressant is required during treatment with tamoxifen.
10. Avoid the use of medications that inhibit the CYP2D6 system.
11. Pregnancy category D. Breastfeeding should be avoided.

TOXICITY 1
Menopausal symptoms, including hot flashes, nausea, vomiting, vaginal bleeding, and menstrual irregularities. Vaginal discharge and vaginal dryness also observed.

TOXICITY 2
Fluid retention and peripheral edema observed in about 30% of patients.

TOXICITY 3
Tumor flare usually occurs within the first 2 weeks of starting therapy. May observe increased bone pain, urinary retention, back pain with spinal cord compression, and/or hypercalcemia.

TOXICITY 4
Headache, lethargy, dizziness occur rarely. Visual disturbances, including cataracts, retinopathy, and decreased visual acuity, have been described.

TOXICITY 5
Skin rash, pruritus, hair thinning, and/or partial hair loss.

TOXICITY 6
Myelosuppression is rare, with transient thrombocytopenia and leukopenia. Usually resolves after the first week of treatment.

TOXICITY 7
Thromboembolic complications, including deep vein thrombosis, pulmonary embolism, and superficial phlebitis. Incidence of thromboembolic events may be increased when tamoxifen is given concomitantly with chemotherapy.

TOXICITY 8
Elevations in serum triglycerides.

TOXICITY 9
Increased incidence of endometrial hyperplasia, polyps, and endometrial cancer.

TAS-102

TRADE NAME	Lonsurf	**CLASSIFICATION**	Antimetabolite
CATEGORY	Chemotherapy drug	**DRUG MANUFACTURER**	Taiho Oncology

MECHANISM OF ACTION
- Composed of trifluridine, a fluorinated pyrimidine nucleoside analog, and tipiracil, a thymidine phosphorylase inhibitor, at a molar ratio of 1:0.5.
- The presence of tipiracil inhibits trifluridine metabolism by thymidine phosphorylase, thereby enhancing trifluridine exposure and subsequent metabolism to the triphosphate metabolite.
- Trifluridine monophosphate inhibits thymidylate synthase, leading to inhibition of thymidylate, a key nucleotide precursor for DNA biosynthesis.
- Trifluridine triphosphate is incorporated into DNA resulting in inhibition of DNA synthesis and function.
- Retains activity in 5-FU resistant model systems.
- Appears to have similar clinical activity in *KRAS*-wt and *KRAS*-mutant colorectal cancer.

MECHANISM OF RESISTANCE
- None well-characterized to date

ABSORPTION
Peak plasma levels of trifluridine are reached in 2 hours. The rate and extent of absorption are reduced by food.

DISTRIBUTION
Trifluridine is mainly bound to serum albumin. Plasma protein binding of tipiracil is less than 10%.

METABOLISM
Trifluridine is primarily eliminated via metabolism by thymidine phosphorylase to form the inactive metabolite 5-trifluromethyluracil (FTY). No other major metabolites have been identified in plasma or urine. Trifluridine and tipiracil are not metabolized by the liver P450 enzymes. Greater than 90% of an administered dose of drug and its metabolites is cleared in the urine. Following a single dose of TAS-102, the mean 48-hour urinary excretion was 1.5% for unchanged trifluridine, 19.2% for FTY, and 29.3% for unchanged tipiracil. The mean elimination half-life of trifluridine is 2.1 hours and of tipiracil is 2.4 hours.

INDICATIONS
FDA-approved for the treatment of patients with metastatic colorectal cancer who have been previously treated with fluoropyrimidine-, oxaliplatin-, and

irinotecan-based chemotherapy, an anti-VEGF biological therapy, and if KRAS wild-type, an anti-EGFR therapy.

DOSAGE RANGE
Recommended dose is 35 mg/m^2 PO bid on days 1–5 and 8–12 of a 28-day cycle.

DRUG INTERACTIONS
Drug-drug interactions studies have not yet been conducted with TAS-102.

SPECIAL CONSIDERATIONS
1. TAS-102 should be taken within 1 hour after completion of morning and evening meals.
2. Use with caution in patients >65 years of age as the incidence of grade 3/4 myelosuppression is increased in this patient population.
3. Closely monitor CBCs prior to and on day 15 of each cycle.
4. TAS-102 should not be initiated until the ANC is >1,500/mm^3, platelets are >75,000/mm^3, and grade 3/4 non-hematologic toxicity has resolved to grade 0 or 1.
5. Within a treatment cycle, TAS-102 should be withheld for any of the following: ANC <500/mm^3, platelets are <50,000/mm^3, and grade 3/4 non-hematologic toxicity.
6. No dose adjustment is necessary in patients with mild liver dysfunction. However, patients should be closely monitored. Hepatic dysfunction studies are on-going to determine the effect of moderate or severe hepatic impairment on drug metabolism.
7. No dose adjustment is recommended in patients with mild to moderate renal dysfunction (baseline CrCl, 30–59 mL/min). However, patients with moderate renal dysfunction should be closely monitored as they may be at greater risk for increased toxicity. Renal dysfunction studies are on-going to determine the effect of moderate or severe renal impairment on drug metabolism.
8. Pregnancy category D. Breastfeeding should be avoided.

TOXICITY 1
Myelosuppression with neutropenia, anemia, and thrombocytopenia.

TOXICITY 2
GI toxicity with diarrhea, abdominal pain, and nausea/vomiting.

TOXICITY 3
Fatigue, asthenia.

TOXICITY 4
Anorexia.

Temozolomide

TRADE NAME	Temodar	CLASSIFICATION	Nonclassic alkylating agent
CATEGORY	Chemotherapy drug	DRUG MANUFACTURER	Merck

MECHANISM OF ACTION

- Imidazotetrazine analog that is structurally and functionally similar to dacarbazine.
- Cell cycle–nonspecific agent.
- Metabolic activation to the reactive compound MTIC is required for antitumor activity.
- Although the precise mechanism of cytotoxicity is unclear, this drug methylates guanine residues in DNA and inhibits DNA, RNA, and protein synthesis. Does not cross-link DNA strands.

MECHANISM OF RESISTANCE

Increased activity of DNA repair enzymes such as AGAT.

ABSORPTION

Widely distributed in body tissues. Rapidly and completely absorbed with an oral bioavailability approaching 100%. Maximum plasma concentrations are reached within 1 hour after administration. Food reduces the rate and extent of drug absorption.

DISTRIBUTION

Because temozolomide is lipophilic, it crosses the blood-brain barrier. Levels in brain and CSF are 30%–40% of those achieved in plasma.

METABOLISM

Metabolized primarily by non-enzymatic hydrolysis at physiologic pH. Undergoes conversion to the metabolite MTIC, which is further hydrolyzed to AIC, a known intermediate in purine de novo synthesis, and methylhydrazine, the presumed active alkylating species. The elimination half-life of the drug is 2 hours. About 40%–50% of the parent drug is excreted in urine within 6 hours of administration, and tubular secretion is the predominant mechanism of renal excretion. No specific guidelines for drug dosing in the setting of hepatic and/or renal dysfunction. However, dose modification should be considered in patients with moderately severe hepatic and/or renal dysfunction.

INDICATIONS

1. FDA-approved for refractory anaplastic astrocytomas at first relapse following treatment with a nitrosourea and procarbazine-containing regimen.
2. FDA-approved for newly diagnosed glioblastoma multiforme (GBM) in combination with radiotherapy and then as maintenance treatment.
3. Metastatic melanoma.

DOSAGE RANGE

- Usual dose is 150 mg/m^2 PO daily for 5 days every 28 days.
- Dose is adjusted to nadir neutrophil and platelet counts. If nadir of ANC is acceptable, the dose may be increased to 200 mg/m^2 PO daily for 5 days. If ANC falls below acceptable levels during any cycle, the next dose should be reduced by 50 mg/m^2 PO daily.
- Temozolomide is given at 75 mg/m^2 PO daily for 42 days along with radiotherapy (60 Gy in 30 fractions) for newly diagnosed GBM. During the maintenance phase, which is started 4 weeks after completion of the combined modality therapy, temozolomide is given on cycle 1 at 150 mg/m^2 PO daily for 5 days followed by 23 days without treatment. For cycles 2–6, the dose of temozolomide may be escalated to 200 mg/m^2 if tolerated.

DRUG INTERACTIONS

None known.

SPECIAL CONSIDERATIONS

1. Temozolomide is a moderately emetogenic agent. Aggressive use of antiemetics prior to drug administration is required to decrease the risk of nausea and vomiting.
2. Patients should be warned to avoid sun exposure for several days after drug treatment.
3. Use with caution in elderly patients (age >65) as they are at increased risk for myelosuppression.
4. Patients should be monitored closely for the development of PCP, and those receiving temozolomide and radiotherapy require PCP prophylaxis.
5. Pregnancy category D. Breastfeeding should be discontinued.

TOXICITY 1

Myelosuppression is dose-limiting. Leukopenia and thrombocytopenia are commonly observed.

TOXICITY 2

Nausea and vomiting. Mild to moderate, usually occurring within 1–3 hours and lasting for up to 12 hours. Aggressive antiemetic therapy strongly recommended.

TOXICITY 3
Headache and fatigue.

TOXICITY 4
Mild elevation in hepatic transaminases.

TOXICITY 5
Photosensitivity.

TOXICITY 6
Teratogenic, mutagenic, and carcinogenic.

Temsirolimus

TRADE NAMES	Torisel, CCI-779	CLASSIFICATION	Signal transduction inhibitor
CATEGORY	Chemotherapy drug	DRUG MANUFACTURER	Pfizer

MECHANISM OF ACTION
- Potent inhibitor of the mammalian target of rapamycin (mTOR) kinase, which is a key component of cellular signaling pathways involved in the growth and proliferation of tumor cells.
- Inhibition of mTOR signaling results in cell cycle arrest, induction of apoptosis, and inhibition of angiogenesis.

MECHANISM OF RESISTANCE
None well characterized to date.

ABSORPTION
Not available for oral use and is administered only by the IV route.

DISTRIBUTION
Widely distributed in tissues. Steady-state drug concentrations are reached in 7–8 days.

METABOLISM
Metabolism in the liver primarily by CYP3A4 microsomal enzymes. The main metabolite is sirolimus, which is a potent inhibitor of mTOR signaling, with the other metabolites accounting for <10% of all metabolites measured. Elimination is mainly hepatic with excretion in the feces, and renal elimination of parent drug and its metabolites accounts for only 5% of an administered dose. The terminal half-life of the parent drug is 17 hours, while that of sirolimus is 55 hours.

INDICATIONS
FDA-approved for the treatment of advanced renal cell cancer.

DOSAGE RANGE
Recommended dose is 25 mg IV administered on a weekly schedule.

DRUG INTERACTION 1
Phenytoin and other drugs that stimulate liver microsomal CYP3A4 enzymes, including carbamazepine, rifampin, phenobarbital, and St. John's wort—These drugs may increase the rate of metabolism of temsirolimus, resulting in its inactivation.

DRUG INTERACTION 2
Drugs that inhibit liver microsomal CYP3A4 enzymes, including ketoconazole, itraconazole, erythromycin, and clarithromycin—These drugs may decrease the rate of metabolism of temsirolimus, resulting in increased drug levels and potentially increased toxicity.

SPECIAL CONSIDERATIONS
1. Use with caution in patients with mild hepatic impairment, and dose reduction to 15 mg/week is recommended.
2. Patients should be premedicated with an H1-antagonist antihistamine (diphenhydramine 25–50 mg IV) 30 minutes before the start of therapy to reduce the incidence of hypersensitivity reactions.
3. Closely monitor serum glucose levels in all patients, especially those with diabetes mellitus.
4. Closely monitor patients for new or progressive pulmonary symptoms, including cough, dyspnea, and fever. Temsirolimus therapy should be interrupted pending further diagnostic evaluation.

5. Patients are at increased risk for developing opportunistic infections while on temsirolimus given its potential immunosuppressive effects.
6. Closely monitor serum triglyceride and cholesterol levels while on therapy.
7. Patients should be advised to report the development of fever, abdominal pain, and/or bloody stools, as temsirolimus may cause bowel perforation on rare occasions.
8. Closely monitor renal function during therapy, as temsirolimus can cause progressive and severe renal failure, especially in patients with pre-existing renal impairment.
9. Use with caution after surgical procedures, as temsirolimus can impair the process of wound healing.
10. Avoid grapefruit and grapefruit products while on temsirolimus.
11. Avoid the use of live vaccines and/or close contact with those who have received live vaccines while on temsirolimus.
12. Pregnancy category D. Breastfeeding should be avoided.

TOXICITY 1
Asthenia and fatigue.

TOXICITY 2
Pruritus, dry skin with mainly a pustular, acneiform skin rash.

TOXICITY 3
Nausea/vomiting, mucositis, and anorexia. On rare occasions, bowel perforations can occur and present as fever, abdominal pain, and bloody stools.

TOXICITY 4
Hyperlipidemia with increased serum triglycerides and/or cholesterol in up to 90% of patients.

TOXICITY 5
Hyperglycemia in up to 80%–90% of patients.

TOXICITY 6
Allergic, hypersensitivity reactions occur in 10% of patients.

TOXICITY 7
Pulmonary toxicity in the form of ILD manifested by increased cough, dyspnea, fever, and pulmonary infiltrates. Observed in less than 1% of patients and more frequent in patients with underlying pulmonary disease.

TOXICITY 8
Renal toxicity with elevation in serum creatinine.

TOXICITY 9
Peripheral edema.

Thalidomide

TRADE NAME	Thalomid	CLASSIFICATION	Immunomodulatory agent, antiangiogenic agent
CATEGORY	Unclassified therapeutic agent, biologic response modifier agent	DRUG MANUFACTURER	Celgene

MECHANISM OF ACTION
- Mechanism of action is not fully characterized.
- Inhibition of TNF-α synthesis and down-modulation of selected cell surface adhesion molecules.
- May exert an antiangiogenic effect through inhibition of bFGF and VEGF as well as through as yet undefined mechanisms.

MECHANISM OF RESISTANCE
None well characterized to date.

ABSORPTION
Oral bioavailability of thalidomide is not known due to poor aqueous solubility. Slowly absorbed from the GI tract with peak plasma levels reached 3–6 hours after oral administration.

DISTRIBUTION
The extent of binding to plasma proteins is not known. Remains unclear whether thalidomide is present in the ejaculate of males.

METABOLISM
Non-enzymatic hydrolysis appears to be the principal mechanism of thalidomide breakdown. However, the exact metabolic pathway(s) has not been fully characterized. The precise route of drug excretion is not well defined.

INDICATIONS
1. FDA-approved in combination with dexamethasone for the treatment of newly diagnosed multiple myeloma.
2. FDA-approved for the treatment of the cutaneous manifestations of erythema nodosum leprosum (ENL).
3. Thalidomide has activity in MDS and in a broad range of solid tumors.

DOSAGE RANGE

No standard dose recommendations for use in cancer patients have been established. When used in combination with chemotherapy, doses are typically titrated up to 400 mg PO daily given as a single bedtime dose. As a single agent, doses have been in the range of 100 mg to 1200 mg daily.

DRUG INTERACTION 1

Barbiturates, chlorpromazine, and reserpine—Sedative effect of thalidomide is enhanced with concurrent use of these medications.

DRUG INTERACTION 2

Alcohol—Sedative effect of thalidomide is enhanced with concurrent use of alcohol.

SPECIAL CONSIDERATIONS

1. Pregnancy category X. Severe fetal malformations can occur if even one capsule is taken by a pregnant woman. All women should have a baseline β-human chorionic gonadotropin before starting therapy with thalidomide. All women of childbearing potential should practice two forms of birth control throughout treatment with thalidomide: one highly effective (intrauterine device, hormonal contraception, partner's vasectomy) and one additional barrier method (latex condom, diaphragm, cervical cap). It is strongly recommended that these precautionary measures begin 4 weeks before initiation of therapy, that they continue while on therapy, and continue for at least 4 weeks after therapy is discontinued.
2. Breastfeeding while on therapy should be avoided given the potential for serious adverse reactions from thalidomide in nursing infants. It remains unknown whether thalidomide is excreted in human milk.
3. Men taking thalidomide must use latex condoms for every sexual encounter with a woman of childbearing potential, since thalidomide may be present in semen.
4. Patients with AIDS should have their HIV mRNA levels monitored after the first and third months after treatment initiation with thalidomide, then every 3 months thereafter, as HIV mRNA levels may be increased while on thalidomide.
5. Instruct patients to avoid operating heavy machinery or driving a car while on thalidomide, as the drug can cause drowsiness.
6. Patients who develop a skin rash during therapy with thalidomide should have prompt medical evaluation. Serious skin reactions, including Stevens-Johnson syndrome, which may be fatal, have been reported.
7. There is an increased risk of thromboembolic complications, including DVT and PE, and prophylaxis with low-molecular weight heparin, warfarin, or aspirin can help to prevent and/or reduce the incidence.

TOXICITY 1

Teratogenic effect is most serious toxicity. Severe birth defects or death to an unborn fetus. Manifested as absent or defective limbs, hypoplasia or absence of bones, facial palsy, absent or small ears, absent or shrunken eyes, congenital heart defects, and GI and renal abnormalities.

TOXICITY 2

General neurologic-related events that occur frequently include fatigue, orthostatic hypotension, and dizziness. Specific peripheral neuropathy in the form of numbness, tingling, and pain in the feet or hands does not appear to be dose- or duration-related. Prior exposure to neurotoxic agents increases the risk of occurrence.

TOXICITY 3

Constipation is most common GI toxicity.

TOXICITY 4

No known direct myelosuppressive effects. Certain patient populations (ENL and HIV) have reported a higher incidence of abnormalities in blood counts.

TOXICITY 5

Skin toxicity in the form of maculopapular skin rash, urticaria, and dry skin. Serious dermatologic reactions, including Stevens-Johnson syndrome, have been reported. Patients who develop a skin rash during therapy with thalidomide should discontinue therapy. Therapy can be restarted with caution if the rash was not exfoliative, purpuric, or bullous, or otherwise suggestive of a serious skin condition.

TOXICITY 6

Daytime sedation or fatigue following an evening dose often associated with larger initial doses. Doses can be reduced until the patient accommodates to the effect.

TOXICITY 7

Increased risk of thromboembolic complications, including DVT and PE.

Thioguanine

TRADE NAMES	6-Thioguanine, 6-TG	CLASSIFICATION	Antimetabolite
CATEGORY	Chemotherapy drug	DRUG MANUFACTURER	GlaxoSmithKline

MECHANISM OF ACTION

- Cell cycle–specific purine analog with activity in the S-phase.
- Parent drug is inactive. Requires intracellular phosphorylation by the enzyme HGPRT to the cytotoxic monophosphate form, which is then eventually metabolized to the triphosphate metabolite form.
- Inhibits de novo purine synthesis by inhibiting PRPP amidotransferase.
- Incorporation of thiopurine triphosphate nucleotides into DNA, resulting in inhibition of DNA synthesis and function.
- Incorporation of thiopurine triphosphate nucleotides into RNA, resulting in alterations in RNA processing and/or translation.

MECHANISM OF RESISTANCE

- Decreased expression of the activating enzyme HGPRT.
- Increased expression of the catabolic enzyme alkaline phosphatase or the conjugating enzyme TPMT.
- Decreased cellular transport of drug.
- Decreased expression of mismatch repair enzymes (e.g., hMLH1, hMSH2).
- Cross-resistance between thioguanine and mercaptopurine.

ABSORPTION

Oral absorption of drug is incomplete and variable. Only 30% of an oral dose is absorbed. Peak plasma levels are reached in 2–4 hours after ingestion.

DISTRIBUTION

Distributes widely into the RNA and DNA of peripheral blood and bone marrow cells. Crosses the placenta but does not appear to cross the blood-brain barrier.

METABOLISM

Metabolized in the liver by the processes of deamination and methylation. Main pathway of inactivation is catalyzed by guanine deaminase (guanase). In contrast with mercaptopurine, metabolism of thioguanine does not involve xanthine oxidase. Metabolites are eliminated in both feces and urine. Plasma half-life is on the order of 80–90 minutes.

INDICATIONS

1. Acute myelogenous leukemia.
2. Acute lymphoblastic leukemia.
3. Chronic myelogenous leukemia.

DOSAGE RANGE

1. Induction: 100 mg/m^2 PO every 12 hours on days 1–5, usually in combination with cytarabine.
2. Maintenance: 100 mg/m^2 PO every 12 hours on days 1–5, every 4 weeks, usually in combination with other agents.
3. Single-agent: 1–3 mg/kg PO daily.

DRUG INTERACTIONS
None known.

SPECIAL CONSIDERATIONS
1. Dose of drug does not need to be reduced in patients with abnormal liver and/or renal function.
2. In contrast with 6-mercaptopurine, dose of drug does not need to be reduced in the presence of concomitant allopurinol therapy.
3. Administer on an empty stomach to facilitate absorption.
4. Use with caution in the presence of other hepatotoxic drugs, as the risk of thioguanine-associated hepatotoxicity is increased.
5. Pregnancy category D. Breastfeeding should be avoided.

TOXICITY 1
Myelosuppression is dose-limiting. Neutropenia tends to precede thrombocytopenia with nadir at 10–14 days and recovery by day 21.

TOXICITY 2
Nausea and vomiting. Dose-related, usually mild.

TOXICITY 3
Mucositis and diarrhea. May be severe, requiring dose reduction.

TOXICITY 4
Hepatotoxicity in the form of elevated serum bilirubin and transaminases. Veno-occlusive disease has been reported rarely.

TOXICITY 5
Immunosuppression with increased risk of bacterial, fungal, and parasitic infections.

TOXICITY 6
Transient renal toxicity.

TOXICITY 7
Mutagenic, teratogenic, and carcinogenic.

Thiotepa

TRADE NAMES	Thiotepa Thioplex	CLASSIFICATION	Alkylating agent
CATEGORY	Chemotherapy drug	DRUG MANUFACTURER	Ben Venue Labs

MECHANISM OF ACTION
- Ethylenimine analog chemically related to nitrogen mustard.
- Functions as an alkylating agent by alkylating the N-7 position of guanine.
- Cell cycle–nonspecific agent.
- Inhibits DNA, RNA, and protein synthesis.

MECHANISM OF RESISTANCE
- Decreased uptake of drug into cell.
- Increased activity of DNA repair enzymes.
- Increased expression of sulfhydryl proteins, including glutathione and glutathione-related proteins.

ABSORPTION
Incomplete and erratic absorption via the oral route. Thiotepa is primarily administered by the IV route. Also given by intravesical route where the absorption from the bladder is variable, ranging from 10%–100% of an administered dose.

DISTRIBUTION
Widely distributed throughout the body. About 40% of drug is bound to plasma proteins.

METABOLISM
Extensively metabolized by the liver microsomal P450 system to both active and inactive metabolites. About 60% of a dose is eliminated in urine within 24–72 hours with only a small amount excreted as parent drug. Elimination half-life is on the order of 2–3 hours.

INDICATIONS
1. Breast cancer.
2. Ovarian cancer.
3. Superficial transitional cell cancer of the bladder.
4. Hodgkin's and non-Hodgkin's lymphoma.
5. High-dose transplant setting for breast and ovarian cancer.

DOSAGE RANGE
1. Usual dose is 10–20 mg/m^2 IV given every 3–4 weeks.
2. High-dose transplant setting: Doses range from 180 to 1100 mg/m^2 IV.
3. Intravesical instillation: Dose for bladder instillation is 60 mg administered in 60 mL sterile water weekly for up to 4 weeks.

DRUG INTERACTIONS

Myelosuppressive agents—Bone marrow toxicity of thiotepa is enhanced when combined with other myelosuppressive anticancer agents.

SPECIAL CONSIDERATIONS

1. Monitor CBC while on therapy, as thiotepa is highly toxic to the bone marrow.
2. Use with caution in regimens including other myelosuppressive agents, as the risk of bone marrow toxicity is significantly increased.
3. Resuscitation equipment and medications should be available during administration of drug, as there is a risk of hypersensitivity reaction.
4. Monitor CBC after intravesical administration of drug into the bladder, as severe bone marrow depression can arise from systemically absorbed drug.
5. Caution patients about the risk of skin changes such as rash, urticaria, bronzing, flaking, and desquamation that can occur following high-dose therapy. Topical skin care should be initiated promptly.
6. Pregnancy category D. Breastfeeding should be avoided.

TOXICITY 1

Myelosuppression is dose-limiting. Leukopenia nadir 7–10 days with recovery by day 21. Platelet count nadir occurs at day 21 with usual recovery by day 28–35.

TOXICITY 2

Nausea and vomiting. Dose-dependent. Usual onset is 6–12 hours after treatment.

TOXICITY 3

Mucositis. May be dose-limiting with high-dose therapy.

TOXICITY 4

Allergic reaction in the form of skin rash, hives, and rarely bronchospasm.

TOXICITY 5

Chemical and/or hemorrhagic cystitis. Occurs rarely following intravesical treatment.

TOXICITY 6

Skin changes with rash and bronzing of skin, erythema, flaking, and desquamation developing after high-dose therapy.

TOXICITY 7

Thiotepa is teratogenic, mutagenic, and carcinogenic. Increased risk of secondary malignancies, usually in the form of acute myelogenous leukemia. Breast cancer and NSCLC have also been reported.

Topotecan

TRADE NAME Hycamtin **CLASSIFICATION** Topoisomerase I inhibitor

CATEGORY Chemotherapy drug **DRUG MANUFACTURER** GlaxoSmithKline

MECHANISM OF ACTION

- Semisynthetic derivative of camptothecin, an alkaloid extract from the *Camptotheca acuminata* tree.
- Inhibits topoisomerase I function. Binds to and stabilizes the topoisomerase I-DNA complex and prevents the religation of DNA after it has been cleaved by topoisomerase I. The collision between this stable cleavable complex and the advancing replication fork results in double-strand DNA breaks and cellular death.
- Antitumor activity of drug requires the presence of topoisomerase I and ongoing DNA synthesis.

MECHANISM OF RESISTANCE

- Decreased expression of topoisomerase I.
- Mutations in topoisomerase I enzyme with decreased binding affinity to drug.
- Increased expression of the multidrug-resistant phenotype with overexpression of P170 glycoprotein. Results in enhanced efflux of drug and decreased intracellular accumulation of drug.
- Decreased accumulation of drug into cells through non–multidrug-resistance-related mechanisms.

ABSORPTION

Topotecan is rapidly absorbed with peak plasma concentrations occurring between 1 and 2 hours following oral administration. The oral bioavailability of topotecan is about 40%. Following a high-fat meal, the extent of exposure is similar in the fed and fasted states, while T_{max} is delayed from 1.5–3 hours (topotecan lactone) and from 3–4 hours (total topotecan), respectively. Topotecan can be given without regard to food.

DISTRIBUTION

Widely distributed in body tissues. Binding to plasma proteins is on the order of 10%–35%. Levels of drug in the CSF are only 30% of those in plasma. Peak drug levels are achieved within 1 hour after drug administration.

METABOLISM

Rapid conversion of topotecan in plasma and in aqueous solution from the lactone ring form to the carboxylate acid form. At acidic pH, topotecan is mainly in the lactone ring, while at physiologic and basic pH, the carboxylate form predominates. Only about 20%–30% of a given dose is present as the active lactone metabolite at 1 hour after drug administration. The major route of elimination of topotecan is renal excretion accounting for 40%–68% of drug clearance. Metabolism in the liver appears to be minimal and is mediated by the liver microsomal P450 system. The elimination half-life is approximately 3 hours.

INDICATIONS

1. Ovarian cancer—FDA-approved in patients with advanced ovarian cancer who failed platinum-based chemotherapy.
2. SCLC—FDA-approved in patients with sensitive disease who progressed on first-line chemotherapy.
3. Cervical cancer—FDA-approved in combination with cisplatin for the treatment of stage IV-B, recurrent, or persistent carcinoma of the cervix that is not amenable to curative treatment with surgery and/or radiation therapy.

DOSAGE RANGE

1. IV: Recommended dose is 1.5 mg/m^2/day IV for 5 consecutive days given every 21 days.
2. Oral: Recommended dose is 2.3 mg/m^2/day for 5 consecutive days given every 21 days.

DRUG INTERACTIONS

None known.

SPECIAL CONSIDERATIONS

1. Use with caution in patients with abnormal renal function. Dose reduction is necessary in this setting. Baseline CrCl is critical, as is periodic monitoring of renal function.
2. Monitor CBC on a weekly basis.
3. Carefully monitor administration of drug, as it is a mild vesicant. The infusion site should be carefully monitored for extravasation, in which case flushing with sterile water, elevation of the extremity, and local application of ice are recommended. In severe cases, a plastic surgeon should be consulted.
4. If granulocyte nadir count is low, begin G-CSF or GM-CSF 24 hours after the completion of topotecan therapy.
5. Pregnancy category D. Breastfeeding should be avoided.

TOXICITY 1

Myelosuppression is dose-limiting, with neutropenia being most commonly observed. Nadir typically occurs at days 7–10 with full recovery by days 21–28.

TOXICITY 2

Nausea and vomiting. Mild to moderate and dose-related. Occurs in 60%–80% of patients. Diarrhea with abdominal pain also observed.

TOXICITY 3

Headache, fever, malaise, arthralgias, and myalgias.

TOXICITY 4

Microscopic hematuria. Seen in 10% of patients.

TOXICITY 5

Alopecia.

TOXICITY 6

Transient elevation in serum transaminases, alkaline phosphatase, and bilirubin.

Toremifene

TRADE NAME	Fareston	CLASSIFICATION	Antiestrogen
CATEGORY	Hormonal agent	DRUG MANUFACTURER	Orion and GTx

MECHANISM OF ACTION

- Synthetic analog of tamoxifen.
- Nonsteroidal antiestrogen that directly binds to estrogen receptors on breast cancer cells. Affinity for estrogen receptor is four- to five-fold higher than tamoxifen. Blocks downstream intracellular signal transduction pathways, leading to inhibition of cell growth and induction of apoptosis.

MECHANISM OF RESISTANCE
Cross-resistance between toremifene, tamoxifen, and other antiestrogen agents.

ABSORPTION
Well-absorbed after oral administration. Food does not interfere with oral absorption.

DISTRIBUTION
Widely distributed to body tissues. Extensive (>99%) binding to plasma proteins, mainly albumin. Steady-state plasma concentrations are reached in 4–6 weeks.

METABOLISM
Extensive metabolism in the liver by the cytochrome P450 system. Major metabolites, N-demethyltoremifene and 4-hydroxytoremifene, have long terminal half-lives of 4–6 days secondary to enterohepatic recirculation. Parent drug and metabolites are excreted mainly in bile and feces. Minimal excretion in urine.

INDICATIONS
Metastatic breast cancer in postmenopausal women with ER1 tumors or in cases where ER status is not known. Not recommended in ER2 tumors.

DOSAGE RANGE
Recommended dose is 60 mg PO daily until disease progression.

DRUG INTERACTION 1
Thiazide diuretics—Decreases renal clearance of calcium and increases the risk of hypercalcemia associated with toremifene.

DRUG INTERACTION 2
Warfarin—Toremifene inhibits liver P450 metabolism of warfarin resulting in an increased anticoagulant effect. Coagulation parameters, PT and INR, should be closely monitored, and dose adjustments made accordingly.

DRUG INTERACTION 3
Phenobarbital, carbamazepine, phenytoin—Liver P450 metabolism of toremifene may be enhanced by phenobarbital, carbamazepine, and phenytoin resulting in reduced blood levels and reduced clinical efficacy.

DRUG INTERACTION 4
Ketoconazole and erythromycin—Liver P450 metabolism of toremifene may be inhibited by ketoconazole and erythromycin, resulting in elevated blood levels and enhanced clinical efficacy.

SPECIAL CONSIDERATIONS
1. Patients with a prior history of thromboembolic events must be carefully monitored while on therapy as toremifene is thrombogenic.
2. Use with caution in the setting of brain and/or vertebral body metastases, as tumor flare with bone and/or muscular pain, erythema, and transient increase in tumor volume can occur upon initiation of therapy.

3. Monitor CBC, LFTs, and serum calcium on a regular basis.
4. Contraindicated in patients with a prior history of endometrial hyperplasia. Increased risk of endometrial cancer associated with therapy. Onset of vaginal bleeding during therapy requires immediate gynecologic evaluation.
5. Baseline and biannual eye exams are recommended as toremifene can lead to cataract formation.
6. Pregnancy category D. Breastfeeding should be avoided. Not known whether toremifene is excreted in breast milk.

TOXICITY 1
Hot flashes, sweating, menstrual irregularity, milk production in breast, and vaginal discharge and bleeding are commonly observed.

TOXICITY 2
Transient tumor flare manifested by bone and/or tumor pain.

TOXICITY 3
Ocular toxicity with cataract formation and xerophthalmia.

TOXICITY 4
Nausea, vomiting, and anorexia.

TOXICITY 5
Myelosuppression is usually mild.

TOXICITY 6
Rare skin toxicity in the form of rash, alopecia, and peripheral edema.

Tositumomab

TRADE NAME	Bexxar	**CLASSIFICATION**	Monoclonal antibody
CATEGORY	Biologic response modifier agent	**DRUG MANUFACTURER**	Corixa and GlaxoSmithKline

MECHANISM OF ACTION
- Radioimmunotherapeutic monoclonal antibody-based regimen composed of the tositumomab monoclonal antibody and the radiolabeled monoclonal antibody I-131 tositumomab, a radio-iodinated derivative of tositumomab that has been covalently linked to I-131.
- The antibody moiety is tositumomab, which targets the CD20 antigen, a 35 kDa cell-surface, non-glycosylated phosphoprotein expressed during

early pre–B cell development until the plasma cell stage. Binding of the antibody to CD20 induces a transmembrane signal that blocks cell activation and cell cycle progression.

- CD20 is expressed on more than 90% of all B-cell non-Hodgkin's lymphomas and leukemias. CD20 is not expressed on early pre–B cells, plasma cells, normal bone marrow stem cells, antigen-presenting dendritic reticulum cells, or other normal tissues.
- Ionizing radiation from the I-131 radioisotope results in cell death.

ABSORPTION
Tositumomab is given only by the IV route.

DISTRIBUTION
Higher clearance, shorter terminal half-life, and larger volumes of distribution observed in patients with higher tumor burden, splenomegaly, and/ or bone marrow involvement.

METABOLISM
Elimination of I-131 occurs by decay and excretion in the urine. The total body clearance is 67% of an administered dose, and nearly 100% of the clearance is accounted for in the urine.

INDICATIONS
Relapsed and/or refractory CD20-positive, follicular non-Hodgkin's lymphoma with and without transformation—disease is refractory to rituximab therapy and has relapsed following chemotherapy.

DOSAGE RANGE
Treatment schema is as follows: Day 0, begin Lugol's solution or oral potassium iodide solution; Day 1, dosimetric dose: 450 mg unlabeled tositumomab, followed by 5 mCi of I-131 tositumomab (35 mg). Measurement of whole body counts and calculation of therapeutic dose; Day 7 up to Day 14, therapeutic dose: 450 mg unlabeled tositumomab, followed by calculated therapeutic dose of I-131 tositumomab to deliver 75 cGy; Days 8–21, continue Lugol's solution or oral potassium iodide solution.

DRUG INTERACTIONS
None characterized to date.

SPECIAL CONSIDERATIONS
1. Contraindicated in patients with known type I hypersensitivity or known hypersensitivity to any component of the Bexxar therapeutic regimen.
2. TSH levels should be monitored before treatment and on an annual basis thereafter.
3. Before receiving the dosimetric dose of I-131, patients must receive at least three doses of SSKI, three doses of Lugol's solution, or one dose of 130 mg potassium iodide (at least 24 hours prior to the dosimetric dose).

4. This therapy should be administered only by physicians and healthcare professionals who are qualified and experienced in the safe use and handling of radioisotopes.

5. Patients should be premedicated with acetaminophen and diphenhydramine before each administration of tositumomab in the dosimetric and therapeutic steps to reduce the incidence of infusion-related reactions.

6. The same IV tubing set and filter must be used throughout the dosimetric and therapeutic step as a change in filter can result in loss of effective drug delivery.

7. Monitor for infusion-related events resulting from tositumomab infusion, which usually occur during or within 48 hours of infusion. Infusion rate should be reduced by 50% for mild-to-moderate allergic reaction and immediately stopped for a severe reaction. Immediate institution of diphenhydramine, acetaminophen, corticosteroids, IV fluids, and/or vasopressors may be necessary. In the setting of a severe reaction, the infusion can be restarted at a reduced rate (50%) once symptoms have completely resolved. Resuscitation equipment should be readily available at bedside.

8. Tositumomab therapy should not be given to patients with >25% involvement of the bone marrow by lymphoma and/or impaired bone marrow reserve or to patients with platelet count <100,000/mm^3 or neutrophil count <1500/mm^3.

9. CBCs and platelet counts should be monitored weekly following tositumomab therapy for up to 10–12 weeks after therapy.

10. The tositumomab regimen should be given only as a single-course treatment.

11. The tositumomab regimen may have direct toxic effects on the male and female reproductive organs, and effective contraception should be used during therapy and for up to 12 months following the completion of therapy.

12. Pregnancy category X. Contraindicated in women who are pregnant.

13. Breastfeeding should be discontinued immediately prior to starting therapy.

TOXICITY 1
Infusion-related symptoms, including fever, chills, urticaria, flushing, fatigue, headache, bronchospasm, rhinitis, dyspnea, angioedema, nausea, and/or hypotension. Usually resolve upon slowing and/or interrupting the infusion and with supportive care.

TOXICITY 2
Myelosuppression is most common side effect with neutropenia, thrombocytopenia, and anemia. The time to nadir is typically 4–7 weeks, and the duration of cytopenias is 30 days. In 5%–7% of patients, severe cytopenias persist beyond 12 weeks after therapy.

TOXICITY 3
Mild asthenia and fatigue occur in up to 40% of patients.

TOXICITY 4

Infections develop in up to 45% of patients. Majority of infection events are viral and relatively minor, but up to 10% of patients experience infections that require hospitalization.

TOXICITY 5

Mild nausea and vomiting.

TOXICITY 6

Hypothyroidism.

TOXICITY 7

Secondary malignancies occur in about 2%–3% of patients. Acute myelogenous leukemia and myelodysplastic syndrome have been reported with a cumulative incidence of 1.4% at 2 years and 4.8% at 4 years following therapy.

TOXICITY 8

Development of HAMAs. Rare event in less than 1%–2% of patients.

Trabectedin

TRADE NAMES	Yondelis	CLASSIFICATION	Alklyating agent
CATEGORY	Chemotherapy drug	DRUG MANUFACTURER	Janssen/Johnson & Johnson

MECHANISM OF ACTION

- Tetrahydroisoquinolone alklyating agent that binds to the N2 position of guanine residues in the minor groove of DNA, leading to formation of DNA adducts and to bending of the DNA helix towards the major groove.
- DNA adduct formation results in single- and double-strand breaks and inhibition of DNA synthesis and function.

- Induces cell-cycle arrest and cell death that is not dependent in p53.
- Antitumor activity may also relate to effects on the tumor microenvironment.
- Has potent immunomodulatory effects, with cytotoxic effects against monocytes and tumor-associated macrophages.
- Inhibits production of pro-inflammatory and pro-angiogenic mediators in the tumor microenvironment.
- Cell cycle-nonspecific. Active in all phases of the cell cycle.

MECHANISM OF RESISTANCE
None well characterized to date.

ABSORPTION
Trabectedin is administered only by the IV route.

DISTRIBUTION
Mean steady-state volume of distribution exceeds 5000 L. Based on *in vitro* testing, about 97% of drug bound to plasma proteins.

METABOLISM
Trabectedin is rapidly and extensively metabolized by CYP3A liver microsomal enzymes. There is negligible unchanged drug in feces and urine following drug administration. Elimination is mainly hepatic with excretion in feces (~58%), with renal elimination accounting for only 6% of an administered dose. The terminal elimination half-life is approximately 175 hours.

INDICATIONS
FDA-approved for the treatment of unresectable or metastatic liposarcoma or leiomyosarcoma following a prior anthracycline-containing regimen.

DOSAGE RANGE
Recommended dose is 1.5 mg/m^2 as a 24-hour infusion every 3 weeks. The drug is to be administered through a central venous line.

DRUG INTERACTION 1
Drugs such as ketoconazole, itraconazole, erythromycin, clarithromycin, atazanavir, indinavir, nefazodone, nelfinavir, ritonavir, saquinavir, telithromycin, and voriconazole may decrease the rate of metabolism of trabectedin, resulting in increased drug levels and potentially increased toxicity.

DRUG INTERACTION 2
Drugs such as rifampin, phenytoin, phenobarbital, carbamazepine, and St. John's wort may increase the rate of metabolism of trabectedin, resulting in its inactivation.

SPECIAL CONSIDERATIONS

1. Use with caution in patients with hepatic dysfunction. Dose reduction is recommended in patients with moderate hepatic dysfunction, and a dose of 0.9 mg/m^2 should be administered. Trabectedin should not be given in the setting of severe hepatic dysfunction.
2. Dose reduction is not required in patients with mild or moderate renal dysfunction. However, trabectedin has not been studied in patients with severe renal dysfunction and end-stage renal disease.
3. Closely monitor CBCs on a periodic basis with a focus on the ANC.
4. Trabectedin should be held for >grade 2 neutropenia.
5. Closely monitor CPK levels prior to each cycle of therapy as rhabdomyolysis and musculoskeletal toxicity can occur.
6. LFTs should be monitored as hepatotoxicity, including hepatic failure, is associated with trabectedin.
7. Baseline and periodic evaluation of LVEF by echocardiogram of MUGA. Trabectedin should be held for LVEF below the lower limit of normal, and permanently discontinued for symptomatic cardiomyopathy or persistent LV dysfunction that does not return to the lower limit of normal within 3 weeks.
8. Trabectedin must be administrered through a central line as drug extravasation can cause tissue necrosis.
9. Pregnancy category D. Breastfeeding should be avoided.

TOXICITY 1
Myelosuppression with neutropenia. Severe and fatal neutropenic sepsis may occur.

TOXICITY 2
Rhabdomyolysis and musculoskeletal toxicity.

TOXICITY 3
Hepatotoxicity with elevations in SGOT, SGPT, bilirubin, and alkaline phosphatase.

TOXICITY 4
Cardiac toxicity with reduction in LVEF, diastolic dysfunction, CHF, and cardiac failure.

TOXICITY 5
GI toxicity with nausea/vomiting, constipation, and diarrhea.

TOXICITY 6
Fatigue and anorexia.

Trametinib

TRADE NAME	Mekinist	CLASSIFICATION	Signal transduction inhibitor
CATEGORY	Chemotherapy drug	DRUG MANUFACTURER	GlaxoSmithKline

MECHANISM OF ACTION
- Reversible inhibitor of mitogen-activated extracellular signal-regulated kinase 1 (MEK1) and kinase 2 (MEK2) activity.
- Results in inhibition of downstream regulators of the extracellular signalregulated kinase (ERK) pathway, leading to inhibition of cellular proliferation.
- Inhibits growth of BRAF-V600 mutation-positive melanoma.

MECHANISM OF RESISTANCE
None characterized to date.

ABSORPTION
Oral bioavailability is on the order of 70%. Peak plasma drug concentrations are achieved in 1.5 hours after oral ingestion. Food with a high fat content reduces C_{max}, T_{max}, and AUC.

DISTRIBUTION
Extensive binding (97.4%) of trametinib to plasma proteins.

METABOLISM
Metabolized mainly via deacetylation alone or with mono-oxygenation or in combination with glucuronidation biotransformation pathways in the liver. The process of deacetylation is mediated by hydrolytic enzymes, such as carboxylesterases or amidases. Elimination is hepatic with excretion in feces (>80%), with renal elimination accounting for <20% of an administered dose. The median terminal half-life of trametinib is approximately 4–5 days.

INDICATIONS

1. FDA-approved as a single agent or in combination with dabrafenib for unresectable or metastatic melanoma with BRAF-V600E or V600K mutations as determined by an FDA-approved diagnostic test.
2. Not recommended for patients who have received prior BRAF-inhibitor therapy.

DOSAGE RANGE

Recommended dose as a single agent or in combination with dabrafenib is 2 mg PO daily. Should be taken at least 1 hour before or at least 2 hours after a meal.

DRUG INTERACTIONS

None well characterized to date.

SPECIAL CONSIDERATIONS

1. Baseline and periodic evaluations of LVEF should be performed while on therapy. Approximately 10% of patients will develop cardiomyopathy at a median time of 63 days. Treatment should be held if the absolute LVEF drops by 10% from pretreatment baseline. Therapy should be permanently stopped for symptomatic cardiomyopathy or persistent, asymptomatic LVEF dysfunction that does not resolve within 4 weeks.
2. Patients should be warned about the possibility of visual disturbances.
3. Careful eye exams should be done at baseline and with any new visual changes to rule out the possibility of retinal detachments or retinal vein occlusion.
4. Monitor patients for pulmonary symptoms. Therapy should be held in patients presenting with new or progressive pulmonary symptoms and should be terminated in patients diagnosed with treatment-related pneumonitis or ILD.
5. Monitor patients for serious skin toxicity and secondary infections, with the median time to onset of 15 days. The median time to resolution of skin toxicity is 48 days.
6. BRAF testing using an FDA-approved diagnostic test to confirm the presence of the BRAF-V600E or –V600K mutations is required for determining which patients should receive trametinib therapy.
7. No dose adjustment is needed for patients with mild hepatic dysfunction. However, caution should be used in patients with moderate-to-severe hepatic dysfunction.
8. No dose adjustment is needed for patients with mild-to-moderate renal dysfunction. Use with caution in patients with severe renal dysfunction.
9. Pregnancy category D. Breastfeeding should be avoided.

TOXICITY 1

Cardiac toxicity in the form of cardiomyopathy.

TOXICITY 2

Opthalmologic side effects, including retinal detachment and retinal vein occlusion.

TOXICITY 3
Pulmonary toxicity in the form of ILD presenting as cough, dyspnea, hypoxia, pleural effusion, or infiltrates. Observed rarely in about 2% of patients.

TOXICITY 4
Skin toxicity with rash, dermatitis, acneiform rash, hand-foot syndrome, erythema, pruritus, and paronychia. Severe skin toxicity observed in 12% of patients.

TOXICITY 5
Diarrhea, mucositis, and abdominal pain are the most common GI side effects.

TOXICITY 6
Hypertension.

TOXICITY 7
Lymphedema.

Trastuzumab

TRADE NAMES	Herceptin, Anti-HER2-antibody	CLASSIFICATION	Monoclonal antibody
CATEGORY	Biologic response modifier agent	DRUG MANUFACTURER	Genentech/Roche

MECHANISM OF ACTION
- Recombinant humanized monoclonal antibody directed against the extracellular domain (IV) of the HER2/neu growth factor receptor. This receptor is overexpressed in several human cancers, including 25%–30% of breast cancers and up to 20% of gastric cancers.
- Precise mechanism(s) of action remains unknown.
- Downregulates expression of HER2/neu receptor.
- Inhibits HER2/neu intracellular signaling pathways.
- Induction of apoptosis through as yet undetermined mechanisms.
- Immunologic mechanisms may also be involved in antitumor activity, and they include recruitment of antibody-dependent cellular cytotoxicity (ADCC) and/or complement-mediated cell lysis.

MECHANISM OF RESISTANCE
- Mutations in the HER2/neu growth factor receptor leading to decreased binding affinity to trastuzumab.
- Decreased expression of HER2/neu receptors.
- Expression of P95HER2, a constitutively active, truncated form of the HER2 receptor.

- Increased expression of HER3.
- Activation/induction of alternative cellular signaling pathways, such as the IGF-1 receptor and/or the c-Met receptor.

DISTRIBUTION
Distribution in body is not well characterized.

METABOLISM
Metabolism of trastuzumab has not been extensively characterized. Half-life is on the order of 6 days with a weekly schedule and 16 days with the every-3-week schedule.

INDICATIONS
1. Metastatic breast cancer—First-line therapy in combination with paclitaxel. Patient's tumor must express HER2/neu protein to be treated with this monoclonal antibody.
2. Metastatic breast cancer—Second- and third-line therapy as a single agent in patients whose tumors overexpress the HER2/neu protein.
3. Early-stage breast cancer—FDA-approved for the adjuvant therapy of node-positive, HER2-overexpressing breast cancer as part of a treatment regimen containing doxorubicin, cyclophosphamide, and either paclitaxel or docetaxel.
4. Metastatic gastric and gastroesophageal junction adenocarcinoma—FDA-approved in combination with cisplatin and capecitabine or 5-FU for the treatment of patients with HER2 overexpressing metastatic gastric or gastroesophageal junction adenocarcinoma who have not received prior treatment for metastatic disease.

DOSAGE RANGE
1. Recommended loading dose of 4 mg/kg IV administered over 90 minutes, followed by maintenance dose of 2 mg/kg IV on a weekly basis. One week following the last weekly dose of trastuzumab, administer trastuzumab at 6 mg/kg as an intravenous infusion over 30–90 minutes every three weeks.
2. Alternative schedule is to give a loading dose of 8 mg/kg IV administered over 30–90 minutes, followed by maintenance dose of 6 mg/kg IV every 3 weeks.
3. Administer trastuzumab, alone or in combination with paclitaxel, at an initial dose of 4 mg/kg as a 90-minute intravenous infusion followed by subsequent once weekly doses of 2 mg/kg as 30-minute intravenous infusions until disease progression.
4. Administer trastuzumab at an initial dose of 8 mg/kg as a 90-minute intravenous infusion followed by subsequent doses of 6 mg/kg as an intravenous infusion over 30–90 minutes every 3 weeks until disease progression.

DRUG INTERACTIONS
Anthracyclines, taxanes—Increased risk of cardiotoxicity when trastuzumab is used in combination with anthracyclines and/or taxanes.

SPECIAL CONSIDERATIONS

1. Caution should be exercised in treating patients with pre-existing cardiac dysfunction. Careful baseline assessment of cardiac function (LVEF) before treatment and frequent monitoring (every 3 months) of cardiac function while on therapy. Trastuzumab should be held for >16% absolute decrease in LVEF from a normal baseline value. Trastuzumab therapy should be stopped immediately in patients who develop clinically significant congestive heart failure. When trastuzumab is used in the adjuvant setting, cardiac function should be assessed every 6 months for at least 2 years following the completion of therapy.

2. Carefully monitor for infusion reactions, which typically occur during or within 24 hours of drug administration. Administer initial loading dose over 90 minutes and then observe patient for 1 hour following completion of the loading dose. May need to treat with diphenhydramine and acetaminophen. Rarely, in severe cases, may need to treat with IV fluids and/or pressors.

3. Maintenance doses are administered over 30 minutes if loading dose was well tolerated without fever and chills. However, if fever and chills were experienced with loading dose, administer over 90 minutes.

4. Pregnancy category D.

TOXICITY 1

Infusion-related symptoms with fever, chills, urticaria, flushing, fatigue, headache, bronchospasm, dyspnea, angioedema, and hypotension. Occur in 40%–50% of patients. Usually mild to moderate in severity and observed most commonly with administration of the first infusion.

TOXICITY 2

Mild GI toxicity in the form of nausea/vomiting and diarrhea.

TOXICITY 3

Cardiotoxicity in the form of dyspnea, peripheral edema, and reduced left ventricular function. Significantly increased risk when used in combination with an anthracycline-based regimen. In most instances, cardiac dysfunction is readily reversible.

TOXICITY 4

Myelosuppression. Increased risk and severity when trastuzumab is administered with chemotherapy.

TOXICITY 5

Generalized pain, asthenia, and headache.

TOXICITY 6

Pulmonary toxicity in the form of increased cough, dyspnea, rhinitis, sinusitis, pulmonary infiltrates, and/or pleural effusions.

Tretinoin

TRADE NAMES	All-*trans*-retinoic acid, ATRA, Vesanoid	CLASSIFICATION	Retinoid
CATEGORY	Differentiating agent	DRUG MANUFACTURER	Roche

MECHANISM OF ACTION
- Precise mechanism of action has not been fully elucidated.
- Induces differentiation of acute promyelocytic cells to normal myelocyte cells, thereby decreasing cellular proliferation.
- Upon entry into cells, tretinoin binds to the cytoplasmic protein, cellular retinoic acid binding protein (CRABP). The retinoid CRABP complex is transported to the nucleus, where it binds to retinoid-dependent receptors known as RAR and/or RXR. This process affects the transcription and subsequent expression of various target cellular genes involved in growth, proliferation, and differentiation.
- Effects on the immune system may also contribute to antitumor activity.
- Induces apoptosis through as yet undetermined mechanisms.

MECHANISM OF RESISTANCE
- Alteration in drug metabolism by the liver P450 system. Tretinoin induces the activity of cytochrome P450 enzymes, which are responsible for its oxidative metabolism. Plasma concentrations decrease to about one-third of their day one values after 1 week of continuous therapy.
- Increased expression of CRABP, which acts to sequester tretinoin within the cell, preventing its subsequent delivery to the nucleus.

ABSORPTION
Well-absorbed by the GI tract, reaching peak plasma concentration between 1 and 2 hours after oral administration.

DISTRIBUTION
Binds extensively (>95%) to plasma proteins, mainly to albumin. The apparent volume of distribution has not been determined.

METABOLISM
Undergoes oxidative metabolism by the liver cytochrome P450 system. Several metabolites have been identified, including 13-*cis* retinoic acid, 4-oxo *trans*-retinoic acid, 4-oxo *cis*-retinoic acid, and 4-oxo *trans*-retinoic acid glucuronide. Excreted in urine (63%) and in feces (31%). The terminal elimination half-life is approximately 40–120 minutes.

INDICATIONS

Acute promyelocytic leukemia (APL)—Induction of remission in patients with APL characterized by the t(15;17) translocation and/or the presence of the PML/RAR-α gene following progression and/or relapse with anthracycline-based chemotherapy or for whom anthracycline-based chemotherapy is contraindicated.

DOSAGE RANGE

Recommended dose is 45 mg/m^2/day PO divided in two daily doses for a minimum of 45 days and a maximum of 90 days.

DRUG INTERACTION 1

Drugs metabolized by liver P450 system—Tretinoin is metabolized by hepatic cytochrome P450 enzymes. Caution should be exercised when using drugs that induce this enzyme system, such as rifampin and phenobarbital, and drugs that inhibit this system, including ketoconazole, cimetidine, erythromycin, verapamil, diltiazem, and cyclosporine.

DRUG INTERACTION 2

Vitamin A supplements—Use of vitamin A supplements may increase toxicity of tretinoin.

SPECIAL CONSIDERATIONS

1. Contraindicated in patients with known hypersensitivity to retinoids.
2. Monitor for new-onset fever, respiratory symptoms, and leukocytosis as 25% of patients develop the retinoic acid syndrome. Tretinoin should be stopped immediately, and high-dose dexamethasone, 10 mg IV q 12 hours should be given for 3 days or until resolution of symptoms. In most cases, therapy can be resumed once the syndrome has completely resolved. Usually occurs during the first month of treatment.
3. Use with caution in patients with pre-existing hypertriglyceridemia and in those with diabetes mellitus, obesity, and/or predisposition to excessive alcohol intake. Serum triglyceride and cholesterol levels should be closely monitored.
4. Monitor CBC, coagulation profile, and LFTs on a frequent basis during therapy.
5. Oral absorption of tretinoin may be increased when taken with food.
6. Pregnancy category D. Breastfeeding should be avoided.

TOXICITY 1

Vitamin A toxicity is nearly universal. Most common side effects are headache, usually occurring in the first week of therapy with improvement; thereafter, fever, dryness of the skin and mucous membranes, skin rash, peripheral edema, mucositis, pruritus, and conjunctivitis.

TOXICITY 2

Retinoic acid syndrome. Can be dose-limiting and occurs in 25% of patients. Varies in severity but has resulted in death. Characterized by fever, leukocytosis, dyspnea, weight gain, diffuse pulmonary infiltrates on chest X-ray, and pleural and/or pericardial effusions. More commonly observed with WBC >10,000/mm^3. Usually observed during the first month of therapy but may follow the initial drug dose.

TOXICITY 3
Flushing, hypotension, hypertension, phlebitis, and congestive heart failure. Cardiac ischemia, myocardial infarction, stroke, myocarditis, pericarditis, and pulmonary hypertension are rarer events, each being reported in less than 3% of patients.

TOXICITY 4
Increased serum cholesterol and triglyceride levels occur in up to 60% of patients. Usually reversible upon completion of treatment.

TOXICITY 5
CNS toxicity in the form of dizziness, anxiety, paresthesias, depression, confusion, and agitation. Hallucinations, agnosia, aphasia, slow speech, asterixis, cerebellar disorders, convulsion, coma, dysarthria, encephalopathy, facial paralysis, hemiplegia, and hyporeflexia are less often seen.

TOXICITY 6
GI toxicity. Relatively common and manifested by abdominal pain, constipation, diarrhea, and GI bleeding. Elevations in serum transaminases and alkaline phosphatase occur in 50%–60% of patients and usually resolve after completion of therapy.

TOXICITY 7
Alterations in hearing sensation with hearing loss. About 25% of patients describe earache or a fullness in the ears.

TOXICITY 8
Renal dysfunction and dysuria occur rarely.

TOXICITY 9
Pseudotumor cerebri. Benign intracranial hypertension with papilledema, headache, nausea and vomiting, and visual disturbances.

TOXICITY 10
Teratogenic.

Vandetanib

TRADE NAME	Caprelsa	**CLASSIFICATION**	Signal transduction inhibitor
CATEGORY	Chemotherapy drug	**DRUG MANUFACTURER**	AstraZeneca

MECHANISM OF ACTION
- Small-molecule inhibitor of tyrosine kinases associated with the EGFR family, VEGFR, rearranged during transfection (RET), protein tyrosine kinase 6 (BRK), Tie-2, EPH receptors, and Src family members.
- Inhibition of these receptor tyrosine kinases results in inhibition of critical signaling pathways involved in proliferation, growth, invasion/metastasis, and angiogenesis.

MECHANISM OF RESISTANCE
- Increased expression of the target receptor tyrosine kinases (RTKs), such as EGFR and VEGFR.
- Alterations in binding affinity of the drug to the RTKs resulting from mutations in the tyrosine kinase domain, e.g., EGFR T790M mutation.
- Activation/induction of alternative cellular signaling pathways, such as IGF-1R and c-Met.

ABSORPTION
Oral absorption is slow, with peak plasma concentrations achieved at a median of 6 hours, and is unaffected by food.

DISTRIBUTION
Vandetanib binds to human serum albumin and α1-acid glycoprotein on the order of 90%. With daily dosing, steady-state blood levels are achieved in about 28 days.

METABOLISM
Following oral administration, parent vandetanib and metabolites, including N-oxide vandetanib and N-desmethyl vandetanib, are detected in plasma, urine, and feces. A glucuronide conjugate is observed as a minor metabolite.

N-desmethyl vandetanib is primarily produced by CYP3A4 and vandetanib N-oxide by flavin-containing monooxygenase enzymes FMO1 and FMO3. Approximately 70% is recovered with 45% in feces and 25% in urine. The terminal half-life is prolonged on the order of >100 hours.

INDICATIONS

FDA-approved for the treatment of symptomatic or progressive medullary thyroid cancer in patients with unresectable locally advanced or metastatic disease.

DOSAGE RANGE

Recommended dose is 300 mg PO daily. Vandetanib may be taken with or without food.

DRUG INTERACTIONS

1. Drugs that stimulate liver microsomal CYP3A4 enzymes, including phenytoin, carbamazepine, rifampin, phenobarbital, and St. John's wort—These drugs may increase the metabolism of vandetanib, resulting in its inactivation.
2. Drugs that inhibit liver microsomal CYP3A4 enzymes, including ketoconazole, itraconazole, erythromycin, and clarithromycin—These drugs may reduce the metabolism of vandetanib, resulting in increased drug levels and potentially increased toxicity.
3. Drugs that are associated with QT prolongation—Certain phenothiazines (chlorpromazine, mesoridazine, and thioridazine), antiarrhythmic drugs (including, but not limited to amiodarone, disopyramide, procainamide, sotalol, dofetilide, quinidine) and other drugs that may prolong the QT interval (including but not limited to chloroquine, clarithromycin, erythromycin, dolasetron, granisetron, haloperidol, methadone, moxifloxacin, and pimozide), pentamidine, posaconazole, saquinavir, sparfloxacin, terfenadine, and troleandomycin.

SPECIAL CONSIDERATIONS

1. Vandetanib is only available through a restricted distribution program. This program is designed to inform healthcare providers about the potential serious risks of QT prolongation, torsades de pointes, and sudden death from vandetanib.
2. Contraindicated in patients with the congenital long QT syndrome.
3. Closely monitor ECG with QTc measurements at baseline and periodically during therapy, as QTc prolongation has been observed. Use with caution in patients with CHF, bradyarrhythmias, concomitant use of drugs that prolong QT interval, and electrolyte abnormalities (hypokalemia and hypomagnesemia). This represents a black-box warning.
4. In the event of corrected QTc (QTcF) interval greater than 500 msec, vandetanib needs to be held until QTcF returns to less than 450 msec, at which time a reduced dose should be administered.
5. Vandetanib is not recommended for patients with moderate (Child-Pugh B) and severe (Child-Pugh C) hepatic impairment.

6. Use with caution in patients with moderate-to-severe (CrCl <30 mL/ min) renal impairment. In this setting, the starting dose should be reduced to 200 mg.

7. Vandetanib tablets should not be crushed. When vandetanib tablets cannot be taken whole, they can be dispensed in a glass containing 2 ounces of non-carbonated water and stirred for approximately 10 minutes until the tablet is dispersed.

8. Closely monitor thyroid function tests, as increases in the dose of thyroid replacement therapy may be required while on vandetanib. Thyroid-stimulating hormone (TSH) levels should be obtained at baseline, at 2 to 4 weeks and 8 to 12 weeks after starting treatment, and every 3 months thereafter.

9. Closely monitor BP while on therapy. Use with caution in patients with uncontrolled hypertension. Should be discontinued in patients who develop hypertensive crisis. Blood pressure is usually well controlled with oral antihypertensive medication.

10. Patients with recent history of hemoptysis of ⩾1/2 teaspoon of red blood should not receive vandetanib. Discontinue vandetanib in patients who develop severe hemorrhage.

11. Vandetanib treatment can result in RPLS, as manifested by headache, seizure, lethargy, confusion, blindness and other visual side effects, as well as other neurologic disturbances. Magnetic resonance imaging is helpful in confirming the diagnosis.

12. Pregnancy category D. Breastfeeding should be avoided.

TOXICITY 1
Mild-to-moderate skin reactions with rash, acne, dry skin, dermatitis, pruritis and other skin reactions (including photosensitivity reactions and palmar-plantar erythrodysesthesia syndrome). Rare cases of severe skin reactions (including Stevens-Johnson syndrome) resulting in deaths have been reported.

TOXICITY 2
Diarrhea and nausea/vomiting.

TOXICITY 3
Fatigue.

TOXICITY 4
Hypertension. In rare cases, heart failure has been observed.

TOXICITY 5
Bleeding complications.

TOXICITY 6
QT prolongation and torsades de pointes.

TOXICITY 7
ILD or pneumonitis.

TOXICITY 8
RPLS with seizures, headache, visual disturbances, confusion, or altered mental function.

Vemurafenib

TRADE NAMES	Zelboraf, PLX4032	CLASSIFICATION	Signal transduction inhibitor
CATEGORY	Chemotherapy drug	DRUG MANUFACTURER	Genentech-Roche

MECHANISM OF ACTION
- Inhibits mutant forms of BRAF serine-threonine kinase, including BRAF-V600E, which results in constitutive activation of MAPK signaling.
- Does not inhibit wild-type BRAF or other Raf kinases, including ARAF and CRAF.

MECHANISM OF RESISTANCE
- Presence of NRAS mutations.
- Presence of MEK1 and MEK2 mutations, leading to increased expression of MAPK signaling.
- Activation/induction of alternative cellular signaling pathways, such as c-Met, FGFR, EGFR, and PI3K/Akt.
- Reactivation of Ras/Raf signaling via mutations in KRAS, NRAS, and BRAF.
- Increased expression of BRAF through gene amplification.
- Loss of tumor suppressor genes stromal antigen 2 (STAG2) and STAG3

ABSORPTION
Oral bioavailability and the potential effect of food on drug absorption have not yet been determined.

DISTRIBUTION

Extensive binding (>99%) of vemurafenib to plasma proteins. Steady-state drug levels are reached in 15 to 22 days following initiation of therapy.

METABOLISM

Metabolized in the liver primarily by CYP3A4 microsomal enzymes to produce its primary active metabolite, which is further metabolized by CYP3A4. Elimination is hepatic with excretion in feces (~94%), with renal elimination accounting for approximately 1% of the administered dose. The median terminal half-life of vemurafenib is approximately 60 hours.

INDICATIONS

1. FDA-approved for unresectable or metastatic melanoma with BRAF-V600E mutation as determined by an FDA-approved test.
2. Not recommended for wild-type BRAF melanoma.

DOSAGE RANGE

Recommended dose is 960 mg PO bid.

DRUG INTERACTION 1

Drugs such as ketoconazole, itraconazole, erythromycin, clarithromycin, atazanavir, indinavir, nefazodone, nelfinavir, ritonavir, saquinavir, telithromycin, and voriconazole may decrease the rate of metabolism of vemurafenib, resulting in increased drug levels and potentially increased toxicity.

DRUG INTERACTION 2

Drugs such as rifampin, phenytoin, phenobarbital, carbamazepine, and St. John's wort may increase the rate of metabolism of vemurafenib, resulting in its inactivation.

SPECIAL CONSIDERATIONS

1. Baseline and periodic evaluations of ECG and electrolyte status should be performed while on therapy. ECGs should be done at day 15, monthly during the first 3 months of therapy, and every 3 months thereafter. If the QTc >500 msec, therapy should be interrupted. Use with caution in patients at risk of developing QT prolongation, including hypokalemia, hypomagnesemia, congenital long QT syndrome, and in patients taking antiarrhythmic medications or any other drugs that may cause QT prolongation.
2. Closely monitor LFTs and serum bilirubin.
3. Careful skin exams should be done at baseline and every 2 months while on therapy, given the increased incidence of cutaneous squamous cell cancers.
4. Monitor for severe dermatologic reactions, such as Stevens-Johnson syndrome and toxic epidermal necrolysis. Therapy should be terminated in patients who experience these skin reactions.
5. Patients should be cautioned to avoid sun exposure while on therapy.
6. Monitor patients for eye reactions, including uveitis, iritis, and retinal vein occlusion.

7. BRAF testing using an FDA-approved test to confirm the presence of the BRAF-V600E mutation is required for determining which patients should receive vemurafenib therapy.
8. No dose adjustment is needed for patients with mild and moderate hepatic and/or renal dysfunction. However, caution should be used in patients with severe hepatic and/or renal dysfunction.
9. Pregnancy category D. Breastfeeding should be avoided.

TOXICITY 1
Cutaneous squamous cell cancers and keratoacanthomas occur in up to 25% of patients. Usually occurs within 7–8 weeks of starting therapy.

TOXICITY 2
Skin reactions, including Stevens-Johnson syndrome and toxic epidermal necrolysis, have been reported.

TOXICITY 3
Cardiac toxicity with QTc prolongation.

TOXICITY 4
Elevations in serum bilirubin and liver transaminases.

TOXICITY 5
Photosensitivity.

TOXICITY 6
Opthalmologic side effects, including uveitis, iritis, photophobia, and retinal vein occlusion.

TOXICITY 7
Fatigue.

Venetoclax

V

TRADE NAMES	Venclexta	CLASSIFICATION	Signal transduction inhibitor
CATEGORY	Chemotherapy drug	DRUG MANUFACTURER	AbbVie; Genentech/Roche

MECHANISM OF ACTION
- Selective small molecule inhibitor of BCL-2, an important anti-apoptotic protein.
- Activity in tumor cells that overexpress BCL-2, such as CLL.
- Restores the process of apoptosis by binding directly to the BCL-2 protein, displacing pro-apoptotic proteins, such as BIM, which then triggers mitochondrial outer membrane permeabilization and subsequent activation of caspases.

MECHANISM OF RESISTANCE
- Increased expression of MCL1.
- Mutations in the BCL2 protein resulting in reduced binding affinity to the drug.
- Increased degradation and/or metabolism of drug.

ABSORPTION
Rapidly absorbed after an oral dose with peak plasma levels achieved within 5–8 hours. Oral bioavailability on the order of 40%–60%. Food with a high fat content reduces oral bioavailability by up to 15%.

DISTRIBUTION
Highly bound (>99%) to plasma proteins. Steady-state drug concentrations are reached in 15 days.

METABOLISM
Metabolized in the liver primarily by CYP3A4 and CYP3A5 microsomal enzymes. The major metabolite is M27, which has BCL-2 inhibitory activity. Elimination is hepatic with excretion in feces (>99.9%), with renal elimination accounting for <0.1% of an administered dose. Unchanged parent drug represents approximately 21% of an administered dose in feces. The terminal half-life of venetoclax is approximately 26 hours.

INDICATIONS
FDA-approved for the treatment of CLL with 17p deletion as detected by an FDA-approved test following at least one prior therapy.

DOSAGE RANGE
Initial therapy starting at 20 mg PO once daily for 7 days following by a weekly ramp-up schedule over 5 weeks to the final recommended dose of 400 mg PO once daily.

DRUG INTERACTION 1

Drugs such as ketoconazole, itraconazole, erythromycin, clarithromycin, atazanavir, indinavir, nefazodone, nelfinavir, ritonavir, saquinavir, telithromycin, and voriconazole may decrease the rate of metabolism of venetoclax, resulting in increased drug levels and potentially increased toxicity. The dose of venetoclax should be reduced by at least 50% if a moderate CYP3A4 inhibitor is used.

DRUG INTERACTION 2

Drugs such as rifampin, phenytoin, phenobarbital, carbamazepine, and St. John's wort may increase the rate of metabolism of venetoclax, resulting in its inactivation.

DRUG INTERACTION 3

Drugs such as amiodarone, azithromycin, captopril, carvedilol, cyclosporine, felodipine, quinidine, ranolazine, and ticagrelor, which are P-glycoprotein inhibitors, may decrease the rate of metabolism of venetoclax, resulting in increased drug levels and potentially increased toxicity. The dose of venetoclax should be reduced by at least 50% if a P-glycoprotein inhibitor is used.

DRUG INTERACTION 4

Warfarin—Patients receiving coumarin-derived anticoagulants should be closely monitored for alterations in their clotting parameters (PT and INR) and/or bleeding, as venetoclax may inhibit the metabolism of warfarin by the liver P450 system. Dose of warfarin may require careful adjustment in the presence of venetoclax therapy.

SPECIAL CONSIDERATIONS

1. Use with caution in patients with hepatic dysfunction. No dose reduction is recommended in patients with mild or moderate hepatic dysfunction although there may be an increased risk of toxicity in patients with moderate hepatic dysfunction. The drug has not been well studied in severe hepatic dysfunction.
2. No dose reduction is recommended for patients with mild or moderate renal dysfunction. The drug has not been well studied in severe renal dysfunction or in patients on dialysis.
3. Closely monitor CBCs and consider using growth factors to support neutrophil count.
4. All patients should be assessed for the possibility of tumor lysis syndrome, with an increased risk in patients with high tumor burden and/or high peripheral white blood cell count. This can occur within 6-8 hours following the first dose of venetoclax.
5. Closely monitor serum chemistries, such as potassium, phosphate, BUN/creatinine, and uric acid for evidence of tumor lysis syndrome.
6. Patients receiving venetoclax along with oral warfarin anticoagulant therapy should have their coagulation parameters (PT and INR) monitored frequently, as elevations in INR and bleeding events have been observed.

7. Venetoclax oral bioavailability is not affected by gastric acid reducing agents, such as proton pump inhibitors, H2-receptor antagonists, and antacids.
8. Venetoclax tablets should be taken with a meal and water and swallowed whole and not chewed, crushed, or broken prior to ingestion.
9. CLL patients without a 17p deletion at the initial time of diagnosis should be re-tested at the time of disease relapse as acquisition of 17p deletion may occur.
10. Avoid Seville oranges, starfruit, pomelos, grapefruit, and grapefruit juice while on venetoclax therapy.
11. Live attenuated vaccines should not be administered prior to, during, or after venetoclax therapy.
12. Pregnancy category D. Breastfeeding should be avoided.

TOXICITY 1
Tumor lysis syndrome, especially in the setting of high tumor burden and high peripheral white blood cell count.

TOXICITY 2
Myelosuppression with neutropenia, anemia, and thrombocytopenia.

TOXICITY 3
GI toxicity with diarrhea, nausea/vomiting, abdominal pain, and reduced appetite.

TOXICITY 4
Constitutional side effects with fatigue, asthenia, anorexia, and headache.

TOXICITY 5
Pulmonary toxicity with cough, URI, sinusitis, and dyspnea.

TOXICITY 6
Infections, which include pneumonia, herpes simplex, urinary tract infections, viral infections, and influenza-like illness.

Vinblastine

TRADE NAME	Velban	CLASSIFICATION	Vinca alkaloid, anti-microtubule agent
CATEGORY	Chemotherapy drug	DRUG MANUFACTURER	Eli Lilly

MECHANISM OF ACTION
- Plant alkaloid extracted from the periwinkle plant *Catharanthus roseus*.
- Cell cycle–specific with activity in the mitosis (M) phase.
- Inhibits tubulin polymerization, disrupting formation of microtubule assembly during mitosis. This results in an arrest in cell division, ultimately leading to cell death.
- May also inhibit DNA, RNA, and protein synthesis.

MECHANISM OF RESISTANCE
- Overexpression of the P170 glycoprotein encoded by the multidrug-resistant gene, resulting in enhanced efflux of drug and decreased intracellular drug accumulation. Cross-resistance may be observed with other natural products, such as taxanes, epipodophyllotoxins, anthracyclines, and actinomycin-D.
- Mutations in α- and β-tubulin proteins with decreased binding affinity to vinblastine.

ABSORPTION
Poorly and erratically absorbed by the oral route.

DISTRIBUTION
Widely and rapidly distributed into most body tissues. Binds extensively to platelets, RBCs, and WBCs within 30 minutes of administration. Poor penetration into the CSF.

METABOLISM
Metabolized in the liver by the cytochrome P450 microsomal system. Small quantities of at least one metabolite, desacetyl vinblastine, may be as active as the parent drug. Majority of vinblastine is excreted in metabolite form via the enterohepatic biliary system. Only about 10% of the parent drug is excreted in feces. Approximately 14% of the drug is eliminated by the kidneys. Plasma terminal half-life of about 25 hours.

INDICATIONS
1. Hodgkin's and non-Hodgkin's lymphoma.
2. Testicular cancer.
3. Breast cancer.
4. Kaposi's sarcoma.
5. Renal cell carcinoma.

DOSAGE RANGE
1. Hodgkin's lymphoma: 6 mg/m^2 IV on days 1 and 15, as part of the ABVD regimen.
2. Testicular cancer: 0.15 mg/kg IV on days 1 and 2, as part of the PVB regimen.

DRUG INTERACTION 1
Drugs metabolized by liver P450 system—Vinblastine should be used cautiously in patients receiving medications that inhibit drug metabolism via the hepatic cytochrome P450 system, including calcium channel blockers, cimetidine, cyclosporine, erythromycin, metoclopramide, and ketoconazole.

DRUG INTERACTION 2
Phenytoin—Vinblastine reduces blood levels of phenytoin through either reduced absorption of phenytoin or an increase in the rate of its metabolism and elimination.

DRUG INTERACTION 3
Bleomycin—Risk of Raynaud's syndrome may be increased with the combination of vinblastine and bleomycin.

SPECIAL CONSIDERATIONS
1. Use with caution in patients with abnormal liver function as toxicity of vinblastine may be significantly enhanced. Dose reduction is recommended in this setting.
2. Vinblastine should be infused as a rapid push in a free-flowing IV line to avoid extravasation. If extravasation occurs, the infusion should be discontinued immediately. Flushing with sterile water, elevation of the involved extremity, and local application of ice are recommended. In severe cases, a plastic surgeon should be consulted.
3. Patients should be warned about the risk of constipation upon starting therapy, and a bowel regimen including a high-fiber diet and a stool softener should be initiated.
4. Observe for hypersensitivity reactions, especially when the drug is administered in association with mitomycin-C.
5. Contamination of the eye may lead to severe irritation and even corneal ulceration. If accidental contamination occurs, the eyes should be immediately and thoroughly washed.
6. Pregnancy category D. Breastfeeding should be avoided.

TOXICITY 1
Myelosuppression is dose-limiting with neutropenia being most commonly observed. Thrombocytopenia and anemia are less common.

TOXICITY 2
Mucositis and stomatitis. More frequently observed with vinblastine than with vincristine. Nausea, vomiting, anorexia, and diarrhea may also occur.

TOXICITY 3
Alopecia is common, usually mild, and reversible.

TOXICITY 4

Hypertension. Most common cardiovascular side effect and occurs as a consequence of autonomic dysfunction.

TOXICITY 5

Neurotoxicity. Occurs much less frequently than with vincristine. Presents with the same manifestations as seen with vincristine: peripheral neuropathy (paresthesias, paralysis, loss of deep tendon reflexes, and constipation) and autonomic nervous system dysfunction (orthostatic hypotension, paralytic ileus, and urinary retention). Less commonly, cranial nerve paralysis, ataxia, cortical blindness, seizures, and coma may occur.

TOXICITY 6

Vesicant. Extravasation may cause local skin damage.

TOXICITY 7

Syndrome of inappropriate antidiuretic hormone secretion (SIADH).

TOXICITY 8

Headache and depression.

TOXICITY 9

Vascular events, such as stroke, MI, and Raynaud's syndrome.

TOXICITY 10

Acute pulmonary edema, bronchospasm, acute respiratory distress, interstitial pulmonary infiltrates, and dyspnea have been reported on rare occasions.

Vincristine

| **TRADE NAMES** | Oncovin, VCR | **CLASSIFICATION** | Vinca alkaloid, antimicrotubule agent |
| **CATEGORY** | Chemotherapy drug | **DRUG MANUFACTURER** | Eli Lilly |

MECHANISM OF ACTION

- Plant alkaloid derived from the periwinkle plant *Catharanthus roseus*.
- Cell cycle–specific with activity in the mitosis (M) phase.
- Inhibits tubulin polymerization, disrupting formation of microtubule assembly during mitosis. This results in an arrest in cell division, ultimately leading to cell death.
- May also inhibit DNA, RNA, and protein synthesis.

MECHANISM OF RESISTANCE

- Overexpression of the P170 glycoprotein encoded by the multidrug-resistant gene, resulting in enhanced efflux of drug and decreased intracellular drug accumulation. Cross-resistance may be observed with other natural products, such as taxanes, epipodophyllotoxins, anthracyclines, and actinomycin-D.
- Mutations in α- and β-tubulin proteins with decreased affinity to vincristine.

ABSORPTION

Not available for oral use and administered only by the IV route.

DISTRIBUTION

Widely and rapidly distributed into body tissues within 30 minutes of administration. Poor penetration across the blood-brain barrier and into the CSF.

METABOLISM

Metabolized in the liver by the cytochrome P450 microsomal system. The majority of vincristine (80%) is excreted in bile and feces. Only 15%–20% of the drug is recovered in urine. Terminal half-life is long, on the order of 85 hours.

INDICATIONS

1. Acute lymphoblastic leukemia.
2. Hodgkin's and non-Hodgkin's lymphoma.
3. Multiple myeloma.
4. Rhabdomyosarcoma.
5. Neuroblastoma.
6. Ewing's sarcoma.
7. Wilms' tumor.
8. Chronic leukemias.
9. Thyroid cancer.
10. Brain tumors.
11. Trophoblastic neoplasms.

DOSAGE RANGE

1. Doses usually vary between 0.5 and 1.4 mg/m^2. The total individual dose should be limited to 2 mg to prevent the development of neurotoxicity.
2. Continuous infusion: 0.4 mg/day IV continuous infusion for 4 days, as part of the VAD regimen for multiple myeloma.

DRUG INTERACTION 1

Drugs metabolized by liver P450 system—Vincristine should be used with caution in patients receiving medications that inhibit drug metabolism via the hepatic cytochrome P450 system.

DRUG INTERACTION 2

Phenytoin—Vincristine reduces the blood levels of phenytoin and its subsequent efficacy through either reduced absorption of phenytoin or an increase in the rate of its metabolism and/or elimination.

DRUG INTERACTION 3

Digoxin—Vincristine reduces the blood levels of digoxin resulting in decreased efficacy.

DRUG INTERACTION 4

Cisplatin and paclitaxel—Concurrent administration of vincristine with other neurotoxic agents such as cisplatin and paclitaxel may increase the risk and severity of neurotoxicity.

DRUG INTERACTION 5

L-Asparaginase—When used in combination with L-asparaginase, vincristine should be administered 12–24 hours before, as L-asparaginase inhibits vincristine clearance.

DRUG INTERACTION 6

Methotrexate—Vincristine increases the cellular uptake of methotrexate, resulting in enhanced antitumor activity and host toxicity.

DRUG INTERACTION 7

Filgrastim—Concurrent use of vincristine with filgrastim may result in severe atypical neuropathy.

SPECIAL CONSIDERATIONS

1. Use with caution in patients with abnormal liver function as increased toxicity may be observed. Dose reduction is necessary in this setting.
2. Vincristine should be infused as a rapid push over 1 minute in a side port of a free-flowing IV line to avoid extravasation. If extravasation occurs, the infusion should be discontinued immediately. Application of ice to the area of leakage along with elevation of involved extremity may minimize discomfort and the possibility of cellulitis. In severe cases, a plastic surgeon should be consulted.

3. Contamination of the eye may lead to severe irritation and even corneal ulceration. If accidental contamination occurs, the eyes should be washed immediately and thoroughly.

4. Patients should be warned about the risk of constipation upon starting therapy, and a bowel regimen including stool softeners and high-fiber diet should be initiated. Patients should be advised to seek medical attention if persistent nausea, vomiting, and abdominal pain develop after beginning therapy.

5. Careful baseline neurologic evaluation should be performed before starting therapy and at the start of each cycle. The onset of severe signs and/or symptoms of neurotoxicity warrants immediate discontinuation of the drug. Avoid the simultaneous use of drugs associated with neurologic toxicity. Risk factors for neurotoxicity include elderly patients and those with pre-existing neuropathies and/or neuromuscular disorders.

6. Overdose of vincristine may be treated with leucovorin 100 mg IV every 3 hours for the first 24 hours and then every 6 hours for 48 hours. Other supportive measures should be considered, including prevention of SIADH; use of anticonvulsants, enemas, or cathartics to prevent ileus; monitoring of the cardiovascular system; and monitoring of CBC.

7. Pregnancy category D. Breastfeeding should be avoided.

TOXICITY 1

Neurotoxicity. Most commonly observed dose-limiting toxicity. Clinical manifestations are variable, and include peripheral neuropathy (paresthesias, paralysis, and loss of deep tendon reflexes), autonomic nervous system dysfunction (orthostasis, sphincter problems, and paralytic ileus), cranial nerve palsies, ataxia, cortical blindness, seizures, and coma. Bone, back, limb, jaw, and parotid gland pain may also occur.

TOXICITY 2

Constipation, abdominal pain, and paralytic ileus are common. A prophylactic bowel regimen for constipation is recommended. Nausea, vomiting, and diarrhea can also occur, but are rare.

TOXICITY 3

Alopecia, skin rash, and fever.

TOXICITY 4

Vesicant. Extravasation may cause local tissue injury, inflammation, and necrosis.

TOXICITY 5

Myelosuppression. Generally mild and much less significant than with vinblastine.

TOXICITY 6

SIADH.

TOXICITY 7
Hypersensitivity reactions.

TOXICITY 8
Azoospermia and amenorrhea.

Vinorelbine

TRADE NAME	Navelbine	CLASSIFICATION	Vinca alkaloid, antimicrotubule agent
CATEGORY	Chemotherapy drug	DRUG MANUFACTURER	GlaxoSmithKline

MECHANISM OF ACTION
- Semisynthetic alkaloid derived from vinblastine.
- Cell cycle–specific with activity in mitosis (M) phase.
- Inhibits tubulin polymerization, disrupting formation of microtubule assembly during mitosis. This results in an arrest in cell division, ultimately leading to cell death.
- Relatively high specificity for mitotic microtubules with lower affinity for axonal microtubules.
- May also inhibit DNA, RNA, and protein synthesis.

MECHANISM OF RESISTANCE
- Overexpression of the P170 glycoprotein encoded by the multidrug-resistant gene, resulting in enhanced efflux of drug and decreased intracellular drug accumulation. Cross-resistance may be observed with other natural products, such as taxanes, epipodophyllotoxins, anthracyclines, and actinomycin-D.
- Mutations in α- and β-tubulin proteins with decreased binding affinity to vinorelbine.

ABSORPTION
Administered only by the IV route.

DISTRIBUTION
Widely and rapidly distributed into most body tissues with a large apparent volume of distribution (>30 L/kg). Extensive binding to plasma proteins (about 80%).

METABOLISM
Metabolized in the liver by the cytochrome P450 microsomal system. Small quantities of at least one metabolite, desacetyl vinorelbine, have antitumor activity similar to that of parent drug. Majority of vinorelbine excreted in feces via the enterohepatic biliary system (50%). About 15%–20% of the drug is eliminated by the kidneys. Prolonged terminal half-life of 27–43 hours secondary to relatively slow efflux of drug from peripheral tissues.

INDICATIONS
1. NSCLC.
2. Breast cancer.
3. Ovarian cancer.

DOSAGE RANGE
Usual dose is 30 mg/m^2 IV on a weekly schedule either as a single agent or in combination with cisplatin.

DRUG INTERACTION 1
Drugs metabolized by the liver P450 system—Vinorelbine should be used cautiously in patients receiving medications that inhibit drug metabolism via the hepatic cytochrome P450 system.

DRUG INTERACTION 2
Phenytoin—Vinorelbine reduces blood levels of phenytoin through either reduced absorption of phenytoin or an increase in the rate of its metabolism and elimination.

DRUG INTERACTION 3
Cisplatin—Risk of myelosuppression increases when vinorelbine is used in combination with cisplatin.

DRUG INTERACTION 4
Mitomycin-C—Increased risk of acute allergic reactions when vinorelbine is used in combination with mitomycin-C.

SPECIAL CONSIDERATIONS
1. Use with caution in patients with abnormal liver function as toxicity of vinorelbine may be significantly enhanced. Dose reduction is recommended in this setting.
2. Use with caution in patients previously treated with chemotherapy and/or radiation therapy, as their bone marrow reserve may be compromised.
3. Vinorelbine should be infused as a rapid push in a free-flowing IV line to avoid extravasation. If extravasation occurs, the infusion should be

discontinued immediately. Flushing with sterile water, elevation of the extremity, and local application of ice are recommended. In severe cases, a plastic surgeon should be consulted.

4. Contamination of the eye may lead to severe irritation and even corneal ulceration. If accidental contamination occurs, the eyes should be immediately and thoroughly washed.
5. Pregnancy category D. Breastfeeding should be avoided.

TOXICITY 1
Myelosuppression. Dose-limiting toxicity. Readily reversible once treatment is stopped. Neutropenia is most commonly observed. Nadirs occur by day 7, with recovery by day 14. Thrombocytopenia and anemia are less common.

TOXICITY 2
Nausea and vomiting. Usually moderate and occur within first 24 hours after treatment.

TOXICITY 3
GI toxicities in the form of constipation (35%), diarrhea (17%), stomatitis (<20%), and anorexia (<20%).

TOXICITY 4
Transient elevation in LFTs, including SGOT and bilirubin. Usually clinically asymptomatic.

TOXICITY 5
Vesicant. Extravasation may cause local tissue injury and inflammation.

TOXICITY 6
Neurotoxicity. Usually mild in severity and occurs much less frequently than with other vinca alkaloids. Vinorelbine has lower affinity for axonal microtubules than observed with vincristine or vinblastine. Increased risk in patients with pre-existing neuromuscular disease.

TOXICITY 7
Alopecia. Observed in 10%–15% of patients.

TOXICITY 8
SIADH.

TOXICITY 9
Hypersensitivity and/or allergic reactions presenting as dyspnea and bronchospasm. Incidence is increased when used in combination with mitomycin-C.

TOXICITY 10
Generalized fatigue. Occurs in 35% of patients and incidence increases with cumulative doses.

V

Vismodegib

TRADE NAME	Erivedge	CLASSIFICATION	Signal transduction inhibitor
CATEGORY	Chemotherapy drug	DRUG MANUFACTURER	Genentech-Roche

MECHANISM OF ACTION
- Small-molecule inhibitor of the Hedgehog pathway.
- Binds to and inhibits smoothened, a transmembrane protein that is involved in Hedgehog signaling.

MECHANISM OF RESISTANCE
- Increased expression of MAPK signaling.
- Activation/induction of alternative cellular signaling pathways, such as c-Met, FGFR, EGFR, and PI3K/Akt.
- Reactivation of Ras/Raf signaling via mutations in KRAS, NRAS, and BRAF.

ABSORPTION
Oral bioavailability is approximately 32%. Food does not affect drug exposure.

DISTRIBUTION
Extensive binding (>99%) of vismodegib to plasma proteins, including albumin and α1-acid glycoprotein.

METABOLISM
Mainly excreted as unchanged drug. Several minor metabolites are produced in the liver primarily by CYP3A4/5 and CYP2C9 microsomal enzymes. Elimination is hepatic with excretion in feces (82%), with renal elimination accounting for only 4.4% of the administered dose. The elimination half-life of vismodegib is approximately 4 days. Population pharmacokinetic analyses show that age, renal function, and sex do not impact on systemic exposure to drug.

INDICATIONS

FDA-approved for metastatic basal cell cancer, locally advanced basal cell cancer that has recurred following surgery, or in patients who are not candidates for surgery and/or radiation.

DOSAGE RANGE

Recommended dose is 150 mg PO on a daily basis.

DRUG INTERACTION 1

Proton pump inhibitors, H2-receptor inhibitors, and antacids—Drugs that alter the pH of the upper GI tract may alter vismodegib solubility, thereby reducing drug bioavailability and decreasing systemic drug exposure.

DRUG INTERACTION 2

P-glycoprotein inhibitors (clarithromycin, erythromycin, azithromycin)—Drugs that inhibit P-glycoprotein may increase systemic exposure of vismodegib, resulting in increased toxicity as vismodegib is a substrate of the P-glycoprotein efflux transport protein.

SPECIAL CONSIDERATIONS

1. Vismodegib may be taken with or without food. Capsules should not be opened or crushed and should be swallowed whole.
2. The safety and efficacy of vismodegib have not been studied in patients with hepatic and/or renal impairment.
3. Patients should be advised not to donate blood or blood products while on vismodegib and for at least 7 months after the last drug dose.
4. The pregnancy status of female patients must be verified prior to the start of vimodegib therapy given the risk of embryo-fetal death and/or severe birth defects. This is a black-box warning.
5. Female and male patients of reproductive potential should be counseled on pregnancy prevention and planning. Female patients should be advised on the need for contraception while males should be advised of the potential risk of drug exposure through semen. Women who have been exposed to vismodegib during pregnancy, either directly or through seminal fluid, should participate in the pregnancy pharmacovigilance program by contacting the Genentech Adverse Event Line at (888-835-2555).
6. Avoid drugs that will alter the pH of the upper GI tract, such as proton pump inhibitors, H2-receptor inhibitors, and antacids while on vismodegib therapy.
7. Pregnancy category D. Breastfeeding should be avoided.

TOXICITY 1

Embryo-fetal deaths and/or severe birth defects.

TOXICITY 2

Muscle spasms and arthralgias.

TOXICITY 3

Decreased appetite, fatigue, and weight loss.

TOXICITY 4
Change in taste and/or loss of taste.

TOXICITY 5
Alopecia.

TOXICITY 6
Nausea/vomiting, constipation, and diarrhea.

Vorinostat

TRADE NAME	Zolinza	**CLASSIFICATION**	Histone deacetylase (HDAC) inhibitor
CATEGORY	Chemotherapy drug	**DRUG MANUFACTURER**	Merck

MECHANISM OF ACTION
- Potent inhibitor of histone deacetylases HDAC1, HDAC2, and HDAC3 (Class I) and HDAC6 (Class II).
- Inhibition of HDAC activity leads to accumulation of acetyl groups on the histone lysine residues, resulting in open chromatin structure and transcriptional activation. Induction of cell cycle arrest and/or apoptosis may then occur.
- The precise mechanism(s) by which vorinostat exerts its antitumor activity has not been fully characterized.

MECHANISM OF RESISTANCE
None well characterized to date.

ABSORPTION
Oral absorption is not significantly affected when administered with food.

DISTRIBUTION
Significant binding (75%) to plasma proteins and extensive tissue distribution. Peak plasma levels are achieved 4 hours after ingestion.

METABOLISM

Metabolism involves glucuronidation and hydrolysis followed by β-oxidation. In vitro studies suggest minimal biotransformation by the cytochrome P450 system. Elimination is mainly via metabolism, and renal elimination of parent drug accounts for <1% of an administered dose. The terminal half-life of the parent drug is 2 hours.

INDICATIONS

FDA-approved for the treatment of patients with CTCL who have progressive, persistent, or recurrent disease on or after two systemic therapies.

DOSAGE RANGE

Recommended dose is 400 mg PO daily.

DRUG INTERACTION 1

Warfarin—Patients receiving coumarin-derived anticoagulants should be closely monitored for alterations in their clotting parameters (PT and INR) and/or bleeding, as prolongation of PT and INR has been observed with concomitant use of vorinostat. The dose of warfarin may require careful adjustment in the presence of vorinostat therapy.

DRUG INTERACTION 2

HDAC inhibitors—Severe thrombocytopenia and GI bleeding have been reported when vorinostat and other HDAC inhibitors, such as valproic acid, are used together. CBC and platelet counts should be monitored every 2 weeks for the first 2 months of therapy.

SPECIAL CONSIDERATIONS

1. Use with caution in patients with hepatic impairment, although no specific dose recommendations have been provided.
2. Patients should be instructed to drink at least 2 L/day of fluids to maintain hydration.
3. Closely monitor CBC and platelet count every 2 weeks during the first 2 months of therapy and at monthly intervals thereafter.
4. Monitor ECG with QT measurement at baseline and periodically during therapy, as QTc prolongation has been observed. Use with caution in patients at risk of developing QT prolongation, including hypokalemia, hypomagnesemia, congenital long QT syndrome, patients taking antiarrhythmic medications or any other products that may cause QT prolongation, and cumulative high-dose anthracycline therapy.
5. Closely monitor serum glucose levels, especially in diabetic patients, as hyperglycemia may develop while on therapy. Alterations in diet and/or therapy for increased glucose may be necessary.
6. Pregnancy category D. Breastfeeding should be avoided.

TOXICITY 1

Nausea/vomiting and diarrhea are the most common GI toxicities.

TOXICITY 2
Myelosuppression with thrombocytopenia and anemia more common than neutropenia.

TOXICITY 3
Fatigue and anorexia.

TOXICITY 4
Cardiac toxicity with QTc prolongation.

TOXICITY 5
Hyperglycemia.

TOXICITY 6
Increased risk of thromboembolic complications, including DVT and PE.

Ziv-aflibercept

TRADE NAME	Zaltrap	**CLASSIFICATION**	Monoclonal antibody, anti-VEGF antibody
CATEGORY	Biologic response modifier agent	**DRUG MANUFACTURER**	Regeneron/ Sanofi-Aventis

MECHANISM OF ACTION
- Recombinant fusion protein made up of portions of the extracellular domains of human VEGFR-1 and VEGFR-2 fused to the Fc portion of the human IgG1 molecule.
- Functions as a soluble receptor that binds to VEGF-A, VEGF-B, and PlGF. Binds with much higher affinity to VEGF-A than bevacizumab.
- Precise mechanism(s) of action remains unknown.
- Binding of VEGF ligands prevents their subsequent interaction with VEGF receptors on the surface of endothelial cells and tumors, and in so doing, results in inhibition of downstream VEGFR-mediated signaling.
- Inhibits formation of new blood vessels in primary tumor and metastatic tumors.
- Inhibits tumor blood vessel permeability and reduces interstitial tumoral pressures, and in so doing, may enhance blood flow delivery within tumor.

MECHANISM OF RESISTANCE
- Increased expression/activity of IL6/STAT3 signaling pathway.
- Increased expression of pro-angiogenic factor ligands, such as bFGF and HGF.
- Recruitment of bone marrow-derived cells, which circumvents the requirement of VEGF signaling and restores neovascularization and tumor angiogenesis.

DISTRIBUTION
Distribution in body is not well characterized. The predicted time to reach steady-state levels is on the order of 14 days.

METABOLISM
Metabolism of ziv-aflibercept has not been extensively characterized. The elimination half-life of free-ziv-aflibercept is on the order of 6 days with minimal clearance by the liver or kidneys. Tissue half-life has not been well-characterized.

INDICATIONS
1. Metastatic colorectal cancer—FDA-approved for use in combination with 5-FU, LV, irinotecan (FOLFIRI) in patients with mCRC that is resistant to or has progressed following an oxaliplatin-based regimen.

DOSAGE RANGE
1. Recommended dose is 4 mg/kg IV every 2 weeks.
2. Can also be administered at 6 mg/kg IV every 3 weeks.

DRUG INTERACTIONS
None well characterized to date.

SPECIAL CONSIDERATIONS
1. Patients should be warned of the increased risk of arterial thromboembolic events, including myocardial infarction and stroke. This represents a black-box warning.
2. Patients should be warned of the potential for serious and sometimes fatal bleeding complications, including GI hemorrhage, hemoptysis, hematuria, and postprocedural hemorrhage. This represents a black-box warning.
3. Ziv-aflibercept treatment can result in the development of GI perforations and wound dehiscence, which in some cases has resulted in death. These events represent a black-box warning for the drug. Use with caution in patients who have undergone recent surgical and/or invasive procedures. Ziv-aflibercept treatment should be held for at least 4 weeks prior to elective surgery and should not be given for at least 28 days after any surgical and/or invasive intervention and until the surgical wound is completely healed.
4. Ziv-aflibercept treatment can result in fistula formation of both GI and non-GI sites.
5. Use with caution in patients with uncontrolled hypertension, as ziv-aflibercept can result in grade 3 hypertension in about 20% of patients. Should be permanently discontinued in patients who develop hypertensive crisis. In most cases, however, hypertension is well-managed with increasing the dose of the antihypertensive medication and/or with the addition of another antihypertensive medication.
6. Monitor older patients for diarrhea and dehydration, as the incidence of diarrhea is increased in patients >65 years of age.
7. Monitor urine for proteinuria by urine dipstick analysis and urinary protein creatinine ratio. A 24-hour urine collection is recommended for patients with a urine protein creatinine ratio >1.
8. Ziv-aflibercept should be terminated in patients who develop the nephrotic syndrome (>3 g/24 hours). Therapy should be interrupted for proteinuria >2 g/24 hours and resumed when <2 g/24 hours.
9. Ziv-aflibercept treatment can result in RPLS, which presents with headache, seizure, lethargy, confusion, blindness and other visual side effects, as well as other neurologic disturbances. Magnetic resonance imaging (MRI) is usually required to confirm the diagnosis.
10. Closely monitor CBC while on therapy.
11. Pregnancy category C. Breastfeeding should be avoided.

TOXICITY 1
Gastrointestinal perforations and wound-healing complications.

TOXICITY 2

Bleeding complications. Serious, life-threatening intracranial and pulmonary hemorrhage/hemoptysis occur in rare cases.

TOXICITY 3

Increased risk of arterial thromboembolic events, including myocardial infarction, angina, and stroke. There is also a slightly increased risk of venous thromboembolic complications, such as DVT and PE.

TOXICITY 4

Hypertension occurs in up to 40% of patients, with grade 3 hypertension observed in 20% of patients. Usually wellcontrolled with oral antihypertensive medication.

TOXICITY 5

Myelosuppression with neutropenia. Febrile neutropenia occurs in about 4% of patients.

TOXICITY 6

Diarrhea and mucositis.

TOXICITY 7

Proteinuria with nephrotic syndrome in up to nearly 10% of patients.

TOXICITY 8

CNS events with dizziness and depression. RPLS occurs rarely, presenting with headache, seizure, lethargy, confusion, blindness, and other visual disturbances.

3

Guidelines for Chemotherapy and Dosing Modifications

M. Sitki Copur, Dawn Tiedemann, Laurie J. Harrold, and Edward Chu

Successful administration of chemotherapy relies on several critical patient factors: age; performance status; co-morbid illnesses; prior therapy; and baseline hematologic, hepatic, and renal status. The dose of a given chemotherapeutic agent should be adjusted accordingly to reflect these parameters, as well as any specific drug-induced toxicities that may have been experienced with prior treatment. This chapter outlines performance scales that have been established to determine functional status; reviews methods to calculate creatinine clearance, body surface area, and drug dose; and provides recommendations for dosing in the setting of hepatic and renal dysfunction. General guidelines for dialyzing chemotherapeutic agents in the setting of drug overdose or renal failure are provided. A more detailed review for each individual drug is provided in Chapter 2. The reader is also advised to refer to the published literature for further details regarding recommendations for specific dose modifications for drug.

Table 1. Performance Scales

Karnofsky

(%)	Performance
100	Normal, no evidence of disease
90	Able to carry on normal activity, minor signs or symptoms of disease
80	Normal activity with effort, some signs or symptoms of disease
70	Unable to perform normal activity, cares for self
60	Requires occasional assistance
50	Requires considerable assistance and frequent medical care
40	Disabled, requires special care and assistance
30	Severely disabled, hospitalization may be required
20	Hospitalization necessary for support, very sick
10	Moribund, rapid progression of disease
0	Dead

ECOG

(%)	Performance
0	Asymptomatic, normal activity
1	Fully ambulatory, symptomatic, able to perform activities of daily living
2	Symptomatic, up and about, in bed less than 50% of time
3	Symptomatic, capable of only limited self-care, in bed more than 50% of time
4	Completely disabled, cannot perform any self-care, bedridden 100% of time
5	Dead

Table 2. Determination of Creatinine Clearance

- The creatinine clearance is determined by the Cockcroft–Gault formula (Cockcroft DW, Gault MH. *Nephron*. 1976;16(1):31–34), which takes into account age, weight, and serum creatinine.

$$\text{Males: Creatinine Clearance (mL/min)} = \frac{\text{weight (kg)}\times(140\text{-age})}{72\times\text{serum creatinine (mg/dL)}}$$

$$\text{Females: Creatinine Clearance (mL/min)} = \frac{\text{weight (kg)}\times(140\text{-age})\times0.85}{72\times\text{serum creatinine (mg/dL)}}$$

- The creatinine clearance can also be determined from a timed urine collection.

$$\text{Creatine Clearance} = \frac{\text{urine creatine}}{\text{serum creatine}} \times \frac{\text{urine volume}}{\text{time}}$$

Table 3. Determination of Target Area Under the Curve (AUC)

AUC refers to the area under the drug concentration × time curve, and it provides a measure of total drug exposure. It is expressed in concentration × units (mg/mL × min).

A formula for quantifying exposure to carboplatin based on dose and renal function was developed by Calvert et al. (Calvert AH, Newell DR, Gumbrell LA, et al. *J Clin Oncol*. 1989;7(11):1748–1756) and is as follows:

Carboplatin Dose (mg) = target AUC (mg/mL × min) × [GFR (mL/min) + 25].

It is important to note that the total dose is in mg and **NOT** mg/m^2. Target AUC is usually between 5 and 7 mg/mL/min for previously untreated patients. In previously treated patients, lower AUCs (between 4 and 6 mg/mL/min) are recommended. AUCs >7 are generally associated with increased toxicity and not improved response rates.

Table 4. Determination of Drug Dose

- Drug doses are usually calculated according to body surface area (BSA, mg/m^2).
- BSA is determined by using a nomogram scale or by using a BSA calculator.
- Once the BSA is determined, multiply the BSA by the amount of drug specified in the regimen to give the total dose of drug to be administered.
- Dosing of obese patients remains controversial. Ideal body weight (IBW), as opposed to the actual body weight, may be used to calculate BSA. It is important to refer to an IBW table to determine the IBW based on the individual's actual height. Once the IBW is determined, add one-third of the IBW to the IBW, which is then used to determine the BSA.
- IBW can be calculated from the following formulas: IBW for men (kg): 50.0 kg + 2.3 kg per inch over = feet; IBW for women (kg): 45.5 kg + 2.3 kg per inch over 5 feet.[1]
- Full weight-based chemotherapy doses may be used in obese patients, especially when the treatment has curative intent.[2]

1. Data from: Olin BR, Hebel SK, Gremp JL, Hulbertt MK, editors. *Drug Facts and Comparisons*. St. Louis, MO: JB Lippincott; 1995; Griggs JJ, Mangu PB, Anderson H, et al. *J Clin Oncol*. 2012;30(13):1553–1561.

2. Griggs JJ, Mangu PB, Anderson H, et al. *J Clin Oncol*. 2012;30:1553–1561.

Table 5. Calculation of Body Surface Area in Adult Amputees

Body Part	% Surface Area of Amputated Part
Hand and five fingers	3.0
Lower part of arm	4.0
Upper part of arm	6.0
Foot	3.0
Lower part of leg	6.0
Thigh	12.0

BSA (m^2) = BSA − [(BSA) × (%BSA$_{part}$)], where BSA = body surface area, BSA = body surface area of amputated part.

Reproduced from: *Am J Hosp Pharm*. by American Society of Hospital Pharmacists.

Reproduced with permission of American Society of Hospital Pharmacists.

Table 6. General Guidelines for Chemotherapy Dosage Based on Hepatic Function

Drug	Recommended Dose Reduction for Hepatic Dysfunction
Afatinib	No dose reduction is necessary in patients with Child–Pugh Class A and B hepatic dysfunction. Has not been studied in patients with Child–Pugh Class C dysfunction, and dose reduction may be necessary in this setting.
Alemtuzumab	N/A
Altretamine	No dose reduction is necessary.
Amifostine	No dose reduction is necessary.
Aminoglutethimide	No dose reduction is necessary.
Amsacrine	Reduce dose by 25% if bilirubin >2.0 mg/dL.
Anastrozole	No formal recommendation for dose reduction.
	Dose reduction may be necessary in patients with hepatic dysfunction.
Arsenic trioxide	No dose reduction is necessary.
Asparaginase	No dose reduction is necessary.
Azacitidine	No dose reduction is necessary.
Bendamustine	Use with caution in patients with mild hepatic dysfunction. Omit in the presence of moderate (SGOT or SGPT 2.5–10 × ULN and total bilirubin >1.5 × ULN) or severe (total bilirubin >3 × ULN) hepatic dysfunction.
Bevacizumab	N/A
Bicalutamide	No formal recommendation for dose reduction.
	Dose reduction may be necessary if bilirubin >3.0 mg/dL.
Bleomycin	No dose reduction is necessary.
Bosutinib	Reduce dose to 200 mg PO daily in patients with mild, moderate, and severe hepatic dysfunction.
Buserelin	No dose reduction is necessary.
Busulfan	No dose reduction is necessary.
Cabozantinib	No dose reduction is necessary for mild hepatic dysfunction.
	Omit in the setting of moderate and severe hepatic dysfunction.
Capecitabine	No formal recommendation for dose reduction.
	Patients need to be closely monitored in the setting of moderate-to-severe hepatic dysfunction.

Table 6 (cont.)

Drug	Recommended Dose Reduction for Hepatic Dysfunction
Carfilzomib	N/A
Carboplatin	No dose reduction is necessary.
Carmustine	No dose reduction is necessary.
Ceritinib	No dose reduction is necessary for mild hepatic dysfunction. Patients need to be closely monitored in the setting of moderate and severe hepatic dysfunction, and dose reduction may be necessary.
Cetuximab	No dose reduction is necessary.
Chlorambucil	No dose reduction is necessary.
Cisplatin	No dose reduction is necessary.
Cladribine	No dose reduction is necessary.
Cyclophosphamide	Reduce by 25% if bilirubin 3.0–5.0 mg/dL or SGOT >180 mg/dL. Omit if bilirubin >5.0 mg/dL.
Cytarabine	No formal recommendation for dose reduction.
Dabrafenib	No dose reduction is necessary with mild hepatic dysfunction. Dose reduction may be necessary with moderate and severe hepatic dysfunction.
Dacarbazine	No dose reduction is necessary.
Dactinomycin	Reduce dose by 50% if bilirubin >3.0 mg/dL.
Daunorubicin	Reduce dose by 25% if bilirubin 1.5–3.0 mg/dL. Reduce dose by 50% if bilirubin >3.0 mg/dL. Omit if bilirubin >5.0 mg/dL.
Decitabine	N/A
Docetaxel	Omit if bilirubin >1.5 mg/dL, SGOT >60 mg/dL, or alkaline phosphatase >2.5 × ULN.
Doxorubicin	Reduce dose by 50% if bilirubin 1.5–3.0 mg/dL. Reduce dose by 75% if bilirubin 3.1–5.0 mg/dL. Omit if bilirubin >5.0 mg/dL.
Doxorubicin liposome	Reduce dose by 50% if bilirubin 1.5–3.0 mg/dL. Reduce dose by 75% if bilirubin 3.1–5.0 mg/dL. Omit if bilirubin >5.0 mg/dL.
Erlotinib	No formal recommendations for dose reduction. Dose reduction or interruption should be considered in patients with severe hepatic dysfunction and/or in those with a bilirubin >3 × ULN.

Table 6 (cont.)

Drug	Recommended Dose Reduction for Hepatic Dysfunction
Estramustine	No dose reduction is necessary.
Etoposide	Reduce dose by 50% if bilirubin 1.5–3.0 mg/dL or SGOT 60–180 mg/dL.
	Omit if bilirubin >3 mg/dL or SGOT >180 mg/dL.
Etoposide phosphate	Reduce dose by 50% if bilirubin 1.5–3.0 mg/dL or SGOT phate 60–180 mg/dL.
	Omit if bilirubin >3 mg/dL or SGOT >180 mg/dL.
Everolimus	Reduce dose to 5 mg/day in setting of moderate hepatic dysfunction (Child–Pugh Class B).
	Omit in setting of severe hepatic dysfunction (Child–Pugh Class C).
Floxuridine	No dose reduction is necessary.
Fludarabine	No dose reduction is necessary.
5-Fluorouracil	No formal recommendations for dose reduction.
	Omit if bilirubin >5.0 mg/dL.
Flutamide	No formal recommendation for dose reduction.
	Dose reduction may be necessary if bilirubin >3.0 mg/dL.
Gefitinib	No formal recommendations for dose reduction.
	Dose reduction or interruption should be considered in patients with severe hepatic dysfunction.
Gemcitabine	No dose reduction is necessary.
Goserelin	No dose reduction is necessary.
Hydroxyurea	No dose reduction is necessary.
Ibrutinib	No formal recommendations for dose reduction in the presence of hepatic dysfunction. Dose reduction may be necessary.
Idarubicin	Reduce dose by 25% if bilirubin 1.5–3.0 mg/dL or SGOT 60–180 mg/dL.
	Reduce dose by 50% if bilirubin 3.0–5.0 or SGOT >180 mg/dL.
	Omit if bilirubin >5.0 mg/dL.
Ifosfamide	No dose reduction is necessary.
Imatinib	Reduce dose from 400 mg to 300 mg or from 600 mg to 400 mg if bilirubin >1.5 or SGOT >2.5 × ULN.
	Omit if bilirubin >3 mg/dL or SGOT >5 × ULN.
Interferon-α	No dose reduction is necessary.

Table 6 (cont.)

Drug	Recommended Dose Reduction for Hepatic Dysfunction
Interleukin–2	Omit if signs of hepatic failure (ascites, encephalopathy, jaundice) are observed. Do **NOT** restart sooner than 7 weeks after recovery from severe hepatic dysfunction.
Irinotecan	No formal recommendation for dose reduction in the presence of hepatic dysfunction. Dose reduction may be necessary.
Isotretinoin	No formal recommendation for dose reduction in the presence of mild or moderate hepatic dysfunction. Dose reduction may be necessary.
Ixabepilone	Omit when used in combination with capecitabine if SGOT or SGPT >2.5 × ULN or bilirubin >1 × ULN.
	When used as monotherapy, dose reduce to 32 mg/m^2 if SGOT or SGPT ≤10 × ULN and bilirubin ≤1.5 × ULN and dose reduce to 20–30 mg/m^2 if SGOT or SGPT ≤10 × ULN and bilirubin >1.5 × ULN to ≤3 × ULN.
Lapatinib	No formal recommendation for dose reduction in the presence of mild or moderate hepatic dysfunction. Reduce dose to 750 mg/day in setting of severe hepatic dysfunction (Child–Pugh Class C).
Lenalidomide	No formal recommendations for dose reduction.
Leuprolide	No dose reduction is necessary.
Lomustine	No dose reduction is necessary.
Mechlorethamine	No dose reduction is necessary.
Megestrol acetate	No dose reduction is necessary.
Melphalan	No dose reduction is necessary.
6–Mercaptopurine	No dose reduction is necessary.
Methotrexate	Reduce dose by 25% if bilirubin 3.1–5.0 mg/dL or SGOT >180 mg/dL.
	Omit if bilirubin >5.0 mg/dL.
Mitomycin–C	No dose reduction is necessary.
Mitotane	No formal recommendation for dose reduction in the presence of hepatic dysfunction. Dose reduction may be necessary.
Mitoxantrone	No formal recommendation for dose reduction in the presence of hepatic dysfunction. Dose reduction may be necessary when bilirubin >3.0 mg/dL.
Nelarabine	N/A
Nilutamide	No formal recommendation for dose reduction.
	Dose reduction may be necessary if bilirubin >3.0 mg/dL.

Table 6 (cont.)

Drug	Recommended Dose Reduction for Hepatic Dysfunction
Ofatumumab	N/A
Oxaliplatin	No dose reduction is necessary.
Paclitaxel	No formal recommendation for dose reduction if bilirubin 1.5–3.0 mg/dL or SGOT 60–180 mg/dL. Omit if bilirubin >5.0 mg/dL or SGOT >180 mg/dL.
Panitumumab	No dose reduction is necessary.
Pazopanib	Reduce dose to 200 mg/day in setting of moderate hepatic dysfunction. No formal guidelines for severe hepatic dysfunction.
Pegasparaginase	No dose reduction is necessary.
Pemetrexed	No dose reduction is necessary.
Pertuzumab	N/A
Pomalidomide	Omit if bilirubin >2.0 mg/dL and SGOT/SGPT >3 × ULN.
Ponatinib	Reduce dose to 30 mg PO daily if SGOT/SGPT >3 × ULN. Omit if SGOT/SGPT ≤ 3 × ULN and bilirubin >2 × ULN and alkaline phosphatase <2 × ULN.
Pralatrexate	N/A
Procarbazine	No formal recommendation for dose reduction in the presence of hepatic dysfunction. Dose reduction may be necessary.
Ramucirumab	N/A
Regorafenib	No dose reduction is necessary in the presence of mild and moderate hepatic dysfunction. Omit in the setting of severe hepatic dysfunction.
Rituximab	No dose reduction is necessary.
Sorafenib	No formal recommendation for dose reduction in the presence of hepatic dysfunction.
Streptozocin	No dose reduction is necessary.
Sunitinib	No dose reduction is necessary in patients with Child–Pugh Class A or B hepatic dysfunction. Dose reduction may be necessary in patients with Child–Pugh Class C hepatic dysfunction, although there are no formal recommendations.
Tamoxifen	No dose reduction is necessary.
Temozolomide	No dose reduction is necessary.
Thalidomide	N/A

Table 6 (cont.)

Drug	Recommended Dose Reduction for Hepatic Dysfunction
Thioguanine	Omit if bilirubin >5.0 mg/dL.
Thiotepa	No formal recommendation for dose reduction in the presence of hepatic dysfunction.
Topotecan	No dose reduction is necessary.
Trametinib	No dose reduction is necessary in the presence of mild hepatic dysfunction. Dose reduction may be necessary in patients with moderate and severe hepatic dysfunction.
Trastuzumab	No dose reduction is necessary.
Tretinoin	Reduce dose to a maximum of 25 mg/m^2 if bilirubin 3.1–5.0 mg/dL or SGOT >180 mg/dL. Omit if bilirubin >5.0 mg/dL.
Vemurafenib	No dose reduction is necessary in the presence of mild and moderate hepatic dysfunction. Dose reduction may be required with severe hepatic dysfunction.
Vinblastine	No dose reduction if bilirubin <1.5 mg/dL and SGOT <60 mg/dL. Reduce by 50% if bilirubin 1.5–3.0 mg/dL and SGOT 60–180 mg/dL. Omit if bilirubin >3.0 mg/dL or SGOT >180 mg/dL.
Vincristine	No dose reduction if bilirubin <1.5 mg/dL and SGOT <60 mg/dL. Reduce by 50% if bilirubin 1.5–3.0 mg/dL and SGOT 60–180 mg/dL. Omit if bilirubin >3.0 mg/dL or SGOT >180 mg/dL.
Vinorelbine	No dose reduction if bilirubin <2.0 mg/dL. Reduce dose by 50% if bilirubin 2.0–3.0 mg/dL. Reduce dose by 75% if bilirubin 3.1–5.0 mg/dL. Omit if bilirubin >5.0 mg/dL.
Vorinostat	N/A

N/A—not available

ULN—upper limit of normal

Table 7. General Guidelines for Chemotherapy Dosage Based on Renal Function

Drug	Recommended Dose Reduction for Renal Dysfunction
Afatinib	No dose reduction is necessary in the presence of mild renal dysfunction. Dose reduction may be necessary with moderate to severe renal dysfunction.
Alemtuzumab	N/A
Altretamine	N/A
Aminoglutethimide	N/A
Anastrozole	No dose reduction is necessary.
Arsenic trioxide	No formal recommendation for dose reduction in the presence of renal dysfunction. Dose reduction may be necessary.
L-Asparaginase	Omit if CrCl <60 mL/min.
Bendamustine	Omit if CrCl <40 mL/min.
Bevacizumab	N/A
Bicalutamide	No dose reduction is necessary.
Bleomycin	No dose reduction if CrCl >60 mL/min.
	Reduce dose by 25% if CrCl 10–60 mL/min.
	Reduce dose by 50% if CrCl <10 mL/min.
Buserelin	N/A
Busulfan	No dose reduction is necessary.
Cabozantinib	No dose reduction is necessary in the presence of mild and moderate renal dysfunction. Omit in the presence of severe renal dysfunction.
Capecitabine	No dose reduction if CrCl >50 mL/min.
	Reduce dose by 25% if CrCl 30–50 mL/min.
	Omit if CrCl <30 mL/min.
Carboplatin	No dose reduction if CrCl >60 mL/min. AUC dose is modified according to CrCl.
Carfilzomib	No dose reduction is necessary.
Carmustine	Omit if CrCl <60 mL/min.
Ceritinib	N/A
Cetuximab	No dose reduction is necessary.
Chlorambucil	No dose reduction is necessary.

Table 7 (cont.)

Drug	Recommended Dose Reduction for Renal Dysfunction
Cisplatin	No dose reduction if CrCl >60 mL/min.
	Reduce dose by 50% if CrCl 30–60 mL/min.
	Omit if CrCl <30 mL/min.
Cladribine	No formal recommendation for dose reduction in the presence of renal dysfunction. Dose reduction may be necessary.
Cyclophosphamide	No dose reduction if CrCl >50 mL/min.
	Reduce dose by 25% if CrCl 10–50 mL/min.
	Reduce dose by 50% if CrCl <10 mL/min.
Cytarabine	No formal recommendation for dose reduction in the presence of renal dysfunction. Dose reduction may be necessary.
Dacarbazine	No formal recommendation for dose reduction in the presence of renal dysfunction. Dose reduction may be necessary.
Dactinomycin	N/A
Dasatinib	No dose reduction is necessary.
Daunorubicin	Reduce dose by 50% if serum creatinine >3.0 mg/dL.
Decitabine	N/A
Docetaxel	No dose reduction is necessary.
Doxorubicin	No dose reduction is necessary.
Doxorubicin liposome	No dose reduction is necessary.
Erlotinib	No dose reduction is necessary.
Estramustine	N/A
Etoposide	No dose reduction if CrCl >50 mL/min.
	Reduce dose by 25% if CrCl 10–50 mL/min.
	Reduce dose by 50% if CrCl <10 mL/min.
Etoposide phosphate	No dose reduction if CrCl >50 mL/min.
	Reduce dose by 25% if CrCl 10–50 mL/min.
	Reduce dose by 50% if CrCl <10 mL/min.
Everolimus	No dose reduction is necessary.
Floxuridine	No dose reduction is necessary.

Table 7 (cont.)

Drug	Recommended Dose Reduction for Renal Dysfunction
Fludarabine	No formal recommendation for dose reduction in the presence of renal dysfunction. Dose reduction may be necessary.
5–Fluorouracil	No dose reduction is necessary.
Flutamide	N/A
Gefitinib	No dose reduction is necessary.
Gemcitabine	No dose reduction is necessary.
Goserelin	No dose reduction is necessary.
Hydroxyurea	Reduce dose by 50% if CrCl 10–50 mL/min.
	Reduce dose by 80% if CrCl <10 mL/min.
Ibrutinib	No dose reduction is necessary in mild to moderate renal dysfunction. Has not been studied in patients with severe renal dysfunction and in those on dialysis.
Idarubicin	No dose reduction is necessary.
Ifosfamide	N/A
Imatinib	No dose reduction is necessary.
Interferon–α	No dose reduction is necessary.
Interleukin–2	Omit or discontinue if serum creatinine >4.5 mg/dL.
Irinotecan	No dose reduction is necessary.
Isotretinoin	N/A
Ixabepilone	No formal recommendation for dose reduction.
Lapatinib	No dose reduction is necessary.
Lenalidomide	No formal recommendation for dose reduction.
	In the setting of moderate–to–severe renal dysfunction, dose reduction may be necessary.
Leuprolide	N/A
Lomustine	Omit if CrCl <60 mL/min.
Mechlorethamine	N/A
Megestrol acetate	N/A
Melphalan	No formal recommendation for dose reduction.
	However, use with caution in the presence of renal dysfunction.
6–Mercaptopurine	No formal recommendation for dose reduction in the presence of renal dysfunction. Adjust for renal dysfunction by either increasing the interval or decreasing the dose.

Table 7 (cont.)

Drug	Recommended Dose Reduction for Renal Dysfunction
Methotrexate	No dose reduction is necessary if CrCl >60 mL/min Reduce by 50% if CrCl 30–60 mL/min. Omit if CrCl <30 mL/min.
Mitomycin–C	No dose reduction is necessary if CrCl >60 mL/min. Reduce dose by 25% if CrCl 10–60 mL/min. Reduce dose by 50% if CrCl <10 mL/min.
Mitotane	N/A
Mitoxantrone	No dose reduction is necessary.
Nelarabine	No formal recommendation for dose reduction. Dose reduction may be necessary in the setting of moderate–to–severe renal dysfunction.
Nilotinib	No dose reduction is necessary.
Nilutamide	No dose reduction is necessary.
Ofatumumab	N/A
Oxaliplatin	No formal recommendation for dose reduction. Omit if CrCl <20 mL/min.
Paclitaxel	No dose reduction is necessary.
Panitumumab	No dose reduction is necessary.
Pazopanib	No dose reduction is necessary.
Pegasparaginase	N/A
Pemetrexed	No dose reduction is necessary when CrCl >40 mL/min. Omit if CrCL <45 mL/min.
Pertuzumab	No dose reduction is necessary in the presence of mild and moderate renal dysfunction. No formal recommendation for dose reduction in the presence of severe renal dysfunction.
Pomalidomide	No dose reduction is necessary in patients with serum creatinine <3.0 mg/dL. Omit if serum creatinine >3.0 mg/dL.
Ponatinib	No dose reduction is necessary in the presence of mild renal dysfunction. Dose reduction may be necessary in the setting of moderate–to–severe renal dysfunction.
Pralatrexate	No formal recommendation for dose reduction. Dose reduction may be necessary in the setting of moderate–to–severe renal dysfunction.
Procarbazine	Omit if CrCl <30 mL/min.

Table 7 (cont.)

Drug	Recommended Dose Reduction for Renal Dysfunction
Ramucirumab	N/A
Regorafenib	No dose reduction is necessary in the presence of mild renal dysfunction. No formal recommendation for dose reduction in the presence of moderate and severe renal dysfunction.
Rituximab	N/A
Sorafenib	No dose reduction is necessary.
Streptozocin	Omit if CrCl <60 mL/min.
Sunitinib	N/A
Tamoxifen	No dose reduction is necessary.
Temozolomide	N/A
Temsirolimus	No dose reduction is necessary.
Thalidomide	No formal recommendation for dose reduction in the presence of renal dysfunction.
Thioguanine	N/A
Thiotepa	No formal recommendation for dose reduction in the presence of renal dysfunction.
Topotecan	No dose reduction is necessary if CrCl >40 mL/min
Reduce dose by 50% if CrCl 20–39 mL/min.
Omit if CrCl <20 mL/min.
Trametinib	No dose reduction is necessary in the presence of mild and moderate renal dysfunction. No formal recommendation for dose reduction in the presence of severe renal dysfunction.
Trastuzumab	N/A
Tretinoin	Give a maximum of 25 mg/m^2 in the presence of renal dysfunction.
Vinblastine	No dose reduction is necessary.
Vincristine	No dose reduction is necessary.
Vinorelbine	No dose reduction is necessary.
Vorinostat	No dose reduction is necessary.

CrCl—creatinine clearance

N/A—not available

Table 8. Guidelines for Dialysis of Chemotherapy Drugs

Drug	Hemodialysis			Peritoneal Dialysis		
	YES	NO	UNKNOWN	YES	NO	UNKNOWN
Afatinib			X			X
Alemtuzumab			X			X
Altretamine			X			X
Aminoglutethimide	X					X
Amsacrine			X			X
Anastrozole			X			X
Arsenic trioxide			X			X
Azacitidine			X			X
Bevacizumab			X			X
Bicalutamide			X			X
Bleomycin		X			X	
Bortezomib			X			X
Bosutinib			X			X
Buserelin			X			X
Busulfan			X			X
Cabozantinib			X			X
Capecitabine			X			X
Carboplatin	X				X	
Carfilzomib			X			X
Carmustine		X			X	X
Ceritinib			X			X
Cetuximab			X			X
Chlorambucil			X			X
Cisplatin	X					X
Cladribine			X			X
Clofarabine			X			X
Cyclophosphamide	X					X
Cytarabine			X		X	
Dabrafenib			X			X
Dacarbazine			X			X
Dactinomycin			X			X
Daunorubicin			X			X

Table 8 (cont.)

Drug	Hemodialysis			Peritoneal Dialysis		
	YES	**NO**	**UNKNOWN**	**YES**	**NO**	**UNKNOWN**
Docetaxel			X			X
Doxorubicin		X				X
Doxorubicin liposome			X			X
Estramustine			X			X
Etoposide	X				X	
Etoposide phosphate		X				X
Floxuridine		X				X
Fludarabine		X				X
5–Fluorouracil		X				X
Flutamide		X				X
Gemcitabine	X		X		X	
Goserelin	X		X			X
Hydroxyurea		X				X
Ibrutinib		X				X
Idarubicin		X				X
Ifosfamide		X				X
Imatinib		X				X
Irinotecan		X				X
Isotretinoin		X				X
Lapatinib			X			X
Lenalidomide			X			X
Leuprolide		X				X
Lomustine	X					X
Mechlorethamine			X			X
Megestrol acetate			X			X
Melphalan			X		X	
6–Mercaptopurine			X			X
Methotrexate		X			X	
Mitomycin–C			X			X
Mitotane			X			X
Mitoxantrone			X			X
Nelarabine			X			X
Nilutamide			X			X

Table 8 (cont.)

Drug	Hemodialysis			Peritoneal Dialysis		
	YES	NO	UNKNOWN	YES	NO	UNKNOWN
Ofatumumab			X			X
Oxaliplatin	X					X
Paclitaxel	X				X	
Pazopanib			X			X
Pemetrexed		X				X
Pentostatin			X			X
Pertuzumab			X			X
Pomalidomide			X			X
Ponatinib	X				X	
Pralatrexate			X			X
Procarbazine			X			X
Ramucirumab			X			X
Regorafenib			X			X
Rituximab			X			X
Sorafenib	X				X	
Streptozocin			X			X
Sunitinib			X			X
Tamoxifen			X			X
Temozolomide			X			X
Temsirolimus			X			X
Thalidomide			X			X
Thioguanine			X			X
Thiotepa			X			X
Topotecan			X			X
Trametinib			X			X
Trastuzumab			X			X
Vemurafenib			X			X
Vinblastine			X			X
Vincristine			X			X
Vinorelbine			X			X
Vorinostat			X			X
Ziv–aflibercept			X			X

Table 9. Classification of Teratogenic Potential and Use in Pregnancy for Chemotherapy Agents

Pregnancy Category A. Controlled studies show no risk in pregnancy.

Controlled studies in pregnant women have not shown an increased risk of fetal abnormalities when the drug is administered during pregnancy. The possibility of fetal harm appears remote when the drug is used during pregnancy.

Pregnancy Category B. No evidence of risk in pregnancy.

(a) Controlled studies in animals have shown that the drug poses a risk to the fetus. However, studies in pregnant women have failed to show such a risk.

(b) Controlled studies in animals do not show evidence of impaired fertility or harm to the fetus. However, similar studies have not been performed in humans. Because animal studies are not entirely predictive of human response, the drug should be used during pregnancy only if clearly needed.

Pregnancy Category C. Risk in pregnancy cannot be ruled out.

Controlled studies either have not been conducted in animals or show that the drug is teratogenic or has an embryocidal effect and/or other adverse effect In animals. However, there are no adequate and well-controlled studies in pregnant women. The drug should be used during pregnancy only if the potential benefit justifies the potential risk to the fetus. The drug can cause fetal harm when administered to a pregnant woman. If the drug is used during pregnancy, or if a patient becomes pregnant while taking this drug, the patient should be informed of the potential hazard to the fetus. However, the potential benefits of treatment may outweigh any potential risk.

Pregnancy Category D. Clear evidence of risk in pregnancy.

The drug can cause fetal harm when administered to a pregnant woman. If the drug is used during pregnancy, or if a patient becomes pregnant while taking this drug, the patient should be informed of the potential hazard to the fetus. However, the potential benefits of treatment may outweigh any potential risk.

Pregnancy Category X. Absolutely contraindicated in pregnancy.

The drug has been shown to cause fetal harm when administered to a pregnant woman. The drug is absolutely contraindicated in women who are or who may become pregnant. If this drug is used during pregnancy or if a patient becomes pregnant while taking this drug, the patient should be informed of the potential hazard to the fetus. In this setting, the potential risk outweighs any potential benefit from treatment.

4

Common Chemotherapy Regimens in Clinical Practice

M. Sitki Copur, Laurie J. Harrold, and Edward Chu

This chapter provides some of the common combination regimens and selected single-agent regimens for solid tumors and hematologic malignancies. They are organized alphabetically by the specific cancer type. In each case, the regimens selected are based on the published literature and are used in clinical practice in the medical oncology community. It should be emphasized that not all of the drugs and dosages in the regimens have been officially approved by the Food and Drug Administration (FDA) for the treatment of a particular tumor. As such, the reader should be aware that some of these treatment regimens may not be approved for reimbursement. This chapter should serve as a quick reference for physicians and healthcare providers actively engaged in the practice of cancer treatment and provides several options for treating an individual tumor type. It is not intended to be an all-inclusive review of current treatments, nor is it intended to endorse and/or prioritize any particular combination or single-agent regimen.

It is important to emphasize that the reader should carefully review the original reference for each of the regimens cited to confirm the specific doses and schedules and to check the complete prescribing information contained within the package insert for each agent.

While considerable efforts have been made to ensure the accuracy of the regimens presented, printing and/or typographical errors may have been made in the preparation of this book. As a result, no liability can be assumed for their use. Moreover, the reader should be reminded that several variations in combination and single-agent regimens exist based on institutional and/or individual experience. Additionally, modifications in dose and schedule may be required according to individual performance status, comorbid illnesses, baseline blood counts, baseline hepatic and/or renal function, development of toxicity, and co-administration of other prescription and non-prescription drugs.

ADRENOCORTICAL CANCER

Combination Regimens

Etoposide + Doxorubicin + Cisplatin + Mitotane

Etoposide:	100 mg/m^2 IV on days 5–7
Doxorubicin:	20 mg/m^2 on days 1 and 8
Cisplatin:	40 mg/m^2 IV on days 1 and 9
Mitotane:	4 g PO daily

Repeat cycle every 21 days [1].

Streptozocin + Mitotane

Streptozocin:	1000 mg IV on days 1–5 for cycle 1 and 2000 mg IV on days 1–5 on subsequent cycles
Mitotane:	4 g PO daily

Repeat cycle every 28 days [1].

ANAL CANCER

Combined Modality Therapy

5-Fluorouracil + Mitomycin-C + Radiation Therapy (RTOG/ECOG regimen)

5-Fluorouracil:	1000 mg/m^2/day IV continuous infusion on days 1–4 and 29–32
Mitomycin-C:	10 mg/m^2 IV (maximum of 20 mg) on days 1 and 29
Radiation therapy:	180 cGy/day, 5 days/week for a total of 5 weeks (total dose, 4500 cGy)

Chemotherapy is given concurrently with radiation therapy [2].

5-Fluorouracil + Mitomycin-C + Radiation Therapy (EORTC regimen)

5-Fluorouracil:	200 mg/m^2/day IV continuous infusion on days 1–26
Mitomycin-C:	10 mg/m^2 IV on day 1
Radiation therapy:	180 cGy/day, 5 days/week for a total of 4 weeks (total dose, 3600 cGy)

Chemotherapy is given concurrently with radiation therapy [3]. There is a 2-week break following the completion of this first treatment, after which the second treatment is initiated with concurrent chemotherapy and radiation therapy.

5-Fluorouracil:	200 mg/m^2/day IV continuous infusion on days 1–17
Mitomycin-C:	10 mg/m^2 IV on day 1
Radiation therapy:	Total dose, 2340 cGy over 17 days

5-Fluorouracil + Cisplatin + Radiation Therapy

5-Fluorouracil:	250 mg/m^2/day IV continuous infusion on days 1–5 of each week of radiation therapy
Cisplatin:	4 mg/m^2/day IV continuous infusion on days 1–5 of each week of radiation therapy
Radiation therapy:	Total dose, 5500 cGy over 6 weeks

Chemotherapy is given concurrently with radiation therapy [4].

or

Phase I (days 1–56)

5-Fluorouracil:	1000 mg/m^2/day IV continuous infusion on days 1–5 and 29–33
Cisplatin:	100 mg/m^2 on days 1 and 29

Phase II (days 57–112)

5-Fluorouracil:	1000 mg/m^2/day IV continuous infusion on days 57–60 and 99–102
Mitomycin-C:	10 mg/m^2 IV on days 57 and 99
Radiation therapy:	180 cGy/day, 5 days/week on days 57–59 and days 99–108 for a total dose of 3060 cGy

Phase III (days 127–131)

5-Fluorouracil:	800 mg/m^2/day IV continuous infusion on days 127–131
Cisplatin:	100 mg/m^2 on day 127
Radiation therapy:	180 cGy/day, 5 days/week on days 127–131

Combined modality therapy for poor prognosis anal cancer [5].

XELOX + Radiation Therapy

Capecitabine:	825 mg/m^2 PO bid on Monday–Friday for 6 weeks
Oxaliplatin:	50 mg/m^2 IV on days 1, 8, 22, 29
Radiation therapy:	180 cGy/day, 5 days/week for a total of 6 weeks

Chemotherapy is given concurrently with radiation therapy [6].

Metastatic Disease and/or Salvage Chemotherapy

Combination Regimens

5-Fluorouracil + Cisplatin

5-Fluorouracil:	1000 mg/m^2/day IV continuous infusion on days 1–5
Cisplatin:	100 mg/m^2 IV on day 2

Repeat cycle every 21–28 days [7].

BASAL CELL CANCER

Single-Agent Regimens

Vismodegib

Vismodegib:	150 mg PO daily

Continue treatment until disease progression [8].

Sonidegib

Sonidegib:	200 mg PO daily

Continue treatment until disease progression [9].

BILIARY TRACT CANCER

Combination Regimens

Gemcitabine + Cisplatin

Gemcitabine:	1250 mg/m^2 IV on days 1 and 8
Cisplatin:	75 mg/m^2 on day 1

Repeat cycle every 21 days [10].

or

Gemcitabine:	1000 mg/m^2 IV on days 1 and 8
Cisplatin:	25 mg/m^2 on days 1 and 8

Repeat cycle every 21 days for 8 cycles [11].

Gemcitabine + Capecitabine

Gemcitabine:	1000 mg/m^2 IV on days 1 and 8
Capecitabine:	650 mg/m^2 PO bid on days 1–14

Repeat cycle every 21 days [12].

Gemcitabine + Oxaliplatin

Gemcitabine:	1000 mg/m^2 IV on day 1
Oxaliplatin·	100 mg/m^2 on day 2

Repeat cycle every 14 days [13].

5-Fluorouracil + Cisplatin

5-Fluorouracil:	400 mg/m^2 IV on day 1, followed by 600 mg/m^2 IV infusion over 22 hours on days 1 and 2
Cisplatin:	50 mg/m^2 IV on day 2

Repeat cycle every 21 days [14].

Capecitabine + Cisplatin

Capecitabine:	1250 mg/m^2 PO bid on days 1–14
Cisplatin:	60 mg/m^2 IV on day 2

Repeat cycle every 21 days [15].

Capecitabine + Oxaliplatin

Capecitabine: 1000 mg/m^2 PO bid on days 1–14

Oxaliplatin: 130 mg/m^2 IV on day 1

Repeat cycle every 21 days [16].

Single-Agent Regimens

Capecitabine

Capecitabine: 1000 mg/m^2 PO bid on days 1–14

Repeat cycle every 21 days [17]. Dose may be reduced to 825–900 mg/m^2 PO bid on days 1–14.

Docetaxel

Docetaxel: 100 mg/m^2 IV on day 1

Repeat cycle every 21 days [18].

Gemcitabine

Gemcitabine: 1000 mg/m^2 IV on days 1 and 8

Repeat cycle every 21 days [19].

BLADDER CANCER

Combination Regimens

ITP

Ifosfamide: 1500 mg/m^2 IV on days 1–3

Paclitaxel: 200 mg/m^2 IV over 3 hours on day 1

Cisplatin: 70 mg/m^2 IV on day 1

Repeat cycle every 21 days [20]. G-CSF support is recommended. Regimen can also be administered every 28 days.

Gemcitabine + Cisplatin

Gemcitabine: 1000 mg/m^2 IV on days 1, 8, and 15

Cisplatin: 75 mg/m^2 IV on day 1

Repeat cycle every 28 days [21].

Gemcitabine + Carboplatin

Gemcitabine: 1000 mg/m^2 IV on days 1 and 8

Carboplatin: AUC of 4, IV on day 1

Repeat cycle every 21 days up to 6 cycles [22].

Gemcitabine + Paclitaxel

Gemcitabine: 1000 mg/m^2 IV on days 1, 8, and 15
Paclitaxel: 200 mg/m^2 IV on day 1
Repeat cycle every 21 days [23].
or
Gemcitabine: 2500 mg/m^2 IV on day 1
Paclitaxel: 150 mg/m^2 IV on day 1
Repeat cycle every 14 days [24].

Gemcitabine + Docetaxel

Gemcitabine: 1000 mg/m^2 IV on days 1, 8, and 15
Docetaxel: 60 mg/m^2 IV on day 1
Repeat cycle every 28 days [25].

Dose-Dense MVAC

Methotrexate: 30 mg/m^2 IV on days 1, 15, and 22
Vinblastine: 3 mg/m^2 IV on days 2, 15, and 22
Doxorubicin: 30 mg/m^2 IV on day 2
Cisplatin: 70 mg/m^2 IV on day 2
Repeat cycle every 28 days [26].

CMV

Cisplatin: 100 mg/m^2 IV on day 2 (give 12 hours after methotrexate)
Methotrexate: 30 mg/m^2 IV on days 1 and 8
Vinblastine: 4 mg/m^2 IV on days 1 and 8
Repeat cycle every 21 days [27].

MCV

Methotrexate: 30 mg/m^2 IV on days 1, 15, and 22
Carboplatin: AUC of 4.5, IV on day 1
Vinblastine: 3 mg/m^2 IV on days 1, 15, and 22
Repeat cycle every 28 days [28].

Docetaxel + Cisplatin

Docetaxel: 75 mg/m^2 IV on day 1
Cisplatin: 75 mg/m^2 IV on day 1
Repeat cycle every 21 days up to 6 cycles [29].

Paclitaxel + Carboplatin

Paclitaxel:	225 mg/m^2 IV over 3 hours on day 1
Carboplatin:	AUC of 6, IV on day 1, given 15 minutes after paclitaxel

Repeat cycle every 21 days [30].

CAP

Cyclophosphamide:	400 mg/m^2 IV on day 1
Doxorubicin:	40 mg/m^2 IV on day 1
Cisplatin:	75 mg/m^2 IV on day 2

Repeat cycle every 21 days [31].

5-Fluorouracil + Mitomycin-C + Radiation Therapy

5-Fluorouracil:	500 mg/m^2/day IV continuous infusion on days 1–5 and 16–20 of radiotherapy
Mitomycin-C:	12 mg/^{2} IV on day 1
Radiation therapy	275 cGy/day, 5 days/week for a total of 4 weeks (total dose, 5500 cGy) or 200 cGy/day for 6.5 weeks (total dose, 6400 cGy)

Chemotherapy is given concurrently with radiation therapy [32].

Single-Agent Regimens

Gemcitabine

Gemcitabine:	1200 mg/m^2 IV on days 1, 8, and 15

Repeat cycle every 28 days [33].

Paclitaxel

Paclitaxel:	250 mg/m^2 IV over 24 hours on day 1

Repeat cycle every 21 days [34].

or

Paclitaxel:	80 mg/m^2 IV weekly for 3 weeks

Repeat cycle every 4 weeks [35].

Pemetrexed

Pemetrexed: 500 mg/m^2 IV on day 1

Repeat cycle every 21 days [36]. Folic acid at 350–1000 μg PO daily beginning 1–2 weeks prior to therapy and vitamin B12 at 1000 μg IM to start 1–2 weeks prior to first dose of therapy and repeated every 3 cycles.

Atezolizumab

Atezolizumab: 1200 mg/day IV on day 1

Repeat cycle every 21 days [37].

BRAIN CANCER

Adjuvant Therapy

Combination Regimens

Temozolomide Radiation Therapy

Radiation therapy: 200 cGy/day for 5 days per week for total of 6 weeks

Temozolomide: 75 mg/m^2 PO daily for 6 weeks with radiation therapy. After a 4-week break, 150 mg/m^2 PO on days 1–5

Repeat temozolomide monotherapy every 28 days for up to 6 cycles [38]. If well tolerated, can increase dose to 200 mg/m^2 on subsequent cycles. Patients should be placed on either inhaled pentamidine or trimethoprim/sulfamethoxazole for PCP prophylaxis during the combined-modality regimen.

PCV

Procarbazine: 60 mg/m^2 PO on days 8–21

Lomustine: 130 mg/m^2 PO on day 1

Vincristine: 1.4 mg/m^2 IV on days 8 and 29

Repeat cycle every 8 weeks for 6 cycles [39].

Single-Agent Regimens

Carmustine

Carmustine: 220 mg/m^2 IV on day 1

Repeat cycle every 6–8 weeks for 1 year [40].

or

Carmustine: 75–100 mg/m^2 IV on days 1 and 2

Repeat cycle every 6–8 weeks [40].

Advanced Disease

Combination Regimens

PCV

Procarbazine:	75 mg/m^2 PO on days 8–21
Lomustine:	130 mg/m^2 PO on day 1
Vincristine:	1.4 mg/m^2 IV on days 8 and 29

Repeat cycle every 8 weeks [41].

Irinotecan + Bevacizumab

Irinotecan:	125 mg/m^2 IV on day 1
Bevacizumab:	10 mg/kg IV on day 1

Repeat cycle every 2 weeks for 6 cycles [42].

Temozolomide + Bevacizumab

Temozolomide:	150 mg/m^2 PO on days 1–5
Bevacizumab:	10 mg/kg IV on days 1 and 14

Repeat cycle every 28 days [43].

Carboplatin + Irinotecan + Bevacizumab

Carboplatin:	AUC of 4, IV on day 1
Irinotecan:	340 mg/m^2 IV on days 1 and 14
Bevacizumab:	10 mg/kg IV on days 1 and 14

Repeat cycle every 28 days [44].

Temozolomide + Lomustine

Temozolomide:	100 mg/m^2 PO on days 2–6
Lomustine:	100 mg/m^2 PO on day 1

Repeat cycle every 28 days up to 6 cycles [45].

Single-Agent Regimens

Carmustine

Carmustine:	200 mg/m^2 IV on day 1

Repeat cycle every 6–8 weeks [46].

Procarbazine

Procarbazine:	150 mg/m^2 PO daily divided into 3 doses

Repeat daily [46].

Temozolomide

Temozolomide: 150 mg/m^2 PO on days 1–5

Repeat cycle every 28 days [47]. If tolerated, can increase dose to 200 mg/m^2.

Irinotecan

Irinotecan: 350 mg/m^2 IV over 90 min on day 1

Repeat cycle every 3 weeks [48].

or

Irinotecan: 125 mg/m^2 IV weekly for 4 weeks

Repeat cycle every 6 weeks [49].

Bevacizumab

Bevacizumab: 15 mg/kg IV on day 1

Repeat cycle every 3 weeks [50].

BREAST CANCER

Neoadjuvant Therapy

Combination Regimens

ACT

Doxorubicin: 60 mg/m^2 IV on day 1

Cyclophosphamide: 600 mg/m^2 IV on day 1

Docetaxel: 100 mg/m^2 IV on day 1

Repeat cycle every 21 days for a total of 4 cycles, followed by surgery [51].

Docetaxel + Carboplatin + Pertuzumab + Trastuzumab

Docetaxel: 75 mg/m^2 IV on day 1

Carboplatin: AUC 6, IV on day 1

Pertuzumab: 840 mg IV loading dose on day 1 and then 420 mg IV every 3 weeks

Trastuzumab: 8 mg/kg IV loading dose on day 1 and then 6 mg/kg IV every 3 weeks

Repeat cycle every 21 days [52].

Adjuvant Therapy

Combination Regimens: HER2-negative disease

AC

Doxorubicin:	60 mg/m^2 IV on day 1
Cyclophosphamide:	600 mg/m^2 IV on day 1

Repeat cycle every 21 days for a total of 4 cycles [53].

AC→T

Doxorubicin:	60 mg/m^2 IV on day 1
Cyclophosphamide:	600 mg/m^2 IV on day 1

Repeat cycle every 21 days for a total of 4 cycles, followed by

Paclitaxel:	175 mg/m^2 IV on day 1

Repeat cycle every 21 days for a total of 4 cycles [54].

AC→T (weekly)

Doxorubicin:	60 mg/m^2 IV on day 1
Cyclophosphamide:	600 mg/m^2 IV on day 1

Repeat cycle every 21 days for a total of 4 cycles, followed by

Paclitaxel:	80 mg/m^2 IV on day 1

Repeat on a weekly schedule for 12 weeks [55].

AC→Docetaxel

Doxorubicin:	60 mg/m^2 IV on day 1
Cyclophosphamide:	600 mg/m^2 IV on day 1

Repeat cycle every 21 days for a total of 4 cycles, followed by

Docetaxel:	100 mg/m^2 IV on day 1

Repeat cycle every 21 days for a total of 4 cycles [56].

AC→Docetaxel (weekly)

Doxorubicin:	60 mg/m^2 IV on day 1
Cyclophosphamide:	600 mg/m^2 IV on day 1

Repeat cycle every 21 days for a total of 4 cycles, followed by

Docetaxel:	35 mg/m^2 IV on day 1

Repeat weekly for a total of 12 weeks [57].

TC

Docetaxel:	75 mg/m^2 IV on day 1

Cyclophosphamide: 600 mg/m^2 IV on day 1

Repeat cycle every 21 days for a total of 4 cycles [58].

TAC

Docetaxel: 75 mg/m^2 IV on day 1

Doxorubicin: 50 mg/m^2 IV on day 1

Cyclophosphamide: 500 mg/m^2 IV on day 1

Repeat cycle every 21 days for a total of 6 cycles [59].

CAF

Cyclophosphamide: 600 mg/m^2 IV on day 1

Doxorubicin: 60 mg/m^2 IV on day 1

5-Fluorouracil: 600 mg/m^2 IV on day 1

Repeat cycle every 28 days for a total of 4 cycles [60].

Epirubicin + CMF

Epirubicin: 100 mg/m^2 IV on day 1

Repeat cycle every 21 days for 4 cycles, followed by

Cyclophosphamide: 600 mg/m^2 IV on day 1

Methotrexate: 40 mg/m^2 IV on day 1

5-Fluorouracil: 600 mg/m^2 IV on day 1

Repeat cycle every 21 days for a total of 4 cycles [61].

FEC

5-Fluorouracil: 500 mg/m^2 IV on day 1

Epirubicin: 100 mg/m^2 IV on day 1

Cyclophosphamide: 500 mg/m^2 IV on day 1

Repeat cycle every 21 days for a total of 6 cycles [62].

FEC→Docetaxel

5-Fluorouracil: 500 mg/m^2 IV on day 1

Epirubicin: 100 mg/m^2 IV on day 1

Cyclophosphamide: 500 mg/m^2 IV on day 1

Repeat cycle every 21 days for a total of 6 cycles [63], followed by

Docetaxel: 100 mg/m^2 IV on day 1

Repeat cycle every 21 days for 3 cycles.

AC→T

Doxorubicin:	60 mg/m^2 IV on day 1
Cyclophosphamide:	600 mg/m^2 IV on day 1

Repeat cycle every 14 days for a total of 4 cycles, followed by

Paclitaxel:	175 mg/m^2 IV on day 1

Repeat cycle every 14 days for a total of 4 cycles [64].

Administer pegfilgrastim 6 mg SC on day 2 of each treatment cycle.

A→T→C

Doxorubicin:	60 mg/m^2 IV on day 1

Repeat cycle every 2 weeks for 4 cycles, followed by

Paclitaxel:	175 mg/m^2 IV on day 1

Repeat cycle every 2 weeks for 4 cycles, followed by

Cyclophosphamide:	600 mg/m^2 IV on day 1

Repeat cycle every 2 weeks for 4 cycles.

Administer filgrastim 5 µg/kg SC on days 3–10 of each treament cycle [65].

AC→Docetaxel

Doxorubicin:	60 mg/m^2 IV on day 1
Cyclophosphamide:	600 mg/m^2 IV on day 1

Repeat cycle every 14 days for a total of 4 cycles, followed by

Docetaxel:	75 mg/m^2 IV on day 1

Repeat cycle every 14 days for a total of 4 cycles [66].

Administer pegfilgrastim 6 mg SC on day 2 of each treatment cycle.

Docetaxel→AC

Docetaxel:	75 mg/m^2 IV on day 1

Repeat cycle every 14 days for a total of 4 cycles, followed by

Doxorubicin:	60 mg/m^2 IV on day 1
Cyclophosphamide:	600 mg/m^2 IV on day 1

Repeat cycle every 14 days for a total of 4 cycles [66].

Administer pegfilgrastim 6 mg SC on day 2 of each treatment cycle.

Combination Regimens: HER2-positive disease

AC→T + Trastuzumab

Doxorubicin:	60 mg/m^2 IV on day 1
Cyclophosphamide:	600 mg/m^2 IV on day 1

Repeat cycle every 21 days for a total of 4 cycles, followed by

Paclitaxel:	80 mg/m^2 IV over 1 hour on day 1
Trastuzumab:	4 mg/kg IV loading dose, then 2 mg/kg IV weekly

Repeat weekly for 12 weeks, followed by

Trastuzumab:	2 mg/kg IV weekly

Repeat weekly for 40 weeks [67].

AC→T + Trastuzumab (dose dense)

Doxorubicin:	60 mg/m^2 IV on day 1
Cyclophosphamide·	600 mg/m^2 IV on day 1

Repeat cycle every 14 days for a total of 4 cycles, followed by

Paclitaxel:	175 mg/m^2 IV on day 1

Repeat cycle every 14 days for a total of 4 cycles.

Trastuzumab:	4 mg/kg IV loading dose along with paclitaxel and then 2 mg/kg IV weekly

Trastuzumab is administered for a total of 1 year [68].

TCH

Docetaxel:	75 mg/m^2 IV on day 1
Carboplatin:	AUC of 6, IV on day 1
Trastuzumab:	4 mg/kg IV loading dose and then 2 mg/kg IV weekly

Repeat chemotherapy every 21 days for a total of 6 cycles. At the completion of chemotherapy, trastuzumab is administered at 6 mg/kg IV every 3 weeks for a total of 1 year [69].

DH→FEC

Docetaxel:	100 mg/m^2 IV on day 1
Trastuzumab	4 mg/kg IV loading dose on day 1 and then 2 mg/kg IV weekly

Repeat cycle every 21 days for 3 cycles, followed by

5-Fluorouracil:	600 mg/m^2 IV on day 1
Epirubicin:	60 mg/m^2 IV on day 1
Cyclophosphamide:	600 mg/m^2 IV on day 1

Repeat cycle every 21 days for 3 cycles [70].

Pertuzumab + + Trastuzumab + Docetaxel

Docetaxel:	75 mg/m^2 IV on day 1
Trastuzumab:	8 mg/kg IV loading dose on day 1 and then 6 mg/kg IV every 3 weeks
Pertuzumab:	840 mg IV loading dose on day 1 and then 420 mg IV every 3 weeks

Repeat cycle every 21 days [71].

Hormonal Regimens

Tamoxifen

| Tamoxifen: | 20 mg PO daily |

Repeat daily for 5 years in patients with ER+ tumors or ER status unknown [72].

Anastrozole

| Anastrozole: | 1 mg PO daily |

Repeat daily for 5 years in patients with ER+ tumors or ER status unknown [73].

Letrozole

| Letrozole: | 2.5 mg PO daily |

Repeat daily for 5 years in patients with ER+ or PR+ tumors [74].

Tamoxifen + Letrozole [75]

| Tamoxifen: | 20 mg PO daily for 5 years, followed by |
| Letrozole: | 2.5 mg PO daily for 5 years |

Tamoxifen + Exemestane [76]

| Tamoxifen: | 20 mg PO daily for 2–3 years, followed by |
| Exemestane: | 25 mg PO daily for the remainder of 5 years |

Tamoxifen + Goserelin + Zoledronic acid

| Tamoxifen: | 20 mg PO daily |
| Goserelin: | 3.6 mg SC every 28 days |

Zoledronic acid: 4 mg IV every 6 months
Continue treatment for a total of 3 years [77].

Anastrozole + Goserelin + Zoledronic acid

Anastrozole: 1 mg PO daily
Goserelin: 3.6 mg SC every 28 days
Zoledronic acid: 4 mg IV every 6 months
Continue treatment for a total of 3 years [77].

Everolimus + Exemestane [78]

Everolimus: 10 mg PO daily
Exemestane: 25 mg PO daily

Metastatic Disease

Combination Regimens: HER2-negative disease

AC

Doxorubicin: 60 mg/m^2 IV on day 1
Cyclophosphamide: 600 mg/m^2 IV on day 1
Repeat cycle every 21 days [53].

AT

Doxorubicin: 50 mg/m^2 IV on day 1
Paclitaxel: 150 mg/m^2 IV over 24 hours on day 1
Repeat cycle every 21 days [79].

or

Doxorubicin: 60 mg/m^2 IV on day 1
Repeat cycle every 21 days up to a maximum of 8 cycles, followed by
Paclitaxel: 175 mg/m^2 IV on day 1
Repeat cycle every 21 days until disease progression [79].
or
Paclitaxel: 175 mg/m^2 IV on day 1
Repeat cycle every 21 days until disease progression, followed by
Doxorubicin: 60 mg/m^2 IV on day 1
Repeat cycle every 21 days up to a maximum of 8 cycles [79].

CAF

Cyclophosphamide:	600 mg/m^2 IV on day 1
Doxorubicin:	60 mg/m^2 IV on day 1
5-Fluorouracil:	600 mg/m^2 IV on day 1

Repeat cycle every 21 days [60].

CEF

Cyclophosphamide:	75 mg/m^2 PO on days 1–14
Epirubicin:	60 mg/m^2 IV on days 1 and 8
5-Fluorouracil:	500 mg/m^2 IV on days 1 and 8

Repeat cycle every 28 days [80].

CMF

Cyclophosphamide:	600 mg/m^2 IV on day 1
Methotrexate:	40 mg/m^2 IV on day 1
5-Fluorouracil:	600 mg/m^2 IV on day 1

Repeat cycle every 21 days [61].

Capecitabine + Docetaxel (XT)

Capecitabine:	1250 mg/m^2 PO bid on days 1–14
Docetaxel:	75 mg/m^2 IV on day 1

Repeat cycle every 21 days [81]. May decrease dose of capecitabine to 825–1000 mg/m^2 PO bid on days 1–14 to reduce the risk of toxicity without compromising clinical efficacy.

Capecitabine + Paclitaxel (XP)

Capecitabine:	825 mg/m^2 PO bid on days 1–14
Paclitaxel:	175 mg/m^2 IV on day 1

Repeat cycle every 21 days [82].

Capecitabine + Navelbine (XN)

Capecitabine:	1000 mg/m^2 PO bid on days 1–14
Navelbine:	25 mg/m^2 IV on days 1 and 8

Repeat cycle every 21 days [82].

Capecitabine + Ixabepilone (XI)

Capecitabine:	1000 mg/m^2 PO bid on days 1–14

Ixabepilone: 40 mg/m^2 IV on day 1
Repeat cycle every 21 days [83].

Docetaxel + Doxorubicin

Docetaxel: 75 mg/m^2 IV on day 1
Doxorubicin: 50 mg/m^2 IV on day 1
Repeat cycle every 21 days [84].

Doxorubicin liposome + Docetaxel

Doxorubicin liposome: 30 mg/m^2 on day 1
Docetaxel: 60 mg/m^2 on day 1
Repeat cycle every 21 days [85].

FEC-100

5-Fluorouracil: 500 mg/m^2 IV on day 1
Epirubicin: 100 mg/m^2 IV on day 1
Cyclophosphamide: 500 mg/m^2 IV on day 1

Repeat cycle every 21 days [86].

FEC-75

5-Fluorouracil: 500 mg/m^2 IV on day 1
Epirubicin: 75 mg/m^2 IV on day 1
Cyclophosphamide: 500 mg/m^2 IV on day 1
Repeat cycle every 21 days [87].

FEC-50

5-Fluorouracil: 500 mg/m^2 IV on day 1
Epirubicin: 50 mg/m^2 IV on day 1
Cyclophosphamide: 500 mg/m^2 IV on day 1
Repeat cycle every 21 days [87].

Gemcitabine + Paclitaxel

Gemcitabine: 1250 mg/m^2 IV on days 1 and 8
Paclitaxel: 175 mg/m^2 IV on day 1
Repeat cycle every 21 days [88].

Carboplatin + Paclitaxel

Carboplatin: AUC of 6, IV on day 1

Paclitaxel: 200 mg/m^2 IV over 3 hours on day 1

Repeat cycle every 21 days [89].

Carboplatin + Docetaxel

Carboplatin: AUC of 6, IV on day 1

Docetaxel: 75 mg/m^2 IV on day 1

Repeat cycle every 21 days [90].

Paclitaxel + Bevacizumab

Paclitaxel: 90 mg/m^2 IV on days 1, 8, and 15

Bevacizumab: 10 mg/kg on days 1 and 15

Repeat cycle every 28 days [91].

Combination Regimens: HER2-positive disease

Pertuzumab + Trastuzumab + Docetaxel

Docetaxel: 75 mg/m^2 IV on day 1

Trastuzumab: 8 mg/kg IV loading dose on day 1 and
                                     then 6 mg/kg IV every 3 weeks

Pertuzumab: 840 mg IV loading dose on day 1 and
                                     then 420 mg IV every 3 weeks

Repeat cycle every 21 days [71].

Trastuzumab + Paclitaxel

Trastuzumab: 4 mg/kg IV loading dose and then
                                     2 mg/kg weekly

Paclitaxel: 175 mg/m^2 IV over 3 hours on day 1

Repeat cycle every 21 days [92].

or

Trastuzumab: 4 mg/kg IV loading dose and then
                                     2 mg/kg weekly

Paclitaxel: 80 mg/m^2 IV weekly

Repeat cycle every 4 weeks [93].

Trastuzumab + Docetaxel

Trastuzumab:	4 mg/kg IV loading dose and then 2 mg/kg IV on days 8 and 15
Docetaxel:	35 mg/m^2 IV on days 1, 8, and 15

First cycle is administered weekly for 3 weeks, with 1-week rest.
For subsequent cycles,

Trastuzumab:	2 mg/kg IV weekly
Docetaxel:	35 mg/m^2 IV weekly

Repeat cycle every 4 weeks [94].

TCH

Carboplatin:	AUC of 6, IV on day 1
Docetaxel:	75 mg/m^2 IV on day 1
Trastuzumab:	4 mg/kg IV loading dose on day 1 and then 2 mg/kg IV on days 8 and 15, 2 mg/kg IV weekly thereafter

Repeat cycle every 21 days [95].

Gemcitabine + Carboplatin + Trastuzumab

Gemcitabine:	1500 mg/m^2 IV on day 1
Carboplatin:	AUC of 2.5, IV on day 1
Trastuzumab:	8 mg/kg IV loading dose on day 1 and then 4 mg/kg IV every 2 weeks

Repeat cycle every 2 weeks [96].

Trastuzumab + Navelbine

Trastuzumab:	4 mg/kg IV loading dose and then 2 mg/kg IV weekly
Navelbine:	25 mg/m^2 IV weekly

Repeat on a weekly basis until disease progression [97].

Trastuzumab + Gemcitabine

Trastuzumab:	4 mg/kg IV loading dose and then 2 mg/kg IV weekly
Gemcitabine:	1200 mg/m^2 IV weekly for 2 weeks

Repeat cycle every 21 days [98].

Trastuzumab + Capecitabine

Trastuzumab: 4 mg/kg IV loading dose and then 2 mg/kg IV weekly

Capecitabine: 1250 mg/m^2 PO bid on days 1–14

Repeat cycle every 21 days [99].

or

Trastuzumab: 8 mg/kg IV loading dose and then 6 mg/kg

IV on day 1 of all subsequent cycles

Capecitabine: 1250 mg/m^2 PO bid on days 1–14

Repeat cycle every 21 days [100].

Trastuzumab + Lapatinib

Trastuzumab: 4 mg/kg IV loading dose and then 2 mg/kg IV weekly

Lapatinib: 1000 mg PO daily

Continue until disease progression [101].

Capecitabine + Lapatinib

Capecitabine: 1000 mg/m^2 PO bid on days 1–14

Lapatinib: 1250 mg PO daily

Repeat cycle every 21 days [102].

Everolimus + Exemestane [78]

Everolimus: 10 mg PO daily

Exemestane: 25 mg PO daily

Palbociclib + Letrozole

Palbociclib: 125 mg PO daily for 21 days

Letrozole: 2.5 mg PO daily

Repeat cycle every 21 days [103].

Palbociclib + Fulvestrant

Palbociclib: 125 mg PO daily for 21 days

Fulvestrant: 500 mg IM loading dose on day 1, then 500 mg IM on days 15 and 29

Repeat cycle every 28 days [104].

Single-Agent Regimens

Tamoxifen

Tamoxifen: 20 mg PO daily [105]

Toremifene

Toremifene: 60 mg PO daily [106]

Exemestane

Exemestane: 25 mg PO daily [107]

Anastrozole

Anastrozole: 1 mg PO daily [108]

Letrozole

Letrozole: 2.5 mg PO daily [109]

Fulvestrant

Fulvestrant: 250 mg IM on day 1
Repeat injection every month [110].

or

Fulvestrant: 500 mg IM loading dose on day 1, then 500 mg IM on days 15 and 29
Continue treatment on a monthly basis until disease progression [111].

Megestrol

Megestrol: 40 mg PO qid [112]

Trastuzumab

Trastuzumab: 4 mg/kg IV loading dose and then 2 mg/kg IV weekly
Repeat cycle weekly for a total of 10 weeks. In the absence of disease progression, continue weekly maintenance dose of 2 mg/kg [113].

or

Trastuzumab: 8 mg/kg IV loading dose, then 6 mg/kg IV every 3 weeks
Continue treatment until disease progression [114].

Ado-trastuzumab emtansine

Ado-trastuzumab: 3.6 mg/kg IV on day 1
Repeat cycle every 21 days [115].

Capecitabine

Capecitabine: 1250 mg/m^2 PO bid for 2 weeks fol-
                                          lowed by 1-week rest period

Repeat cycle every 21 days [116]. May decrease dose to 850–1000 mg/m^2
PO bid on days 1–14 to reduce risk of toxicity without compromising clinical
efficacy.

Docetaxel

Docetaxel: 100 mg/m^2 IV on day 1
Repeat cycle every 21 days [117].

or

Docetaxel: 35–40 mg/m^2 IV weekly for 6 weeks
Repeat cycle every 8 weeks [118].

Paclitaxel

Paclitaxel: 175 mg/m^2 IV over 3 hours on day 1
Repeat cycle every 21 days [119].
or
Paclitaxel: 80–100 mg/m^2 IV weekly for 3 weeks
Repeat cycle every 4 weeks [120].

Ixabepilone

Ixabepilone: 40 mg/m^2 IV on day 1
Repeat cycle every 21 days [121].

Vinorelbine

Vinorelbine: 30 mg/m^2 IV on day 1
Repeat cycle every 7 days [122].

Doxorubicin

Doxorubicin: 20 mg/m^2 IV on day 1
Repeat cycle every 7 days [123].

Gemcitabine

Gemcitabine: 725 mg/m^2 IV weekly for 3 weeks
Repeat cycle every 28 days [124].

Doxorubicin liposome:

Doxorubicin liposome: 40 mg/m^2 IV on day 1
Repeat cycle every 28 days [125].

Abraxane

Abraxane: 260 mg/m^2 IV on day 1
Repeat cycle every 21 days [126].
or
Abraxane: 125 mg/m^2 IV on days 1, 8, and 15
Repeat cycle every 28 days [127].

Eribulin

Eribulin: 1.4 mg/m^2 IV on days 1 and 8
Repeat cycle every 21 days [128].

CANCER OF UNKNOWN PRIMARY

Combination Regimens

PCE

Paclitaxel: 200 mg/m^2 IV over 1 hour on day 1
Carboplatin: AUC of 6, IV on day 1
Etoposide: 50 mg alternating with 100 mg PO on
                                                 days 1–10

Repeat cycle every 21 days [129].

EP

Etoposide: 100 mg/m^2 IV on days 1–5
Cisplatin: 100 mg/m^2 IV on day 1
Repeat cycle every 21 days [130].

PEB

Cisplatin:	20 mg/m^2 IV on days 1–5
Etoposide:	100 mg/m^2 IV on days 1–5
Bleomycin:	30 units IV on days 1, 8, and 15

Repeat cycle every 21 days [131].

GCP

Gemcitabine:	1000 mg/m^2 IV on days 1 and 8
Carboplatin:	AUC of 5, IV on day 1
Paclitaxel:	200 mg/m^2 IV on day 1

Repeat cycle every 21 days for 4 cycles [132]. This is to be followed by paclitaxel at 70 mg/m^2 IV every week for 6 weeks with a 2-week rest. Repeat for a total of 3 cycles.

Gemcitabine + Cisplatin + Paclitaxel

Gemcitabine:	1000 mg/m^2 IV on days 1 and 8
Cisplatin:	75 mg/m^2 IV on day 1
Paclitaxel:	175 mg/m^2 IV on day 1

Repeat cycle every 21 days [133].

Gemcitabine + Irinotecan

Gemcitabine:	1000 mg/m^2 IV on days 1 and 8
Irinotecan:	100 mg/m^2 IV on days 1 and 8

Repeat cycle every 21 days [134].

Capecitabine + Oxaliplatin

Capecitabine:	1000 mg/m^2 PO on days 1–14
Oxaliplatin:	130 mg/m^2 IV on day 1

Repeat cycle every 21 days [135].

Bevacizumab + Erlotinib

Bevacizumab:	10 mg/kg IV on day 1
Erlotinib:	150 mg PO daily

Continue until disease progression [136].

CARCINOID TUMORS AND NEUROENDOCRINE TUMORS

Combination Regimens

5-Fluorouracil + Streptozocin

5-Fluorouracil:	400 mg/m^2/day IV on days 1–5
Streptozocin:	500 mg/m^2/day IV on days 1–5

Repeat cycle every 6 weeks [137].

Doxorubicin + Streptozocin

Doxorubicin:	50 mg/m^2 IV on days 1 and 22
Streptozocin:	500 mg/m^2/day IV on days 1–5

Repeat cycle every 6 weeks [137].

Cisplatin + Etoposide

Cisplatin:	45 mg/m^2/day IV continuous infusion on days 2 and 3
Etoposide:	130 mg/m^2/day IV continuous infusion on days 1–3

Repeat cycle every 21 days [138].

Everolimus + Octreotide LAR

Everolimus:	10 mg PO daily
Octreotide LAR:	30 mg IM on day 1

Repeat cycle every 28 days [139].

Capecitabine + Temozolomide

Capecitabine:	750 mg/day PO on days 1–14
Temozolomide:	200 mg/m^2/day PO on days 10–14

Repeat cycle every 28 days [140].

Single-Agent Regimens

Octreotide

Octreotide:	150–250 μg SC tid

Continue until disease progression [141].

Lanreotide

Lanreotide:	120 mg SC on day 1

Repeat cycle every 21 days [142].

Sunitinib

Sunitinib:	50 mg PO daily for 4 weeks

Repeat cycle every 6 weeks [143].

Everolimus

Everolimus:	10 mg PO daily

Continue treatment until disease progression [144].

CERVICAL CANCER

Combination Regimens

Cisplatin + Radiation Therapy

Radiation therapy:	1.8 to 2 Gy per fraction (total dose, 45 Gy)
Cisplatin:	40 mg/m^2 IV weekly (maximal dose, 70 mg per week)

Cisplatin is given 4 hours before radiation therapy on weeks 1–6 [145].

Paclitaxel + Cisplatin

Paclitaxel:	135 mg/m^2 IV over 24 hours on day 1
Cisplatin:	75 mg/m^2 IV on day 2

Repeat cycle every 21 days [146].

Cisplatin + Topotecan

Cisplatin:	50 mg/m^2 IV on day 1
Topotecan:	0.75 mg/m^2/day IV on days 1–3

Repeat cycle every 21 days [147].

Paclitaxel + Topotecan

Paclitaxel:	175 mg/m^2 IV on day 1
Topotecan:	0.75 mg/m^2 IV on days 1-3

Repeat cycle every 21 days [148].

Paclitaxel + Topotecan + Bevacizumab

Paclitaxel:	175 mg/m^2 IV on day 1
Topotecan:	0.75 mg/m^2/day IV on days 1–3
Bevacizumab:	15 mg/kg IV on day 1

Repeat cycle every 21 days [148].

Cisplatin + Paclitaxel + Bevacizumab

Cisplatin:	50 mg/m^2 IV on day 1
Paclitaxel:	135–175 mg/m^2 IV on day 1
Bevacizumab:	15 mg/kg IV on day 1

Repeat cycle every 21 days [148].

BIP

Bleomycin:	30 U IV over 24 hours on day 1
Ifosfamide:	5000 mg/m^2 IV over 24 hours on day 2
Mesna:	6000 mg/m^2 IV over 36 hours on day 2
Cisplatin:	50 mg/m^2 IV on day 2

Repeat cycle every 21 days [149].

BIC

Bleomycin:	30 U IV on day 1
Ifosfamide:	2000 mg/m^2 IV on days 1–3
Mesna:	400 mg/m^2 IV, 15 minutes before ifosfamide dose, then 400 mg/m^2 IV at 4 and 8 hours following ifosfamide
Carboplatin:	200 mg/m^2 IV on day 1

Repeat cycle every 21 days [150].

Cisplatin + 5-Fluorouracil

Cisplatin:	75 mg/m^2 IV on day 1
5-Fluorouracil:	1000 mg/m^2/day IV continuous infusion on days 2–5

Repeat cycle every 21 days [151].

Cisplatin + Vinorelbine

Cisplatin:	80 mg/m^2 IV on day 1
Vinorelbine:	25 mg/m^2 IV on days 1 and 8

Repeat cycle every 21 days [152].

Cisplatin + Irinotecan

Cisplatin:	60 mg/m^2 IV on day 1
Irinotecan:	60 mg/m^2 IV on days 1, 8, and 15

Repeat cycle every 28 days [153].

Cisplatin + Gemcitabine

Cisplatin:	50 mg/m^2 IV on day 1
Gemcitabine:	1000 mg/m^2 IV on days 1 and 8

Repeat cycle every 21 days for up to 6 cycles [154].

or.

Cisplatin:	30 mg/m^2 IV on day 1
Gemcitabine:	800 mg/m^2 IV on days 1 and 8

Repeat cycle every 28 days [155].

Carboplatin + Docetaxel

Carboplatin:	AUC of 6, IV on day 1
Docetaxel:	60 mg/m^2 IV on day 1

Repeat cycle every 21 days [156].

Cisplatin + Pemetrexed

Cisplatin:	50 mg/m^2 IV on day 1
Pemetrexed:	500 mg/m^2 IV on day 1

Repeat cycle every 21 days [157]. Folic acid at 350–1000 μg PO q day and vitamin B12 at 1000 μg IM to start 1 week prior to first dose of pemetrexed and repeated every 3 cycles.

Single-Agent Regimens

Docetaxel

Docetaxel:	100 mg/m^2 IV on day 1

Repeat cycle every 21 days [158].

Paclitaxel

Paclitaxel:	175 mg/m^2 IV over 3 hours on day 1

Repeat cycle every 21 days [159].

Irinotecan

Irinotecan:	125 mg/m^2 IV weekly for 4 weeks

Repeat cycle every 6 weeks [160].

Topotecan

Topotecan: 1.5 mg/m^2/day on days 1–5

Repeat cycle every 21 days [161].

Pemetrexed

Pemetrexed: 500 mg/m^2 IV on day 1

Repeat cycle every 21 days [162]. Folic acid at 350–1000 μg PO q day and vitamin B12 at 1000 μg IM to start 1 week prior to first dose of therapy and repeated every 3 cycles.

Gemcitabine

Gemcitabine: 800 mg/m^2 IV on days 1, 8, and 15

Repeat cycle every 28 days [163].

COLORECTAL CANCER

Neoadjuvant Combined Modality Therapy for Rectal Cancer

Combination Regimens

5-Fluorouracil + Radiation Therapy (German AIO regimen)

5-Fluorouracil: 1000 mg/m^2/day IV continuous infusion on days 1–5

Repeat infusional 5-FU on weeks 1 and 5.

Radiation therapy: 180 cGy/day for 5 days per week (total dose, 5040 cGy)

Followed by surgical resection and then adjuvant chemotherapy with 5-FU at 500 mg/m^2 IV for 5 days every 28 days for a total of 4 cycles [164].

Infusion 5-FU + Radiation Therapy

5-Fluorouracil: 225 mg/m^2/day IV continuous infusion throughout entire course of radiation therapy

Radiation therapy: 180 cGy/day for 5 days per week (total dose, 5040 cGy)

Followed by surgical resection and then adjuvant chemotherapy with capecitabine, 5-FU/LV, or FOLFOX4 for a total of 4 months [165].

Capecitabine + Radiation Therapy

Capecitabine:	825 mg/m^2 PO bid throughout the entire course of radiation therapy or 900–1000 mg/m^2 PO bid on days 1–5 of each week of radiation therapy
Radiation therapy:	180 cGy/day for 5 days per week (total dose, 5040 cGy)

Followed by surgical resection and then adjuvant chemotherapy with capecitabine, 5-FU, or 5-FU/LV for a total of 4 cycles [166].

5-FU/LV Oxaliplatin + Radiation Therapy

5-Fluorouracil:	200 mg/m^2/day IV continuous infusion throughout entire course of radiation therapy
Oxaliplatin:	60 mg/m^2 IV on days 1, 8, 15, 22, 29, and 36
Radiation therapy:	180 cGy/day for 5 days each week (total dose, 5040 cGy)

Followed by surgical resection 4–6 weeks after completion of chemoradiotherapy and then adjuvant chemotherapy [167].

XELOX + Radiation Therapy

Capecitabine:	825 mg/m^2 PO bid on days 1–14 and 22–35
Oxaliplatin:	50 mg/m^2 IV on days 1, 8, 22, and 29
Radiation therapy:	180 cGy/day for 5 days per week (total dose, 5040 cGy)

Followed by surgical resection and then adjuvant chemotherapy with

Capecitabine:	1000 mg/m^2 PO bid on days 1–14
Oxaliplatin:	130 mg/m^2 IV on day 1

Repeat cycle every 3 weeks for 4 cycles [168].

Adjuvant Therapy

Combination Regimens

5-Fluorouracil + Leucovorin (Mayo Clinic schedule)

5-Fluorouracil:	425 mg/m^2 IV on days 1–5
Leucovorin:	20 mg/m^2 IV on days 1–5, administered before 5-fluorouracil

Repeat cycle every 4–5 weeks for a total of 6 cycles [169].

5-Fluorouracil + Leucovorin (weekly schedule, high dose)

5-Fluorouracil:	500 mg/m^2 IV weekly for 6 weeks
Leucovorin:	500 mg/m^2 IV over 2 hours weekly for 6 weeks, administered before 5-fluorouracil

Repeat cycle every 8 weeks for a total of 4 cycles (32 weeks total) [170].

5-Fluorouracil + Leucovorin (weekly schedule, low dose)

5-Fluorouracil:	500 mg/m^2 IV weekly for 6 weeks
Leucovorin:	20 mg/m^2 IV weekly for 6 weeks, administered before 5-fluorouracil

Repeat cycle every 8 weeks for a total of 4 or 6 cycles (32 or 48 weeks total) [171].

Oxaliplatin + 5-Fluorouracil + Leucovorin (FOLFOX4)

Oxaliplatin:	85 mg/m^2 IV on day 1
5-Fluorouracil:	400 mg/m^2 IV bolus, followed by 600 mg/m^2 IV continuous infusion for 22 hours on days 1 and 2
Leucovorin:	200 mg/m^2 IV on days 1 and 2 as a 2-hour infusion before 5-fluorouracil

Repeat cycle every 2 weeks for a total of 12 cycles (6 months total) [172].

Oxaliplatin + 5-Fluorouracil + Leucovorin (mFOLFOX7)

Oxaliplatin:	100 mg/m^2 IV on day 1
5-Fluorouracil:	3000 mg/m^2 IV continuous infusion on days 1 and 2 for 46 hours
Leucovorin:	200 mg/m^2 IV on day 1 as a 2-hour infusion before 5-fluorouracil

Repeat cycle every 2 weeks for a total of 12 cycles (6 months total) [173].

FLOX

5-Fluorouracil:	500 mg/m^2 IV weekly for 6 weeks, administered 1 hour after LV infusion begun
Leucovorin:	500 mg/m^2 IV over 2 hours weekly for 6 weeks, administered before 5-fluorouracil
Oxaliplatin:	85 mg/m^2 IV administered before 5-fluorouracil and LV and on days 1, 15, and 29

Repeat cycle every 8 weeks for a total of 3 cycles (6 months total) [174].

Oxaliplatin + Capecitabine (XELOX)

Oxaliplatin: 130 mg/m^2 IV on day 1

Capecitabine: 1000 mg/m^2 PO bid on days 1–14

Repeat cycle every 3 weeks for a total of 8 cycles (6 months total) [175]. Dose may be decreased to 850 mg/m^2 PO bid days 1–14 to reduce risk of toxicity without compromising efficacy.

LV5FU2 (deGramont regimen)

5-Fluorouracil: 400 mg/m^2 IV bolus, followed by 600 mg/m^2 IV continuous infusion for 22 hours on days 1 and 2

Leucovorin: 200 mg/m^2 IV on days 1 and 2 as a 2-hour infusion before 5-fluorouracil

or

L-Leucovorin: 100 mg/m^2 IV on days 1 and 2 as a 2-hour infusion before 5-fluorouracil

Repeat cycle every 2 weeks for a total of 12 cycles [172].

Capecitabine

Capecitabine: 1250 mg/m^2 PO bid on days 1–14

Repeat cycle every 21 days for a total of 8 cycles [176]. Dose may be decreased to 850–1000 mg/m^2 PO bid on days 1–14 to reduce risk of toxicity without compromising clinical efficacy.

Metastatic Disease

Combination Regimens

Irinotecan + 5-Fluorouracil + Leucovorin (IFL Saltz regimen)

Irinotecan: 125 mg/m^2 IV over 90 minutes weekly for 4 weeks

5-Fluorouracil: 500 mg/m^2 IV weekly for 4 weeks

Leucovorin: 20 mg/m^2 IV weekly for 4 weeks

Repeat cycle every 6 weeks [177].

Irinotecan 5-Fluorouracil Leucovorin (IFL Saltz regimen) + Bevacizumab (BV)

Irinotecan: 125 mg/m^2 IV over 90 minutes weekly for 4 weeks

5-Fluorouracil: 500 mg/m^2 IV weekly for 4 weeks

Leucovorin: 20 mg/m^2 IV weekly for 4 weeks

Bevacizumab: 5 mg/kg IV every 2 weeks

Repeat cycle every 6 weeks [178].

Irinotecan + 5-Fluorouracil + Leucovorin (Modified IFL Saltz regimen)

Irinotecan:	125 mg/m^2 IV over 90 minutes weekly for 2 weeks
5-Fluorouracil:	500 mg/m^2 IV weekly for 2 weeks
Leucovorin:	20 mg/m^2 IV weekly for 2 weeks

Repeat cycle every 3 weeks [179].

Irinotecan + 5-Fluorouracil + Leucovorin (Douillard regimen)

Irinotecan:	180 mg/m^2 IV on day 1
5-Fluorouracil:	400 mg/m^2 IV bolus, followed by 600 g/m^2 IV continuous infusion for 22 hours on days 1 and 2
Leucovorin:	200 mg/m^2 IV on days 1 and 2 as a 2-hour infusion prior to 5-fluorouracil

Repeat cycle every 2 weeks [180].

Irinotecan + 5-Fluorouracil + Leucovorin (FOLFIRI regimen)

Irinotecan:	180 mg/m^2 IV on day 1
5-Fluorouracil:	400 mg/m^2 IV bolus on day 1, followed by 2400 mg/m^2 IV continuous infusion for 46 hours
Leucovorin:	200 mg/m^2 IV on day 1 as a 2-hour infusion prior to 5-fluorouracil

Repeat cycle every 2 weeks [181].

Oxaliplatin + 5-Fluorouracil + Leucovorin (FOLFOX4)

Oxaliplatin:	85 mg/m^2 IV on day 1
5-Fluorouracil:	400 mg/m^2 IV bolus, followed by 600 mg/m^2 IV continuous infusion for 22 hours on days 1 and 2
Leucovorin:	200 mg/m^2 IV on days 1 and 2 as a 2-hour infusion before 5-fluorouracil

or

L-Leucovorin:	100 mg/m^2 IV on days 1 and 2 as a 2-hour infusion before 5-fluorouracil

Repeat cycle every 2 weeks [182].

Oxaliplatin + 5-Fluorouracil + Leucovorin (FOLFOX6)

Oxaliplatin:	100 mg/m^2 IV on day 1

| 5-Fluorouracil: | 400 mg/m^2 IV bolus on day 1, followed by 2400 mg/m^2 IV continuous infusion for 46 hours |
| Leucovorin: | 400 mg/m^2 IV on day 1 as a 2-hour infusion before 5-fluorouracil |

Repeat cycle every 2 weeks [183].

Oxaliplatin + 5-Fluorouracil + Leucovorin (FOLFOX7)

Oxaliplatin:	130 mg/m^2 IV on day 1
5-Fluorouracil:	2400 mg/m^2 IV continuous infusion on days 1 and 2 for 46 hours
Leucovorin:	400 mg/m^2 IV on day 1 as a 2-hour infusion before 5-fluorouracil

or

| L-Leucovorin: | 200 mg/m^2 IV on days 1 and 2 as a 2-hour infusion before 5-fluorouracil |

Repeat cycle every 2 weeks [184].

Oxaliplatin + 5-Fluorouracil + Leucovorin (mFOLFOX7)

Oxaliplatin:	100 mg/m^2 IV on day 1
5-Fluorouracil:	3000 mg/m^2 IV continuous infusion on days 1 and 2 for 46 hours
Leucovorin:	200 mg/m^2 IV on day 1 as a 2-hour infusion before 5-fluorouracil

Repeat cycle every 2 weeks [185].

FOLFOXIRI

Irinotecan:	165 mg/m^2 IV on day 1
Oxaliplatin:	85 mg/m^2 IV on day 1
5-Fluorouracil:	3200 mg/m^2 IV continuous infusion for 46 hours on days 1 and 2
Leucovorin:	200 mg/m^2 IV on day 1 as a 2-hour infusion prior to 5-fluorouracil

Repeat cycle every 2 weeks for a total of 12 cycles [186].

FOLFOXIRI + Bevacizumab

Irinotecan:	165 mg/m^2 IV on day 1
Oxaliplatin:	85 mg/m^2 IV on day 1
5-Fluorouracil:	3200 mg/m^2 IV continuous infusion for 46 hours on days 1 and 2

| Leucovorin: | 200 mg/m^2 IV on day 1 as a 2-hour infusion prior to 5-fluorouracil |
| Bevacizumab: | 5 mg/kg IV on day 1 |

Repeat cycle every 2 weeks [187].

FOLFOXIRI + Panitumumab

Irinotecan:	150 mg/m^2 IV on day 1
Oxaliplatin:	85 mg/m^2 IV on day 1
5-Fluorouracil:	3000 mq/m^2 IV continuous infusion for 46 hours on days 1 and 2
Leucovorin:	200 mg/m^2 IV on day 1 as a 2-hour infusion prior to 5-fluorouracil
Panitumumab:	6 mg/kg IV on day 1

Repeat cycle every 2 weeks [188].

Cetuximab + Irinotecan

| Cetuximab: | 400 mg/m^2 IV loading dose, then 250 mg/m^2 IV weekly |
| Irinotecan: | 350 mg/m^2 IV on day 1 |

Repeat cycle every 21 days [189].

or

| Cetuximab: | 400 mg/m^2 IV loading dose, then 250 mg/m^2 IV weekly |
| Irinotecan: | 180 mg/m^2 IV on day 1 |

Repeat cycle every 14 days [189].

Capecitabine + Oxaliplatin (XELOX)

| Capecitabine: | 1000 mg/m^2 PO bid on days 1–14 |
| Oxaliplatin: | 130 mg/m^2 IV on day 1 |

Repeat cycle every 21 days [190]. May decrease dose of capecitabine to 850 mg/m^2 PO bid and dose of oxaliplatin to 100 mg/m^2 IV to reduce risk of toxicity without compromising clinical efficacy.

or

| Capecitabine: | 1750 mg/m^2 PO bid on days 1–7 |
| Oxaliplatin: | 85 mg/m^2 IV on day 1 |

Repeat cycle every 14 days [190]. May decrease dose of capecitabine to 1000–1250 mg/m^2 PO bid to reduce risk of toxicity without compromising clinical efficacy.

Capecitabine + Irinotecan (XELIRI)

Capecitabine:	1000 mg/m^2 PO bid on days 1–14
Irinotecan:	250 mg/m^2 IV on day 1

Repeat cycle every 21 days [191]. May decrease dose of capecitabine to 850 mg/m^2 PO bid and dose of irinotecan to 200 mg/m^2 IV to reduce risk of toxicity without compromising clinical efficacy.

or

Capecitabine:	1500 mg/m^2 PO bid on days 2–8
Irinotecan:	150 mg/m^2 IV on day 1

Repeat cycle every 14 days [192].

Capecitabine + Mitomycin-C

Capecitabine:	1000 mg/m^2 PO bid on days 1–14
Mitomycin-C:	7 mg/m^2 IV on day 1

Repeat capecitabine every 3 weeks and mitomycin-C every 6 weeks [193].

Oxaliplatin + Irinotecan (IROX regimen)

Oxaliplatin:	85 mg/m^2 IV on day 1
Irinotecan:	200 mg/m^2 IV on day 1

Repeat cycle every 3 weeks [194].

5-Fluorouracil + Leucovorin (Mayo Clinic schedule)

5-Fluorouracil:	425 mg/m^2 IV on days 1–5
Leucovorin:	20 mg/m^2 IV on days 1–5, administered before 5-fluorouracil

Repeat cycle every 4–5 weeks [195].

5-Fluorouracil + Leucovorin (Roswell Park schedule, high dose)

5-Fluorouracil:	500 mg/m^2 IV weekly for 6 weeks
Leucovorin:	500 mg/m^2 IV weekly for 6 weeks, administered before 5-fluorouracil

Repeat cycle every 8 weeks [196].

5-Fluorouracil + Leucovorin + Bevacizumab

5-Fluorouracil:	500 mg/m^2 IV weekly for 6 weeks
Leucovorin:	500 mg/m^2 IV weekly for 6 weeks, administered before 5-fluorouracil

Bevacizumab: 5 mg/kg IV every 2 weeks

Repeat cycle every 8 weeks [197].

5-Fluorouracil + Leucovorin (German schedule, low dose)

5-Fluorouracil: 600 mg/m^2 IV weekly for 6 weeks

Leucovorin: 20 mg/m^2 IV weekly for 6 weeks, administered before 5-fluorouracil

Repeat cycle every 8 weeks [198].

5-Fluorouracil + Leucovorin (de Gramont regimen)

5-Fluorouracil: 400 mg/m^2 IV and then 600 mg/m^2 IV for 22 hours on days 1 and 2

Leucovorin: 200 mg/m^2 IV on days 1 and 2 as a 2-hour infusion before 5-fluorouracil

Repeat cycle every 2 weeks [199].

FOLFOX4 + Bevacizumab

Oxaliplatin: 85 mg/m^2 IV on day 1

5-Fluorouracil: 400 mg/m^2 IV bolus, followed by 600 mg/m^2 IV continuous infusion on days 1 and 2

Leucovorin: 200 mg/m^2 IV on days 1 and 2 as a 2-hour infusion before 5-fluorouracil

Bevacizumab: 10 mg/kg IV every 2 weeks

Repeat cycle every 2 weeks [200].

LV5FU2 + Mitomycin-C

5-Fluorouracil: 400 mg/m^2 IV bolus, followed by 600 mg/m^2 IV continuous infusion on days 1 and 2

Leucovorin: 200 mg/m^2 IV on days 1 and 2 as a 2-hour infusion before 5-fluorouracil

Mitomycin-C: 7 mg/m^2 IV on day 1

Repeat 5-FU/LV every 2 weeks and mitomycin-C every 4 weeks [201].

Capecitabine + Oxaliplatin (XELOX) + Bevacizumab

Capecitabine: 850 mg/m^2 PO bid on days 1–14

Oxaliplatin: 130 mg/m^2 IV on day 1

Bevacizumab: 7.5 mg/kg every 3 weeks

Repeat cycle every 21 days [202].

Cetuximab + Bevacizumab + Irinotecan

Cetuximab: 400 mg/m^2 IV loading dose, then 250 mg/m^2 IV weekly

Bevacizumab: 5 mg/kg IV every 2 weeks

Irinotecan: 180 mg/m^2 IV on day 1

Repeat cycle every 2 weeks [203].

Cetuximab + Bevacizumab

Cetuximab: 400 mg/m^2 IV loading dose, then 250 mg/m^2 IV weekly

Bevacizumab: 5 mg/kg IV every 2 weeks

Repeat cycle every 2 weeks [203].

Irinotecan + Cetuximab

Irinotecan: 125 mg/m^2 IV weekly for 4 weeks

Cetuximab: 400 mg/m^2 IV loading dose, then 250 mg/m^2 IV weekly

Repeat cycle every 6 weeks [204].

or

Irinotecan: 350 mg/m^2 IV on day 1

Cetuximab: 400 mg/m^2 IV loading dose, then 250 mg/m^2 IV weekly

Repeat cycle every 3 weeks [205].

FOLFIRI + Cetuximab

Irinotecan: 180 mg/m^2 IV on day 1

5-Fluorouracil: 400 mg/m^2 IV bolus followed by 2400 mg/m^2 IV continuous infusion for 46 hours on days 1 and 2

Leucovorin: 400 mg/m^2 IV on day 1 as a 2-hour infusion prior to 5-fluorouracil

Cetuximab: 400 mg/m^2 IV loading dose, then 250 mg/m^2 IV weekly

Repeat cycle every 2 weeks [206].

FOLFOX4 + Cetuximab

Oxaliplatin: 85 mg/m^2 IV on day 1

5-Fluorouracil:	400 mg/m^2 IV bolus followed by 600 mg/m^2 IV continuous infusion for 22 hours on days 1 and 2
Leucovorin:	200 mg/m^2 IV on days 1 and 2 as a 2-hour infusion prior to 5-fluorouracil
Cetuximab:	400 mg/m^2 IV loading dose, then 250 mg/m^2 IV weekly

Repeat cycle every 2 weeks [207].

FOLFOX6 + Cetuximab

Oxaliplatin:	85 mg/m^2 IV on day 1
5-Fluorouracil:	400 mg/m^2 IV bolus on day 1, followed by 2400 mg/m^2 IV continuous infusion over 46 hours on days 1 and 2
Leucovorin:	400 mg/m^2 IV on day 1 as a 2-hour infusion before 5-fluorouracil
Cetuximab:	400 mg/m^2 IV loading dose and then 250 mg/m^2 IV weekly

Repeat cycle every 2 weeks [208].

FOLFOX4 + Panitumumab

Oxaliplatin:	85 mg/m^2 IV on day 1
5-Fluorouracil:	400 mg/m^2 IV bolus followed by 600 mg/m^2 IV continuous infusion for 22 hours on days 1 and 2
Leucovorin:	200 mg/m^2 IV on days 1 and 2 as a 2-hour infusion before 5-fluorouracil
Panitumumab:	6 mg/kg IV on day 1

Repeat cycle every 2 weeks [209].

FOLFIRI + Panitumumab

Irinotecan:	180 mg/m^2 IV on day 1
5-Fluorouracil:	400 mg/m^2 IV bolus on day 1, followed by 2400 mg/m^2 IV continuous infusion for 46 hours on days 1 and 2
Leucovorin:	400 mg/m^2 IV on day 1 as a 2-hour infusion before 5-fluorouracil
Panitumumab:	6 mg/kg IV on day 1

Repeat cycle every 2 weeks [210].

FOLFIRI + Bevacizumab

Irinotecan:	180 mg/m^2 IV on day 1
5-Fluorouracil:	400 mg/m^2 IV bolus on day 1, followed by 2400 mg/m^2 IV continuous infusion for 46 hours on days 1 and 2
Leucovorin:	400 mg/m^2 IV on day 1 as a 2-hour infusion prior to 5-fluorouracil
Bevacizumab:	5 mg/kg IV every 2 weeks

Repeat cycle every 2 weeks [211].

FOLFIRI + Ziv-aflibercept

Irinotecan:	180 mg/m^2 IV on day 1
5-Fluorouracil:	400 mg/m^2 IV bolus on day 1, followed by 2400 mg/m^2 IV continuous infusion for 46 hours on days 1 and 2
Leucovorin:	400 mg/m^2 IV on day 1 as a 2-hour infusion prior to 5-fluorouracil
Ziv-aflibercept:	4 mg/kg IV on day 1

Repeat cycle every 2 weeks [212].

FOLFIRI + Ramucirumab

Irinotecan:	180 mg/m^2 IV on day 1
5-Fluorouracil:	400 mg/m^2 IV bolus on day 1, followed by 2400 mg/m^2 IV continuous infusion for 46 hours on days 1 and 2
Leucovorin:	400 mg/m^2 IV on day 1 as a 2-hour infusion prior to 5-fluorouracil
Ramucirumab:	8 mg/kg IV on day 1

Repeat cycle every 2 weeks [213].

Hepatic Artery Infusion
Floxuridine

Floxuridine (FUDR):	0.3 mg/kg/day HAI on days 1–14
Dexamethasone:	20 mg HAI on days 1–14
Heparin:	50,000 U HAI on days 1–14

Repeat cycle every 14 days [214].

Single-Agent Regimens

Capecitabine

Capecitabine: 1250 mg/m^2 PO bid on days 1–14

Repeat cycle every 21 days [215]. Dose may be decreased to 850–1000 mg/m^2 PO bid on days 1–14 to reduce risk of toxicity without compromising clinical efficacy.

CPT-11 (weekly schedule)

CPT-11:   125 mg/m^2 IV over 90 minutes weekly for 4 weeks

Repeat cycle every 6 weeks [216].

or

CPT-11:   125 mg/m^2 IV over 90 minutes weekly for 2 weeks

Repeat cycle every 3 weeks.

or

CPT-11:   175 mg/m^2 IV on days 1 and 10

Repeat cycle every 3 weeks [217].

CPT-11 (monthly schedule)

CPT-11:   350 mg/m^2 IV on day 1

Repeat cycle every 3 weeks [218].

Cetuximab

Cetuximab: 400 mg/m^2 IV loading dose, then 250 mg/m^2 IV weekly

Repeat cycle on a weekly basis [219].

or

Cetuximab: 500 mg/m^2 IV every 2 weeks (no loading dose is necessary)

Repeat cycle every 2 weeks [220].

Panitumumab

Panitumumab: 6 mg/kg every 2 weeks

Repeat cycle every 2 weeks [221].

5-Fluorouracil (continuous infusion)

5-Fluorouracil:	2600 mg/m^2 IV over 24 hours weekly

Repeat cycle weekly for 4 weeks [222].

or

5-Fluorouracil:	1000 mg/m^2/day IV continuous infusion on days 1–4

Repeat cycle every 21–28 days [223].

or

5-Fluorouracil:	200 mg/m^2/day IV continuous infusion on days 1–4
L-Leucovorin:	5 mg/m^2/day IV on days 1–14

Repeat cycle every 28 days [224].

Regorafenib

Regorafenib:	160 mg PO daily on days 1–21

Repeat cycle every 28 days [225].

TAS-102

TAS-102:	35 mg/m^2 PO bid on days 1–5 and 8–12

Repeat cycle every 28 days [226].

ENDOMETRIAL CANCER

Combination Regimens

Paclitaxel + Carboplatin

Paclitaxel:	175 mg/m^2 IV over 3 hours on day 1
Carboplatin:	AUC of 5–7, IV on day 1

Repeat cycle every 28 days [227].

AC

Doxorubicin:	60 mg/m^2 IV on day 1
Cyclophosphamide:	500 mg/m^2 IV on day 1

Repeat cycle every 21 days [228].

AP

Doxorubicin:	50 mg/m^2 IV on day 1

Cisplatin: 50 mg/m^2 IV on day 1
Repeat cycle every 21 days [229].

Doxorubicin + Paclitaxel

Doxorubicin: 50 mg/m^2 IV on day 1
Paclitaxel: 150 mg/m^2 IV on day 1
Repeat cycle every 21 days [230].

Cisplatin + Doxorubicin + Paclitaxel

Cisplatin: 50 mg/m^2 IV on day 1
Doxorubicin: 45 mg/m^2 IV on day 1
Paclitaxel: 160 mg/m^2 IV over 3 hours on day 2
Filgrastim: 5 µg/kg SC on days 3–12
Repeat cycle every 21 days [231].

CAP

Cyclophosphamide: 500 mg/m^2 IV on day 1
Doxorubicin: 50 mg/m^2 IV on day 1
Cisplatin: 50 mg/m^2 IV on day 1
Repeat cycle every 21 days [232].

Carboplatin + Doxorubicin liposome:

Carboplatin: AUC of 5, IV on day 1
Doxorubicin liposome: 40 mg/m^2 IV on day 1
Repeat cycle every 28 days [233].

Paclitaxel + Ifosfamide (carcinosarcoma)

Paclitaxel: 135 mg/m^2 IV over 3 hours on day 1
Ifosfamide: 1600 mg/m^2/day IV on days 1–3
Repeat cycle every 21 days for up to 8 cycles [234]. Mesna to be given as either IV
or PO. G-CSF support at 5 µg/kg/day SC to be started on day 4.

Cisplatin + Ifosfamide (carcinosarcoma)

Cisplatin: 20 mg/m^2/day IV on days 1-4
Ifosfamide: 1500 mg/m^2/day IV on day 1
Mesna: 120 mg/m^2 IV (loading dose) followed by
                                          1500 mg/m^2/day for 24 hours
Repeat cycle every 21 days for 3 cycles [235].

Gemcitabine + Docetaxel

Gemcitabine:	900 mg/m^2 IV on days 1 and 8
Docetaxel:	100 mg/m^2 IV on day 8

Repeat cycle every 21 days [236].

Single-Agent Regimens

Doxorubicin

Doxorubicin:	60 mg/m^2 IV on day 1

Repeat cycle every 21 days [237].

Megestrol

Megestrol:	160 mg PO daily

Repeat on a daily basis [238].

Paclitaxel

Paclitaxel:	200 mg/m^2 IV over 3 hours on day 1

Repeat cycle every 21 days [239]. Reduce dose to 175 mg/m^2 IV for patients with prior pelvic radiation therapy.

Topotecan

Topotecan:	1.0 mg/m^2/day IV on days 1–5

Repeat cycle every 21 days [240]. Reduce dose to 0.8 mg/m^2/day IV on days 1–3 in patients with prior radiation therapy.

Temsirolimus

Temsirolimus:	25 mg IV on day 1

Repeat cycle every 28 days [241].

ESOPHAGEAL CANCER

Neoadjuvant Combined Modality Therapy

5-Fluorouracil + Cisplatin + Radiation Therapy (Herskovic regimen)

5-Fluorouracil:	1000 mg/m^2/day IV continuous infusion on days 1–4
Cisplatin:	75 mg/m^2 IV on day 1

Repeat on weeks 1, 5, 8, and 11 [242].

Radiation therapy:	200 cGy/day for 5 days per week (total dose, 1000 cGy), followed by a boost to the field of 1000 cGy.

5-Fluorouracil + Cisplatin + Radiation Therapy (FFD French regimen)

5-Fluorouracil:	800 mg/m^2/day IV continuous infusion on days 1–5
Cisplatin:	15 mg/m^2 IV on days 1–5. Administer on days 1, 22, 43, 64, and 92
Radiation therapy:	200 cGy/day for 5 days per week to a total dose of 6600 cGy over 6.5 weeks

Chemotherapy is given concurrently with radiation therapy, followed by surgical resection [243].

Preoperative Chemoradiation

5-Fluorouracil + Cisplatin + Radiation Therapy (Hopkins/Yale regimen)

5-Fluorouracil:	225 mg/m^2/day IV continuous infusion on days 1–30
Cisplatin:	20 mg/m^2/day IV on days 1–5 and 26–30
Radiation therapy:	200 cGy/day to a total dose of 4400 cGy

Chemotherapy is given concurrently with radiation therapy. Followed by esophagectomy and then adjuvant chemotherapy in patients who had total gross removal of disease with negative margins.

Adjuvant Chemotherapy

Paclitaxel:	135 mg/m^2 IV for 24 hours on day 1
Cisplatin.	75 mg/m^2 IV on day 2

Adjuvant chemotherapy is given 8–12 weeks after esophagectomy, and each cycle is given every 21 days for a total of 3 cycles [244].

MAGIC Trial

Preoperative ECF Chemotherapy

Epirubicin:	50 mg/m^2 IV on day 1
Cisplatin:	60 mg/m^2 IV on day 1
5-Fluorouracil:	200 mg/m^2/day IV continuous infusion on days 1–21

Repeat cycle every 21 days for 3 cycles [245].

Followed by esophagectomy and then adjuvant chemotherapy in patients who had total gross removal of disease with negative margins.

Adjuvant Chemotherapy

Epirubicin:	50 mg/m^2 IV on day 1
Cisplatin:	60 mg/m^2 IV on day 1
5-Fluorouracil:	200 mg/m^2/day IV continuous infusion on days 1–21

Repeat cycle every 21 days for 3 cycles [245].

Metastatic Disease

Combination Regimens

5-Fluorouracil + Cisplatin

5-Fluorouracil:	1000 mg/m^2/day IV continuous infusion on days 1–5
Cisplatin:	100 mg/m^2 IV on day 1

Repeat cycle on weeks 1, 5, 8, and 11 [246].

Irinotecan + Cisplatin

Irinotecan:	65 mg/m^2 IV weekly for 4 weeks
Cisplatin:	30 mg/m^2 IV weekly for 4 weeks

Repeat cycle every 6 weeks [246a].

Paclitaxel + Cisplatin

Paclitaxel:	200 mg/m^2 IV over 24 hours on day 1
Cisplatin:	75 mg/m^2 IV on day 2

Repeat cycle every 21 days [247]. G-CSF support is recommended.

Capecitabine + Oxaliplatin

Capecitabine:	1000 mg/m^2 PO bid on days 1–14
Oxaliplatin:	130 mg/m^2 IV on day 1

Repeat cycle every 21 days [248].

ECF

Epirubicin:	50 mg/m^2 IV on day 1
Cisplatin:	60 mg/m^2 IV on day 1
5-Fluorouracil:	200 mg/m^2/day IV continuous infusion

Repeat cycle every 21 days [249].

EOF

Epirubicin:	50 mg/m^2 IV on day 1
Oxaliplatin:	130 mg/m^2 IV on day 1
5-Fluorouracil:	200 mg/m^2/day IV continuous infusion

Repeat cycle every 21 days [249].

ECX

Epirubicin:	50 mg/m^2 IV on day 1
Cisplatin:	60 mg/m^2 IV on day 1
Capecitabine:	625 mg/m^2 PO bid continuously

Repeat cycle every 21 days [249].

EOX

Epirubicin:	50 mg/m^2 IV on day 1
Oxaliplatin:	130 mg/m^2 IV on day 1
Capecitabine:	625 mg/m^2 PO bid continuously

Repeat cycle every 21 days [249].

Single-Agent Regimens

Paclitaxel

Paclitaxel:	250 mg/m^2 IV over 24 hours on day 1

Repeat cycle every 21 days [250]. G-CSF support is recommended.

GASTRIC CANCER

Adjuvant Therapy

One cycle of chemotherapy is administered as follows:

5-Fluorouracil:	425 mg/m^2 IV on days 1–5
Leucovorin:	20 mg/m^2 IV on days 1–5

Chemoradiotherapy is then started 28 days after the start of the initial cycle of chemotherapy as follows:

Radiation therapy:	180 cGy/day to a total dose of 4500 cGy, starting on day 28
5-Fluorouracil:	400 mg/m^2 IV on days 1–4 and days 23–25 of radiation therapy
Leucovorin:	20 mg/m^2 IV on days 1–4 and days 23–25 of radiation therapy

Chemoradiotherapy is followed by 2 cycles of chemotherapy that are given 1 month apart and include [251]:

5-Fluorouracil:	425 mg/m^2 IV on days 1–5
Leucovorin:	20 mg/m^2 IV on days 1–5

Capecitabine + Oxaliplatin

Capecitabine: 1000 mg/m^2 PO bid on days 1–14

Oxaliplatin: 130 mg/m^2 IV on day 1

Repeat cycle every 21 days for 6 months [252].

Metastatic Disease

Combination Regimens

DCF

Docetaxel: 75 mg/m^2 IV on day 1

Cisplatin: 75 mg/m^2 IV on day 1

5-Fluorouracil: 750 mg/m^2/day IV continuous infusion
                                 on days 1–5

Repeat cycle every 21 days [253].

CF

Cisplatin: 100 mg/m^2 IV on day 1

5-Fluorouracil: 1000 mg/m^2/day IV continuous infusion
                                 on days 1–5

Repeat cycle every 28 days [254].

ECF

Epirubicin: 50 mg/m^2 IV on day 1

Cisplatin: 60 mg/m^2 IV on day 1

5-Fluorouracil: 200 mg/m^2/day IV continuous infusion

Repeat cycle every 21 days [249].

EOF

Epirubicin: 50 mg/m^2 IV on day 1

Oxaliplatin: 130 mg/m^2 IV on day 1

5-Fluorouracil: 200 mg/m^2/day IV continuous infusion

Repeat cycle every 21 days [249].

ECX

Epirubicin: 50 mg/m^2 IV on day 1

Cisplatin: 60 mg/m^2 IV on day 1

Capecitabine: 625 mg/m^2 PO bid continuously

Repeat cycle every 21 days [249].

EOX

Epirubicin:	50 mg/m^2 IV on day 1
Oxaliplatin:	130 mg/m^2 IV on day 1
Capecitabine:	625 mg/m^2 PO bid continuously

Repeat cycle every 21 days [249].

IP

Irinotecan:	70 mg/m^2 IV on days 1 and 15
Cisplatin:	80 mg/m^2 IV on day 1

Repeat cycle every 28 days [255].

IPB

Irinotecan:	65 mg/m^2 IV on days 1 and 8
Cisplatin:	30 mg/m^2 IV on days 1 and 8
Bevacizumab:	15 mg/kg IV on day 1

Repeat cycle every 21 days [256].

Docetaxel + Cisplatin

Docetaxel:	85 mg/m^2 IV on day 1
Cisplatin:	75 mg/m^2 IV on day 1

Repeat cycle every 21 days [257].

IDO

Irinotecan:	150 mg/m^2 IV on day 1
Docetaxel:	60 mg/m^2 IV on day 1
Oxaliplatin:	85 mg/m^2 IV on day 2

Repeat cycle every 21 days [258].

Capecitabine + Cisplatin

Capecitabine:	1000 mg/m^2 PO bid on days 1–14
Cisplatin:	80 mg/m^2 IV on day 1

Repeat cycle every 21 days [259].

XP + Trastuzumab

Capecitabine:	1000 mg/m^2 PO bid on days 1–14
Cisplatin:	80 mg/m^2 IV on day 1

Trastuzumab: 8 mg/kg IV loading dose, then 6 mg/kg
                                      IV every 3 weeks

Repeat cycle every 21 days [260].

FP + Trastuzumab

5-Fluorouracil: 800 mg/m^2 IV continuous infusion on
                                      days 1–5

Cisplatin: 80 mg/m^2 IV on day 1
Trastuzumab: 8 mg/kg IV loading dose, then 6 mg/kg
                                      IV every 3 weeks

Repeat cycle every 21 days [260].

FLO

5-Fluorouracil: 2600 mg/m^2 IV on day 1 as a continuous
                                      infusion over 24 hours

Leucovorin: 200 mg/m^2 IV on day 1 as a 2-hour
                                      infusion

Oxaliplatin: 85 mg/m^2 IV on day 1
Repeat cycle every 14 days [261].

mFOLFOX6

Oxaliplatin: 100 mg/m^2 IV on day 1
5-Fluorouracil: 2400 mg/m^2 IV infusion for 46 hours
                                      starting on day 1

Leucovorin: 100 mg/m^2 IV on day 1 as a 2-hour
                                      infusion prior to 5-FU

Repeat cycle every 2 weeks [262].

Paclitaxel + Ramucirumab

Paclitaxel: 80 mg/m^2 IV on days 1, 8, and 15
Ramucirumab: 8 mg/kg IV on days 1 and 15
Repeat cycle every 28 days [263].

Single-Agent Regimens

5-Fluorouracil

5-Fluorouracil: 500 mg/m^2 IV on days 1–5
Repeat cycle every 28 days [264].

5-Fluorouracil + Leucovorin

5-Fluorouracil: 370 mg/m^2 IV on days 1–5

Leucovorin: 200 mg/m^2 IV on days 1–5

Repeat cycle every 21 days [265].

Docetaxel

Docetaxel: 100 mg/m^2 IV on day 1

Repeat cycle every 21 days [266].

or

Docetaxel: 36 mg/m^2 IV weekly for 6 weeks

Repeat cycle every 8 weeks [267].

Ramucirumab

Ramucirumab: 8 mg/kg IV on day 1

Repeat cycle every 14 days [268].

GASTROINTESTINAL STROMAL TUMOR (GIST)

Adjuvant Therapy

Imatinib

Imatinib: 400 mg/day PO

Continue treatment for a total of 3 years [269].

Metastatic Disease

Single-Agent Regimens

Imatinib

Imatinib: 400 mg/day PO

Continue treatment until disease progression [270]. May increase dose to 600 mg/day if no response is seen. In patients with KIT exon 9 (or exon 11) mutation, use dose of 800 mg/day (400 mg bid).

Nilotinib

Nilotinib: 400 mg PO bid

Continue treatment until disease progression [271].

Sunitinib

Sunitinib:	50 mg/day PO for 4 weeks

Repeat cycle every 6 weeks [272].

Sorafenib

Sorafenib:	400 mg/day PO bid

Continue treatment until disease progression [273].

Regorafenib

Regorafenib:	160 mg/day PO for 21 days

Repeat cycle every 28 days [274].

HEAD AND NECK CANCER

Combined Modality Therapy

Cetuximab + Radiation Therapy

Cetuximab:	400 mg/m^2 IV loading dose, 1 week before radiation therapy, then 250 mg/m^2 IV weekly
Radiation therapy:	200 cGy/day for 5 days per week (total dose, 7000 cGy)

Cetuximab is given concurrently with radiation therapy [275].

TPF Induction Chemotherapy Followed by Carboplatin + Radiation Therapy

Docetaxel:	75 mg/m^2 IV on day 1
Cisplatin:	75–100 mg/m^2 IV on day 1
5-Fluorouracil:	1000 mg/m^2/day IV continuous infusion on days 1–4

Repeat cycle every 3 weeks for 3 cycles followed by:

Carboplatin:	AUC of 1.5, IV weekly for 7 weeks during radiation therapy
Radiation therapy:	200 cGy/day to a total dose of 7400 cGy

At the completion of chemoradiotherapy, surgical resection as indicated [276].

Combination Regimens

TIP

Paclitaxel:	175 mg/m^2 IV over 3 hours on day 1

Mesna: 400 mg/m^2 IV before ifosfamide and
                                                200 mg/m^2 IV, 4 hours after ifosfamide
Cisplatin: 60 mg/m^2 IV on day 1
Repeat cycle every 21–28 days [277].

TPF

Docetaxel: 75 mg/m^2 IV on day 1
Cisplatin: 75–100 mg/m^2 IV over 24 hours on day 1
5-Fluorouracil: 1000 mg/m^2 over 24 hours on days 1–4
Repeat cycle every 21 days [278].

TIC

Paclitaxel: 175 mg/m^2 IV over 3 hours on day 1
Ifosfamide: 1000 mg/m^2 IV over 2 hours on days
                                                1–3
Mesna: 400 mg/m^2 IV before ifosfamide and
                                                200 mg/m^2 IV, 4 hours after ifosfamide
Carboplatin: AUC of 6, IV on day 1
Repeat cycle every 21–28 days [279].

Paclitaxel + Carboplatin

Paclitaxel: 175 mg/m^2 IV over 3 hours on day 1
Carboplatin: AUC of 6, IV on day 1
Repeat cycle every 21 days [280].

Paclitaxel + Cisplatin

Paclitaxel: 175 mg/m^2 IV over 3 hours on day 1
Cisplatin: 75 mg/m^2 IV on day 2
G-CSF: 5 μg/kg/day SC on days 4–10
Repeat cycle every 21 days [281].

PF

Cisplatin: 100 mg/m^2 IV on day 1
5-Fluorouracil: 1000 mg/m^2/day IV continuous infusion
                                                on days 1–5
Repeat cycle every 21–28 days [282].

Carboplatin + 5-FU

Carboplatin:	AUC of 5, IV on day 1
5-Fluorouracil:	1000 mg/m^2/day IV continuous infusion on days 1–4

Repeat cycle every 21 days [283].

PF + Cetuximab

Cisplatin:	100 mg/m^2 IV on day 1
5-Fluorouracil:	1000 mg/m^2/day IV continuous infusion on days 1–4
Cetuximab:	400 mg/m^2 IV loading dose, then 250 mg/m^2 IV weekly

Repeat cycle every 21 days for up to 6 cycles. If no evidence of disease progression at the end of 6 cycles, can continue with weekly cetuximab [284].

Carboplatin + 5-FU + Cetuximab

Carboplatin:	AUC of 5, IV on day 1
5-Fluorouracil:	1000 mg/m^2/day IV continuous infusion on days 1–4
Cetuximab:	400 mg/m^2 IV loading dose, then 250 mg/m^2 IV weekly

Repeat cycle every 21 days for up to 6 cycles. If no evidence of disease progression at the end of 6 cycles, can continue with weekly cetuximab [284].

Cisplatin + Cetuximab

Cisplatin:	100 mg/m^2 IV on day 1
Cetuximab:	400 mg/m^2 IV loading dose, then 250 mg/m^2 IV weekly

Repeat cycle every 21 days [285].

PF-Larynx Preservation

Cisplatin:	100 mg/m^2 IV on day 1
5-Fluorouracil:	1000 mg/m^2/day IV continuous infusion on days 1–5
Radiation therapy:	6600–7600 cGy in 180–200 cGy fractions

Repeat cycle every 21–28 days for 3 cycles [286].

Concurrent Chemoradiation Therapy for Laryngeal Preservation

Cisplatin:	100 mg/m^2 IV on days 1, 22, and 43

Radiation therapy:	7000 cGy in 200 cGy fractions

Administer cisplatin concurrently with radiation therapy [287].

Chemoradiotherapy for Nasopharyngeal Cancer

Cisplatin:	100 mg/m^2 IV on days 1, 22, and 43 during radiotherapy
Radiation therapy:	Total dose of 7000 cGy in 180–200 cGy fractions

At the completion of chemoradiotherapy, chemotherapy is administered as follows:

Cisplatin:	80 mg/m^2 IV on day 1
5-Fluorouracil:	1000 mg/m^2/day IV continuous infusion on days 1–4

Repeat cycle every 28 days for a total of 3 cycles [288].

VP

Vinorelbine:	25 mg/m^2 IV on days 1 and 8
Cisplatin:	80 mg/m^2 IV on day 1

Repeat cycle every 21 days [289].

Single-Agent Regimens

Docetaxel

Docetaxel:	100 mg/m^2 IV on day 1

Repeat cycle every 21 days [290].

Paclitaxel

Paclitaxel:	250 mg/m^2 IV over 24 hours on day 1

Repeat cycle every 21 days [291].

or

Paclitaxel:	137–175 mg/m^2 IV over 3 hours on day 1

Repeat cycle every 21 days [291].

Methotrexate

Methotrexate:	40 mg/m^2 IV or IM weekly

Repeat cycle every week [292].

Vinorelbine

Vinorelbine: 30 mg/m^2 IV weekly
Repeat cycle every week [293].

Cetuximab

Cetuximab: 400 mg/m^2 IV loading dose, then
                                      250 mg/m^2 IV weekly

Repeat cycle every week [294].

Pembrolizumab

Pembrolizumab: 200 mg IV on day 1
Repeat cycle every 3 weeks [295].

HEPATOCELLULAR CANCER

Combination Regimens

GEMOX

Gemcitabine: 1000 mg/m^2 IV on day 1
Oxaliplatin: 100 mg/m^2 IV on day 2
Repeat cycle every 2 weeks [296].

FOLFOX4

Oxaliplatin: 85 mg/m^2 IV on day 1
5-Fluorouracil: 400 mg/m^2 IV bolus, followed by
                                      600 mg/m^2 IV continuous infusion for
                                      22 hours on days 1 and 2

Leucovorin: 200 mg/m^2 IV on days 1 and 2 as a
                                      2-hour infusion before 5-fluorouracil

Repeat cycle every 2 weeks [297].

Bevacizumab + Erlotinib

Bevacizumab: 10 mg/kg IV on days 1 and 14
Erlotinib: 150 mg PO daily
Repeat cycle every 28 days [298].

Single-Agent Regimens

Sorafenib

Sorafenib: 400 mg PO bid

Continue until disease progression [299]. Dose may be reduced to 400 mg once daily or 400 mg every 2 days.

Doxorubicin

Doxorubicin: 20–30 mg/m^2 IV weekly
Repeat cycle every week [300].

Cisplatin

Cisplatin. 80 mg/m^2 IV on day 1
Repeat cycle every week [301].

Capecitabine

Capecitabine: 1000 mg/m^2 PO bid on days 1–14

Repeat cycle every 21 days [302]. Dose may be reduced to 825–900 mg/m^2 PO bid on days 1–14. This dose reduction may decrease risk of toxicity without compromising clinical efficacy.

Bevacizumab

Bevacizumab: 10 mg/kg IV on day 1
Repeat cycle every 14 days [303].

KAPOSI'S SARCOMA

Combination Regimens

BV

Bleomycin: 10 U/m^2 IV on days 1 and 15
Vincristine: 1.4 mg/m^2 IV on days 1 and 15 (maximum, 2 mg)

Repeat cycle every 2 weeks [304].

ABV

Doxorubicin: 40 mg/m^2 IV on day 1
Bleomycin: 15 U/m^2 IV on days 1 and 15

| Vinblastine: | 6 mg/m^2 IV on day 1 |

Repeat cycle every 28 days [305].

Single-Agent Regimens

Daunorubicin liposome

| Daunorubicin liposome: | 40 mg/m^2 IV on day 1 |

Repeat cycle every 14 days [306].

Doxorubicin liposome:

| Doxorubicin liposome: | 20 mg/m^2 IV on day 1 |

Repeat cycle every 21 days [307].

Paclitaxel

| Paclitaxel: | 135 mg/m^2 IV over 3 hours on day 1 |

Repeat cycle every 21 days [308].

or

| Paclitaxel: | 100 mg/m^2 IV over 3 hours on day 1 |

Repeat cycle every 2 weeks [309].

Docetaxel

| Docetaxel: | 25 mg/m^2 IV weekly for 8 weeks, then every other week |

Continue until disease progression [310].

Etoposide

| Etoposide: | 50 mg PO daily on days 1–7 |

Repeat cycle every 2 weeks [311].

Vinorelbine

| Vinorelbine: | 30 mg/m^2 IV on day 1 |

Repeat cycle every 2 weeks [312].

Interferon-α

| Interferon α-2a: | 36 million IU/m^2 SC or IM, daily for 8–12 weeks [313] |
| Interferon α-2b: | 30 million IU/m^2 SC or IM, 3 times weekly [314] |

LEUKEMIA

Acute Lymphocytic Leukemia

Induction Therapy

Linker Regimen [315, 316]

Daunorubicin:	50 mg/m^2 IV every 24 hours on days 1–3
Vincristine:	2 mg IV on days 1, 8, 15, and 22
Prednisone:	60 mg/m^2 PO divided into 3 doses on days 1–28
L-Asparaginase:	6000 U/m^2 IM on days 17–28

If bone marrow on day 14 is positive for residual leukemia,

Daunorubicin:	50 mg/m^2 IV on day 15

If bone marrow on day 28 is positive for residual leukemia,

Daunorubicin:	50 mg/m^2 IV on days 29 and 30
Vincristine:	2 mg IV on days 29 and 36
Prednisone:	60 mg/m^2 PO on days 29–42
L-Asparaginase:	6000 U/m^2 IM on days 29–35

Consolidation Therapy

Linker Regimen [315, 316]

Treatment A (cycles 1, 3, 5, and 7)

Daunorubicin:	50 mg/m^2 IV on days 1 and 2
Vincristine:	2 mg IV on days 1 and 8
Prednisone:	60 mg/m^2 PO on days 1–14
L-Asparaginase:	12,000 U/m^2 on days 2, 4, 7, 9, 11, and 14

Treatment B (cycles 2, 4, 6, and 8)

Teniposide:	165 mg/m^2 IV on days 1, 4, 8, and 11
Cytarabine:	300 mg/m^2 IV on days 1, 4, 8, and 11

Treatment C (cycle 9)

Methotrexate:	690 mg/m^2 IV over 42 hours
Leucovorin:	15 mg/m^2 IV every 6 hours for 12 doses beginning at 42 hours

Maintenance Therapy

Linker Regimen [315, 316]

Methotrexate:	20 mg/m^2 PO weekly

| 6-Mercaptopurine: | 75 mg/m^2 PO daily |

Continue for a total of 30 months of complete response.

CNS Prophylaxis

| Cranial irradiation: | 1800 cGy in 10 fractions over 12–14 days |
| Methotrexate: | 12 mg IT weekly for 6 weeks |

Begin within 1 week of complete response.

In patients with documented CNS involvement at time of diagnosis, intrathecal chemotherapy should begin during induction chemotherapy.

| Methotrexate: | 12 mg IT weekly for 10 doses |
| Cranial irradiation: | 2800 cGy |

Induction Therapy

Larson Regimen [317]

Induction (weeks 1–4)

Cyclophosphamide:	1200 mg/m^2 IV on day 1
Daunorubicin:	45 mg/m^2 IV on days 1–3
Vincristine:	2 mg IV on days 1, 8, 15, and 22
Prednisone:	60 mg/m^2/day PO on days 1–21
L-Asparaginase:	6000 U/m^2 SC on days 5, 8, 11, 15, 18, 22

Early Intensification (weeks 5–12)

Methotrexate:	15 mg IT on day 1
Cyclophosphamide:	1000 mg/m^2 IV on day 1
6-Mercaptopurine:	60 mg/m^2/day PO on days 1–14
Cytarabine:	75 mg/m^2 IV on days 1–4 and 8–11
Vincristine:	2 mg IV on days 15 and 22
L-Asparaginase:	6000 U/m^2 SC on days 15, 18, 22, and 25

Repeat the early intensification cycle once.

CNS Prophylaxis and Interim Maintenance (weeks 13–25)

Cranial irradiation:	2400 cGy on days 1–12
Methotrexate:	15 mg IT on days 1, 8, 15, 22, and 29
6-Mercaptopurine:	60 mg/m^2/day PO on days 1–70
Methotrexate:	20 mg/m^2 PO on days 36, 43, 50, 57, and 64

Late Intensification (weeks 26–33)

Doxorubicin:	30 mg/m^2 IV on days 1, 8, and 15
Vincristine:	2 mg IV on days 1, 8, and 15
Dexamethasone:	10 mg/m^2/day PO on days 1–14
Cyclophosphamide:	1000 mg/m^2 IV on day 29
6-Thioguanine:	60 mg/m^2/day PO on days 29–42
Cytarabine:	75 mg/m^2 on days 29, 32, 36–39

Prolonged Maintenance (continue until 24 months after diagnosis)

Vincristine:	2 mg IV on day 1
Prednisone:	60 mg/m^2/day PO on days 1–5
Methotrexate:	20 mg/m^2 PO on days 1, 8, 15, and 22
6-Mercaptopurine:	80 mg/m^2/day PO on days 1–28

Repeat maintenance cycle every 28 days.

Hyper-CVAD Regimen

Cyclophosphamide:	300 mg/m^2 IV every 12 hours for 6 doses on days 1–3
Mesna:	600 mg/m^2 IV over 24 hours on days 1–3 ending 6 hours after the last dose of cyclophosphamide
Vincristine:	2 mg IV on days 4 and 11
Doxorubicin:	50 mg/m^2 IV on day 4
Dexamethasone:	40 mg PO or IV on days 1–4 and 11–14

Alternate cycles every 21 days with the following:

Methotrexate:	200 mg/m^2 IV over 2 hours, followed by 800 mg/m^2 IV over 24 hours on day 1
Leucovorin:	15 mg IV every 6 hours for 8 doses, starting 24 hours after the completion of methotrexate infusion
Cytarabine:	3000 mg/m^2 IV every 12 hours for 4 doses on days 2–3
Methylprednisolone:	50 mg IV bid on days 1–3

Alternate 4 cycles of hyper-CVAD with 4 cycles of high-dose methotrexate and cytarabine therapy [318].

CNS Prophylaxis

Methotrexate:	12 mg IT on day 2

| Cytarabine: | 100 mg IT on day 8 |

Repeat with each cycle of chemotherapy, depending on the risk of CNS disease.

Supportive Care

Ciprofloxacin:	500 mg PO bid
Fluconazole:	200 mg/day PO
Acyclovir:	200 mg PO bid
G-CSF:	10 μg/kg/day starting 24 hours after the end of chemotherapy (i.e., on day 5 of hyper-CVAD therapy and on day 4 of high-dose methotrexate and cytarabine therapy)

Single-Agent Regimens

Clofarabine

| Clofarabine: | 52 mg/m^2 IV for 5 days |

Repeat cycle every 2–6 weeks [319].

Nelarabine

| Nelarabine: | 1.5 g/m^2/day IV on days 1, 3, and 5 |

Repeat cycle every 28 days up to a total of 4 cycles [320].

Imatinib

| Imatinib: | 600 mg PO daily |

Continue until disease progression [321].

Dasatinib

| Dasatinib: | 70 mg PO bid |

Continue until disease progression [322].

Nilotinib

| Nilotinib: | 400–600 mg PO bid |

Continue until disease progression [323].

Blinatumomab

| Blinatumomab: | 9 μg IV on days 1-7 and 28 μg IV on days 8-28 on cycle 1; 28 μg on days 1-28 on all subsequent cycles |

Repeat cycle every 42 days [324].

ACUTE MYELOGENOUS LEUKEMIA

Induction Regimens

Ara-C + Daunorubicin (7 + 3) [325]

Cytarabine:	100 mg/m^2/day IV continuous infusion on days 1–7
Daunorubicin:	45 mg/m^2 IV on days 1–3

Ara-C + Idarubicin [326]

Cytarabine:	100 mg/m^2/day IV continuous infusion on days 1–7
Idarubicin:	12 mg/m^2 IV on days 1–3

Ara-C + Doxorubicin [327]

Cytarabine:	100 mg/m^2/day IV continuous infusion on days 1–7
Doxorubicin:	30 mg/m^2 IV on days 1–3

Ara-C + Clofarabine

Clofarabine:	40 mg/m^2 IV over 1 hour on days 2–6
Cytarabine:	1000 mg/m^2 IV over 2 hours on days 1–5

Repeat cycles every 4–6 weeks for up to a total of 3 cycles [328].

AIDA (acute promyelocytic leukemia only) [329]

ATRA:	45 mg/m^2 PO daily
Idarubicin:	12 mg/m^2 IV on days 2, 4, 6, and 8

Tretinoin + Daunorubicin + Cytarabine (acute promyelocytic leukemia) [330]

ATRA:	45 mg/m^2 PO daily
Daunorubicin:	60 mg/m^2 IV on days 1–3
Cytarabine:	200 mg/m^2 IV on days 1–7

Tretinoin + Arsenic trioxide (acute promyelocytic leukemia) [331]

ATRA:	45 mg/m^2 PO daily
Arsenic trioxide:	0.15 mg/kg/day IV starting on day 10

Continue treatment until CR [331]. Once in CR, patients receive the following:

ATRA:	45 mg/m^2 PO daily on weeks 1–2, 5–6, 9–10, 13–14, 17–18, 21–22, and 25–26

Arsenic trioxide: 0.15 mg/kg/day IV on Monday–Friday on
                                      weeks 1–4, 9–12, 17–20, and 25–28

Therapy should be terminated 28 weeks after the CR date.

Mitoxantrone + Etoposide (salvage regimen) [332]

Mitoxantrone: 10 mg/m^2/day IV on days 1–5

Etoposide: 100 mg/m^2/day IV on days 1–5

FLAG

Fludarabine: 30 mg/m^2 IV on days 1–5

Cytarabine: 2000 mg/m^2/day IV over 4 hours on
                                      days 1–5 starting 3.5 hours after
                                      fludarabine

G-CSF: 5 μg/kg/day SC starting 24 hours
                                      before chemotherapy

An additional cycle may be given in the setting of a partial response [333].

Consolidation Regimens

Ara-C + Daunorubicin (5 + 2) [334]

Cytarabine: 100 mg/m^2/day IV continuous infusion
                                      on days 1–5

Daunorubicin: 45 mg/m^2 IV on days 1 and 2

Ara-C + Idarubicin [335]

Cytarabine: 100 mg/m^2 IV continuous infusion on
                                      days 1–5

Idarubicin: 13 mg/m^2 IV on days 1 and 2

Repeat cycle every 21–28 days.

Single-Agent Regimens

Cladribine [336]

Cladribine: 0.1 mg/kg/day IV continuous infusion
                                      on days 1–7

High-Dose Cytarabine

Cytarabine: 1500–3000 mg/m^2 IV over 3 hours,
                                      every 12 hours on days 1, 3, and 5

Repeat cycle every 28 days [337].

Clofarabine

Clofarabine: 40 mg/m^2 IV on days 1–5
Repeat cycle every 3–6 weeks [338].

Tretinoin (acute promyelocytic leukemia only) [339]
Tretinoin: 45 mg/m^2 PO daily in 1–2 divided doses

Arsenic trioxide (acute promyelocytic leukemia only)
Arsenic trioxide: 0.15 mg/kg IV daily [340]

Continue until bone marrow remission up to a maximum of 60 doses. Patients who meet the criteria for clinical CR can receive an additional course of arsenic trioxide as consolidation beginning 3–4 weeks after completion of induction therapy up to a cumulative total of 25 doses [341].

Sorafenib
Sorafenib: 200–400 mg PO bid

Continue until disease progression or stem cell transplant [342].

Azacitidine
Azacitidine: 75 mg/m^2 SC daily for 7 days
Repeat cycle every 28 days for at least 6 cycles [343].

Decitabine
Decitabine: 20 mg/m^2 IV on days 1–5
Repeat cycle every 4 weeks [344].

CHRONIC LYMPHOCYTIC LEUKEMIA

Combination Regimens
CVP

Cyclophosphamide: 400 mg/m^2 PO on days 1–5 (or 800 mg/m^2 IV on day 1)

Vincristine: 1.4 mg/m^2 IV on day 1 (maximum dose, 2 mg)

Prednisone: 100 mg/m^2 PO on days 1–5
Repeat cycle every 21 days [345].

CF

Cyclophosphamide:	1000 mg/m^2 IV on day 1
Fludarabine:	20 mg/m^2 IV on days 1–5

Trimethoprim/sulfamethoxazole (Bactrim DS) 1 tablet PO bid
Repeat cycle every 21–28 days [346].

FP

Fludarabine:	30 mg/m^2 IV on days 1–5
Prednisone:	30 mg/m^2 IV on days 1–5

Repeat cycle every 28 days [347].

CP

Chlorambucil:	30 mg/m^2 PO on day 1
Prednisone:	80 mg PO on days 1–5

Repeat cycle every 28 days [345].

FR

Fludarabine:	25 mg/m^2 IV on days 1–5
Rituximab:	375 mg/m^2 IV on days 1 and 4 of cycle 1 and then on day 1 thereafter

Repeat cycle every 28 days for 6 cycles [348, 349].

FCR

Fludarabine:	25 mg/m^2 IV on days 1–3
Cyclophosphamide:	250 mg/m^2 IV on days 1–3
Rituximab:	375 mg/m^2 IV on day 1

Repeat cycle every 28 days for 6 cycles [350]. On cycles 2–6, rituximab is given at 500 mg/m^2.

PCR

Pentostatin:	2 mg/m^2 IV on day 1
Cyclophosphamide:	600 mg/m^2 IV on day 1
Rituximab:	375 mg/m^2 IV on day 1

Repeat cycle every 21 days [351].

Bendamustine + Rituximab

Bendamustine:	90 mg/m^2 IV on days 1 and 2
Rituximab:	375 mg/m^2 IV on day 0 of cycle 1, then 500 mg/m^2 IV on day 1 of cycles 2–6

Repeat cycle every 28 days for up to 6 cycles [352].

Idelasib + Rituximab [353]

Idelasib:	150 mg PO bid
Rituximab:	375 mg/m^2 IV on day 1, then 500 mg/m^2 IV every 2 weeks for 4 doses and then every 4 weeks for 3 doses for a total of 8 doses

Obinutuzumab + Chlorambucil

Obinutuzumab:	100 mg IV on day 1, cycle 1 900 mg IV on day 2, cycle1 1000 mg IV on days 8 and 15 of cycle 1 1000 mg IV on day 1 of cycles 2-6
Chlorambucil:	0.5 mg/kg PO on days 1 and 15

Repeat cycle every 28 days [354].

Single-Agent Regimens

Alemtuzumab

Alemtuzumab:	30 mg/day IV, 3 times per week

Repeat weekly for up to a maximum of 23 weeks [355]. Premedicate with diphenhydramine 50 mg PO and acetaminophen 625 mg PO 30 minutes before drug infusion. Patients should be placed on trimethoprim/sulfamethoxazole (Bactrim DS) PO bid and famciclovir 250 mg PO bid from day 8 through 2 months following completion of therapy.

Chlorambucil

Chlorambucil:	6–14 mg/day PO as induction therapy and then 0.7 mg/kg PO for 2–4 days

Repeat cycle every 21 days [356].

Cladribine

Cladribine:	0.09 mg/kg/day IV continuous infusion on days 1–7

Repeat cycle every 28–35 days [357].

Fludarabine

Fludarabine: 20–30 mg/m^2 IV on days 1–5
Repeat cycle every 28 days [358].

Prednisone

Prednisone: 20–30 mg/m^2/day PO for 1–3 weeks
                                      [358a].

Rituximab

Rituximab: 375 mg/m^2 IV weekly for 4 weeks
Repeat cycle every 6 months for a total of 4 courses [359].

Ofatumumab

Ofatumumab: 300 mg IV initial dose followed 1 week
                                      later by 2000 mg IV weekly dose for
                                      7 doses, followed 4 weeks later by 2000
                                      mg IV every 4 weeks for 4 doses.
A total of 12 doses is recommended [360]

Pentostatin

Pentostatin: 4 mg/m^2 IV on day 1
Repeat cycle every 14 days [361].

Bendamustine

Bendamustine: 100 mg/m^2 IV on days 1 and 2
Repeat cycle every 28 days for up to 6 cycles [362].
or
Bendamustine: 60 mg/m^2 IV on days 1–5
Repeat cycle every 28 days [363]. In patients >70 years, use dose of 50 mg/m^2.

Lenalidomide

Lenalidomide: 10 mg PO daily on days 1–28
Increase dose by 5 mg every 28 days up to a maximum of 25 mg daily until disease progression or toxicity [364].

Ibrutinib

Ibrutinib: 560 mg PO daily
Continue treatment until disease progression [365].

Venetoclax

Venetoclax:

20 mg/day PO on days 1-7
50 mg/day PO on days 8-14
100 mg/day PO on days 15-21
200 mg/day PO on days 22-28
and then 400 mg/day PO daily

Continue treatment until disease progression [366].

CHRONIC MYELOGENOUS LEUKEMIA

Combination Regimens

Interferon + Cytarabine

Interferon α-2b: 5 million U/m^2 SC daily

Cytarabine: 20 mg/m^2 SC daily for 10 days

Repeat cytarabine on a monthly basis [367]. The dose of interferon should be reduced by 50% when the neutrophil count drops below 1500/mm^3, the platelet count drops below 100,000/m^3, or both. Interferon and cytarabine should both be discontinued when the neutrophil count drops below 1000/mm^3, platelet count drops below 50,000/mm^3, or both.

Single-Agent Regimens

Imatinib

Imatinib: 400 mg/day PO (chronic phase);
                   600 mg/day PO (accelerated phase
                   blast crisis) [368]

Dasatinib

Dasatinib: 70 mg PO bid [369]
or
Dasatinib: 100 mg PO daily [370]

Nilotinib

Nilotinib: 400 mg PO bid [371]
or
Nilotinib: 300 mg PO bid [372]

Bosutinib

Bosutinib: 500 mg PO daily [373]

Ponatinib

Ponatinib: 45 mg PO bid [374]

Busulfan

Busulfan: 1.8 mg/m^2/day PO [375]

Hydroxyurea

Hydroxyurea: 1–5 g/day PO [376]

Interferon α-2α

Interferon α-2α: 9 million U/day SC [377]

Omacetaxine

Omacetaxine: 1.25 mg/m^2 SC bid on days 1–14 for
                                      first cycle and induction phase followed
                                      by 1.25 mg/m^2 SC bid on days 1–7 as
                                      maintenance phase

Repeat cycle every 28 days [378].

HAIRY CELL LEUKEMIA

Single-Agent Regimens

Cladribine

Cladribine: 0.09 mg/kg/day IV continuous infusion
                                      on days 1–7

Administer one cycle [379].

Pentostatin

Pentostatin: 4 mg/m^2 IV on day 1

Repeat cycle every 14 days for 6 cycles [380].

Interferon α-2a

Interferon α-2a: 3 million U SC or IM, 3 times per week

Continue treatment for up to 1 to 1.5 years [381].

LUNG CANCER

Non–Small Cell Lung Cancer

Combined Modality Therapy

Cisplatin + Etoposide + Radiation Therapy

Cisplatin:	50 mg/m^2 IV on days 1, 8, 29, and 36
Etoposide:	50 mg/m^2 IV on days 1–5 and 29–33
Radiation therapy:	180 cGy/day for a total dose of 4500 cGy

Chemotherapy is given concurrently with radiation therapy [382].

Weekly Carboplatin + Paclitaxel + Radiation Therapy

Paclitaxel:	45 mg/m^2 IV weekly for 7 weeks
Carboplatin:	AUC of 2, IV weekly for 7 weeks
Radiation therapy:	200 cGy/day for a total dose of 6300 cGy over 7 weeks

Chemotherapy is given concurrently with radiation therapy [383]. Three to four weeks after the completion of chemoradiotherapy, 2 additional cycles of the following chemotherapy are given:

Paclitaxel:	200 mg/m^2 IV on day 1
Carboplatin:	AUC of 6, IV on day 1

Repeat cycle every 21 days for 2 cycles.

Adjuvant Therapy

Combination Regimens

Paclitaxel + Carboplatin

Paclitaxel:	175 mg/m^2 IV over 3 hours on day 1
Carboplatin:	AUC of 6, IV on day 1

Repeat cycle every 21 days for 4 cycles [384].

Vinorelbine + Cisplatin

Vinorelbine:	25 mg/m^2 IV weekly for 16 weeks
Cisplatin:	50 mg/m^2 IV on days 1 and 8

Repeat cycle every 28 days for 4 cycles [385].

Cisplatin + Vinblastine

Cisplatin:	100 mg/m^2 IV on day 1

| Vinblastine: | 4 mg/m^2 IV on days 1, 8, 15, 22, and 29, then every 2 weeks after day 43 |

Repeat cycle every 28 days for 4 cycles [386].

Etoposide + Cisplatin

| Etoposide: | 100 mg/m^2 IV on days 1–3 |
| Cisplatin: | 100 mg/m^2 IV on day 1 |

Repeat cycle every 28 days for 4 cycles [386].

Pemetrexed + Cisplatin

| Pemetrexed: | 500 mg/m^2 IV on day 1 |
| Cisplatin: | 80 mg/m^2 IV on day 1 |

Repeat cycle every 21 days for 6 cycles [387]. Folic acid at 350–1000 μg PO q day beginning 1 week prior to therapy and vitamin B12 at 1000 μg IM beginning 1–2 weeks prior to first dose of therapy and repeated every 9 weeks. Dexamethasone at 4 mg PO bid on the day before, the day of, and the day after pemetrexed.

Metastatic Disease

Combination Regimens

Carboplatin + Paclitaxel (PC)

| Carboplatin: | AUC of 6, IV on day 1 |
| Paclitaxel: | 200 mg/m^2 IV over 3 hours on day 1 |

Repeat cycle every 21 days [388].

Carboplatin + Nab-Paclitaxel

| Carboplatin: | AUC of 6, IV on day 1 |
| Nab-Paclitaxel: | 100 mg/m^2 IV weekly on days 1, 8, and 15 |

Repeat cycle every 21 days [389].

Carboplatin + Paclitaxel (weekly regimen)

| Carboplatin: | AUC of 6, IV on day 1 |
| Paclitaxel: | 100 mg/m^2 IV weekly for 3 weeks |

Repeat cycle every 4 weeks up to 4 cycles [390]. If response or stable disease, may then treat with maintenance chemotherapy of:

| Paclitaxel: | 70 mg/m^2 IV weekly for 3 weeks |

Continue until disease progression.

Carboplatin + Paclitaxel + Bevacizumab (PCB)

Carboplatin:	AUC of 6, IV on day 1
Paclitaxel:	200 mg/m^2 IV on day 1
Bevacizumab:	15 mg/kg IV on day 1

Repeat cycle every 21 days [388].

Gemcitabine + Cisplatin + Bevacizumab (GCB)

Gemcitabine:	1250 mg/m^2 IV on days 1 and 8
Cisplatin:	80 mg/m^2 IV on day 1
Bevacizumab:	7.5 or 15 mg/kg IV on day 1

Repeat cycle every 21 days for a total of 6 cycles [391].

Cisplatin + Paclitaxel

Cisplatin:	80 mg/m^2 IV on day 1
Paclitaxel:	175 mg/m^2 IV over 3 hours on day 1

Repeat cycle every 21 days [392].

Docetaxel + Carboplatin

Docetaxel:	75 mg/m^2 IV on day 1
Carboplatin:	AUC of 6, IV on day 1

Repeat cycle every 21 days [393].

Docetaxel + Cisplatin

Docetaxel:	75 mg/m^2 IV on day 1
Cisplatin:	75 mg/m^2 IV on day 1

Repeat cycle every 21 days [394].

Docetaxel + Gemcitabine

Docetaxel:	100 mg/m^2 IV on day 8
Gemcitabine:	1100 mg/m^2 IV on days 1 and 8

Repeat cycle every 21 days [395]. G-CSF support is required from day 9 to day 15.

Gemcitabine + Cisplatin

Gemcitabine:	1000 mg/m^2 IV on days 1, 8, and 15
Cisplatin:	100 mg/m^2 IV on day 1

Repeat cycle every 21 days [396].

Gemcitabine + Carboplatin

Gemcitabine: 1000 mg/m^2 IV on days 1 and 8

Carboplatin: AUC of 5, IV on day 1

Repeat cycle every 21 days [397].

Gemcitabine + Vinorelbine

Gemcitabine: 1200 mg/m^2 IV on days 1 and 8

Vinorelbine: 30 mg/m^2 IV on days 1 and 8

Repeat cycle every 21 days [398].

Vinorelbine + Cisplatin

Vinorelbine: 30 mg/m^2 IV on days 1, 8, and 15

Cisplatin: 120 mg/m^2 IV on day 1

Repeat cycle every 28 days [399].

Vinorelbine + Cisplatin + Cetuximab

Vinorelbine: 25 mg/m^2 IV on days 1 and 8

Cisplatin: 80 mg/m^2 IV on day 1

Cetuximab: 400 mg/m^2 IV loading dose, then
                250 mg/m^2 IV weekly

Repeat cycle every 3 weeks up to 6 cycles [400].

Vinorelbine + Carboplatin

Vinorelbine: 25 mg/m^2 IV on days 1 and 8

Carboplatin: AUC of 6, IV on day 1

Repeat cycle every 28 days [401].

Pemetrexed + Cisplatin

Pemetrexed: 500 mg/m^2 IV on day 1

Cisplatin: 75 mg/m^2 IV on day 1

Repeat cycle every 21 days up to 6 cycles [402]. Folic acid at 350–1000 μg PO q day beginning 1 week prior to therapy and vitamin B12 at 1000 μg IM beginning 1–2 weeks prior to first dose of therapy and repeated every 9 weeks. Dexamethasone at 4 mg PO bid on the day before, the day of, and the day after pemetrexed.

Pemetrexed + Carboplatin

Pemetrexed: 500 mg/m^2 IV on day 1

Carboplatin: AUC of 5, IV on day 1

Repeat cycle every 21 days up to 4 cycles [403]. Folic acid at 350–1000 μg PO q day beginning 1 week prior to therapy and vitamin B12 at 1000 μg IM beginning 1–2 weeks prior to first dose of therapy and repeated every 9 weeks. Dexamethasone at 4 mg PO bid on the day before, the day of, and the day after pemetrexed.

EP

Etoposide: 120 mg/m^2 IV on days 1–3

Cisplatin: 60 mg/m^2 IV on day 1

Repeat cycle every 21–28 days [404].

EP + Docetaxel

Cisplatin: 50 mg/m^2 IV on days 1, 8, 29, and 36

Etoposide: 50 mg/m^2 IV on days 1–5 and 29–33

Administer concurrent thoracic radiotherapy, followed 4–6 weeks after the completion of combined modality therapy by

Docetaxel: 75 mg/m^2 IV on day 1

Repeat cycle every 21 days for 3 cycles [405]. Dose of docetaxel can be escalated to 100 mg/m^2 IV on subsequent cycles in the absence of toxicity.

Docetaxel + Bevacizumab

Docetaxel: 75 mg/m^2 IV on day 1

Bevacizumab: 15 mg/kg IV on day 1

Repeat cycle every 21 days [406].

Pemetrexed + Carboplatin + Bevacizumab

Pemetrexed: 500 mg/m^2 IV on day 1

Carboplatin: AUC of 6, IV on day 1

Bevacizumab: 15 mg/kg IV on day 1

Repeat cycle every 21 days up to 6 cycles [407]. Folic acid at 350–1000 μg PO q day beginning 1 week prior to therapy and vitamin B12 at 1000 μg IM beginning 1–2 weeks prior to first dose of therapy and repeated every 9 weeks. Dexamethasone at 4 mg PO bid on the day before, the day of, and the day after pemetrexed.

Cisplatin + Vinorelbine + Cetuximab

Cisplatin: 80 mg/m^2 IV on day 1

Vinorelbine: 25 mg/m^2 IV continuous on days 1 and 8

Cetuximab: 400 mg/m^2 IV loading dose, then 250 mg/m^2 IV weekly

Repeat cycle every 21 days up to 6 cycles [408].

Platinum-Based Chemotherapy + Maintenance Pemetrexed (non-squamous histology)

Platinum-based chemotherapy × 4 cycles, followed by:

Pemetrexed: 500 mg/m^2 IV on day 1

Repeat cycle every 21 days up to 6 cycles [409]. Folic acid at 350–1000 μg PO q day beginning 1 week prior to therapy and vitamin B12 at 1000 μg IM beginning 1–2 weeks prior to first dose of therapy and repeated every 9 weeks. Dexamethasone at 4 mg PO bid on the day before, the day of, and the day after pemetrexed.

Nab-Paclitaxel + Carboplatin

Nab-Paclitaxel: 100 mg/m^2 IV on days 1, 8, and 15

Carboplatin: AUC of 6, IV on day 1

Repeat cycle every 21 days [410].

Docetaxel + Ramucirumab

Docetaxel: 75 mg/m^2 IV on day 1

Ramucirumab: 10 mg/kg IV on day 1

Repeat cycle every 21 days [411].

Gemcitibine + Cisplatin + Necitumumab

Gemcitabine: 1250 mg/m^2 IV on days 1 and 8

Cisplatin: 75 mg/m^2 IV on day 1

Necitumumab: 800 mg IV on days 1 and 8

Repeat cycle every 21 days [411a].

Single-Agent Regimens

Paclitaxel

Paclitaxel: 225 mg/m^2 IV over 3 hours on day 1

Repeat cycle every 21 days [412].

or

Paclitaxel: 80–100 mg/m^2 IV weekly for 3 weeks

Repeat cycle every 28 days after 1-week rest [413].

Nab-Paclitaxel

Nab-Paclitaxel: 125 mg/m^2 IV on days 1, 8, and 15

Repeat cycle every 28 days [414].

Docetaxel

Docetaxel: 75 mg/m^2 IV on day 1

Repeat cycle every 21 days [415].

or

Docetaxel: 36 mg/m^2 IV weekly for 6 weeks

Repeat cycle every 8 weeks after 2-week rest [416]. Premedicate with dexameth-asone 8 mg PO at 12 hours and immediately before docetaxel infusion and 12 hours after each dose.

Pemetrexed

Pemetrexed: 500 mg/m^2 IV on day 1

Repeat cycle every 21 days [417]. Folic acid at 350–1000 μg PO q day beginning 1 week prior to therapy and vitamin B12 at 1000 μg IM beginning 1–2 weeks prior to first dose of therapy and repeated every 3 cycles.

Gemcitabine

Gemcitabine: 1000 mg/m^2 IV on days 1, 8, and 15

Repeat cycle every 28 days [418].

Vinorelbine

Vinorelbine: 25 mg/m^2 IV on day 1

Repeat cycle every 7 days [418a].

Gefitinib

Gefitinib: 250 mg/day PO

Continue treatment until disease progression [419].

Erlotinib

Erlotinib: 150 mg/day PO

Continue treatment until disease progression [420].

Afatinib

Afatinib: 40 mg/day PO

Continue treatment until disease progression [421].

Sunitinib

Sunitinib: 50 mg/day PO for 4 weeks

Repeat cycle every 6 weeks [422].

Cetuximab

Cetuximab: 400 mg/m^2 IV loading dose, then
250 mg/m^2 IV weekly

Repeat cycle every week [423].

Nivolumab

Nivolumab: 240 mg IV on day 1

Repeat cycle every 2 weeks [424].

Crizotinib

Crizotinib: 250 mg PO bid

Continue treatment until disease progression [425].

Ceritinib

Ceritinib: 750 mg/day PO

Continue treatment until disease progression [426].

Alectinib

Alectinib: 600 mg PO bid

Continue treatment until disease progression [427].

Osimertinib

Osimertinib: 80 mg/day PO

Continue treatment until disease progression [428].

Pembrolizumab

Pembrolizumab: 200 mg IV on day 1

Repeat cycle every 3 weeks [429].

SMALL CELL LUNG CANCER

Combination Regimens

EP

Etoposide: 80 mg/m^2 IV on days 1–3
Cisplatin: 80 mg/m^2 IV on day 1

Repeat cycle every 21 days [430].

EC

Etoposide:	100 mg/m^2 IV on days 1–3
Carboplatin:	AUC of 6, IV on day 1

Repeat cycle every 28 days [431].

Irinotecan + Cisplatin

Irinotecan:	60 mg/m^2 IV on days 1, 8, and 15
Cisplatin:	60 mg/m^2 IV on day 1

Repeat cycle every 28 days [432].

Topotecan + Cisplatin

Topotecan:	1.7 mg/m^2/day PO on days 1–5
Cisplatin:	60 mg/m^2 IV on day 5

Repeat cycle every 21 days up to 4 cycles or 2 cycles beyond best response [433].

Carboplatin + Paclitaxel + Etoposide

Carboplatin:	AUC of 6, IV on day 1
Paclitaxel:	200 mg/m^2 IV over 1 hour on day 1
Etoposide:	50 mg alternating with 100 mg PO on days 1–10

Repeat cycle every 21 days [434].

Carboplatin + Paclitaxel

Carboplatin:	AUC of 2, IV on days 1, 8, and 15
Paclitaxel:	80 mg/m^2 IV on days 1, 8, and 15

Repeat cycle every 28 days for 6 cycles [435].

CAV

Cyclophosphamide:	1000 mg/m^2 IV on day 1
Doxorubicin:	40 mg/m^2 IV on day 1
Vincristine:	1 mg/m^2 IV on day 1 (maximum, 2 mg)

Repeat cycle every 21 days [436].

CAE

Cyclophosphamide:	1000 mg/m^2 IV on day 1
Doxorubicin:	45 mg/m^2 IV on day 1

Etoposide: 50 mg/m^2 IV on days 1–5
Repeat cycle every 21 days [437].

Single-Agent Regimens

Etoposide

Etoposide: 160 mg/m^2 PO on days 1–5
Repeat cycle every 28 days [438].

or

Etoposide: 50 mg/m^2/day PO on days 1–21
Repeat cycle as tolerated [439].

Paclitaxel

Paclitaxel: 80–100 mg/m^2 IV weekly for 3 weeks
Repeat cycle every 28 days [440].

Topotecan

Topotecan: 1.5 mg/m^2 IV on days 1–5
Repeat cycle every 21 days [441].

Gemcitabine

Gemcitabine: 1000 mg/m^2 PO on days 1, 8, and 15
Repeat cycle every 28 days [442].

LYMPHOMA

HODGKIN'S LYMPHOMA

Combination Regimens

ABVD

Doxorubicin: 25 mg/m^2 IV on days 1 and 15
Bleomycin: 10 U/m^2 IV on days 1 and 15
Vinblastine: 6 mg/m^2 IV on days 1 and 15
Dacarbazine: 375 mg/m^2 IV on days 1 and 15
Repeat cycle every 28 days [443].

MOPP

Nitrogen mustard:	6 mg/m^2 IV on days 1 and 8
Vincristine:	1.4 mg/m^2 IV on days 1 and 8
Procarbazine:	100 mg/m^2 PO on days 1–14
Prednisone:	40 mg/m^2 PO on days 1–14

Repeat cycle every 28 days [444].

MOPP/ABVD Hybrid

Nitrogen mustard:	6 mg/m^2 IV on days 1 and 8
Vincristine:	1.4 mg/m^2 IV on day 1 (maximum dose, 2 mg)
Procarbazine:	100 mg/m^2 PO on days 1–14
Prednisone:	40 mg/m^2 PO on days 1–14
Doxorubicin:	35 mg/m^2 IV on day 8
Bleomycin:	10 U/m^2 IV on day 8
Hydrocortisone:	100 mg IV given before bleomycin
Vinblastine:	6 mg/m^2 IV on day 8

Repeat cycle every 28 days [445].

MOPP Alternating with ABVD

See MOPP and ABVD regimens outlined above.

Stanford V

Nitrogen mustard:	6 mg/m^2 IV on day 1
Doxorubicin:	25 mg/m^2 IV on days 1 and 15
Vinblastine:	6 mg/m^2 IV on days 1 and 15
Vincristine:	1.4 mg/m^2 IV on days 8 and 22
Bleomycin:	5 U/m^2 IV on days 8 and 22
Etoposide:	60 mg/m^2 IV on days 15 and 16
Prednisone:	40 mg PO every other day

Repeat cycle every 28 days [446]. In patients >50 years of age, vinblastine dose reduced to 4 mg/m^2 and vincristine dose reduced to 1 mg/m^2 on weeks 9 and 12. Dose of prednisone tapered starting on week 10. Patient should be placed on prophylactic trimethoprim/sulfamethoxazole (Bactrim DS) PO bid and acyclovir 200 mg PO tid.

EVA

Etoposide:	100 mg/m^2 IV on days 1–3
Vinblastine:	6 mg/m^2 IV on day 1
Doxorubicin:	50 mg/m^2 IV on day 1

Repeat cycle every 28 days for up to 6 cycles [447].

EVAP

Etoposide:	120 mg/m^2 IV on days 1, 8, and 15
Vinblastine:	4 mg/m^2 IV on days 1, 8, and 15
Cytarabine:	30 mg/m^2 IV on days 1, 8, and 15
Cisplatin:	40 mg/m^2 IV on days 1, 8, and 15

Repeat cycle every 28 days [448].

Mini-BEAM

Carmustine:	60 mg/m^2 IV on day 1
Etoposide:	75 mg/m^2 IV on days 2–5
Ara-C:	100 mg/m^2 IV every 12 hours on days 2–5
Melphalan:	30 mg/m^2 IV on day 6

Repeat cycle every 4–6 weeks [449].

BEACOPP

Bleomycin:	10 mg/m^2 IV on day 8
Etoposide:	100 mg/m^2 IV on days 1–3
Doxorubicin:	25 mg/m^2 IV on day 1
Cyclophosphamide:	650 mg/m^2 IV on day 1
Vincristine:	1.4 mg/m^2 IV on day 8 (maximum, 2 mg)
Procarbazine:	100 mg/m^2 PO on days 1–7
Prednisone:	40 mg/m^2 PO on days 1–14

Repeat cycle every 21 days [450].

BEACOPP Escalated

Bleomycin:	10 mg/m^2 IV on day 8
Etoposide:	200 mg/m^2 IV on days 1–3
Doxorubicin:	35 mg/m^2 IV on day 1
Cyclophosphamide:	1200 mg/m^2 IV on day 1

Vincristine:	1.4 mg/m^2 IV on day 8 (maximum dose, 2 mg)
Procarbazine:	100 mg/m^2 PO on days 1–7
Prednisone:	40 mg/m^2 PO on days 1–14

Repeat cycle every 21 days [451]. G-CSF support, at dose of 5 μg/kg/day SC, starting on day 8 and continue until neutrophil recovery.

GVD

For transplant-naïve patients:

Gemcitabine:	1000 mg/m^2 IV on days 1 and 8
Vinorelbine:	20 mg/m^2 IV on days 1 and 8
Doxil:	15 mg/m^2 IV on days 1 and 8

Repeat cycle every 21 days [452].

or

For post-transplant patients:

Gemcitabine:	800 mg/m^2 IV on days 1 and 8
Vinorelbine:	15 mg/m^2 IV on days 1 and 8
Doxil:	10 mg/m^2 IV on days 1 and 8

Repeat cycle every 21 days [452].

Single-Agent Regimens

Gemcitabine

| Gemcitabine: | 1250 mg/m^2 IV on days 1, 8, and 15 |

Repeat cycle every 28 days [453].

Rituximab

| Rituximab: | 375 mg/m^2 IV on day 1 |

Repeat weekly for 4 weeks [454].

Brentuximab

| Brentuximab: | 1.8 mg/kg IV on day 1 |

Repeat cycle every 3 weeks for up to 16 cycles [455].

Nivolumab

| Nivolumab: | 3 mg/kg IV on day 1 |

Repeat cycle every 2 weeks [456].

Non-Hodgkin's Lymphoma

Low-Grade

Combination Regimens

CVP

Cyclophosphamide:	400 mg/m^2 PO on days 1–5 (or 800 mg/m^2 IV on day 1)
Vincristine:	1.4 mg/m^2 IV on day 1 (maximum, 2 mg)
Prednisone:	100 mg/m^2 PO on days 1–5

Repeat cycle every 21 days [457].

CHOP

Cyclophosphamide:	750 mg/m^2 IV on day 1
Doxorubicin:	50 mg/m^2 IV on day 1
Vincristine:	1.4 mg/m^2 IV on day 1 (maximum, 2 mg)
Prednisone:	100 mg/m^2 PO on days 1–5

Repeat cycle every 21 days [458].

CNOP

Cyclophosphamide:	750 mg/m^2 IV on day 1
Mitoxantrone:	10 mg/m^2 IV on day 1
Vincristine:	1.4 mg/m^2 IV on day 1 (maximum, 2 mg)
Prednisone:	50 mg/m^2 PO on days 1–5

Repeat cycle every 21 days [459].

FND

Fludarabine:	25 mg/m^2 IV on days 1–3
Mitoxantrone:	10 mg/m^2 IV on day 1
Dexamethasone:	20 mg PO on days 1–5
Trimethoprim/sulfamethoxazole (Bactrim DS):	1 tablet PO bid, 3 times per week

Repeat cycle every 21 days [460].

FC

Fludarabine:	20 mg/m^2 IV on days 1–5
Cyclophosphamide:	1000 mg/m^2 IV on day 1

Trimethoprim/sulfamethoxazole (Bactrim DS): 1 tablet PO bid

Repeat cycle every 21–28 days [461].

FCR

Fludarabine:	25 mg/m^2 IV on days 1–3
Cyclophosphamide:	300 mg/m^2 IV on days 1–3
Rituximab:	375 mg/m^2 IV on day 1

Repeat cycle every 21 days for 4 cycles [462].

R-CHOP

Cyclophosphamide:	750 mg/m^2 IV on day 1
Doxorubicin:	50 mg/m^2 IV on day 1
Vincristine:	1.4 mg/m^2 IV on day 1 (maximum, 2 mg)
Prednisone:	100 mg/day PO on days 1–5

Repeat cycle every 21 days up to 6 cycles [463]. Patients who experience a response to therapy can then receive maintenance therapy with

Rituximab:	375 mg/m^2 IV on day 1

Repeat cycle every 3 months up to a maximum of 2 years.

R-FCM

Rituximab:	375 mg/m^2 IV on day 0
Fludarabine:	25 mg/m^2 IV on days 1–3
Cyclophosphamide:	200 mg/m^2 IV on days 1–3
Mitoxantrone:	8 mg/m^2 IV on day 1

Repeat cycle every 4 weeks for a total of 4 cycles [464]. Patients who experience a response can then receive maintenance therapy at 3 and 9 months after completion of therapy with

Rituximab:	375 mg/m^2 IV weekly for 4 weeks

Bendamustine + Rituximab

Bendamustine:	90 mg/m^2 IV on days 1 and 2
Rituximab:	375 mg/m^2 IV on day 1

Repeat cycle every 28 days for 4 cycles [465].

or

Rituximab:	375 mg/m^2 IV on day 1
Bendamustine:	90 mg/m^2 IV on days 2 and 3

Repeat cycle every 28 days for 4–6 cycles [466]. An additional dose of rituximab is administered 1 week prior to the first cycle and 4 weeks after the last cycle.

Bortezomib (mantle cell lymphoma)

Bortezomib: 1.3 mg/m² IV or SC on days 1, 4, 8, and 11
Repeat cycle every 21 days for up to 17 cycles [467].

Ibrutinib (mantle cell lymphoma)

Ibrutinib: 560 mg/day PO
Continue treatment until disease progression [468].

Bendamustine + Obinutuzumab

Bendamustine: 90 mg/m² IV on days 1 and 2
Obinutuzumab: 1000 mg IV on days 1, 8, and 15
First cycle is administered over 28 days followed by
Bendamustine: 90 mg/m² IV on days 1 and 2
Obinutuzumab: 1000 mg IV on day 1
Repeat cycle every 28 days for a total of 5 cycles [469].

Intermediate-Grade

CHOP

Cyclophosphamide: 750 mg/m² IV on day 1
Doxorubicin: 50 mg/m² IV on day 1
Vincristine: 1.4 mg/m² IV on day 1 (maximum, 2 mg)
Prednisone: 100 mg PO on days 1–5
Repeat cycle every 21 days [470].

CHOP + Rituximab

Cyclophosphamide: 750 mg/m² IV on day 1
Doxorubicin: 50 mg/m² IV on day 1
Vincristine: 1.4 mg/m² IV on day 1 (maximum, 2 mg)
Prednisone: 40 mg/m² PO on days 1–5
Rituximab: 375 mg/m² IV on day 1
Repeat cycle every 21 days [471]. Rituximab is to be administered first, followed by cyclophosphamide, doxorubicin, and vincristine.

or

R-CHOP-14

Cyclophosphamide: 750 mg/m² IV on day 1
Doxorubicin: 50 mg/m² IV on day 1

Vincristine:	1.4 mg/m^2 IV on day 1 (maximum, 2 mg)
Prednisone:	100 mg/day PO on days 1–5
Rituximab:	375 mg/m^2 IV on day 1

Repeat cycle every 2 weeks up to 6 cycles [472]. G-CSF support to start on day 4 of each cycle.

CNOP

Cyclophosphamide:	750 mg/m^2 IV on day 1
Mitoxantrone:	10 mg/m^2 IV on day 1
Vincristine:	1.4 mg/m^2 IV on day 1 (maximum, 2 mg)
Prednisone:	100 mg PO on days 1–5

Repeat cycle every 21 days [473].

EPOCH

Etoposide:	50 mg/m^2/day IV continuous infusion on days 1–4
Prednisone:	60 mg/m^2 PO on days 1–5
Vincristine:	0.4 mg/m^2/day IV continuous infusion on days 1–4
Cyclophosphamide:	750 mg/m^2 IV on day 5, begin after infusion
Doxorubicin:	10 mg/m^2/day IV continuous infusion on days 1–4
Trimethoprim/sulfamethoxazole (Bactrim DS):	1 tablet PO bid, 3 times per week

Repeat cycle every 21 days [474].

EPOCH + Rituximab

Etoposide:	50 mg/m^2/day IV continuous infusion on days 1–4
Prednisone:	60 mg/m^2 PO bid on days 1–5
Vincristine:	0.4 mg/m^2/day IV continuous infusion on days 1–4
Cyclophosphamide:	750 mg/m^2 IV on day 5, begin after infusion
Doxorubicin:	10 mg/m^2/day IV continuous infusion on days 1–4

Rituximab: 375 mg/m^2 IV on day 1

Repeat cycle every 21 days [475]. Rituximab is to be administered first followed by infusions of etoposide, doxorubicin, and vincristine. Prophylaxis with tri-methoprim/sulfamethoxazole (Bactrim DS) 1 tablet PO bid, 3 times per week to reduce the risk of *Pneumocystis carinii* infection.

MACOP-B

Methotrexate: 400 mg/m^2 IV on weeks 2, 6, and 10

Leucovorin: 15 mg/m^2 PO every 6 hours for 6 doses, beginning 24 hours after methotrexate

Doxorubicin: 50 mg/m^2 IV on weeks 1, 3, 5, 7, 9, and 11

Cyclophosphamide: 350 mg/m^2 IV on weeks 1, 3, 5, 7, 9, and 11

Vincristine: 1.4 mg/m^2 IV on weeks 2, 4, 6, 8, 10, and 12

Prednisone: 75 mg/day PO for 12 weeks with taper over the last 2 weeks

Bleomycin: 10 U/m^2 IV on weeks 4, 8, and 12

Bactrim DS: 1 tablet PO bid

Ketoconazole: 200 mg/day PO

Administer one cycle [476].

m-BACOD

Methotrexate: 200 mg/m^2 IV on days 8 and 15

Leucovorin: 10 mg/m^2 PO every 6 hours for 8 doses, beginning 24 hours after methotrexate

Bleomycin: 4 U/m^2 IV on day 1

Doxorubicin: 45 mg/m^2 IV on day 1

Cyclophosphamide: 600 mg/m^2 IV on day 1

Vincristine: 1 mg/m^2 IV on day 1 (maximum, 2 mg)

Dexamethasone: 6 mg/m^2 PO on days 1–5

Repeat cycle every 21 days [477].

ProMACE/CytaBOM

Prednisone: 60 mg/m^2 PO on days 1–14

Doxorubicin: 25 mg/m^2 IV on day 1

Cyclophosphamide: 650 mg/m^2 IV on day 1

Etoposide: 120 mg/m^2 IV on day 1

Cytarabine:	300 mg/m^2 IV on day 8
Bleomycin:	5 U/m^2 IV on day 8
Vincristine:	1.4 mg/m^2 IV on day 8
Methotrexate:	120 mg/m^2 IV on day 8
Leucovorin rescue:	25 mg/m^2 PO every 6 hours for 6 doses, beginning 24 hours after methotrexate
Trimethoprim/sulfamethoxazole	1 tablet PO bid on days 1–21

Repeat cycle every 21 days [478].

ESHAP (salvage regimen)

Etoposide:	40 mg/m^2 IV on days 1–4
Methylprednisolone:	500 mg IV on days 1–4
Cisplatin:	25 mg/m^2/day IV continuous infusion on days 1–4
Cytarabine:	2000 mg/m^2 IV on day 5 after completion of cisplatin and etoposide

Repeat cycle every 21 days [479].

DHAP (salvage regimen)

Cisplatin:	100 mg/m^2 IV continuous infusion over 24 hours on day 1
Cytarabine:	2000 mg/m^2 IV over 3 hours every 12 hours for 2 doses on day 2 after completion of cisplatin infusion
Dexamethasone:	40 mg PO or IV on days 1–4

Repeat cycle every 3–4 weeks [480].

ICE (salvage regimen)

Ifosfamide:	5000 mg/m^2 IV continuous infusion for 24 hours on day 2
Etoposide:	100 mg/m^2 IV on days 1–3
Carboplatin:	AUC of 5, IV on day 2
Mesna:	5000 mg/m^2 IV in combination with ifosfamide dose

Repeat cycle every 14 days [481]. G-CSF support is administered at 5 μg/kg/day on days 5–12.

RICE (salvage regimen)

Rituximab:	375 mg/m^2 IV on day 1
Ifosfamide:	5000 mg/m^2 IV continuous infusion for 24 hours on day 4
Etoposide:	100 mg/m^2 IV on days 3–5
Carboplatin:	AUC of 5, IV on day 4
Mesna:	5000 mg/m^2 IV in combination with ifosfamide dose

Repeat cycle every 14 days [482]. Rituximab is also given at 48 hours before the start of the first cycle. G-CSF is administered at 5 μg/kg/day SC on days 7–14 after the first 2 cycles and at 10 μg/kg/day SC after the third cycle.

MINE (salvage regimen)

Mesna:	1330 mg/m^2 IV administered at same time as ifosfamide on days 1–3, then 500 mg IV 4 hours after ifosfamide on days 1–3
Ifosfamide:	1330 mg/m^2 IV on days 1–3
Mitoxantrone:	8 mg/m^2 IV on day 1
Etoposide:	65 mg/m^2 IV on days 1–3

Repeat cycle every 21 days [483].

R-GemOx (salvage regimen)

Rituximab:	375 mg/m^2 IV on day 1
Gemcitabine:	1000 mg/m^2 IV on day 2
Oxaliplatin:	50 mg/m^2 IV on day 2

Repeat cycle every 2 weeks for a total of 8 cycles [484].

High-Grade

Magrath Protocol (Burkitt's lymphoma)

Cyclophosphamide:	1200 mg/m^2 IV on day 1
Doxorubicin:	40 mg/m^2 IV on day 1
Vincristine:	1.4 mg/m^2 IV on day 1 (maximum, 2 mg)
Prednisone:	40 mg/m^2 PO on days 1–5
Methotrexate:	300 mg/m^2 IV on day 10 for 1 hour, then 60 mg/m^2 IV on days 10 and 11 for 41 hours
Leucovorin rescue:	15 mg/m^2 IV every 6 hours for 8 doses, starting 24 hours after methotrexate on day 12

| Intrathecal ara-C: | 30 mg/m^2 IT on day 7, cycle 1 only; 45 mg/m^2 IT on day 7, all subsequent cycles |
| Intrathecal methotrexate: | 12.5 mg IT on day 10, all cycles |

Repeat cycle every 28 days [485].

or

Regimen A (CODOX-M) [486]

Cyclophosphamide:	800 mg/m^2 IV on day 1 and 200 mg/m^2 IV on days 2–5
Doxorubicin:	40 mg/m^2 IV on day 1
Vincristine:	1.5 mg/m^2 IV on days 1 and 8 in cycle 1 and on days 1, 8, and 15 in cycle 3
Methotrexate:	1200 mg/m^2 IV over 1 hour, followed by 240 mg/m^2/hour for the next 23 hours on day 10
Leucovorin:	192 mg/m^2 IV starting at hour 36 after the start of the infusion and 12 mg/m^2 IV every 6 hours thereafter until serum methotrexate levels <50 nM

CNS Prophylaxis

| Cytarabine: | 70 mg IT on days 1 and 3 |
| Methotrexate: | 12 mg IT on day 15 |

Regimen B (IVAC)

Ifosfamide:	1500 mg/m^2 IV on days 1–5
Etoposide:	60 mg/m^2 IV on days 1–5
Cytarabine:	2 g/m^2 IV every 12 hours on days 1 and 2 for a total of 4 doses
Methotrexate:	12 mg IT on day 5

Stanford Regimen (small noncleaved cell and Burkitt's lymphoma)

Cyclophosphamide:	1200 mg/m^2 IV on day 1
Doxorubicin:	40 mg/m^2 IV on day 1
Vincristine:	1.4 mg/m^2 IV on day 1 (maximum, 2 mg)
Prednisone:	40 mg/m^2 PO on days 1–5
Methotrexate:	3 g/m^2 IV over 6 hours on day 10

Leucovorin rescue:	25 mg/m² IV or PO every 6 hours for 12 doses, beginning 24 hours after methotrexate
Intrathecal methotrexate:	12 mg IT on days 1 and 10

Repeat cycle every 21 days [487].

Hyper-CVAD/Methotrexate-Ara-C

Cyclophosphamide:	300 mg/m² IV every 12 hours for 6 doses on days 1–3
Mesna:	600 mg/m²/day continuous infusion on days 1–3 to start 1 hour before cyclophosphamide until 12 hours after completion of cyclophosphamide
Vincristine:	2 mg IV on days 4 and 11
Doxorubicin:	50 mg/m² IV over 24 hours on day 4
Dexamethasone:	40 mg PO or IV on days 1–4 and days 11–14

Administer every 3–4 weeks on cycles 1, 3, 5, and 7 [488].

Methotrexate:	200 mg/m² IV over 2 hours followed by 800 mg/m² continuous infusion over 22 hours on day 1
Cytarabine:	3000 mg/m² IV over 2 hours every 12 hours for 4 doses on days 2–3 (1 g/m² for patients >60 years old)
Leucovorin:	50 mg IV every 6 hours starting 12 hours after completion of methotrexate until methotrexate level <50 nM

Administer every 3–4 weeks on cycles 2, 4, 6, and 8

Intrathecal Chemotherapy Prophylaxis:	
Methotrexate:	12 mg IT on day 2 of each cycle for a total of 3–4 treatments
Cytarabine:	100 mg IT on day 8 of each cycle for a total of 3–4 treatments
Intrathecal Chemotherapy:	Administer intrathecal chemotherapy twice a week with methotrexate 12 mg and cytarabine 100 mg, respectively, until no more cancer cells in CSF, then decrease intrathecal chemotherapy to once a week for 4 weeks, followed by methotrexate 12 mg on day 2 and cytarabine 100 mg on day 8 for the remaining chemotherapy cycles.

Single-Agent Regimens

Rituximab

Rituximab: 375 mg/m^2 IV on days 1, 8, 15, and 22
Repeat one additional cycle [489].
or
Rituximab: 375 mg/m^2 IV on days 1, 8, 15, and 22
followed by 375 mg/m^2 IV at week 12 and
at months 5, 7, and 9 [489a]

Ibritumomab Tiuxetan Regimen

Rituximab: 250 mg/m^2 IV on days 1 and 8
^{111}In-Ibritumomab tiuxetan: 5 mCi of ^{111}In, 1.6 mg of ibritumomab
tiuxetan IV on day 1
^{90}Y-Ibritumomab tiuxetan: 0.4 mCi/kg IV over 10 min on day 8 after
the day 8 rituximab dose

The dose of ^{90}Y-ibritumomab tiuxetan is capped at 32 mCi [490].

Fludarabine

Fludarabine: 25 mg/m^2 IV on days 1–5
Repeat cycle every 28 days [491]

Cladribine

Cladribine: 0.5–0.7 mg/kg SC on days 1–5 or 0.1 mg/kg
IV on days 1–7
Repeat cycle every 28 days [492].

Bendamustine

Bendamustine: 120 mg/m^2 IV on days 1 and 2
Repeat cycle every 21 days up to 8 cycles [493].

Vorinostat (peripheral T-cell lymphoma)

Vorinostat: 400 mg PO daily
Continue therapy until disease progression [494]. If toxicity is observed, dose
may be reduced to 300 mg PO daily.

Pralatrexate

Pralatrexate: 30 mg/m^2 IV weekly for 6 weeks

Repeat cycle every 7 weeks [495]. Folic acid at 1–1.25 mg PO q day beginning 10 days prior to therapy and vitamin B12 at 1 mg IM beginning no more than 10 weeks prior to first dose of therapy and repeated every 8–10 weeks.

Brentuximab

Brentuximab: 1.8 mg/kg IV on day 1

Repeat cycle every 3 weeks for up to 16 cycles [496].

Romidepsin (peripheral T-cell lymphoma)

Romidespsin: 14 mg/m^2 IV on days 1, 8, and 15

Repeat cycle every 28 days [497].

Belinostat (peripheral T-cell lymphoma)

Belinostat: 1000 mg/m^2 IV on days 1-5

Repeat cycle every 21 days [498].

Bortezomib (mantle cell lymphoma)

Bortezomib: 1.3–1.5 mg/m^2 IV on days 1, 4, 8, and 11

Repeat cycle every 21 days [499].

Lenalidomide (mantle cell lymphoma)

Lenalidomide: 25 mg/day PO on days 1–21

Repeat cycle every 28 days for up to 52 weeks [500].

PRIMARY CNS LYMPHOMA

Combination Regimens

Methotrexate:	3500 mg/m^2 IV over 2 hours every other week for 5 doses
Intrathecal methotrexate:	12 mg IT weekly every other week after IV methotrexate
Leucovorin:	10 mg IV every 6 hours for 12 doses starting 24 hours after IV methotrexate; 10 mg IV every 12 hours for 8 doses starting 24 hours after IT methotrexate
Vincristine:	1.4 mg/m^2 IV every other week along with IV methotrexate

| Procarbazine: | 100 mg/m^2/day PO for 7 days on first, third, and fifth cycle of IV methotrexate |

Once chemotherapy is completed, whole-brain radiation therapy is administered to a total dose of 45 cGy [501].

R-MPV + Radiation Therapy + Cytarabine

Rituximab:	500 mg/m^2 IV on day 1
Methotrexate:	3500 mg/m^2 IV on day 2
Leucovorin:	20–25 mg every 6 hours starting 24 hours after methotrexate infusion for 72 hours or until serum methotrexate level, 1×10^{-8} mg/dL.

Increase leucovorin to 40 mg every 4 hours IV, if methotrexate level > 1×10^{-8} mg/dL at 48 hours or > 1×10^{-8} mg/dL at 72 hours

| Vincristine: | 1.4 mg/m^2 (maximum, 2.8 mg) IV on day 2 |
| Procarbazine: | 100 mg/m^2 PO on days 1–7 of odd-numbered cycles only |

If positive CSF cytology, administer 12 mg methotrexate IT between days 5 and 12 of each cycle

Repeat cycle every 2 weeks for 5 cycles [502].

After 5 cycles of R-MPV:

If CR, whole-brain radiotherapy (WBRT) 180 cGy/day for 13 days to a total of 2340 cGy beginning 3–5 weeks after the completion of R-MPV.

If PR, administer 2 additional cycles of R-MPV. If CR is achieved after 7 cycles of R-MPV, administer WBRT 180 cGy/day × 13 days to a total of 2340 cGy beginning 3–5 weeks after completion of R-MPV.

If persistent disease exists after 7 cycles of R-MPV, administer WBRT 180 cGy/day × 25 days to a total of 4500 cGy beginning 3–5 weeks after the completion of R-MPV.

If stable or progressive disease after 5 cycles of R-MPV, administer WBRT 180 cGy/day for 25 days to a total of 4500 cGy beginning 3–5 weeks after the completion of R-MPV. Three weeks after the completion of WBRT, consolidation therapy is given with cytarabine 3 g/m^2/day (maximum, 6 g) IV over 3 hours for 2 days. A second cycle of cytarabine is given 1 month later.

Single-Agent Regimens

High-Dose Methotrexate

| Methotrexate: | 8000 mg/m^2 IV on day 1 |

Repeat cycle every 2 weeks up to 8 cycles, followed by 8000 mg/m^2 IV on day 1 every month up to 100 months [503].

Temozolomide

Temozolomide: 150 mg/m^2/day PO on days 1–5
Repeat cycle every 4 weeks [504].

Topotecan

Topotecan: 1.5 mg/m^2 IV on days 1–5
Repeat cycle every 3 weeks [505].

MALIGNANT MELANOMA

Adjuvant Therapy

Interferon α-2b

Interferon α-2b: 20 million U/m^2 IV, 5 times weekly for
4 weeks, then 10 million IU/m^2 SC,
3 times weekly for 48 weeks

Treatment is for a total of 1 year [506].

Peg-Interferon α-2b

Peg-Interferon α-2b: 6 μg/kg SC weekly for 8 weeks, then
3 μg/kg SC weekly for up to 5 years

Treatment is for up to a total of 5 years [507].

Ipilimumab

Ipilimumab: 10 mg/kg IV on day 1

Repeat cycle every 3 weeks for 4 doses followed by 10 mg/kg on day 1 every 12 weeks for up to 3 years [507a].

Metastatic Disease

Combination Regimens

DTIC + Carmustine + Cisplatin

Dacarbazine: 220 mg/m^2 IV on days 1–3

Carmustine: 150 mg/m^2 IV on day 1

Cisplatin: 25 mg/m^2 IV on days 1–3

Repeat cycle with dacarbazine and cisplatin every 21 days and carmustine every 42 days [508].

IFN + DTIC

Interferon α-2b: 15 million IU/m^2 IV on days 1–5, 8–12, and 15–19 as induction therapy

Interferon α-2b: 10 million IU/m^2 SC 3 times weekly after induction therapy

Dacarbazine: 200 mg/m^2 IV on days 22–26

Repeat cycle every 28 days [509].

Temozolomide + Thalidomide

Temozolomide: 75 mg/m^2/day PO for 6 weeks

Thalidomide: 200 mg/day PO for 6 weeks

Repeat cycle every 8 weeks [510]. Consider dose escalation to 400 mg/day for patients <70 years and starting at a lower dose of 100 mg/day with dose escalation to 250 mg/day for patient >70 years.

Dabrafenib + Trametinib

Dabrafenib: 150 mg PO bid

Trametinib: 2 mg PO daily

Continue treatment until disease progression [511].

Cobimetinib + Vemurafenib

Cobimetinib: 60 mg/day PO on days 1-21

Vemurafenib: 960 mg PO bid daily

Repeat cycle every 28 days [512].

Nivolumab + Ipilumumab

Ipilumumab: 1 mg/kg IV on day 1

Nivolumab: 1 mg/kg IV on day 1

Repeat cycle every 21 days for 4 cycles followed by

Nivolumab: 240 mg IV on day 1

Repeat cycle every 14 days until disease progression [513].

Single-Agent Regimens

Dacarbazine

Dacarbazine: 250 mg/m^2 IV on days 1–5

Repeat cycle every 21 days [514].

or

Dacarbazine: 850 mg/m^2 IV on day 1

Repeat cycle every 3–6 weeks [515].

Interferon-α

Interferon α-2b: 20 million IU/m^2 IM, 3 times weekly for
                                         12 weeks [516].

Aldesleukin

Aldesleukin (IL-2):   720,000 IU/kg IV every 8 hours on days
                                         1–5 and 15–19

Repeat cycle in 6- to 12-week intervals [517].

or

Aldesleukin (IL-2):   100,000 IU/kg IV every 4 hours on days
                                         1–5 and 15–19

Repeat cycle in 12-week intervals up to a total of 3 cycles [518].

or

Aldesleukin (IL-2):   720,000 IU/kg IV at 8 am and 6 pm on
                                         days 1–5 and 15–19

Treat up to a maximum of 8 total doses on days 1–5 and repeat on days 15–19.
Repeat cycle in 8- to 12-week intervals [519].

Ipilumumab

Ipilumumab: 3 mg/kg IV on day 1

Repeat cycle every 3 weeks for a total of 4 doses [520].

Pembrolizumab

Pembrolizumab: 2 mg/kg IV on day 1

Repeat cycle every 3 weeks [521].

Nivolumab

Nivolumab: 240 mg IV on day 1

Repeat cycle every 2 weeks [522].

Temozolomide

Temozolomide: 150 mg/m^2 PO on days 1–5

Repeat cycle every 28 days [523]. If tolerated, can increase dose to 200 mg/m^2 PO
on days 1–5.

Vemurafenib

Vemurafenib: 960 mg PO bid
Continue treatment until disease progression [524].

Dabrafenib

Dabrafenib: 150 mg PO bid
Continue treatment until disease progression [525].

Trametinib

Trametinib: 2 mg PO daily
Continue treatment until disease progression [526].

MALIGNANT MESOTHELIOMA

Combination Regimens

Doxorubicin + Cisplatin

Doxorubicin: 60 mg/m^2 IV on day 1
Cisplatin: 60 mg/m^2 IV on day 1
Repeat cycle every 21–28 days [527].

CAP

Cyclophosphamide: 500 mg/m^2 IV on day 1
Doxorubicin: 50 mg/m^2 IV on day 1
Cisplatin: 80 mg/m^2 IV on day 1
Repeat cycle every 21 days [528].

Gemcitabine + Cisplatin

Gemcitabine: 1000 mg/m^2 IV on days 1, 8, and 15
Cisplatin: 100 mg/m^2 IV on day 1
Repeat cycle every 28 days [529].

Gemcitabine + Carboplatin

Gemcitabine: 1000 mg/m^2 IV on days 1, 8, and 15
Carboplatin: AUC of 5, IV on day 1
Repeat cycle every 28 days [530].

Pemetrexed + Cisplatin

Pemetrexed: 500 mg/m^2 IV on day 1

Cisplatin: 75 mg/m^2 IV on day 1

Repeat cycle every 21 days [531]. Folic acid at 350–1000 μg PO q day beginning 1 week prior to therapy and vitamin B12 at 1000 μg IM to start 1–2 weeks prior to first dose of therapy and repeated every 3 cycles.

Gemcitabine + Vinorelbine

Gemcitabine: 1000 mg/m^2 IV on days 1 and 8

Vinorelbine: 25 mg/m^2 IV on days 1 and 8

Repeat cycle every 21 days [532].

Pemetrexed + Gemcitabine

Pemetrexed: 500 mg/m^2 IV on day 8

Gemcitabine: 1250 mg/m^2 IV on days 1 and 8

Repeat cycle every 21 days [533]. Folic acid at 350–1000 μg PO q day beginning 1–2 weeks prior to therapy and vitamin B12 at 1000 μg IM to start 1–2 weeks prior to first dose of therapy and repeated every 3 cycles.

Single-Agent Regimens

Pemetrexed

Pemetrexed: 500 mg/m^2 IV on day 1

Repeat cycle every 21 days [534]. Folic acid at 350–1000 μg PO q day beginning 1 week prior to therapy and vitamin B12 at 1000 μg IM to start 1–2 weeks prior to first dose of therapy and repeated every 3 cycles.

Dexamethasone 4 mg PO bid on the day before, day of, and day after each dose of pemetrexed.

Vinorelbine

Vinorelbine: 30 mg/m^2 IV weekly

One cycle consists of 6 weekly injections. Continue until disease progression [535].

MULTIPLE MYELOMA

Combination Regimens

MP

Melphalan: 8–10 mg/m^2 PO on days 1–4

| Prednisone: | 60 mg/m^2 on days 1–4 |

Repeat cycle every 42 days [536].

MPT

Melphalan:	0.25 mg/kg PO on days 1–4
Prednisone:	1.5 mg/kg PO on days 1–4
Thalidomide:	50–100 mg/day PO q day

Repeat cycle every 28 days [537].

or

Melphalan:	0.25 mg/kg/day PO on days 1–4
Prednisone:	2 mg/kg/day PO on days 1–4
Thalidomide:	100–400 mg PO q day

Repeat cycle every 42 days [538].

MPL

Melphalan:	0.18 mg/kg PO on days 1–4
Prednisone:	2 mg/kg PO on days 1–4
Lenalidomide:	10 mg/day PO on days 1–21

Repeat cycle every 28 days [539].

VAD

Vincristine:	0.4 mg/day IV continuous infusion on days 1–4
Doxorubicin:	9 mg/m^2/day IV continuous infusion on days 1–4
Dexamethasone:	40 mg PO on days 1–4, 9–12, and 17–20

Repeat cycle every 28 days [540].

Thalidomide + Dexamethasone

| Thalidomide: | 200 mg/day PO |
| Dexamethasone: | 40 mg/day PO on days 1–4, 9–12, and 17–20 for first 4 cycles and then 40 mg/day PO on days 1–4 |

Repeat cycle every 28 days [541].

Lenalidomide + Dexamethasone

| Lenalidomide: | 25 mg/day PO on days 1–21 |

| Dexamethasone: | 40 mg/day PO on days 1–4, 9–12, and 17–20 (first 4 cycles) and then 40 mg/day PO on days 1–4 with future cycles |

Repeat cycles every 28 days [542].

or

| Lenalidomide: | 25 mg/day PO on days 1–21 |
| Dexamethasone: | 40 mg/m²/day PO on days 1, 8, 15, and 22 |

Repeat cycle every 28 days [543].

RVD

Lenalidomide:	25 mg/day PO on days 1–14
Bortezomib:	1.3 mg/m² IV or SC on days 1, 4, 8, and 11
Dexamethasone:	20 mg/day PO on days 1, 2, 4, 5, 8, 9, 11, and 12

Repeat cycle every 21 days for 8 cycles [544].

Panobinostat + Bortezomib + Dexamethasone

Panobinostat:	20 mg/day PO on days 1, 3, 5, 8, 10, and 12
Bortezomib:	1.3 mg/m² IV on days 1, 4, 8, and 11
Dexamethasone:	20 mg/day PO on days 1, 2, 4, 5, 8, 9, 11, and 12

Repeat cycle every 21 days [545].

PD

| Pomalidomide: | 4 mg/day PO on days 1–21 |
| Dexamethasone: | 40 mg/day PO on day 1 |

Repeat cycle every 28 days [546].

or

| Pomalidomide: | 2 mg/day PO on days 1–21 |
| Dexamethasone: | 40 mg/day PO on days 1, 8, 15, and 22 |

Repeat cycle every 28 days [547].

DVD

| Doxorubicin liposome: | 40 mg/m² IV on day 1 |
| Vincristine: | 2 mg IV on day 1 |

Dexamethasone: 40 mg PO on days 1–4
Repeat cycles every 28 days [548].

Bortezomib + Doxorubicin liposome:

Bortezomib: 1.3 mg/m^2 IV or SC on days 1, 4, 8, and 11

Doxorubicin liposome: 30 mg/m^2 IV infusion on day 4
Repeat cycle every 21 days [549].

Bortezomib + Melphalan

Bortezomib: 1.0 mg/m^2 IV or SC on days 1, 4, 8, and 11

Melphalan: 0.10 mg/kg PO on days 1–4
Repeat cycle every 28 days up to 8 cycles [550].

BMP

Bortezomib: 1.3 mg/m^2 IV or SC on days 1, 4, 8, 11, 22, 25, 29, and 32

Melphalan: 9 mg/m^2 PO on days 1–4

Prednisone: 60 mg/m^2 PO on days 1–4
Repeat cycle every 6 weeks for 4 cycles [551], then

Bortezomib: 1.3 mg/m^2 IV on days 1, 8, 22, and 29

Melphalan: 9 mg/m^2 PO on days 1–4

Prednisone: 60 mg/m^2 PO on days 1–4
Repeat cycle every 6 weeks for 5 cycles.

BMPT

Bortezomib: 1–1.3 mg/m^2 IV or SC on days 1, 4, 15, and 22

Melphalan: 6 mg/m^2 PO on days 1–5

Prednisone: 60 mg/m^2 PO on days 1–5

Thalidomide: 50 mg PO daily
Repeat cycle every 5 weeks for 6 cycles [552].

RMPT

Lenalidomide: 10 mg PO on days 1–21

Melphalan: 0.18 mg/kg PO on days 1–4

Prednisone: 2 mg/kg PO on days 1–4

| Thalidomide: | 50 mg PO daily on days 1–28 |

Repeat cycle every 28 days for 6 cycles followed by maintenance lenalidomide 10 mg PO on days 1–21 until progression or toxicity [553].

Carfilzomib + Lenalidomide + Dexamethasone (CLD)

Carfilzomib:	20 mg/m^2 IV on days 1 and 2 of cycle 1, and if tolerated, then 27 mg/m^2 IV on days 8, 9, 15, and 16 during cycles 1 through 12 and 27 mg/m^2 IV on days 1, 2, 15, and 16 during cycles 13 through 18 after which carfilzomib is discontinued
Lenalidomide:	25 mg PO on days 1-21
Dexamethasone:	40 mg PO on days 1, 8, 15, and 22

Repeat cycle every 28 days for up to 9 cycles [554].

Lenalidomide + Dexamethasone + Ixazomib

Lenalidomide:	25 mg/day PO on days 1-21
Dexamethasone:	40 mg/day PO on days 1, 8, 15, and 22
Ixazomib:	4 mg/day PO on days 1, 8, and 15

Repeat cycle every 28 days until disease progression [555].

Daratumumab + Bortezomib + Dexamethasone

Daratumumab:	16 mg/kg IV weekly on cycles 1-3
	16 mg/kg IV on day 1 of cycles 4-8
	16 mg/kg IV on day 1 of cycles 9+
Bortezomib:	1.3 mg/m^2 IV on days 1, 4, 8, and 11 on cycles 1-8
Dexamethasone:	20 mg PO on days 1, 2, 4, 5, 8, 9, 11, and 12 on cycles 1-8

Continue treatment until disease progression or toxicity [556].

Elotuzumab + Lenalidomide + Dexamethasone

Elotuzumab:	10 mg/kg IV on days 1, 8, 15, and 22
Lenalidomide:	25 mg PO on days 1-21
Dexamethasone:	8 mg IV prior to elotuzumab infusion and 28 mg PO on days 1, 8, 15, and 22 and 40 mg PO on day 28

Repeat cycle every 28 days for two cycles followed by:

| Elotuzumab: | 10 mg/kg IV on days 1and 15 |
| Lenalidomide: | 25 mg PO on days 1-21 |

| Dexamethasone: | 8 mg IV prior to elotuzumab infusion and 28 mg PO on days 1, 15, and 40 mg PO on days 22 and 28 |

Repeat cycle every 28 days until disease progression [557].

Single-Agent Regimens

Dexamethasone

| Dexamethasone: | 40 mg IV or PO on days 1–4, 9–12, and 17–20 |

Repeat cycle every 21 days [558].

Melphalan

| Melphalan: | 90–140 mg/m^2 IV on day 1 |

Repeat cycle every 28–42 days [559].

Thalidomide

| Thalidomide: | 200–800 mg PO daily |

Continue treatment until disease progression or undue toxicity [560].

Lenalidomide

| Lenalidomide: | 30 mg PO daily on days 1–21 |

Repeat cycle every 28 days until disease progression or undue toxicity [561].

Bortezomib

| Bortezomib: | 1.3 mg/m^2 IV or SC on days 1, 4, 8, and 11 |

Repeat cycle every 21 days [562].

Carfilzomib

| Carfilzomib: | 20 mg/m^2 IV on days 1, 2, 8, 9, 15, and 16. After cycle 1, increase dose to 27 mg/m^2 IV |

Repeat cycle every 28 days for up to 12 cycles [563].

Daratumumab

| Daratumumab: | 16 mg/kg IV on days 1, 8, 15, 22, 29, 36, 42, and 49; followed by once every 2 weeks for 16 weeks; followed by once every 4 weeks |

Continue treatment until disease progression [564].

Ibrutinib

Ibrutinib: 420 mg/day PO daily

Continue treatment until disease progression [565].

MYELODYSPLASTIC SYNDROME

Single-Agent Regimens

Azacitidine

Azacitidine: 75 mg/m^2 SC daily for 7 days

Repeat cycle every 4 weeks. Patients should be treated for at least 4 cycles [566].

Decitabine

Decitabine: 15 mg/m^2 IV continuous infusion over 3 hours every 8 hours for 3 days

Repeat cycle every 4 weeks. Patients should be treated for at least 4 cycles [567].

or

Decitabine: 20 mg/m^2 IV continuous infusion over 1 hour for 5 days

Repeat cycle every 4–6 weeks. Patients should be treated for at least 4 cycles [568].

Lenalidomide

Lenalidomide: 10 mg PO daily

Continue until disease progression [569].

or

Lenalidomide: 10 mg PO daily for 21 days

Repeat cycle every 28 days [569].

Imatinib

Imatinib: 400 mg PO daily

Continue until disease progression [570].

Antithymocyte globulin (ATG) + Cyclosporine

ATG: 15 mg/kg IV on days 1–5

Cyclosporine: 5–6 mg/kg PO bid

Adjust cyclosporine dose to maintain blood levels between 100–300 ng/mL [571].

OSTEOGENIC SARCOMA

Combination Regimens

Etoposide + Ifosfamide

Etoposide: 100 mg/m^2/day IV on days 1–5

Ifosfamide: 3500 mg/m^2/day IV on days 1–5

Mesna: 700 mg/m^2 IV with first ifosfamide dose, then 3, 6, and 9 hours later on days 1–5

Repeat cycle every 21 days for 2 cycles [572]. Start G-CSF support at 5 µq/kq/day SC to start on day 6. Followed by surgical resection of primary tumor and then intensive maintenance chemotherapy.

Methotrexate: 1200 mg/m^2 IV on weeks 1, 2, 6, 7, 11, 12, 16, 17, 30, and 31

Leucovorin: 15 mg IV every 6 hours for 10 doses starting 24 hours after start of high-dose methotrexate

or

L-Leucovorin: 7.5 mg IV every 6 hours for 10 doses starting 24 hours after start of high-dose methotrexate

Doxorubicin: 37.5 mg/m^2/day IV on days 1–2 on weeks 3, 13, 21, 27, and 32

Cisplatin: 60 mg/m^2/day IV on days 1–2 on weeks 3, 13, 21, and 27

Ifosfamide: 2400 mg/m^2/day IV on days 1–5 on weeks 8, 18, and 24

Administer G-CSF support at 5 µg/kg/day SC on weeks 8, 18, and 24.

Cisplatin + Doxorubicin + High-Dose Methotrexate

Doxorubicin: 25 mg/m^2/day IV on days 1–3 on weeks 0 and 5

Cisplatin: 120 mg/m^2 IV on day 1 on weeks 0 and 5

| Methotrexate: | 1200 mg/m^2 IV on day 1 on weeks 3, 4, 8, and 9 |
| Leucovorin: | 10 mg IV every 6 hours for 10 doses starting 24 hours after start of high-dose methotrexate |

or

| L-Leucovorin: | 7.5 mg IV every 6 hours for 10 doses starting 24 hours after start of high-dose methotrexate |

Induction chemotherapy is followed by surgical resection of primary tumor and then maintenance chemotherapy to begin on week 12 and continuing until week 31 [573].

Doxorubicin:	25 mg/m^2/day IV on days 1–3 on weeks 12, 17, 22, and 27
Cisplatin:	120 mg/m^2 IV on day 1 on weeks 12 and 17
Methotrexate:	1200 mg/m^2 IV on day 1 on weeks 15, 16, 20, 21, 25, 26, 30, and 31
Leucovorin:	10 mg IV every 6 hours for 10 doses starting 24 hours after start of high-dose methotrexate

or

| L-Leucovorin: | 7.5 mg IV every 6 hours for 10 doses starting 24 hours after start of high-dose methotrexate |

OVARIAN CANCER (EPITHELIAL)

Combination Regimens

CC

| Carboplatin: | 300 mg/m^2 IV on day 1 |
| Cyclophosphamide: | 600 mg/m^2 IV on day 1 |

Repeat cycle every 28 days [574].

CP

| Cisplatin: | 100 mg/m^2 IV on day 1 |
| Cyclophosphamide: | 600 mg/m^2 IV on day 1 |

Repeat cycle every 28 days [575].

CT

Cisplatin:	75 mg/m^2 IV on day 2
Paclitaxel:	135 mg/m^2 IV over 24 hours on day 1

Repeat cycle every 21 days [576].

Carboplatin + Paclitaxel

Carboplatin:	AUC of 6–7.5, IV on day 1
Paclitaxel:	175 mg/m^2 IV over 3 hours on day 1

Repeat cycle every 21 days [577].

or

Carboplatin:	AUC of 2, IV on days 1, 8, and 15
Paclitaxel:	60 mg/m^2 IV on days 1, 8, and 15

Repeat cycle every 28 days [578].

Carboplatin + Paclitaxel + Bevacizumab

Carboplatin:	AUC of 6, IV on day 1
Paclitaxel:	175 mg/m^2 IV over 3 hours on day 1
Bevacizumab:	15 mg/kg IV on day 1

Repeat cycle every 21 days for 6 cycles, then maintenance bevacizumab for cycles 7–22 [579].

Carboplatin + Docetaxel

Carboplatin:	AUC of 6, IV on day 1
Docetaxel:	60 mg/m^2 IV on day 1

Repeat cycle every 21 days [580].

Carboplatin + Doxorubicin liposome:

Carboplatin:	AUC of 5, IV on day 1
Doxorubicin liposome:	30 mg/m^2 IV on day 1

Repeat cycle every 28 days [581].

Gemcitabine + Doxorubicin liposome:

Gemcitabine:	1000 mg/m^2 IV on days 1 and 8
Doxorubicin liposome:	30 mg/m^2 IV on day 1

Repeat cycle every 21 days [582].

Gemcitabine + Cisplatin

Gemcitabine:	800–1000 mg/m^2 IV on days 1 and 8
Cisplatin:	30 mg/m^2 IV on days 1 and 8

Repeat cycle every 21 days [583].

Gemcitabine + Carboplatin

Gemcitabine:	1000 mg/m^2 IV on days 1 and 8
Carboplatin:	AUC of 4, IV on day 1

Repeat cycle every 21 days [584].

Paclitaxel + IP Cisplatin + IP Paclitaxel

Paclitaxel:	135 mg/m^2 IV over 24 hours on day 1
Cisplatin:	100 mg/m^2 IP on day 2
Paclitaxel:	60 mg/m^2 IP on day 8

Repeat cycle every 21 days up to
6 cycles [585].

Pemetrexed + Carboplatin

Pemetrexed:	500 mg/m^2 IV on day 1
Carboplatin:	AUC of 5, IV on day 1

Repeat cycle every 21 days [586]. Folic acid at 350–1000 μg PO q day beginning
1–2 weeks prior to therapy and vitamin B12 at 1000 μg IM to start 1–2 weeks
prior to first dose of therapy and repeated every 3 cycles. Dexamethasone 4 mg
PO bid on the day before, day of, and day after each dose of pemetrexed.

Single-Agent Regimens

Altretamine

Altretamine:	260 mg/m^2/day PO in 4 divided doses after meals and at bedtime

Repeat cycle every 14–21 days [587].

Doxorubicin liposome:

Doxorubicin liposome:	40–50 mg/m^2 IV over 1 hour on day 1

Repeat cycle every 28 days [588].

Paclitaxel

Paclitaxel:	135 mg/m^2 IV over 3 hours on day 1

Repeat cycle every 21 days [589].

Ixabepilone

Ixabepilone: 20 mg/m^2 IV on days 1, 8, and 15
Repeat cycle every 28 days [590].

Topotecan

Topotecan: 1.5 mg/m^2 IV on days 1–5
Repeat cycle every 21 days [591].

Gemcitabine

Gemcitabine: 800 mg/m^2 IV weekly for 3 weeks
Repeat cycle every 4 weeks [592].

Etoposide

Etoposide: 50 mg/m^2/day PO on days 1–21
Repeat cycle every 28 days [593].

Vinorelbine

Vinorelbine: 30 mg/m^2 IV on days 1 and 8
Repeat cycle every 21 days [594].

Pemetrexed

Pemetrexed: 900 mg/m^2 IV on day 1
Repeat cycle every 21 days [595]. Folic acid at 350–1000 μg PO q day beginning 1 week prior to therapy and vitamin B12 at 1000 μg IM to start 1–2 weeks prior to first dose of therapy and repeated every 3 cycles. Dexamethasone 4 mg PO bid on the day before, day of, and day after each dose of pemetrexed.

Bevacizumab

Bevacizumab: 15 mg/kg IV on day 1
Repeat cycle every 21 days [596].

Capecitabine

Capecitabine: 1000 mg/m^2 PO bid on days 1–14
Repeat cycle every 21 days [597].

Olaparib

Olaparib: 400 PO bid
Repeat cycle every 28 days [598].

OVARIAN CANCER (GERM CELL)

Combination Regimens

BEP

Bleomycin:	30 U IV on days 2, 9, and 16
Etoposide:	100 mg/m^2 IV on days 1–5
Cisplatin:	20 mg/m^2 IV on days 1–5

Repeat cycle every 21 days [599].

PANCREATIC CANCER

Adjuvant Therapy

Single-Agent Regimens

5-Fluorouracil + Leucovorin

5-Fluorouracil:	425 mg/m^2 IV on days 1–5
Leucovorin:	20 mg/m^2 IV on days 1–5

Repeat cycle every 28 days for a total of 6 cycles [600].

Gemcitabine

Gemcitabine:	1000 mg/m^2 IV on days 1, 8, and 15

Repeat cycle every 28 days for a total of 6 cycles [601].

Locally Advanced Disease

Combination Regimens

5-Fluorouracil + Radiation Therapy (GITSG regimen)

5-Fluorouracil:	500 mg/m^2/day IV on days 1–3 and 29–31, then weekly beginning on day 71
Radiation therapy:	Total dose, 4000 cGy

Chemotherapy and radiation therapy started on the same day and given concurrently [602].

RTOG Chemoradiation Regimen

Gemcitabine:	1000 mg/m^2 IV on days 1, 8, and 15

Followed by concurrent chemoradiation:

5-Fluorouracil:	250 mg/m^2/day IV continuous infusion during radiation therapy
Radiation therapy:	180 cGy/day to a total dose of 5040 cGy

Chemotherapy and radiation therapy started on the same day and given concurrently.

After chemoradiation:

Gemcitabine:	1000 mg/m^2 IV on days 1, 8, and 15

Repeat cycle every 4 weeks for a total of 3 cycles [603].

Gemcitabine + Radiation Therapy (ECOG regimen)

Gemcitabine:	600 mg/m^2 IV weekly for 6 weeks
Radiation therapy:	180 cGy/day to a total dose of 5040 cGy Chemotherapy and radiation therapy started on the same day and given concurrently.

Four weeks after the completion of chemoradiation:

Gemcitabine:	1000 mg/m^2 IV on days 1, 8, and 15

Repeat cycle every 4 weeks for a total of 5 cycles [604].

Metastatic Disease

Combination Regimens

5-Fluorouracil + Leucovorin

5-Fluorouracil:	425 mg/m^2 IV on days 1–5
Leucovorin:	20 mg/m^2 IV on days 1–5

Repeat cycle every 28 days [605].

Gemcitabine + Capecitabine (GEM-CAP)

Gemcitabine:	1000 mg/m^2 IV on days 1 and 8
Capecitabine:	650 mg/m^2 PO bid on days 1–14

Repeat cycle every 21 days [606].

or

Gemcitabine:	1000 mg/m^2 IV on days 1, 8, and 15
Capecitabine:	830 mg/m^2 PO bid on days 1–21

Repeat cycle every 28 days [607].

Gemcitabine + Docetaxel + Capecitabine (GTX)

Gemcitabine:	750 mg/m^2 IV over 75 minutes on days 4 and 11
Docetaxel:	30 mg/m^2 IV on days 4 and 11
Capecitabine:	750 mg/m^2 PO bid on days 1–14

Repeat cycle every 3 weeks [608].

Gemcitabine + Oxaliplatin

Gemcitabine:	1000 mg/m^2 IV over 100 minutes on day 1
Oxaliplatin:	100 mg/m^2 over 2 hours on day 2

Repeat cycle every 2 weeks [609].

or

Gemcitabine:	1000 mg/m^2 IV over 100 minutes on day 1
Oxaliplatin:	100 mg/m^2 over 2 hours on day 1

Repeat cycle every 2 weeks [610].

Gemcitabine + Erlotinib

Gemcitabine:	1000 mg/m^2 IV weekly for 7 weeks, then 1-week rest; subsequent cycles 1000 mg/m^2 IV weekly for 3 weeks with 1-week rest
Erlotinib:	100 mg PO daily

Repeat 3-week cycles every 28 days [611].

Capecitabine + Erlotinib

Capecitabine:	1000 mg/m^2 PO bid on days 1–14
Erlotinib:	150 mg PO daily

Repeat cycle every 21 days [612].

FOLFIRINOX

Oxaliplatin:	85 mg/m^2 IV on day 1
Irinotecan:	180 mg/m^2 IV on day 1
Leucovorin:	400 mg/m^2 IV on day 1
5-Fluorouracil:	400 mg/m^2 IV on day 1
5-Fluorouracil:	2400 mg/m^2 IV continuous infusion over 46 hours on days 1 and 2

Repeat cycle every 2 weeks [613].

Nab-Paclitaxel + Gemcitabine

Nab-Paclitaxel:	125 mg/m^2 IV on days 1, 8, and 15
Gemcitabine:	1000 mg/m^2 IV on days 1, 8, and 15

Repeat cycle every 28 days [614].

Liposomal Irinotecan + 5-Fluorouracil + Leucovorin

Liposomal Irinotecan:	70 mg/m^2 IV on day 1
5-Fluorouracil:	2400 mg/m^2 IV continuous infusion over 46 hours on days 1 and 2
Leucovorin:	400 mg/m^2 IV on day 1

Repeat cycle every 2 weeks [615].

Single-Agent Regimens

Gemcitabine

Gemcitabine:	1000 mg/m^2 IV weekly for 7 weeks, then 1 week rest; subsequent cycles 1000 mg/m^2 IV weekly for 3 weeks with 1-week rest

Repeat 3-week cycle every 28 days [616].

or

Gemcitabine:	1000 mg/m^2 IV over 100 min at 10 mg/m^2/min on days 1, 8, and 5

Repeat cycle every 28 days [617].

Capecitabine

Capecitabine:	1250 mg/m^2 PO bid on days 1–14

May decrease dose to 850–1000 mg/m^2 PO bid on days 1–14 to reduce the risk of toxicity without compromising clinical efficacy.

Repeat cycle every 21 days [618].

PROSTATE CANCER

Combination Regimens

Flutamide + Leuprolide [619]

Flutamide:	250 mg PO tid
Leuprolide:	7.5 mg IM every 28 days or 22.5 mg IM every 12 weeks

Flutamide + Goserelin [620]

Flutamide:	250 mg PO tid
Goserelin:	10.8 mg SC every 12 weeks

Estramustine + Etoposide

Estramustine: 15 mg/kg/day PO in 4 divided doses on days 1–21

Etoposide: 50 mg/m^2/day PO in 2 divided doses on days 1–21

Repeat cycle every 28 days [621].

Estramustine + Vinblastine

Estramustine: 600 mg/m^2 PO daily on days 1–42

Vinblastine: 4 mg/m^2 IV weekly for 6 weeks

Repeat cycle every 8 weeks [622].

Paclitaxel + Estramustine

Paclitaxel: 120 mg/m^2 IV continuous infusion on days 1–4

Estramustine: 600 mg/m^2 PO daily, starting 24 hours before paclitaxel

Repeat cycle every 21 days [623].

or

Paclitaxel: 90 mg/m^2 IV weekly for 3 weeks

Estramustine: 140 mg PO tid, starting day before, day of, and day after paclitaxel

Repeat cycle every 28 days [624].

Mitoxantrone + Prednisone

Mitoxantrone: 12 mg/m^2 IV on day 1

Prednisone: 5 mg PO bid daily

Repeat cycle every 21 days [625].

Docetaxel + Estramustine

Docetaxel: 35 mg/m^2 IV on day 2 of weeks 1 and 2

Estramustine: 420 mg PO for the first 4 doses and 280 mg PO for the next 5 doses on days 1–3 of weeks 1 and 2

Repeat cycle every 21 days [626]. Dexamethasone is administered at 4 mg PO bid on days 1–3 of weeks 1 and 2.

or

Docetaxel: 60 mg/m^2 IV on day 2

| Estramustine: | 280 mg PO tid on days 1–5 |

Repeat cycle every 21 days [627].

Docetaxel + Prednisone

| Docetaxel: | 75 mg/m^2 IV on day 1 |
| Prednisone: | 5 mg PO bid |

Repeat cycle every 21 days for up to a
total of 10 cycles [628].

Docetaxel + Prednisone + Bevacizumab

Docetaxel:	75 mg/m^2 IV on day 1
Prednisone:	5 mg PO bid
Bevacizumab:	15 mg/kg IV on day 1

Repeat cycle every 21 days [629].

Cabazitaxel + Prednisone

| Cabazitaxel: | 25 mg/m^2 IV on day 1 |
| Prednisone: | 10 mg PO daily |

Repeat cycle every 21 days [630].

Abiraterone + Prednisone

| Abiraterone: | 1000 mg PO daily |
| Prednisone: | 5 mg PO bid |

Continue until disease progression [631].

Docetaxel + Leuprolide

| Docetaxel: | 75 mg/m^2 IV on day 1 every 28 days |
| Leuprolide: | 7.5 mg IM on day 1 every 21 days |

Continue until disease progression [632].

Single-Agent Regimens

Paclitaxel

| Paclitaxel: | 135–170 mg/m^2 IV as a 24-hour infusion on day 1 |

Repeat cycle every 3 weeks [633].

or

Paclitaxel: 150 mg/m^2 IV as a 1-hour infusion
                                                   weekly for 6 weeks

Repeat cycle every 8 weeks [634].

Docetaxel

Docetaxel: 75 mg/m^2 IV on day 1

Repeat cycle every 21 days [635].

or

Docetaxel: 20–40 mg/m^2 weekly for 3 weeks

Repeat cycle every 4 weeks [636].

Estramustine

Estramustine: 14 mg/kg/day PO in 3–4 divided doses
                                                   [636a]

Goserelin

Goserelin: 3.6 mg SC on day 1

Repeat cycle every 28 days [637].

or

Goserelin: 10.8 mg SC on day 1

Repeat cycle every 12 weeks [637].

Goserelin (adjuvant therapy)

Goserelin: 3.6 mg SC on day 1

Repeat cycle every 28 days for 24 months [638].

Degarelix

Degarelix: 240 mg SC starting dose followed
                                                   28 days later by the first maintenance
                                                   dose of 80 mg SC

Repeat maintenance dose every 28 days [639].

Leuprolide

Leuprolide: 7.5 mg IM on day 1

Repeat cycle every 28 days [640].

or

Leuprolide: 22.5 mg IM on day 1
Repeat cycle every 12 weeks [641].

or

Leuprolide: 30 mg IM on day 1
Repeat cycle every 16 weeks [642].

Bicalutamide

Bicalutamide: 50 mg PO daily
In patients refractory to other antiandrogen agents, may start with a higher dose of 150 mg PO daily [643].

Flutamide

Flutamide.   250 mg PO tid [644]

Nilutamide

Nilutamide: 300 mg PO on days 1–30, then 150 mg PO daily [645]

Prednisone

Prednisone: 5 mg PO bid [646]
or
Prednisone: 5 mg PO qid [647]

Ketoconazole

Ketoconazole: 1200 mg PO daily [648]

Aminoglutethimide

Aminoglutethimide: 250 mg PO qid, if tolerated may increase to 500 mg PO qid [649]

Sipuleucel-T

Sipuleucel-T   Administer contents of infusion bag IV over 60 minutes on day 1
Repeat cycle every 2 weeks for a total of 3 doses [650].

Enzalutamide

Enzalutamide:	160 mg PO daily [651]

RENAL CELL CANCER

Combination Regimens

Bevacizumab + Interferon-α

Bevacizumab:	10 mg/kg IV every 2 weeks
Interferon α-2a:	9 million U SC, 3 times per week, for 1 year

Continue treatment until disease progression [652].

Interferon-α + IL-2

Interferon α-2a:	9 million U SC on days 1–4, weeks 1–4
Interleukin-2:	12 million U SC on days 1–4, weeks 1–4

Repeat cycle every 6 weeks [653].

Lenvatinib + Everolimus

Lenvatinib:	18 mg/day PO daily
Everolimus:	5 mg/day PO daily

Continue treatment until disease progression [654].

Single-Agent Regimens

Bevacizumab

Bevacizumab:	10 mg/kg IV on day 1

Repeat cycle every 2 weeks [655].

Sunitinib

Sunitinib:	50 mg PO daily for 4 weeks

Repeat cycle every 6 weeks [656].

Sorafenib

Sorafenib:	400 mg PO bid

Continue treatment until disease progression [657].

Pazopanib

Pazopanib: 800 mg PO daily

Continue treatment until disease progression [658].

Axitinib

Axitinib: 5 mg PO bid; after 2 weeks may
                                          increase dose to 7 mg PO bid; after
                                          2 weeks may increase dose to 10 mg
                                          PO bid

Continue cycle every 6 weeks [659].

Temsirolimus

Temsirolimus: 25 mg IV weekly

Continue treatment disease progression [660].

Everolimus

Everolimus: 10 mg PO daily

Continue treatment until disease progression [661].

Aldesleukin

Interleukin-2:   720,000 IU/kg IV every 8 hours on days
                                          1–5 and 15–19

Repeat cycles in 6- to 12-week intervals up to a total of 3 cycles [662].

or

Interleukin-2:   720,000 IU/kg IV at 8 am and 6 pm on
                                          days 1–5 and 15–19

Treat up to a maximum of 8 total doses on days 1–5 and repeat on days 15–19.

Repeat cycles in 8- to 12-week intervals [519].

Interferon-α

Interferon α-2a: 5–15 million U SC daily or 3–5 times
                                          per week [663].

Cabozantinib

Cabozantinib: 60 mg PO daily

Continue treatment until disease progression [664].

Nivolumab

Nivolumab: 240 mg IV on day 1

Repeat cycle every 2 weeks [665].

SOFT TISSUE SARCOMAS

Combination Regimens

AD

Doxorubicin: 15 mg/m^2/day IV continuous infusion on days 1–4

Dacarbazine: 250 mg/m^2/day IV continuous infusion on days 1–4

Repeat cycle every 21 days [666].

AI

Doxorubicin: 20 mg/m^2/day IV continuous infusion on days 1–3

Ifosfamide: 1500 mg/m^2/day IV continuous infusion on days 1–4

Mesna: 225 mg/m^2 IV over 1 hour before ifosfamide and at 4 and 8 hours after ifosfamide

Repeat cycle every 21 days [667]. On day 5, G-CSF support should be started at 5 μg/kg/day for 10 days starting on day 5.

MAID

Mesna: 2500 mg/m^2/day IV continuous infusion on days 1–4

Doxorubicin: 20 mg/m^2/day IV continuous infusion on days 1–3

Ifosfamide: 2500 mg/m^2/day IV continuous infusion on days 1–3

Dacarbazine: 300 mg/m^2/day IV continuous infusion on days 1–3

Repeat cycle every 21 days [668].

CYVADIC

Cyclophosphamide: 500 mg/m^2 IV on day 1

Vincristine:	1.5 mg/m^2 IV on day 1 (maximum, 2 mg)
Doxorubicin:	50 mg/m^2 IV on day 1
Dacarbazine:	750 mg/m^2 IV on day 1

Repeat cycle every 21 days [669].

Gemcitabine + Docetaxel

Gemcitabine:	900 mg/m^2 IV over 90 minutes on days 1 and 8
Docetaxel:	100 mg/m^2 IV on day 8

Repeat cycle every 21 days [670].

Gemcitabine + Navelbine

Gemcitabine:	800 mg/m^2 IV over 90 minutes on days 1 and 8
Vinorelbine:	25 mg/m^2 IV on days 1 and 8

Repeat cycle every 21 days [671].

CAV Alternating with IE (Ewing's sarcoma)

Cyclophosphamide:	1200 mg/m^2 IV on day 1
Doxorubicin:	75 mg/m^2 IV on day 1
Vincristine:	2 mg IV on day 1
Ifosfamide:	1800 mg/m^2 IV on days 1–5
Etoposide:	100 mg/m^2 IV on days 1–5

Alternate CAV with IE every 21 days for a total of 17 cycles [672]. When the cumulative dose of doxorubicin reaches 375 mg/m^2, switch to dactinomycin at 1.25 mg/m^2.

Single-Agent Regimens

Doxorubicin

Doxorubicin:	75 mg/m^2 IV on day 1

Repeat cycle every 21 days [669].

Gemcitabine

Gemcitabine:	1200 mg/m^2 IV on days 1 and 8

Repeat cycle every 21 days [670].

Ifosfamide

Ifosfamide: $\qquad$ 3000 mg/m^2/day IV on days 1–3
Repeat cycle every 21 days [673].

Doxorubicin Liposome

Doxorubicin liposome: $\qquad$ 50 mg/m^2 IV on day 1
Repeat cycle every 28 days [674].

Pazopanib

Pazopanib: $\qquad$ 800 mg PO daily
Continue treatment until disease progression [675].

Trabectedin

Trabectedin: $\qquad$ 1.5 mg/kg IV on day 1
Repeat cycles every 21 days [676].

Eribulin

Eribulin: $\qquad$ 1.4 mg/m^2 IV on days 1 and 8
Repeat cycles every 21 days [677].

TESTICULAR CANCER

Adjuvant Therapy
PEB

Cisplatin: $\qquad$ 20 mg/m^2/day IV on days 1–5

Etoposide: $\qquad$ 100 mg/m^2/day IV on days 1–5

Bleomycin: $\qquad$ 30 U IV on days 2, 9, and 16

Repeat cycle every 28 days for a total of 2 cycles [678]. Adjuvant therapy of stage II testicular cancer treated with orchiectomy and retroperitoneal lymph node dissection.

Carboplatin

Carboplatin: $\qquad$ AUC of 7, IV on day 1
Administer one dose for adjuvant therapy of stage I seminoma [679].

Advanced Disease

BEP

Bleomycin:	30 U IV on days 1, 8, and 15
Etoposide:	100 mg/m^2/day IV on days 1–5
Cisplatin:	20 mg/m^2/day IV on days 1–5

Repeat cycle every 21 days [680].

EP

Etoposide:	100 mg/m^2/day IV on days 1–5
Cisplatin:	20 mg/m^2/day IV on days 1–5

Repeat cycle every 21 days [681].

PVB

Cisplatin:	20 mg/m^2/day IV on days 1–5
Vinblastine:	0.15 mg/kg IV on days 1 and 2
Bleomycin:	30 U IV on days 2, 9, and 16

Repeat cycle every 21 days [682].

VAB-6

Vinblastine:	4 mg/m^2 IV on day 1
Dactinomycin:	1 mg/m^2 IV on day 1
Bleomycin:	30 U IV on day 1, then 20 U/m^2 continuous infusion on days 1–3
Cisplatin:	20 mg/m^2 IV on day 4
Cyclophosphamide:	600 mg/m^2 IV on day 1

Repeat cycle every 21 days [683].

VeIP (salvage regimen)

Vinblastine:	0.11 mg/kg IV on days 1 and 2
Ifosfamide:	1200 mg/m^2/day IV on days 1–5
Cisplatin:	20 mg/m^2/day IV on days 1–5
Mesna:	400 mg/m^2 IV, given 15 minutes before first ifosfamide dose, then 1200 mg/m^2/day IV continuous infusion for 5 days

Repeat cycle every 21 days [684].

VIP (salvage regimen)

Etoposide (VP-16):	75 mg/m^2/day IV on days 1–5
Ifosfamide:	1200 mg/m^2/day IV on days 1–5
Cisplatin:	20 mg/m^2/day IV on days 1–5
Mesna:	400 mg/m^2 IV, given 15 minutes before first ifosfamide dose, then 1200 mg/m^2/day IV continuous infusion for 5 days

Repeat cycle every 21 days [684].

TIP (salvage regimen)

Paclitaxel:	250 mg/m^2 IV over 24 hours on day 1
Ifosfamide:	1500 mg/m^2/day IV on days 2–5
Cisplatin:	25 mg/m^2/day IV on days 1–5
Mesna:	500 mg/m^2 IV, given before ifosfamide dose, and at 4 and 8 hours after ifosfamide on days 2–5

Repeat cycle every 21 days for a total of 4 cycles [685]. G-CSF support at 5 μg/kg/day SC should be given on days 7–18.

Paclitaxel + Gemcitabine

Paclitaxel:	100 mg/m^2 IV on days 1, 8, and 15
Gemcitabine:	1000 mg/m^2 IV on days 1, 8, and 15

Repeat cycle every 28 days for a total of 6 cycles [686].

THYMOMA

CAP

Cyclophosphamide:	500 mg/m^2 IV on day 1
Doxorubicin:	50 mg/m^2 IV on day 1
Cisplatin:	50 mg/m^2 IV on day 1

Repeat cycle every 21 days [687].

Cisplatin + Etoposide

Cisplatin:	60 mg/m^2 IV on day 1
Etoposide:	120 mg/m^2 IV on days 1–3

Repeat cycle every 21 days [688].

ADOC

Cisplatin:	50 mg/m^2 IV on day 1
Doxorubicin:	40 mg/m^2 IV on day 1
Vincristine:	0.6 mg/m^2 IV on day 3
Cyclophosphamide:	700 mg/m^2 IV on day 4

Repeat cycle every 28 days [689].

VIP

Etoposide.	75 mg/m^2 IV on days 1–4
Ifosfamide:	1200 mg/m^2 IV on days 1–4
Cisplatin:	20 mg/m^2 IV on days 1–4
Mesna:	240 mg/m^2 IV before first ifosfamide dose, then 4 and 8 hours later on days 1–4

Repeat cycle every 21 days for a total of 4 cycles [690]. G-CSF support at 5 µg/kg/day should be given on days 5–15.

Gemcitabine + Topotecan

Gemcitabine:	1000 mg/m^2 IV on days, 1, 8, and 15
Topotecan:	0.75–1.5 mg/m^2 IV on days, 1, 8, and 15

Repeat cycle every 21 days [691].

Carboplatin + Paclitaxel

Carboplatin:	AUC of 6, IV on day 1
Paclitaxel:	225 mg/m^2 IV on day 1

Repeat cycle every 21 days [692].

THYROID CANCER

Combination Regimens

Doxorubicin + Cisplatin

Doxorubicin:	60 mg/m^2 IV on day 1

Cisplatin:	40 mg/m^2 IV on day 1

Repeat cycle every 21 days 693].

Single-Agent Regimens

Doxorubicin

Doxorubicin:	60 mg/m^2 IV on day 1

Repeat cycle every 21 days [693].

Sorafenib

Sorafenib:	400 mg PO bid

Continue treatment until disease progression [694].

Sunitinib

Sunitinib:	50 mg PO bid

Continue treatment until disease progression [695].

Pazopanib

Pazopanib:	800 mg PO daily

Continue treatment until disease progression [696].

Vandetanib (medullary carcinoma of the thyroid)

Vandetanib:	300 mg PO daily

Continue treatment until disease progression [697].

Cabozantinib (medullary carcinoma of the thyroid)

Cabozantinib:	140 mg PO daily

Continue treatment until disease progression [698].

Lenvatinib

Lenvatinib:	24 mg PO daily

Continue treatment until disease progression [699].

References

1.   Fassnacht M, et al. N Engl J Med 2012;366:2189–2197.
2.   Flam M, et al. J Clin Oncol 1996;14:2527–2539.
3.   Bosset JF, et al. Eur J Cancer 2003;39:45–51.
4.   Hung A, et al. Cancer 2003;97:1195–1202.

5. Meropol NJ, et al. J Clin Oncol 2008;26:3229–3214.
6. Eng C, et al. J Clin Oncol 2009;27:15S (abstract 4116).
7. Flam MS, et al. J Clin Oncol 1996;16:227–253.
8. Seklulic A, et al. N Engl J Med 2012;366:2171–2179.
9. Migden MR, et al. Lancet Oncol 2015;16:716–728.
10. Thongprasert S, et al. Ann Oncol 2005;16:279–281.
11. Valle JW, et al. N Engl J Med 2010;362:1273–1281.
12. Knox JJ, et al. J Clin Oncol 2005;23:2332–2338.
13. Andre T, et al. Ann Oncol 2004;15:1339–1343.
14. Taieb J, et al. Ann Oncol 2002;13:1192–1196.
15. Hong YS, et al. Cancer Chemother Pharmacol 2007;60:321–328.
16. Nehls O, et al. Br J Cancer 2008;98:309–315.
17. Patt YZ, et al. Cancer 2004;101:578–586.
18. Papakostas P, et al. Eur J Cancer 2001;37:1833–1838.
19. Park JS, et al. Jpn J Clin Oncol 2005;35:68–73.
20. Bajorin DF, et al. Cancer 2000;88:1671–1678.
21. Kaufman D, et al. J Clin Oncol 2000;18:1921–1927.
22. Linardou H, et al. Urology 2004;64:479–484.
23. Meluch AA, et al. J Clin Oncol 2001;19:3018–3024.
24. Sternberg CN, et al. Cancer 2001;92:2993–2998.
25. Gitlitz BJ, et al. Cancer 2003;98:1863–1869.
26. Sternberg CN, et al. Cancer 1989;64:2448–2458.
27. Harker WG, et al. J Clin Oncol 1985;3:1463–1470.
28. Santis MD, et al. J Clin Oncol 2009;27:5634–5638.
29. Garcia del Muro X, et al. Br J Cancer 2002;86:326–330.
30. Vaughn D, et al. Cancer 2002;95:1022–1027.
31. Dreicer R, et al. J Clin Oncol 2000;18:1058–1061.
32. James ND, et al. N Engl J Med 2012;366:1477–1488.
33. Moore MJ, et al. J Clin Oncol 1997;15:3441–3445.
34. Roth BJ, et al. J Clin Oncol 1994;12:2264–2270.
35. Vaughn D, et al. J Clin Oncol 2002;20:937–940.
36. Sweeney CJ, et al. J Clin Oncol 2006;24:3451–3457.
37. Rosenberg JE, et al. Lancet 2016;387:1909-1920.
38. Stupp R, et al. N Engl J Med 2005;352:987–995.
39. Levin VA, et al. Int J Radiat Oncol Biol Phys 1990;18:321–324.
40. DeAngelis LM, et al. Ann Neurol 1998;44:691–695.
41. Buckner JC, et al. J Clin Oncol 2003;21:251–255.
42. Vredenburgh JJ, et al. J Clin Oncol 2007;25:4722–4729.
43. Nicholas MK, et al. J Clin Oncol 2009;27:15S (abstract 2016).
44. Reardon DA, et al. Cancer 2011;26:188–193.
45. Glas M, et al. J Clin Oncol, 2009;27:1257–1261.

46.   Yung A, et al. Proc Am Soc Clin Oncol 1999;18:139a.

47.   Yung A, et al. J Clin Oncol 1999;17:2762–2771.

48.   Raymond E, et al. Ann Oncol 2003;14:603–614.

49.   Friedman H, et al. J Clin Oncol 1999;17:1516–1525.

50.   Beal K, et al. Radiat Oncol 2011;6:2–15.

51.   Bear H, et al. J Clin Oncol 2003;21:4165–4174.

52.   Schneeweiss A, et al. Ann Oncol 2013;24:2278–2284.

53.   Fisher B, et al. J Clin Oncol 2000;8:1483–1496.

54.   Hudis C, et al. J Clin Oncol 1999;17:93–100.

55.   Sparano JA, et al. N Engl J Med 2008;358:1663–1671.

56.   Sparano J, et al. San Antonio Breast Cancer Symposium 2005 (abstract 48).

57.   Jones S, et al. J Clin Oncol 2006;24:5381–5387.

58.   Martin M, et al. N Engl J Med 2005;352:2302–2313.

59.   Budman DR, et al. J Natl Cancer Inst 1998;90:1205–1211.

60.   Weiss RB, et al. Am J Med 1987;83:455–463.

61.   Poole CJ, et al. N Engl J Med 2006;355:1851–1862.

62.   Coombes RC, et al. J Clin Oncol 1996;14:35–45.

63.   Roche H, et al. J Clin Oncol 2006;24:5664–5671.

64.   Burstein HJ, et al. J Clin Oncol 2005;23:8340–8347.

65.   Citron M, et al. J Clin Oncol 2003;21:1431–1439.

66.   Puhalla S, et al. J Clin Oncol 2008;26:1691–1697.

67.   Romond EH, et al. N Engl J Med. 2005;353:1673–1684.

68.   Dang C, et al. J Clin Oncol 2006;24:17S (abstract 582).

69.   Slamon D, et al. San Antonio Breast Cancer Symposium 2006 (abstract 52).

70.   Joensuu H, et al. N Engl J Med 2006;354:809–820.

71.   Baselga J, et al. N Engl J Med 2012;366:109–119.

72.   Fisher B, et al. J Natl Cancer Inst 1997;89:1673–1682.

73.   Howell A, et al. Lancet 2005;365:60–62.

74.   BIG I-98 Collaborative Group, et al. N Engl J Med 2009;361:766–776.

75.   Goss PE, et al. J Natl Cancer Inst 2005;97:1262–1271.

76.   Coombes RC, et al. N Engl J Med 2004;350:1081–1092.

77.   Gnant M, et al. N Engl J Med 2009;360:679–691.

78.   Baselga J, et al. N Engl J Med 2012;366:520–529.

79.   Sledge GE, et al. J Clin Oncol 2003;21:588–592.

80.   Levine MN, et al. J Clin Oncol 1998;16:2651–2658.

81.   O'Shaughnessy J, et al. J Clin Oncol 2002;20:2812–2823.

82.   Biganzoli L, et al. Oncologist 2002;7 (Suppl):29–35.

83.   Thomas ES, et al. J Clin Oncol 2007;25:5210–5217.

84.   Dieras V. Oncology 1997;11:31–33.

85.   Brufman G, et al. Ann Oncol 1997;8:155–162.

86.   Sparano JA, et al. J Clin Oncol 2001;19:3117–3125.

87. The French Epirubicin Study Group. J Clin Oncol 1991;9:305–312.

88. O'Shaughnessy J, et al. Proc Am Soc Clin Oncol 2003;22:7 (abstract 25).

89. Perez EA, et al. Cancer 2000;88:124–131.

90. Fitch V, et al. Proc Am Soc Clin Oncol 2003;22:23 (abstract 90).

91. Miller K, et al. N Engl J Med 2007;35:2666–2676.

92. Slamon DJ, et al. N Engl J Med 2001;344:783–792.

93. Goldenberg MM, et al. Clin Ther 1999;21:309–318.

94. Francisco E, et al. J Clin Oncol 2002;20:1800–1808.

95. Pegram M, et al. Proc Am Soc Clin Oncol 2007;25 (LBA1008).

96. Loesch D, et al. Clin Breast Cancer 2008;8:178–186.

97. Burstein HJ, et al. J Clin Oncol 2001;19:2722–2730.

98. O'Shaughnessy J, et al. Clin Breast Cancer 2004;5:142–147.

99. Schaller G, et al. J Clin Oncol 2007;25:3246–3250.

100. Bartsch R, et al. J Clin Oncol 2007;25:3853–3858.

101. Blackwell KL, et al. J Clin Oncol 2010;28:1124–1130.

102. Geyer CE, et al. N Engl J Med 2006;355:2733–2743.

103. Finn RS, et al. Lancet Oncol 2015;16;25–35.

104. Turner NC, et al. N Engl J Med 2015;373:209–219.

105. Jaiyesimi IA, et al. J Clin Oncol 1995;13:513–529.

106. Hayes DF, et al. J Clin Oncol 1995;13:2556 2566.

107. Lonning PE, et al. J Clin Oncol 2000;18:2234–2244.

108. Buzdar A, et al. J Clin Oncol 1996;14:2000–2011.

109. Dombernowsky P, et al. J Clin Oncol 1998;16:453–461.

110. Howell A. Clin Cancer Res 2001;7 (Suppl 12):4402s–4410s.

111. Di Leo A, et al. J Clin Oncol 2010;28:4594–4600.

112. Kimmick GG, et al. Cancer Treat Res 1998;94:231–254.

113. Baselga J, et al. Semin Oncol 1999;26 (Suppl 12):78–83.

114. Baselga J, et al. J Clin Oncol 2005;23:2162–2171.

115. Verma S, et al. N Engl J Med 2012;367:1783–1791.

116. Blum JL, et al. J Clin Oncol 1999;17:485–493.

117. Chan S. Oncology 1997;11 (Suppl 8):19–24.

118. Baselga J and Tabernero JM. Oncologist 2001;6 (Suppl 3):26–29.

119. Holmes FA, et al. J Natl Cancer Inst 1991;83:1797–1805.

120. Perez EA. Oncologist 1998;3:373–389.

121. Perez EA, et al. J Clin Oncol 2007;25:3407–3414.

122. Fumoleau P, et al. Semin Oncol 1995;22 (Suppl 5):22–28.

123. Torti FM, et al. Ann Intern Med 1983;99:745–749.

124. Carmichael J, et al. Semin Oncol 1996;23 (Suppl 10):77–81.

125. Al-Batran SE, et al. Oncol 2006;70:141–146.

126. O'Shaughnessy JA, et al. Breast Cancer Res Treat 2003;82:Suppl 1 (abstract 43).

127. O'Shaughnessy JA, et al. Breast Cancer Res Treat 2004;88:Suppl 1 (abstract 1070).

128. Cortes J, et al. Lancet 2011;377:914–923.

129. Hainsworth JD, et al. J Clin Oncol 1997;15:2385–2393.

130. Longeval E, et al. Cancer 1982;50:2751–2756.

131. Hainsworth JD, et al. J Clin Oncol 1992;10:912–922.

132. Greco FA, et al. J Clin Oncol 2002;20:1651–1656.

133. Moller AK, et al. Acta Oncol 2010;49:423–430.

134. Hainsworth JD, et al. Cancer J 2010;16:70–75.

135. Hainsworth JD, et al. Cancer 2010;116:2448–2454.

136. Hainsworth JD, et al. J Clin Oncol 2007;25:1747–1752.

137. Moertel CG, et al. N Engl J Med 1992;326:519–526.

138. Moertel CG, et al. Cancer 1991;68:227–232.

139. Pavel ME, et al. Lancet 2011;378:2005–2012.

140. Strosberg JR, et al. Cancer 2011;117:268–275.

141. Saltz L, et al. Cancer 1993;72:244.

142. Coplin ME, et al. N Engl J Med 2014;371:224–233.

143. Kulke MH, et al. J Clin Oncol 2008;26:3403–3410.

144. Yao JC, et al. N Engl J Med 2011;364:514–523.

145. Rose PG, et al. N Engl J Med 1995;15:1144.

146. Morris M, et al. N Engl J Med 1999;340:1137–1143.

147. Fiorica J, et al. Gynecol Oncol 2002;85:89–94.

148. Tewari KS, et al. J Clin Oncol 2013;31:Suppl (abstract 3).

149. Buxton EJ, et al. J Natl Cancer Inst 1989;81:359–361.

150. Murad AM, et al. J Clin Oncol 1994;12:55–59.

151. Whitney CW, et al. J Clin Oncol 1999;17:1339–1348.

152. Pignata S, et al. J Clin Oncol 1999;17:756–760.

153. Chitapanarux I, et al. Gynecol Oncol 2003;89:402–407.

154. Monk BJ, et al. Proc Am Soc Clin Oncol 2008;26:(LBA5504).

155. Brewer CA, et al. Gynecol Oncol 2006;100:385–388.

156. Nagao S, et al. Gynecol Oncol 2005;96:805–809.

157. Miller DS, et al. J Clin Oncol 2014;32:2744–2749.

158. Levy T, et al. Proc Am Soc Clin Oncol 1996;15:292a.

159. Thigpen T, et al. Semin Oncol 1997;24 (Suppl 2):41–46.

160. Verschraegen CF, et al. J Clin Oncol 1997;15:625–631.

161. Muderspach LI, et al. Gynecol Oncol 2001;81:213–215.

162. Lorusso D, et al. Ann Oncol 2010;21:61–66.

163. Schilder RJ, et al. Gynecol Oncol 2005;95:103–107.

164. Sauer R, et al. N Engl J Med 2004;351:1731–1740.

165. Minsky BD. Oncology 1994;6:53–58.

166. Minsky BD. Clin Colorectal Cancer 2004;4 (Suppl 1):S29–36.

167. Ryan DP, et al. J Clin Oncol 2006;24:2557–2562.

168. Rodel C, et al. J Clin Oncol 2007;25:110–117.

169. O'Connell MJ, et al. J Clin Oncol 1997;15:246–250.

170. Wolmark N, et al. J Clin Oncol 1993;11:1879–1887.

171. Benson AB, et al. Oncology 2000;14:203–212.

172. Andre, T et al. N Engl J Med 2004;350:2343–2351.

173. Chung KY and Saltz LB. Cancer J 2007;13:192–197.

174. Kuebler JP, et al. J Clin Oncol 2007;25:2198–2204.

175. Schmoll HJ, et al. J Clin Oncol 2007;25:102–109.

176. Twelves C, et al. N Engl J Med 2005;352:2696–2704.

177. Saltz LB, et al. N Engl J Med 2000;343:905–914.

178. Hurwitz H, et al. N Engl J Med 2004;350:2335–2342.

179. Hwang JJ, et al. Am J Oncol Rev 2003;2 (Suppl 5):15–25.

180. Douillard JY, et al. Lancet 2000;355:1041–1047.

181. Andre T, et al. Eur J Cancer 1999;35:1343–1347.

182. de Gramont A, et al. J Clin Oncol 2000;18:2938–2947.

183. Tournigand C, et al. J Clin Oncol 2004;22:229–237.

184. Andre T, et al. Proc Am Soc Clin Oncol 2003;22:253 (abstract 1016).

185. Maindrault-Goebel F, et al. J Clin Oncol 2006;24 (June 20 Supplement):3504.

186. Falcone A. et al. J Clin Oncol 2007;25:1670–1676.

187. Loupakis F, et al. N Engl J Med 2014;371:1609–1618.

188. Fornaro L, et al. Ann Oncol 2013;24:2062–2067.

189. Cunningham D, et al. N Engl J Med 2004;351:337–345.

190. Scheithauer W, et al. J Clin Oncol 2003;21:1307–1312.

191. Kerr D. Oncology 2002;16 (Suppl 14):12–15.

192. Borner MM, et al. Ann Oncol 2005;16:282–288.

193. Lim DH, et al. Cancer Chemother Pharmacol 2005;56:10–14.

194. Goldberg RM, et al. J Clin Oncol 2004;22:23–30.

195. Poon MA, et al. J Clin Oncol 1989;7:1407–1418.

196. Petrelli N, et al. J Clin Oncol 1989;7:1419–1426.

197. Kabbinavar F, et al. J Clin Oncol 2005;23:3697–3705.

198. Jager E, et al. J Clin Oncol 1996;14:2274–2279.

199. de Gramont A, et al. J Clin Oncol 1997;15:808–815.

200. Giantonio BJ, et al. J Clin Oncol 2007;25:1539–1544.

201. Dimou A, et al. Expert Opin Investing Drugs 2010;19:723–735.

202. Hochster HS, et al. J Clin Oncol 2008;26:3523–3529.

203. Saltz L, et al. J Clin Oncol 2007;22:4557–4561.

204. Cunningham D, et al. N Engl J Med 2004;351:537–545.

205. Sobrero AF, et al. J Clin Oncol 2008;26:2311–2319.

206. van Cutsem EV, et al. N Engl J Med 2009;360:1408–1417.

207. Bokemeyer C, et al. J Clin Oncol 2009;27:663–671.

208. Scott J, et al. J Clin Oncol 2005;23:16S (abstract 3705).

209. Doullard JY, et al. J Clin Oncol 2010;28:4697–4705.

210. Peeters M, et al. J Clin Oncol 2010;28:4706–4713.

211. Kopetz S, et al. J Clin Oncol 2007;25:18S (abstract 4027).

212. van Cutsem EE, et al. J Clin Oncol 2012;30:3499–3506.
213. Tabernero J, et al. Lancet Oncol 2015;16:499–508.
214. Kemeny N, et al. J Clin Oncol 1994;12:2288–2295.
215. Hoff P, et al. J Clin Oncol 2001;15:2282–2292.
216. Pitot HC, et al. J Clin Oncol 1997;15:2910–2919.
217. Ulrich-Pur H, et al. Ann Oncol 2001;12:1269–1272.
218. Rougier P, et al. J Clin Oncol 1997;15:251–260.
219. Saltz LB, et al. J Clin Oncol 2004;22:1201–1208.
220. Tabernero J, et al. J Clin Oncol 2006;24:18S (abstract 3085).
221. van Cutsem EV, et al. J Clin Oncol 2007;25:1658–1664.
222. Leichman CG, et al. J Clin Oncol 1995;13:1303–1311.
223. Leichman CG. Oncology 1999;13 (Suppl 3):26–32.
224. Falcone A, et al. Cancer Chemother Pharmacol 1999;44:159–163.
225. Grothey A, et al. J Clin Oncol 2012; Suppl 4 (abstract LBA385).
226. Mayer RJ, et al. N Engl J Med 2015;20:1909–1919.
227. Hoskins PJ, et al. J Clin Oncol 2001;19:4048–4053.
228. Thigpen JT, et al. J Clin Oncol 1994;12:1408–1414.
229. Deppe G, et al. Eur J Gynecol Oncol 1994;15:263–266.
230. Fiorica JV. Oncologist 2002;7 (Suppl 5):36–45.
231. Fleming GF, et al. J Clin Oncol 2004;22:2159–2165.
232. Burke TW, et al. Gynecol Oncol 1994;55:47–50.
233. Pignata S, et al. Br J Cancer 2007;96:1639–1643.
234. Homesley HD, et al. J Clin Oncol 2007;25:526–531.
235. Wolfson AH, et al. J Clin Oncol 2006;24(18S):5001.
236. Hensley ML, et al. Gynecol Oncol 2008;109:329–334.
237. Muss HB. Semin Oncol 1994;21:107–113.
238. Thigpen JT, et al. J Clin Oncol 1999;17:1736–1744.
239. Ball H, et al. Gynecol Oncol 1996;62:278–282.
240. Wadler S, et al. J Clin Oncol 2003;21:2110–2114.
241. Oza AM, et al. J Clin Oncol 2011;29:3278–3285.
242. Herskovic A, et al. N Engl J Med 1992;326:1593–1598.
243. Bedenne L, et al. J Clin Oncol 2007;25:1160–1168.
244. Heath El, et al. J Clin Oncol 2000;18:868–876.
245. Cunningham D, et al. N Engl J Med 2006;355:11–20.
246. Kies MS, et al. Cancer 1987;60:2156–2160.
246a. Ilson DH, et al. J Clin Oncol 1999;17:3270–3275.
247. Ilson DH, et al. J Clin Oncol 1998;16:1826–1834.
248. van Meerten E, et al. Br J Cancer 2007;96:1348–1352.
249. Cunningham D, et al. N Engl J Med 2008;358:36–46.
250. Ajani JA, et al. Semin Oncol 1995;22 (Suppl 6):35–40.
251. MacDonald JS, et al. N Engl J Med 2001;345:725–730.
252. Bang Y, et al. J Clin Oncol 2011;29:185 (LBA4002).

253. Ajani JA, et al. J Clin Oncol 2007;25:3205–3209.

254. Wilke M, et al. J Clin Oncol 1989;7:1318–1326.

255. Shirao K, et al. J Clin Oncol 1997;15:921–927.

256. Shah MA, et al. J Clin Oncol 2006;24:5201–5206.

257. Ajani JA, et al. Proc Am Soc Clin Oncol 2000;20:165a (abstract 657).

258. Di Lauro L, et al. Br J Cancer 2007;97:593–599.

259. Kang Y, et al. J Clin Oncol 2006;24:18S (LBA4018).

260. van Cutsem EV, et al. J Clin Oncol 2009;27:18s (LBA4509).

261. Al-Batran SE, et al. J Clin Oncol 2008;26:1435–1442.

262. Keam B, et al. BMC Cancer 2008;8:148.

263. Wilke H, et al. Lancet Oncol 2014;11;1224–1235.

264. Cullinan SA, et al. J Clin Oncol 1994;12:412–416.

265. Cascinu S, et al. J Chemother 1992;4:185–188.

266. O'Connell MJ. J Clin Oncol 1985;3:1032–1039.

267. Ajani JA. Oncology 2002;16 (suppl 6):89–96.

268. Fuchs CS, et al. Lancet 2014;383:31–39.

269. Joensu H, et al. J Clin Oncol 2011;29:18S (LBA1).

270. Demetri GD, et al. N Engl J Med 2002;347:472–480.

271. Montemurro M, et al. Eur J Cancer 2009;45:2293–2297.

272. Demetri GD, et al. Proc GI ASCO 2006 (abstract 8).

273. Italiano A, et al. Ann Surg Oncol 2012;19:1551–1559.

274. Demetri GD, et al. Lancet 2013;381:295–302.

275. Bonner JA, et al. N Engl J Med 2006;354:567–578.

276. Posner MR, et al. N Engl J Med 2007;357:1705–1715.

277. Shin DS, et al. J Clin Oncol 1998;16:1325–1330.

278. Posner M, et al. J Clin Oncol 2001;19:1096–1104.

279. Shin DM, et al. Cancer 1999;91:1316–1323.

280. Fountzilas G, et al. Semin Oncol 1997;24 (Suppl 2):65–67.

281. Hitt R, et al. Semin Oncol 1995;22 (Suppl 15):50–54.

282. Kish JA, et al. Cancer 1984;53:1819–1824.

283. Vokes EE, et al. Cancer 1989;63 (Suppl 6):1048–1053.

284. Vermorken JB, et al. N Engl J Med 2008;359:1116–1127.

285. Burtness B, et al. J Clin Oncol 2005;23:8646–8654.

286. Veterans Affairs Laryngeal Cancer Study Group. N Engl J Med 1991;324:1685–1690.

287. Forastiere AA, et al. N Engl J Med 2003;349:2091–2098.

288. Al-Sarraf M, et al. J Clin Oncol 1998;16:1310–1317.

289. Gebbia V, et al. Am J Clin Oncol 1995;18:293–296.

290. Dreyfuss A, et al. Proc Am Soc Clin Oncol 1995;14:875a.

291. Forastiere AA, et al. Ann Oncol 1994;5 (Suppl 6):51–54.

292. Hong WK, et al. N Engl J Med 1983;308:75–79.

293. Degardin M, et al. Ann Oncol 1998;9:1103–1107.

294. Vermorken JB, et al. J Clin Oncol 2007;25:2171–2177.

295. Bauml J, et al. J Clin Oncol 2016;34:abstract 6011.

296. Taieb J, et al. Cancer 2003;98:2664–2670.

297. Qin S, et al. J Clin Oncol 2010:28; 303S (abstract 408).

298. Thomas MB, et al. J Clin Oncol 2009;27:843–850.

299. Llovet J, et al. N Engl J Med 2008;359:378–390.

300. Venook AP, et al. J Clin Oncol 1994;12:1323–1334.

301. Okada S, et al. Oncology 1993;50:22–26.

302. Patt YZ, et al. Cancer 2004;101:578–586.

303. Siegel AB, et al. J Clin Oncol 2008;26:2992–2998.

304. Ireland-Gill A, et al. Semin Oncol 1992;19 (Suppl 5):32–37.

305. Laubenstein LL, et al. J Clin Oncol 1984;2:1115–1120.

306. Gill PS, et al. J Clin Oncol 1996;14:2353–2364.

307. Northfelt DW, et al. J Clin Oncol 1997;15:653–659.

308. Gill PS, et al. J Clin Oncol 1999;17:1876–1880.

309. Gill PS, et al. Cancer 2002;95:147–154.

310. Lim ST, et al. Cancer 2005;103:417–421.

311. Evans SR, et al. J Clin Oncol 2002;20:3236–3241.

312. Nasti G, et al. J Clin Oncol 2000;18:1550–1557.

313. Real FX, et al. J Clin Oncol 1986;4:544–551.

314. Groopman JE, et al. Ann Intern Med 1984;100:671–676.

315. Linker CA, et al. Blood 1987;69:1242–1248.

316. Linker CA, et al. Blood 1991;78:2814–2822.

317. Larson R, et al. Blood 1995;85:2025–2037.

318. Kantarjian HM, et al. J Clin Oncol 2000;18:547–561.

319. Faderl S, et al. Cancer 2005;103:1985–1995.

320. DeAngelo DJ, et al. Blood 2007;109:5136–5142.

321. Ottman OG, et al. Blood 2002;100:1965–1971.

322. Talpaz M, et al. N Engl J Med 2006;354:2531–2541.

323. Kantarjian HM, et al. N Engl J Med 2006;354:2542–2551.

324. Topp MS, et al. Lancet Oncol 2015;16:57–66.

325. Yates JW, et al. Cancer Chemother Rep 1973;57:485–488.

326. Preisler H, et al. Blood 1987;69:1441–1449.

327. Preisler H, et al. Cancer Treat Rep 1977;61:89–92.

328. Faderi S, et al. Blood 2006;108:45–51.

329. Amadori S, et al. J Clin Oncol;34:972–979.

330. Sanz MA, et al. Blood 2010;115:5137–5146.

331. Estey E, et al. Blood 2006;107:3469–3473.

332. Ho AD, et al. J Clin Oncol 1988;6:213–217.

333. Montillo M, et al. Am J Hematol 1998;58:105–109.

334. Wiernik PH, et al. Blood 1992;79:313–319.

335. Tallman MS, et al. Blood 2005;106:1154–1163.

336. Santana VM, et al. J Clin Oncol 1992;10:364–369.

337. Gardin C, et al. Blood 2007;109:5129–5132.

338. Kantarjian HM, et al. Blood 2003;102:2379–2386.

339. Degos L, et al. Blood 1995;85:2643–2653.

340. Soignet SL, et al. J Clin Oncol 2001;19:3852–3860.

341. Sievers EL, et al. Blood 1999;11:3678–3684.

342. Man CH, et al. Blood 2012;119:5133-5143.

343. Fenaux P, et al. J Clin Oncol 2010;28:562–569.

344. Kantarjian HM, et al. J Clin Oncol 2012;30:2670–2677.

345. Raphael B, et al. J Clin Oncol 1991;9:770–776.

346. Keating MJ, et al. Blood 1998;92:1165–1171.

347. O'Brien S, et al. Blood 1993;82:1695–1700.

348. Byrd JC, et al. Blood 2003;101:6–14

349. Byrd JC, et al. J Clin Oncol 2011;29:1349-1355.

350. Keating M, et al. J Clin Oncol 2005;22:4079–4088.

351. Kay NE, et al. Blood 2004;104 (abstract 339).

352. Byrd JC, et al. J Clin Oncol 2014;32:3039-3047.

353. Furman RR, et al. N Engl J Med 2014;370:997–1007.

354. Goede V, et al. N Engl J Med 2014;370:1101–1110.

355. Osterborg A, et al. J Clin Oncol 1997;15:1567–1574.

356. Dighiero G, et al. N Engl J Med 1998;338:1506–1514.

357. Saven A, et al. J Clin Oncol 1995;13:570–574.

358. Keating MJ, et al. Blood 1988;92:1165–1171.

358a. Sawitsky A, et al. Blood 1977;50:1049.

359. Hainsworth JD, et al. J Clin Oncol 2003;21:1746–1751.

360. Wierda WG, et al. J Clin Oncol 2010;28:1749–1755.

361. Grever MR, et al. J Clin Oncol 1985;3:1196–1201.

362. Alvado M, et al. Semin Oncol 2002;29(4 Suppl 13):19–22.

363. Kath R, et al. J Cancer Res Clin Oncol 2001;127:48–54.

364. Ferrajoli A, et al. Blood 2008;111:5291–5297.

365. Byrd JC, et al. N Engl J Med 2014;369:32–42.

366. Stilgenbauer S, et al. Lancet Oncol 2016;17:768-778.

367. Guilhot F, et al. N Engl J Med 1997;337:223–229.

368. Druker BJ, et al. N Engl J Med 2001;344:1031–1037.

369. Kantarjian HM, et al. Blood 2007;110:3540–3546.

370. Kantarjian HM, et al. N Engl J Med 2010;362:2260–2270.

371. Kantarjian HM, et al. Blood 2007;109:5143–5150.

372. Saglio G, et al. N Engl J Med 2010;362:2251–2259.

373. Khoury HJ, et al. Blood 2012;119:3403–3412.

374. Kantarjian HM, et al. Blood 2012;120 (abstract 915).

375. Hehlmann R, et al. Blood 1993;82:398–407.

376. Hehlmann R, et al. Blood 1994;84:4064–4077.

377. The Italian Cooperative Study Group on Chronic Myelogenous Leukemia. N Engl J Med 1994;330:820–825.

378. Cortes J, et al. Blood 2012;120:2573–2581.

379. Saven A, et al. Blood 1992;79:111–1120.

380. Cassileth PA, et al. J Clin Oncol 1991;9:243–246.

381. Ratain MJ, et al. Blood 1985;65:644–648.

382. Gandara DR, et al. J Clin Oncol 2003;21:2004–2010.

383. Belani CP, et al. J Clin Oncol 2005;23:5883–5891.

384. Strauss GM, et al. J Clin Oncol 2004; 621S (abstract 7019).

385. Winton T, et al. N Engl J Med 2005;352:2589–2597.

386. Arriagada R, et al. N Engl J Med 2004:350:351–360.

387. Kreuter M, et al. Ann Oncol 2012;24:986–992.

388. Sandler AB, et al. N Engl J Med 2006;355:2542–2560.

389. Socinski ME, et al. J Clin Oncol 2012; 30:2055–2062.

390. Belani CP, et al. J Clin Oncol 2008;26:468–473.

391. Manegold C, et al. Proc Am Soc Clin Oncol 2007;25 (LBA7514).

392. Giaccone G, et al. J Clin Oncol 1998;16:2133–2141.

393. Fossella F, et al. J Clin Oncol 2003;21:3016–3024.

394. Belani CP, et al. Clin Lung Cancer 1999;1:144–150.

395. Georgoulias V, et al. Lancet 2001;357:1478–1484.

396. Abratt RP, et al. J Clin Oncol 1997;15:744–749.

397. Langer CJ, et al. Semin Oncol 1999;26 (Suppl 4):12–18.

398. Frasci G, et al. J Clin Oncol 2000;18:2529–2536.

399. Smith TJ, et al. J Clin Oncol 1995;13:2166–2173.

400. Pirker R, et al. Proc Am Soc Clin Oncol 2008;26 (abstract 3).

401. Cremonesi M, et al. Oncology 2003;64:97–101.

402. Scagliotti GV, et al. J Clin Oncol 2008;21:3543–3551.

403. Scagliotti GV. Semin Oncol 2005;32 (2 Suppl 2):S5–S8.

404. Longeval E, et al. Cancer 1982;50:2751–2756.

405. Gandara D, et al. J Clin Oncol 2003;21:2004–2010.

406. Herbst RS, et al. J Clin Oncol 2007;25:4734–4750.

407. Patel JD, et al. J Clin Oncol 2009;27:3284–3289.

408. Pirker R, et al. Lancet 2009;373:1525–1531.

409. Belani CP, et al. J Clin Oncol 2009;27:18S (abstract CRA8000).

410. Socinski MA, et al. J Clin Oncol 2012;30:2055–2062.

411. Garon EB, et al. Lancet 2014;384:665–673.

411a. Thatcher N, et al. Lancet Oncol 2015;16:763-774.

412. Lilenbaum RC, et al. J Clin Oncol 2005;23:190–196.

413. Tester WJ, et al. Cancer 1997;79:724–729.

414. Rizvi NA, et al. J Clin Oncol 2008;26:639–643.

415. Miller VA, et al. Semin Oncol 2000;27 (Suppl 3):3–10.

416. Hainsworth JD, et al. Cancer 2000;89:328–333.

417. Hanna N, et al. J Clin Oncol 2004;22:1589–1597.

418. Manegold C, et al. Ann Oncol 1997;8:525–529.

418a. Furuse K, et al. Ann Oncol 1996;7:815–820.

419. Herbst RS. Semin Oncol 2003;30 (Suppl 1):30–38.

420. Shepherd FA, et al. J Clin Oncol 2004;22 (Suppl 1):14S (abstract 7022).

421. Sequist LV, et al. J Clin Oncol 2013;27:3327–3334.

422. Socinski MA, et al. J Clin Oncol 2008;26:650–656.

423. Hanna N, et al. J Clin Oncol 2006;24:5253–5258.

424. Brahmer J, et al. N Engl J Med 2015;373:123–135.

425. Kwak EL, et al. N Engl J Med 2010;363:1693–1703.

426. Shaw AT, et al. N Engl J Med 2014;370:1189–1197.

427. Shaw AT, et al. Lancet Oncol 2016;17:234–242.

428. Yang J, et al. J Thorac Oncl 2016;11:S152-153.

429. Mok T, et al. J Thorac Oncol 2016;11:S142.

430. Ihde DC, et al. J Clin Oncol 1994;12:2022–2034.

431. Viren M, et al. Acta Oncol 1994;33:921–924.

432. Noda K, et al. N Engl J Med 2002;346:85–91.

433. Eckardt JR, et al. J Clin Oncol 2006;24:2044–2051.

434. Hainsworth JD, et al. J Clin Oncol 1997;15:3464–3470.

435. Neubauer M, et al. J Clin Oncol 2004;22:1872–1877.

436. Roth BJ, et al. J Clin Oncol 1992;10:282–291.

437. Aisner J, et al. Semin Oncol 1986;(Suppl 3):54–62.

438. Johnson DH. Semin Oncol 1993;20:315–325.

439. Johnson DH, et al. J Clin Oncol 1990;8:1013–1017.

440. Hainsworth JD, et al. Semin Oncol 1999;26 (Suppl 2):60–66.

441. Ardizzoni A, et al. J Clin Oncol 1997;15:2090–2096.

442. Masters GA, et al. J Clin Oncol 2003;21:1550–1555.

443. Bonadonna G, et al. Cancer 1975;36:252–259.

444. DeVita VT Jr, et al. Ann Intern Med 1970;73:881–895.

445. Klimo P, et al. J Clin Oncol 1985;3:1174–1182.

446. Bartlett NL, et al. J Clin Oncol 1995;13:1080–1088.

447. Canellos GP, et al. Ann Oncol 2003;14:268–272.

448. Longo DL. Semin Oncol 1990;17:716–735.

449. Colwill R, et al. J Clin Oncol 1995;13:396–402.

450. Diehl V, et al. J Clin Oncol 1998;16:3810–3821.

451. Tesch H, et al. Blood 1998;15:4560–4567.

452. Bartlett NL, et al. Ann Oncol 2007;18:1071–1079.

453. Santoro A, et al. J Clin Oncol 2000;18:2615–2619.

454. Schulz H, et al. Blood 2008;111:109–111.

455. Younes A, et al. J Clin Oncol 2012;30:2183–2189.

456. Ansell Sm, et al. N Engl J Med 2015;372:311-318.

457. Bagley CM Jr, et al. Ann Intern Med 1972;76:227–234.

458. Urba WJ, et al. J Natl Cancer Inst Monogr 1990;10:29–37.
459. Sonnevald P, et al. J Clin Oncol 1995;13:2530–2539.
460. McLaughlin P, et al. J Clin Oncol 1996;14:1262–1268.
461. Hochster H, et al. Blood 1994;84 (Suppl 1):383a.
462. Sacchi S, et al. Cancer 2007;110:121–128.
463. van Oers MHJ, et al. Blood 2006;108:3295–3301.
464. Forstpointer R, et al. Blood 2006;108:4003–4008.
465. Rummel MJ, et al. J Clin Oncol 2005;23:3383–3389.
466. Robinson KS, et al. J Clin Oncol 2008;26:4473–4479.
467. Fisher RI, et al. J Clin Oncol 2006;24:4867–4874.
468. Wang ML, et al. N Engl J Med 2013;369:507–516.
469. Sehn LH, et al. J Clin Oncol 2015;33:LBA8502.
470. Klimo P, et al. J Clin Oncol 1985;3:1174–1182.
471. Coiffier B, et al. N Engl J Med 2002;346:235–242.
472. Pfreundschuh M, et al. Lancet Oncol 2008;9:105–116.
473. Vose JM, et al. Leuk Lymphoma 2002;43:799–804.
474. Wilson WH, et al. J Clin Oncol 1993;11:1573–1582.
475. Wilson WH. Semin Oncol 2000;27 (Suppl 12):30–36.
476. Klimo P, et al. Ann Intern Med 1985;102:596–602.
477. Shipp MA, et al. Ann Intern Med 1986;104:757–765.
478. Longo DL, et al. J Clin Oncol 1991;9:25–38.
479. Velasquez WS, et al. J Clin Oncol 1994;12:1169–1176.
480. Velasquez WS, et al. Blood 1988;71:117–122.
481. Moskowitz C, et al. J Clin Oncol 1999;17:3776–3785.
482. Kewairamani T, et al. Blood 2004;103; 3684–3688.
483. Rodriguez MA, et al. Ann Oncol 1995;6:609–611.
484. El Gnaoui T, et al. Ann Oncol 2007;18:1363–1368.
485. Magrath I, et al. Blood 1984;63:1102–1111.
486. Magrath I, et al. J Clin Oncol 1996;14:925.
487. Berstein JI, et al. J Clin Oncol 1986;4:847–858.
488. Thomas DA, et al. Blood 2004;104:1624–1630.
489. McLaughlin P, et al. J Clin Oncol 1998;16:2825–2833.
489a. Ghielmini M, et al. Blood 2004;103:4416–4423.
490. Witzig TE, et al. J Clin Oncol 2002;20:2453–2463.
491. Falkson CI. Am J Clin Oncol 1996;19:268–270.
492. Betticher DC, et al. J Clin Oncol 1998;16:850–858.
493. Friedberg JW, et al. J Clin Oncol 2008;26:204–210.
494. Mann BS, et al. Oncologist 2007;12:1247–1252.
495. O'Connor OA, et al. J Clin Oncol 2009;27:4357–4364.
496. Pro B, et al. J Clin Oncol 2012;30:2190–2196.
497. Piekarz RI, et al. Blood 2011;117:5827–5834.
498. O'Connor OA, et al. J Clin Oncol 2015;33:2492–2499.

499. Strauss SJ, et al. J Clin Oncol 2006;24:2105–2112.

500. Habermann TM, et al. Br J Haematol 2009;145:344–349.

501. Abrey LE, et al. J Clin Oncol 2002;18:3144–3150.

502. Shah GD, et al. J Clin Oncol 2007;25:4730–4735.

503. Batchelor T, et al. J Clin Oncol 2003;21:1044–1049.

504. Reni M, et al. Br J Cancer 2007;96:864–867.

505. Fischer L, et al. Ann Oncol 2006;17:1141–1145.

506. Kirkwood JM, et al. J Clin Oncol 1996;14:7–17.

507. Eggermont AM, et al. Lancet 2008;372:117–126.

507a. Eggermont AM, et al. Lancet Oncol 2015;16:522-530.

508. Creagen ET, et al. J Clin Oncol 1999;17:1884–1890.

509. Falkson CI, et al. J Clin Oncol 1998;16:1743–1751.

510. Hwu WJ, et al. J Clin Oncol 2003;21:3351–3356.

511. Flaherty KT, et al. N Engl J Med 2012;367:1694–1703.

512. Larkin J, et al. N Engl J Med 2014;371:1867-1876.

513. Larkin J, et al. N Engl J Med 2015;373:23-34.

514. Luce JK, et al. Cancer Chemother Rep 1970;54:119–124.

515. Pritchard KI, et al. Cancer Treat Rep 1980;64:1123–1126.

516. Kirkwood JM, et al. Semin Oncol 1997;24 (Suppl 4):1–48.

517. Atkins MB, et al. J Clin Oncol 1999;17:2105–2116.

518. Parkinson DR, et al. J Clin Oncol 1990;8:1650–1656.

519. Acquavella N, et al. J Immunother 2008;31:569–576.

520. Wolchok JD, et al. Lancet Oncology 2010;11:155–164.

521. Robert C, et al. N Engl J Med 2015;372:2521–2532.

522. Weber JS, et al. Lancet Oncol 2015;16:375–384.

523. Middleton MR, et al. J Clin Oncol 2000;18:158–166.

524. Sosman JA, et al. N Engl J Med 2012;366:707–714.

525. Falchook GS, et al. Lancet 2012;379:1893–1901.

526. Kim KB, et al. J Clin Oncol 2013;31:482–489.

527. Ardizzoni A, et al. Cancer 1991;67:2984–2987.

528. Shin DM, et al. Cancer 1995;76:2230–2236.

529. Nowak AK, et al. Br J Cancer 2002;87:491–496.

530. Favaretto AG, et al. Cancer 2003;97:2791–2797.

531. Vogelzang NJ, et al. J Clin Oncol 2003;21:2636–2644.

532. Zucali PA, et al. Cancer 2008;112:1555–1561.

533. Simon GR, et al. J Clin Oncol 2008;21:3567–3572.

534. Jassem J, et al. J Clin Oncol 2008;26:1698–1704.

535. Steele JPC, et al. J Clin Oncol 2000;18:3912–3917.

536. Southwest Oncology Group Study. Arch Intern Med 1975;135:147–152.

537. Palumbo A, et al. Lancet 2006;367:835.

538. Facon T, et al. Proc Am Soc Clin Oncol 2006;24 (abstract 1).

539. Palumbo A, et al. J Clin Oncol 2007;25:4459–4465.

540. Barlogie B, et al. N Engl J Med 1984;310:1353–1356.

541. Rajkumar SV, et al. J Clin Oncol 2002;20:4319–4323.

542. Richardson PG, et al. Blood 2006;108:3458–3464.

543. Rajkumar SV, et al. Proc Am Soc Clin Oncol 2007;25 (LBA8025).

544. Richardson PG, et al. Blood 2010;116:679–686.

545. San-Miguel JF, et al. Lancet Oncol 2014;15:1195–1206.

546. Leleu X, et al. Blood 2013;121:1968–1975.

547. Lacy MQ, et al. Blood 2009;27:5008–5014.

548. Hussein MA, et al. Cancer 2002;95:2160–2168.

549. Orlowski RZ, et al. Proc Am Soc Hematol 2006 (abstract 404).

550. Berenson JR, et al. J Clin Oncol 2006;24:937–944.

551. San Miguel JF, et al. N Engl J Med 2008;359:906–917.

552. Palumbo A, et al. Blood 2007;109:2757–2762.

553. Palumbo A, et al. Leukemia 2010;24:1037–1042.

554. Stewart AK, et al. N Engl J Med 2015;372:142-152.

555. Moreau P, et al. Blood 2015;126:727.

556. Lokhorst HM, et al. N Engl J Med 2015;373:1207-1219.

557. Lonial S, et al. N Engl J Med 2015;373:621-631

558. Alexanian R, et al. Ann Intern Med 1986;105:8–11.

559. Cunningham D, et al. J Clin Oncol 1994;12:764–768.

560. Singhal S, et al. N Engl J Med 1999;341:1565–1571.

561. Richardson PG, et al. Blood 2006;108:3458–3464.

562. Richardson P, et al. N Engl J Med 2003;348:2609–2617.

563. Vij R, et al. Blood 2012;119:5661–5670.

564. Lonial S, et al. Lancet 2016;387:1551-1560.

565. Treon SP, et al. N Engl J Med 2015;372:1430-1400.

566. Silverman LR, et al. J Clin Oncol 2006;24:3895–3903.

567. Kantarjian HM, et al. Cancer 2006;106:1794–1803.

568. Kantarjian HM, et al. Semin Hematology 2005;32 (Suppl 2): S17–S22.

569. Galili N, et al. Expert Opin Investig Drugs 2006;15:805–813.

570. David M, et al. Blood 2007;109:61–64.

571. Passweg JR, et al. J Clin Oncol 2011;29:303–309.

572. Goorin A, et al. Med Pediatr Oncol 1995;24:362–367.

573. Meyers PA, et al. J Clin Oncol 2005;23:2004–2011.

574. Swenerton K, et al. J Clin Oncol 1992;10:718–726.

575. Alberts D, et al. J Clin Oncol 1992;10:706–717.

576. McGuire WP, et al. N Engl J Med 1996;334:1–6.

577. Ozols RE. Semin Oncol 1995;22 (Suppl 15):1–6.

578. Pignata S, et al. Crit Rev Oncol Hematol 2008;66:229–236.

579. Burger RA, et al. J Clin Oncol 2010:28:946S (LBA1).

580. Markman M, et al. J Clin Oncol 2001;19:1901–1905.

581. Pignant S, et al. J Clin Oncol 2009;27:18S (LBA5509).

582. D'Agostino G, et al. Br J Cancer 2003;89:1180–1184.

583. Nagourney RA, et al. Gynecol Oncol 2003;88:35–39.

584. Thigpen T. Semin Oncol 2006;33 (Suppl 6):S26–S32.

585. Armstrong DK, et al. N Engl J Med 2006;354:34–43.

586. Matulonis UA, et al. J Clin Oncol 2008;26:5761–5766.

587. Markman M. Gynecol Oncol 1998;69:226–229.

588. Rose PG, et al. Gynecol Oncol 2001;82:323–328.

589. McGuire WP, et al. Ann Intern Med 1989;111:273–279.

590. DeGeest K, et al. J Clin Oncol 2010;28:149–153.

591. Kudelka AP, et al. J Clin Oncol 1996;14:1552–1557.

592. Lund B, et al. J Natl Cancer Inst 1994;86:1530–1533.

593. Ozols RF. Drugs 1999;58 (Suppl 3):43–49.

594. Sorensen P, et al. Gynecol Oncol 2001;81:58–62.

595. Miller DS, et al. J Clin Oncol 2009;27:2686–2691.

596. Burger RA, et al. J Clin Oncol 2007;25:5165–5171.

597. Wolf JK, et al. Gynecol Oncol 2006;102:468–474.

598. Ledermann J, et al. Lancet Oncol 2014;15:852–861.

599. Dimopoulos MA, et al. Gynecol Oncol 2004;95:695–700.

600. Neoptolemos J, et al. J Clin Oncol 2009;27:18S (abstract LBA4505).

601. Oettle H, et al. JAMA 2007;297:267–277.

602. Gastrointestinal Tumor Study Group. Int J Radiat Oncol Biol Phys 1979;5:1643–1647.

603. Regine WF, et al. Proc Am Soc Clin Oncol 2006;25 (abstract 4007).

604. Loehrer PJ, et al. Proc Am Soc Clin Oncol 2008;26 (abstract 4506).

605. DeCaprio JA, et al. J Clin Oncol 1991;9:2128–2133.

606. Hess V, et al. J Clin Oncol 2003;21:66–68.

607. Cunningham D, et al. Proc. ECCO 2005;13 (abstract 11).

608. Fine RL, et al. Cancer Chemother Pharmacol 2008;61:167–175.

609. Louvet C, et al. J Clin Oncol 2002;20:1512–1518.

610. Louvet C, et al. Proc Am Soc Clin Oncol 2007;25:18S (abstract 4592).

611. Moore MJ, et al. J Clin Oncol 2005;23:16S (abstract 1).

612. Kulke MH, et al. J Clin Oncol 2007;25:4787–4792.

613. Conroy T, et al. J Clin Oncol 2010;28:302S (abstract 4010).

614. Von Hoff DD, et al N Engl J Med 2013;369:1691–1703.

615. Wang-Gilam A, et al. Lancet 2016;387:545–557.

616. Burris HA, et al. J Clin Oncol 1997;15:2403–2413.

617. Brand R, et al. Invest New Drugs 1997;15:331–341.

618. Cartwright TH, et al. J Clin Oncol 2002;20:160–164.

619. Eisenberger MA, et al. Semin Oncol 1994;21:613–619.

620. Jurincic CD, et al. Semin Oncol 1991;18 (Suppl 6):21–25.

621. Pienta KJ, et al. J Clin Oncol 1994;12:2005–2012.

622. Hudes GR, et al. J Clin Oncol 1992;11:1754–1761.

623. Hudes GR, et al. J Clin Oncol 1997;15:3156–3163.

624. Vaughn DJ, et al. Cancer 2004;100:746–750.
625. Tannock IF, et al. J Clin Oncol 1996;14:1756–1764.
626. Copur MS, et al. Semin Oncol 2001;28:16–21.
627. Petrylak DP, et al. N Engl J Med 2004;351:1513–1520.
628. Tannock IF, et al. N Engl J Med 2004;351:1502–1512.
629. Halabi S, et al. J Clin Oncol 2010;28:951S (LBA 4511).
630. DeBono JS, et al. J Clin Oncol 2010;28:344S (abstract 4508).
631. DeBono JS, et al. N Engl J Med 2011;364:1995–2005.
632. Sweeney C, et al. J Clin Oncol 2014;32:5S (LBA2).
633. Roth BJ, et al. Cancer 1993;72:2457–2460.
634. Ahmed S, et al. Proc Am Soc Clin Oncol 1998;17:325a.
635. Petrylak DP. Semin Oncol 2000;27 (Suppl 3):24–29.
636. Dreicer R. Hematol Oncol Clin North Am 2006;20:935–946.
636a. Murphy GP, et al. Urology 1984;23:54–63.
637. Dijkman GA, et al. Eur Urol 1995;27:43–46.
638. Hanks GE, et al. J Clin Oncol 2003;21:3972–3978.
639. Klotz L, et al. BJU Int 2008;10:1531–1538.
640. The Leuprolide Study Group. N Engl J Med 1984;311:1281–1286.
641. Sharifi R, et al. Clin Ther 1996;18:647–657.
642. Please see package insert for Lupron Depot and go to http://www
.lupronadvancedprostatecancer.com/about-lupron-depot.cfm (accessed Sept. 2013).
643. Schellhammer PF, et al. Urology 1997;50:330–336.
644. McLeod DG, et al. Cancer 1993;72:3870–3873.
645. Janknegt RA, et al. J Urol 1993;149:77–82.
646. Tannock IF, et al. J Clin Oncol 1989;7:590–597.
647. Fossa SD, et al. J Clin Oncol 2001;19:62–71.
648. Johnson DE, et al. Urology 1988;31:132–134.
649. Havlin KA, et al. Cancer Treat Res 1988;39:83–96.
650. Kantoff PW, et al. N Engl J Med 2010;363:411–422.
651. Scher HI, et al. N Engl J Med 2012;367:1187–1197.
652. Escudier B, et al. Lancet 2007;370:2103–2111.
653. Atzpodien J, et al. Semin Oncol 1993;20 (Suppl 9):22.
654. Motzer RJ, et al. Lancet Oncol 2015;16:1473–1482.
655. Yang JC, et al. N Engl J Med 2003;349:427–434.
656. Motzer RJ, et al. J Clin Oncol 2006;24:16–24.
657. Ratain MJ, et al. J Clin Oncol 2006;24:2505–2512.
658. Sternberg CN, et al. J Clin Oncol 2010;28:1061–1068.
659. Rini Bl, et al., et al. Lancet 2011;378:1931–1939.
660. Hudes G, et al. N Engl J Med 2007;356:2271–2281.
661. Motzer RJ, et al. Lancet 2008;372:449–456.
662. Fyfe G, et al. J Clin Oncol 1995;13:688–696.
663. Minasian LM, et al. J Clin Oncol 1993;11:1368–1375.

664. Choueiri TK, et al. N Engl J Med 2015:373:1814-1822.

665. Motzer RJ et al. Lancet Oncol 2015;16:1473-1482.

666. Antman K, et al. J Clin Oncol 1993;11:1276–1285.

667. Worden FP, et al. J Clin Oncol 2005;23:105–112.

668. Elias A, et al. J Clin Oncol 1989;7:1208–1216.

669. Santoro A, et al. J Clin Oncol 1995;13:1537–1545.

670. Maki RG, et al. J Clin Oncol 2007;25:2755–2763.

671. Dileo P, et al. Cancer 2007;109:1863–1869.

672. Holcombe E, et al. N Engl J Med 2003;348:694–701.

673. van Oosterom AT, et al. Eur J Cancer 2002;38:2397–2406.

674. Judson I, et al. Eur J Cancer 2001;37:870–877.

675. van Der Graaf, et al. J Clin Oncol 2011;29:18S (LBA 10002).

676. Demetri GD, et al. J Clin Oncol 2016;34:786-793.

677. Schoffski P, et al. Lancet 2016;387:1629-1637.

678. Einhorn LH, et al. J Clin Oncol 1989;7:387–391.

679. Oliver RT, et al. Lancet 2005;366:293–300.

680. Nichols CR, et al. J Clin Oncol 1998;16:1287–1295.

681. Bosl G, et al. J Clin Oncol 1988;6:1231–1238.

682. Einhorn LH, et al. Ann Intern Med 1977;87:293–298.

683. Vugrin D, et al. Ann Intern Med 1981;95:59–61.

684. Loehrer PJ, et al. Ann Intern Med 1988;109:540–546.

685. Kondagunat GV, et al. J Clin Oncol 2005;23:6549–6555.

686. Einhorn LH, et al. J Clin Oncol 2007;25:513–516.

687. Loehrer PJ, et al. J Clin Oncol 1994;12:1164–1168.

688. Giaccone G, et al. J Clin Oncol 1996;14:814–820.

689. Fornasiero A, et al. Cancer 1991;68:30–33.

690. Loehrer PJ, et al. Cancer 2001;91:2010–2015.

691. William WN, et al. Am J Clin Oncol 2009;32:15–19.

692. Lemma GL, et al. J Clin Oncol 2011;29:2060–2065.

693. Shimaoka K, et al. Cancer 1985;56:2155–2160.

694. Gupta-Abramson V, et al. J Clin Oncol 2008;26:2010–2015.

695. Cabanillas ME, et al. J Clin Endocrinol Metab 2010;95:2588–2595.

696. Bible KC, et al. Lancet Oncol 2010;11:962–972.

697. Wells SA, et al. J Clin Oncol 2010;28:767–772.

698. Kurzrock R, et al. J Clin Oncol 2011;29:2660–2666.

699. Schlumberger M, et al. N Engl J Med 2015; 372:621–630.

5

Antiemetic Agents for the Treatment of Chemotherapy-Induced Nausea and Vomiting

M. Sitki Copur, Laurie J. Harrold, and Edward Chu

This chapter presents an overview of the common antiemetic agents as well as selected regimens for the treatment of chemotherapy-induced nausea and vomiting. The various regimens selected are used in clinical practice in the medical oncology community. It should be emphasized that not all of the drugs and dosages in the regimens have been officially approved by the Food and Drug Administration (FDA). This chapter should serve as a quick reference for physicians and healthcare professionals, and it provides several options for treating both acute and delayed nausea and vomiting. It is not intended to be an all-inclusive review of all the antiemetic treatment regimens, nor is it intended to endorse and/or prioritize any particular drug or regimen.

COMMON ANTIEMETIC REGIMENS FOR CHEMOTHERAPY-INDUCED NAUSEA AND VOMITING:

Mildly Emetogenic Chemotherapy (Levels 1 and 2):

1. Prochlorperazine 10–25 mg PO, 5–25 mg IV, or 25 mg PR before chemotherapy and then 10–25 mg PO every 4–6 hours as needed.

2. Thiethylperazine 10 mg PO, 10 mg IM, or 10 mg PR every 4–6 hours as needed.
3. Ondansetron 8 mg PO bid with the first dose 30 minutes before the start of chemotherapy and a subsequent dose 8 hours after the first dose or 32 mg IV.
4. Dexamethasone 4–8 mg PO or 10–20 mg IV before chemotherapy and every 4–6 hours as needed.
5. Prochlorperazine 10–25 mg PO, 5–25 mg IV, or 25 mg PR before chemotherapy and then 10–25 mg PO every 6 hours as needed; dexamethasone 4 mg PO or 10–20 mg IV before chemotherapy and continue with 4 mg PO every 6 hours up to a total of four doses as needed.
6. Prochlorperazine 10–25 mg PO, 5–25 mg IV, or 25 mg PR before chemotherapy and then 10–25 mg PO every 6 hours as needed; dexamethasone 4 mg PO or 10–20 mg IV before chemotherapy and continue with 4 mg PO every 6 hours up to a total of four doses as needed; and lorazepam 1.5 mg/m^2 IV administered 45 minutes before chemotherapy.
7. Metoclopramide 20–40 mg PO and diphenhydramine 25–50 mg PO every 4–6 hours as needed.
8. Metoclopramide 1–2 mg/kg IV and diphenhydramine 25–50 mg IV every 4–6 hours as needed.
9. Dolasetron 100 mg PO daily.
10. Granisetron 1–2 mg (total dose) PO daily.
11. Ondansetron 8–16 mg PO daily.

Moderately Emetogenic Chemotherapy (Level 3):

1. Ondansetron 32 mg IV and dexamethasone 4–8 mg PO or 10–20 mg IV given 30 minutes before chemotherapy. In the next 1–2 mornings, give ondansetron 16 mg PO and dexamethasone 8 mg PO along with prochlorperazine 10 mg PO every 6 hours as needed.
2. Dolasetron 100 mg PO or IV and dexamethasone 8 mg IV 30 minutes before chemotherapy. In the next 1–2 mornings, give dolasetron 100 mg PO and dexamethasone 8 mg PO along with prochlorperazine 10 mg PO every 6 hours as needed.
3. Granisetron 1–2 mg PO one hour before chemotherapy and dexamethasone 8 mg IV 30 minutes before chemotherapy. In the next 1–2 mornings, give granisetron 1 mg PO and dexamethasone 8 mg PO along with prochlorperazine 10 mg PO every 6 hours as needed.
4. Aprepitant 125 mg PO taken 60 minutes before chemotherapy; dexamethasone 12 mg PO and ondansetron 32 mg IV given 30 minutes before chemotherapy.
5. Aprepitant 125 mg PO taken 60 minutes before chemotherapy; dexamethasone 12 mg PO and granisetron 1–2 mg PO or 10 mg/kg IV given 30 minutes before chemotherapy.
6. Aprepitant 115 mg IV taken 30 minutes before chemotherapy; dexamethasone 12 mg PO and granisetron 1–2 mg PO or 10 mg/kg IV given 30 minutes before chemotherapy.
7. Dexamethasone 4–8 mg PO or 10–20 mg IV for one dose before chemotherapy; lorazepam 1.5 mg/m^2 IV before chemotherapy; and prochlorperazine 5–25 mg PO or IV before chemotherapy.

8. Palonosetron 0.25 mg IV given 30 minutes before chemotherapy.
9. Palonosetron 0.25 mg IV given 30 minutes before chemotherapy; aprepitant 125 mg PO taken 60 minutes before chemotherapy on day 1, and 80 mg PO on days 2–3; dexamethasone 12 mg PO taken 30 minutes before chemotherapy on day 1, and 8 mg PO on days 2–3.
10. Rolapitant 180 mg PO 1–2 hours before chemotherapy, granisetron 1–2 mg PO one hour before chemotherapy, and dexamethasone 20 mg IV 30 minutes before chemotherapy. Dexamethasone on days 2–4 is not necessary.
11. Netupitant 300 mg/0.5 mg palonosetron PO 1 hour before chemotherapy and dexamethasone 12 mg PO taken 30 minutes before chemotherapy on day 1. Admininstration of dexamethasone on days 2–4 is not necessary.
12. Fosaprepitant 150 mg IV 30 minutes before chemotherapy on days 1, dexamethasone 12 mg PO taken 30 minutes before chemotherapy on day 1, and 5-HT3 inhibitor on day 1.
13. Granisetron transdermal patch (34.3 mg of granisetron) applied to the upper outer arm at a minimum of 24 hours before chemotherapy. The patch should be removed a minimum of 24 hours after the completion of chemotherapy and may be worn for up to 7 days depending on the duration of the chemotherapy regimen. May also consider including dexamethasone on days 2–4 and/or may include a 5-HT3 inhibitor, such as dolasetron 100 mg PO on days 2–4 or ondansetron 8 mg PO on days 2–4.
14. Olanzapine 10 mg PO on day 1, palonosetron 0.25 mg IV on day 1, dexamethasone 20 mg IV on day 1 and olanzapine 10 mg PO on days 2 and 3

Highly Emetogenic Chemotherapy (Levels 4 and 5):

1. Ondansetron 32 mg IV and dexamethasone 10–20 mg IV plus lorazepam 1 mg PO or IV given 30 minutes before chemotherapy and then every 6 hours as needed. Ondansetron 16 mg PO and dexamethasone 8 mg PO in the next 2–3 mornings along with prochlorperazine 10 mg PO every 6 hours as needed.
2. Dolasetron 100 mg IV and dexamethasone 10–20 mg IV 30 minutes before chemotherapy or the same doses given orally 1 hour before chemotherapy. Dolasetron 100 mg PO and dexamethasone 8 mg PO in the next 2–3 mornings along with prochlorperazine 10 mg PO every 6 hours as needed.
3. Dolasetron 200 mg PO and dexamethasone 20 mg PO 30 minutes before chemotherapy.
4. Granisetron 1 mg or 10 mg/kg IV and dexamethasone 10–20 mg IV 30 minutes before chemotherapy. Granisetron 1 mg PO and dexamethasone 8 mg PO in the next 2–3 mornings along with prochlorperazine 10 mg PO every 6 hours as needed.
5. Aprepitant 125 mg PO taken 60 minutes before chemotherapy on day 1 and 80 mg PO on days 2–3; dexamethasone 12 mg PO and ondansetron 32 mg IV given 30 minutes before chemotherapy.
6. Aprepitant 125 mg PO taken 60 minutes before chemotherapy on day 1 and 80 mg PO on days 2–3; dexamethasone 12 mg PO and granisetron 1–2 mg PO or 10 mg/kg IV given 30 minutes before chemotherapy.

7. Aprepitant 115 mg IV taken 30 minutes before chemotherapy on day 1 and 80 mg PO on days 2–3; dexamethasone 12 mg PO and granisetron 1–2 mg PO or 10 mg/kg IV given 30 minutes before chemotherapy.

8. Metoclopramide 2–3 mg/kg IV, dexamethasone 10–20 mg IV; and diphenhydramine 25–50 mg IV to be given 1 hour before chemotherapy or orally at the same doses 30 minutes before chemotherapy. Metoclopramide 20–40 mg PO, dexamethasone 8 mg PO in the next 2–3 mornings along with prochlorperazine 10 mg PO every 6 hours as needed.

9. Metoclopramide 2–3 mg/kg IV before chemotherapy and then 2 hours post chemotherapy; dexamethasone 10–20 mg IV; diphenhydramine 25–50 mg IV; and lorazepam 1–2 mg IV.

10. Palonosetron 0.25 mg IV given 30 minutes before chemotherapy.

11. Palonosetron 0.25 mg IV given 30 minutes before chemotherapy; aprepitant 125 mg PO taken 60 minutes before chemotherapy on day 1, and 80 mg PO on days 2–3; dexamethasone 12 mg PO taken 30 minutes before chemotherapy on day 1, and 8 mg PO on days 2–3.

12. Rolapitant 180 mg PO 1–2 hours before chemotherapy, granisetron 1–2 mg PO one hour before chemotherapy, and dexamethasone 20 mg IV 30 minutes before chemotherapy. On days 2–4, give dexamethasone 8 mg PO bid with no additional antiemetic therapy.

13. Rolapitant 180 mg PO 1–2 hours before chemotherapy, ondansetron 16–24 mg PO 30 minutes before chemotherapy, and dexamethasone 12 mg PO taken 30 minutes before chemotherapy on day 1. On days 2–4, give dexamethasone 8 mg PO bid with no additional antiemetic therapy.

14. Rolapitant 180 mg PO 1–2 hours before chemotherapy, palonosetron 0.5 mg IV given 30 minutes before chemotherapy, dexamethasone 12 mg PO taken 30 minutes before chemotherapy on day 1. On days 2–4, give dexamethasone 8 mg PO bid with no additional antiemetic therapy.

15. Rolapitant 180 mg PO 1–2 hours before chemotherapy, dolasetron 100 mg PO 30 minutes before chemotherapy, and, dexamethasone 12 mg PO taken 30 minutes before chemotherapy on day 1. On days 2–4, give dexamethasone 8 mg PO bid with no additional antiemetic therapy.

16. Netupitant 300 mg/0.5 mg palonosetron PO 1 hour before chemotherapy and dexamethasone 12 mg PO taken 30 minutes before chemotherapy on day 1. Admininstration of dexamethasone 8 mg once daily on days 2–4.

17. Fosaprepitant 150 mg IV 30 minutes before chemotherapy on day 1, dexamethasone 12 mg PO taken 30 minutes before chemotherapy on day 1 and 8 mg PO on days 2–4, and ondansetron 16–24 mg PO on day 1.

18. Fosaprepitant 150 mg IV 30 minutes before chemotherapy on day 1, dexamethasone 12 mg PO taken 30 minutes before chemotherapy on day 1 and 8 mg PO on days 2–4, and palonosetron 0.5 mg IV on day 1.

19. Fosaprepitant 150 mg IV 30 minutes before chemotherapy on day 1, dexamethasone 12 mg PO taken 30 minutes before chemotherapy on day 1 and 8 mg PO on days 2–4, and dolasetron 100 mg PO on day 1.

20. Fosaprepitant 150 mg IV 30 minutes before chemotherapy on day 1, dexamethasone 12 mg PO taken 30 minutes before chemotherapy on day 1 and 8 mg PO on days 2–4, and, granisetron 1–2 mg PO on day 1.

21. Olanzapine 10 mg PO 1–2 hours before chemotherapy on day 1, palonosetron 0.25 mg IV on day 1, dexamethasone 20 mg IV on day 1, and olanzapine 10 mg PO on days 2–4.
22. Granisetron transdermal patch (34.3 mg of granisetron) applied to the upper outer arm at a minimum of 24 hours before chemotherapy. The patch should be removed a minimum of 24 hours after the completion of chemotherapy and may be worn for up to 7 days depending on the duration of the chemotherapy regimen. May also consider including dexamethasone on days 2–4 and/or may include a 5-HT3 inhibitor, such as dolasetron 100 mg PO on days 2–4 or ondansetron 8 mg PO on days 2–4.

COMMON REGIMENS FOR DELAYED AND/OR BREAKTHROUGH NAUSEA AND VOMITING:

1. Metoclopramide 40 mg PO every 4–6 hours and dexamethasone 4–8 mg PO every 4–6 hours for 4 days.
2. Metoclopramide 40 mg PO every 4–6 hours; dexamethasone 4–8 mg PO every 4–6 hours; and prochlorperazine 10–25 mg PO every 4–6 hours.
3. Aprepitant 80 mg PO and dexamethasone 8–12 mg PO once daily on days 2 and 3.
4. Aprepitant 80 mg PO daily, dexamethasone 8–12 mg PO daily, and ondansetron 8 mg PO bid on days 2 and 3.
5. Aprepitant 80 mg PO daily, dexamethasone 8–12 mg PO daily, and granisetron 1 mg PO bid on days 2 and 3.
6. Aprepitant 80 mg PO daily, dexamethasone 8–12 mg PO daily, and dolasetron 100 mg PO daily on days 2 and 3.
7. Olanzapine 10 mg PO on day 1, palonosetron 0.25 mg IV on day 1, dexamethasone 20 mg IV on day 1 and olanzapine 10 mg PO on days 2–4
8. Olanzapine 10 mg PO on days 1–4, aprepitant or fosaprepitant, and a 5-HT3 inhibitor
9. Ondansetron 8 mg PO bid for up to 2–3 days after chemotherapy.
10. Ondansetron (orally dissolving tablets) 8 mg sublingual every 8 hours as needed.
11. Metoclopramide 20–40 mg PO and diphenhydramine 50 mg PO every 3–4 hours.
12. Prochlorperazine suppository 25 mg PR every 12 hours.
13. Dolasetron 100 mg PO daily.
14. Nabilone 1–2 mg PO bid.
15. Dronabinol 5–10 mg PO every 4–6 hours.
16. Granisetron 1–2 mg PO daily or 1 mg PO bid or 0.01 mg/kg (maximum 1 mg) IV daily or transdermal patch every 7 days
17. Scopolamine transdermal patch every 72 hours
18. Haloperidol 0.5–2 mg PO or IV every 4–6 hours
19. Lorazepam 0.5–2 mg PO, sublingual, or IV every 6 hours

Table 1. Emetogenic Potential of Intravenous Chemotherapy Agents

Level	Frequency of Emesis (%)	Agent
5	>90	AC regimen (doxorubicin plus cyclophosphamide) Actinomycin-D Altretamine Carmustine >250 mg/m^2 Cisplatin ⩾50 mg/m^2 Cyclophosphamide >1500 mg/m^2 Dacarbazine >500 mg/m^2 Ifosfamide ⩾2 g/m^2 Mechlorethamine Pentostatin Procarbazine Streptozocin
4	60–90	Carboplatin Carmustine 250 mg/m^2 Cisplatin <50 mg/m^2 Cyclophosphamide 750–1500 mg/m^2 Cytarabine >1000 mg/m^2 Doxorubicin >60 mg/m^2 Irinotecan Melphalan (IV) Methotrexate >1000 mg/m^2
3	30–60	Aldesleukin >12–15 million IU/m^2 Arsenic trioxide Azacitidine Cyclophosphamide ⩽750 mg/m^2 Cyclophosphamide (oral) Cytarabine >200 mg/m^2 Doxorubicin 20–60 mg/m^2 Epirubicin ⩽90 mg/m^2 5–Fluorouracil >1000 mg/m^2 Idarubicin Ifosfamide Imatinib Methotrexate 250–1000 mg/m^2 Mitoxantrone <15 mg/m^2 Temozolomide
2	10–30	Albumin-bound paclitaxel Aldesleukin <12 million IU/m^2 Bexarotene Capecitabine Cetuximab

Table 1 (cont.)

2	10–30	Cytarabine 100–200 mg/m²
		Daunorubicin
		Docetaxel
		Doxorubicin <20 mg/m²
		Doxorubicin liposome
		Etoposide
		5-Fluorouracil <1000 mg/m²
		Gemcitabine
		Lomustine
		Methotrexate 50–250 mg/m²
		Mitomycin-C
		Paclitaxel
		Pemetrexed
		Thiotepa
		Topotecan
		Vorinostat
1	<10	Alemtuzumab
		Asparaginase
		Bevacizumab
		Bleomycin
		Bortezomib
		Busulfan
		Cetuximab
		Chlorambucil (oral)
		Cladribine
		Dasatinib
		Decitabine
		Denileukin diftitox
		Erlotinib
		Fludarabine
		Gefitinib
		Gemtuzumab
		Hydroxyurea
		Interferon-α
		Ipilumumab
		Lapatinib
		Lenalidomide
		Melphalan (oral)
		6-Mercaptopurine
		Methotrexate ≤50 mg/m²
		Nelarabine
		Nilotinib
		Ofatumumab
		Panitumumab
		Peg-interferon
		Rituximab
		Sorafenib

Table 2 (cont.)

1	<10	Sunitinib
		Temsirolimus
		Thalidomide
		6–Thioguanine (oral)
		Trastuzumab
		Tretinoin
		Vinblastine
		Vincristine
		Vinorelbine

Data from: Hesketh PJ, et al. *J Clin Oncol,* 1997;15:103–109; Gralla RJ, et al. *J Clin Oncol,* 1999;17:2971–2994; Grunberg SM, et al. *Support Care Cancer,* 2005;13:80–84; and NCCN Clinical Practice Guidelines in Oncology, V.1.2015. Antiemesis. NCCN 2015.

Single agents are divided into five different levels of emetogenic potential. They are as follows:

1. Level 1: <10% of patients experience acute (<24 hours after chemotherapy) emesis without antiemetic prophylaxis.
2. Level 2: 10%–30% of patients experience acute emesis without antiemetic prophylaxis.
3. Level 3: 30%–60% of patients experience acute emesis without antiemetic prophylaxis.
4. Level 4: 60%–90% of patients experience acute emesis without antiemetic prophylaxis.
5. Level 5: >90% of patients experience acute emesis without antiemetic prophylaxis.

With regard to combination regimens, the emetogenic levels are determined by identifying the most emetogenic agent in the combination and then assessing the relative contribution of the other agents based on the following:

1. Level 1 agents do not contribute to the emetogenic potential of the combination.
2. The presence of one or more level 2 agents increases the emetogenic potential of the combination by one level greater than the most emetogenic agent in the combination.
3. The presence of level 3 or level 4 agents increases the emetogenic potential of the combination by one level per given agent.

Index

A

abirasterone, 6, 559
abiraterone acetate, 5–7
Abraxane, 13, 14, 465
ABV, 499
ABVD, 522
AC, 452, 454–455, 457, 484
acetaminophen, 48, 69, 339
ACT, 451
Actinomycin-D, 122, 403, 406, 409
acute lymphocytic leukemia, 501–504
acute myelogenous leukemia, 268, 505–507
acute promyelocytic leukemia (APL), 30, 392
acute toxicity, 155, 204, 269, 296
acyclovir, 503
AD, 564
Adcetris, 65
adjuvant chemotherapy, 2, 487
ado-trastuzumab emtansine, 8–10, 464
ADOC, 569
adrenal insufficiency, 26
adrenocortical cancer, 442
Adriamycin, 144
afatinib, 10–12, 425, 431, 436, 519
Afinitor, 170
AG-13736, 37
AI, 564
AIDA, 505
albumin-bound paclitaxel, 13–15
alcohol, 370
aldesleukin (IL-2), 15–17, 540, 563
aldesleukin, 563
Alecensa, 18
alectinib, 18–20
alemtuzumab, 20–22, 425, 431, 436, 509
Alimta, 314
ALK testing, 90, 110
Alkeran, 253
all-*trans*-retinoic acid, 391
allopurinol, 203, 209, 257
α-Interferon, 214
altretamine, 23–24, 425, 431, 436, 552
Amethopterin, 258
amifostine, 425
aminoglutethimide, 25–26, 252, 425, 431, 436, 561
aminoglycosides, 98
amiodarone, 395, 401
AMN107, 274
amphotericin B, 30, 87, 98

amsacrine, 425, 436
anal cancer, 442–444
anastrozole, 27–29, 425, 431, 436, 456, 463
androgen receptor (AR), 151
antacids, 413
anthracyclines, 141, 146, 155, 389, 403, 406, 409
Anti-HER-2-antibody, 317, 388
antiarrhythmic drugs, 395
anticoagulants, 78, 112
antidiabetic agents, 329
antiemetic agents, for chemotherapy-induced nausea and vomiting, 589–596
antiestrogen agents, 379
antihistamines, 329
antihypertensives, 16
antipsychotics, 360
antiretroviral agents, 196
antithymocyte globulin (ATG), 549
AP, 484–485
AP24534, 322
APC8015, 343
APL. *See* acute promyelocytic leukemia
aprepitant, 64, 590, 591, 592
Ara-C, 114, 117, 505, 524
ara-G, 272
arbitrary reduction, 3
area under the curve (AUC), determination of, 423
Arimidex, 27
Aromasin, 173
Arranon, 272
arsenic trioxide (As$_2$O$_3$), 29–31, 425, 431, 436, 505–507
arthralgias, 28
Arzerra, 284
ASCT. *See* autologous stem cell transplant
asparaginase, 32–34, 425
aspirin, 259, 316, 326
asthenia, 28
AT, 457
atazanavir, 19, 38, 43, 72, 109, 119, 226, 310, 341, 354, 384, 398, 401
atezolizumab, 34–37
ATG. *See* antithymocyte globulin
atomoxetine, 307
ATRA, 391
autologous stem cell transplant (ASCT), 66
Avastin, 46
axitinib, 37–39, 563

azacitidine, 40–41, 425, 436, 507, 548
azithromycin, 401, 413

B

Bactrim DS, 529
barbiturates, 266, 370
basal cell cancer, 444
BAY 43-9006, 347
BAY 73-4506, 334
BCL-2, 400
BCNU, 86
BEACOPP, 524
BEACOPP escalated, 524
Beleodaq, 42
belinostat, 42–44, 536
bendamustine, 44–46, 425, 431, 509, 527, 535
BEP, 554, 567
bevacizumab (BV), 46–49, 417, 425, 431, 436,
        450, 451, 460, 466, 469, 474, 477–480,
        491, 498, 514, 517, 551, 553, 559, 562
bexarotene, 50–52
Bexxar, 380
BIC, 469
bicalutamide, 52–53, 425, 431, 436, 561
biliary tract cancer, 445–446
BIP, 469
Bischloroethylnitrosourea, 86
bispecific T-cell engaging (BiTE) antibody, 57
bladder cancer, 446–449
bladder toxicity, 112
Blenoxane, 54
bleomycin, 54–56, 67, 98, 404, 425, 431, 436,
        466, 469, 499, 503, 523–524, 554, 567
blinatumomab, 57–59, 504
Blincyto, 57
BMP, 545
BMPT, 545
BMS-247550, 228
BMS-354825, 127
BMS-936558, 279
body surface area, calculation of, 424
bortezomib, 60–63, 436, 528, 536, 544–547
Bosulif, 63
bosutinib, 63–65, 425, 436, 510
brain cancer, 449
breast cancer, 78, 91, 111, 142, 154, 181, 191,
        263, 451–465
brentuximab, 55, 65–68, 525, 536
bupropion, 360
Burkitt's lymphoma, 532–534
buserelin, 425, 431, 436
busulfan, 68–70, 425, 431, 436, 512
Busulfex, 68
BV, 499

C

cabazitaxel, 71–73, 559
cabozantinib, 73–76, 425, 431, 436, 570

CAE, 521
CAF, 453, 458
calcium channel blockers, 360, 404
calcium/magnesium infusions, 296
Campath, 20
Camptosar, 221
Camptotheca acuminate, 224
camptothecin, 376
cancer chemotherapy, principles of
    combination chemotherapy, 3–4
    overview of, 1
    role of, 2–3
CAP, 448, 485, 541, 568
capecitabine, 76–81, 425, 431, 436, 444–446,
        458, 462, 464, 466, 471–472, 477–479,
        483, 488–491, 499, 553, 555–557
capillary leak syndrome (CLS), 16, 104
Caprelsa, 394
captopril, 401
carbamazepine, 11, 19, 38, 64, 74, 89, 106, 109,
        119, 128, 160, 171, 173, 189, 206, 212,
        222, 225, 229, 231, 234, 239, 243, 275,
        288, 292, 302, 307, 310, 323, 335, 341,
        346, 354, 367, 379, 384, 395, 398, 401
carboplatin, 14, 81–83, 299, 426, 431, 436,
        446, 448, 450, 451, 455, 460–461, 466,
        469, 485, 494–496, 513–518, 521, 531,
        541, 550–552, 566, 569
carcinoid tumors, 467–468
cardiac arrhythmias, 324
cardiac toxicity, 15
cardiotoxicity, 132, 134, 147, 150, 389
    risk of, 146, 155
carfilzomib, 84–86, 426, 431, 436,
        546, 547
carmustine, 86–88, 426, 431, 436, 449,
        450, 524, 538
carvedilol, 401
Casodex, 52
CAV, 521, 565
CBDCA, 81
CC-5013, 236
CC, 550
CCI-779, 366
CCNU, 246
CD20, 337, 380
CD52 antigen, 20
CDDP, 96
CEF, 458
celecoxib, 80
cellular retinoic acid binding protein
        (CRABP), 391
cephalosporins, 259, 326
ceritinib, 88–91, 426, 431, 436, 520
Cerubidine, 130
cervical cancer, 47, 377, 468–471
cetuximab, 91–93, 426, 431, 436, 477,
        480–483, 494, 496, 516, 517, 520
CF, 490, 508
chemoradiation, 554

chemoradiotherapy, 489
  for nasopharyngeal cancer, 497
chemotherapy, 487, 513, 555
  in treatment of cancer, role of, 2–3
  dosage, guidelines for
    hepatic function, 425–430
    renal function, 431–435
chemotherapy-induced nausea and vomiting,
    treatment for
  common antiemetic regimens for, 589–593
  common regimens for delayed and/or
    breakthrough, 593–596
chest X-ray, 55
chlorambucil, 94–96, 282, 426, 431, 436,
    508–509
chloroquine, 395
chlorpromazine, 370, 395
CHOP, 526, 528
chromophore moiety, 123
chronic lymphocytic leukemia, 507–511
chronic myelogenous leukemia, 511–512
chronic toxicity, 269, 296
cimetidine, 24, 87, 154, 209, 229, 247, 254,
    360, 392, 404
ciprofloxacin, 64, 504
cisplatin, 48, 55, 96–100, 179, 191, 192, 209,
    229, 295, 299, 407, 410, 426, 432, 436,
    442–448, 466–470, 485–492, 494–498,
    499, 513–518, 521, 524, 531, 538, 541,
    542, 549–550, 554, 566–570
cladribine, 100–102, 426, 432, 436, 506, 509,
    512, 535
clarithromycin, 11, 19, 38, 64, 72, 106,
    109, 119, 128, 157, 160, 171, 173,
    189, 201, 206, 212, 222, 226, 228,
    234, 240, 243, 275, 289, 292, 302,
    307, 310, 323, 335, 341, 346, 354,
    367, 384, 395, 398, 401, 413
clofarabine, 102–104, 436, 504, 507
clofarabine triphosphate, 103
Clolar, 103
clopidogrel (Plavix), 243
CLS. See capillary leak syndrome
CMF, 453, 458
CMV, 447
CNOP, 526
CNS depressants, 329
CNS lymphoma, 536–538
CNS prophylaxis, 502, 533
CNS toxicity, 393
cobimetinib, 105–107
CODOX-M, 533
colorectal cancer, 176, 181, 222, 471–484
combination chemotherapy, principles of, 3–4
Cometriq, 73
consolidation therapy, 501
corticosteroids, 16, 339
Cosmegen, 122
Cotellic, 105
CP, 508

CPT-11, 221, 483
CRABP. See cellular retinoic acid binding
    protein
cranial irradiation, 502
cranial magnetic resonance imaging (MRI), 58
creatinine clearance, determination of, 423
crizotinib, 108–110, 520
CTX, 110
CVP, 507, 526
cyclophosphamide, 110–113, 146, 154,
    179, 266, 299, 360, 426, 432, 436, 448,
    451–459, 458–459, 502–503, 507–508,
    521, 524–531, 533, 541, 550, 565,
    568–569
cyclosporine, 142, 254, 360, 392, 401,
    404, 549
CYP17, inhibition of, 6
CYP2C8, 152
CYP2D6, 360
CYP3A4, 152, 159, 160, 170, 171, 173, 188,
    189, 353
  enzymes, 341, 367, 395
  inducers, 61
  inhibitors, 346
  microsomal enzymes, 11
Cyramza, 331
Cytadren, 25
cytarabine, 113–117, 179, 426, 432, 436,
    501–506, 504–506, 511, 524, 531,
    533–534, 537
cytidine deaminase, 136
cytochrome P450 system, 50
Cytosine arabinoside, 114
cytotoxic oxygen free radicals, formation of, 130
Cytoxan, 110
CYVADIC, 564

D

DAB389, 139
dabrafenib, 118–120, 426, 436, 539, 541
dacarbazine, 120–122, 426, 432, 436, 522,
    539, 564–565
Dacogen, 135
dactinomycin, 426, 432, 436, 565, 567
dactinomycin-D, 122–124
daratumumab, 124–127, 547
Darzalex, 125
dasatinib, 127–129, 432, 504, 511
Daunomycin, 130
daunorubicin, 130–132, 426, 432, 436, 459,
    502, 505, 506
daunorubicin liposome, 133–135, 500
DaunoXome, 133
DCF, 490
decitabine, 135–137, 426, 432, 507, 548
degarelix, 137–138, 560
denileukin diftitox, 139–140
Depsipeptide, 340
desipramine, 307

dexamethasone, 26, 131, 146, 171, 231, 503, 526, 531, 534, 542–547, 553, 590
dexrazoxane, 131, 146, 156
dextromethorphan, 307
DHAP, 531
dialysis, of chemotherapy drugs, guidelines for, 436–438
Diaminocyclohexane platinum, 295
diarrhea, 12, 80, 140, 223–224, 227, 235
DIC, 120
difluorodeoxycytidine diphosphate (dFdCDP), 191
digoxin, 25, 64, 87, 112, 115, 407
dilantin, 189
diltiazem, 64, 80, 171, 392
diphenhydramine, 21, 48, 339
disopyramide, 395
docetaxel, 141–144, 426, 432, 437, 446, 451–456, 458–461, 464, 470, 486, 491, 494, 497, 500, 515, 551, 555, 558–560, 565
dofetilide, 395
dolasetron, 395, 590, 591, 593
Doxil, 148, 525
doxorubicin, 32, 112, 144–147, 299, 426, 432, 437, 442, 447, 448, 451–455, 458, 459, 465, 467, 485, 499, 500, 503, 505, 521–524, 526–530, 533–534, 541, 543, 549–550, 564–569, 568
doxorubicin liposome, 148–150, 426, 432, 437, 459, 465, 485, 500, 544, 551, 552, 566
dronabinol, 593
drug dose, determination of, 424
DTIC, 539
DTIC-dome, 120
duloxetine, 360
DVD, 544
dysesthesias, 296

E

E7080, 238
early-stage breast cancer, 28, 389
early-stage colon cancer, 296
EC, 521
ECF, 488, 490
ECOG regimen, 555
ECX, 489, 490
Efudex, 180
EGFR tyrosine kinase, 159
Ellence, 153
Eloxatin, 295
Elspar, 32
Emcyt, 162
endometrial cancer, 484–486
enzalutamide, 151–153, 562
EOF, 488, 490
EOX, 489
EP, 465, 517, 567
epidermal growth factor receptor (EGFR), 91

epipodophyllotoxins, 403, 406, 409
epirubicin, 153–156, 453, 458–459, 487, 488, 489
EPOCH, 529
ErbB tyrosine kinases, inhibition of, 11
Erbitux, 91
eribulin, 156–158, 465
Erivedge, 412
erlotinib, 158–161, 426, 432, 466, 498, 519, 556
erythromycin, 11, 19, 38, 51, 64, 106, 109, 119, 128, 142, 157, 160, 161, 171, 173, 189, 201, 206, 212, 222, 226, 228, 234, 240, 243, 275, 289, 292, 302, 307, 323, 341, 346, 354, 360, 367, 379, 384, 392, 395, 398, 401, 404, 413
ESHAP, 531
esophageal cancer, 486–489
Estracyte, 162
estramustine, 162–163, 427, 432, 437, 558–560
estramustine-resistant cells, 162
ethylenimine, 374
Etopophos, 167
etoposide, 98, 164–166, 427, 432, 437, 442, 466, 467, 500, 506, 513, 517, 520–524, 529, 531–533, 553, 553–554, 558, 565–569
etoposide phosphate, 167–169, 427, 432, 437
Eulexin, 183
EVA, 524
EVAP, 524
everolimus, 169–172, 427, 432, 457, 462, 467, 468, 563
exemestane, 172–174, 457, 462, 463
extravasation, 146, 156

F

Fareston, 378
Farydak, 306
Faslodex, 185
fatal hepatotoxicity, 43
FC, 526–527
FCR, 508, 527
FEC, 453, 455
FEC-50, 459
FEC-75, 459
FEC-100, 459
felodipine, 401
Femara, 242
filgrastim, 407
Firmagon, 137
5-aza-2'-deoxycytidine, 135
5-fluoro-2'-deoxyuridine, 175
5-fluorocytosine, 115
5-fluorouracil (5-FU), 146, 154, 180–183, 196, 259, 315, 427, 433, 437, 442–445, 448, 453, 458–459, 467, 469, 471–482, 486–498, 554–557

5-FU/LV oxaliplatin, 472
FLAG, 506
FLO, 492
FLOX, 473
floxuridine, 175–177, 427, 432, 437, 482
fluconazole, 22, 64, 171, 228, 504
Fludara, 178
fludarabine, 116, 177–180, 427, 433, 437, 506, 508, 510, 526, 527, 535
fluid retention syndrome, 143
fluoropyrimidine, 335
fluoxetine, 360
flutamide, 183–185, 427, 433, 437, 557, 561
FND, 526
FOLFIRI, 417, 480–482
FOLFIRINOX, 556
FOLFOX4, 479–481, 498
FOLFOX6, 481
FOLFOXIRI, 476
folic acid supplements, 260
Folotyn, 325
4-demethoxydaunorubicin, 202
4 epi-doxorubicin, 153
fosaprepitant, 591, 592
FP, 492, 508
FR, 508
FUDR, 175
fulvestrant, 185–187, 463

G

G-CSF, 495, 504, 506
gastric cancer, 142, 154, 263, 489–493
gastroesophageal junction
    adenocarcinoma, 389
gastrointestinal stromal tumor (GIST), 3, 493–494
gastrointestinal toxicity, 65
Gazyva, 282
GCB, 515
GCP, 466
gefitinib, 188–190, 427, 433, 519
gemcitabine, 190–193, 427, 433, 437, 445–448, 459, 461, 465, 470, 471, 486, 498, 515, 516, 518, 522, 525, 532, 541, 552–557, 565, 568, 569
gemfibrozil, 43, 51, 226
GEMOX, 498
Gemzar, 190
gentamicin, 115
GI adenocarcinoma, 176
Gilotrif, 10
GIST. See gastrointestinal stromal tumor
GITSG regimen, 554
Gleevec, 210
glioblastoma, 48
glucarpidase, 261
goserelin, 193–194, 427, 433, 437, 457, 557, 560
granisetron, 395, 590, 591, 593

GTX, 555
GVD, 525
GW572016, 233
gynecomastia, 163

H

H2-receptor inhibitors, 413
hairy cell leukemia, 470
Halaven, 156
haloperidol, 395, 593
hand-foot syndrome, 80, 117, 183
HDAC inhibitors, 415
head and neck cancer, 92, 97, 142, 494–498
hemolytic-uremic syndrome, 264
heparin, 121, 131, 146, 154, 203, 268
hepatic dysfunction, 104
hepatic toxicity, 12
hepatic veno-occlusive disease, 265
hepatocellular cancer, 498–499
hepatotoxicity, 10, 17, 20, 176
hepatoveno-occlusive disease, 70, 124
HER2-targeted antibody-drug, 8
HER2 testing, 9
Herceptin, 388
Hexalen, 23
Hexamethylmelamine (HMM), 23
histone deacetylase (HDAC) inhibitors, 414
HMM. See Hexamethylmelamine
Hodgkin's lymphoma, 121, 250, 280, 522–525
HSR. See hypersensitivity reaction
human teratogen, 237
humanized IgG4 antibody, 34
HuMax-CD20, 284
Hycamtin, 376
hydrazine, 328
Hydrea, 195
hydrocortisone, 121, 523
Hydroxydaunorubicin, 144
hydroxyurea, 116, 195–196, 427, 433, 437, 512
hyper-CVAD/methotrexate-ara-C, 534
hypercholesterolemia, 51
hyperpigmentation of skin, 69
hypersensitivity reaction (HSR), 33, 56, 72–73, 83, 99, 113, 140
hypertension, 311, 333, 354
hypertriglyceridemia, 51
hypomagnesemia, 272

I

Ibrance, 301
ibritumomab, 197–199
ibritumomab tiuxetan regimen, 535
ibrutinib, 200–202, 427, 433, 437, 510, 528, 548
ICE, 531
Iclusig, 322
Idamycin, 202
idarubicin, 202–204, 427, 433, 437, 505, 506

IDEC-Y2B8, 197
idelalisib, 205–207
idelasib, 509
IDO, 491
Ifex, 207
IFL saltz regimen, 474
IFN, 539
IFN-α, 214
ifosfamide, 98, 207–210, 427, 433,
        437, 446, 469, 485, 495, 531,
        533, 549, 564–569
IL-2, 562
imatinib, 210–214, 427, 433, 437, 493, 504,
        511, 548
Imbruvica, 200
IMC-1121B, 331
Imidazole Carboxamide, 120
imidazotetrazine, 364
Imlygic, 356
immunologic mechanisms, 20, 91
immunologic-mediated mechanisms, 8
indinavir, 19, 38, 72, 109, 119, 226, 310, 341,
        354, 384, 398, 401
induction therapy, 459, 501–502
infusion 5-FU, 471
infusion-related symptoms, 333, 339
Inlyta, 37
interferon, 511
interferon-α, 214–217
interferon α-2a, 214, 470, 562, 563
interferon α-2b, 427, 433, 500, 538–540,
        562, 563
interleukin-2 (IL-2), 15, 428, 433, 562, 563
interstitial lung disease (ILD), 93
interstitial pneumonitis, 264
intradermal skin test, 33
intrathecal ara-C, 533
intrathecal chemotherapy, 534
intrathecal methotrexate, 534, 536
intravenous chemotherapy agents, emetogenic
        potential of, 594–596t
Intron A, 214
IP, 491
IP cisplatin, 552
IP paclitaxel, 552
IPB, 491
ipilimumab, 217–220, 538
Iressa, 188
irinotecan, 220–224, 335, 428, 433,
        437, 450, 466, 470, 474–478,
        488, 491, 521, 556
irinotecan liposome, 224–227
iron-chelating agent dexrazoxane
        (ICRF-187), 146
Isophosphamide, 207
isotretinoin, 428, 433, 437
Istodax, 340
ITP, 446

itraconazole, 11, 19, 38, 51, 69, 72, 106, 109,
        119, 128, 160, 171, 173, 189, 201, 206,
        212, 222, 226, 228, 234, 240, 243, 275,
        289, 292, 302, 307, 310, 323, 335, 341,
        346, 354, 367, 384, 395, 398, 401
IV fluids, 339
IVAC, 533
ixabepilone, 227–230, 428, 433, 459, 464, 553
ixazomib, 230–232
Ixempra, 228

J

Jevtana, 71

K

Kadcyla, 8
Kaposi's sarcoma, 149, 499–500
keratitis, 12
ketoconazole, 11, 19, 38, 51, 61, 64, 72,
        106, 109, 119, 128, 142, 160, 171,
        173, 189, 201, 206, 212, 222, 226,
        228, 234, 240, 243, 275, 289, 292,
        302, 307, 310, 323, 335, 341, 346,
        354, 367, 379, 384, 392, 395, 398,
        401, 404, 530, 561
Keytruda, 312
Kyprolis, 84

L

L-asparaginase, 32–34, 116, 260, 407, 431,
        459–460
L-leucovorin, 474, 549, 550
L-PAM, 253
lanreotide, 468
lapatinib, 233–235, 428, 433, 437, 462
LBH 589, 306
left ventricular ejection fraction (LVEF), 9, 318
lenalidomide, 231, 235–238, 319, 428, 433,
        437, 510, 536, 543–548, 547
lenvatinib, 238–241, 570
Lenvima, 238
letrozole, 242–244, 456, 463
leucovorin, 79, 176, 182, 260, 315, 326, 459,
        472–482, 489, 492, 498, 503, 530, 531,
        533, 534, 536, 549, 550, 554–557
leucovorin rescue, 532, 534
leukemia, 501–512
Leukeran, 94
leukocytosis, 31
leuprolide, 244–246, 428, 433, 437,
        557, 559, 560
Leustatin, 100
levodopa, 329
LFTs. See liver function tests
lidocaine, 121

liposomal doxorubicin, 149
liposomal irinotecan, 557
liver function tests (LFTs), 9
liver P450-mediated mechanisms, 85
lomustine, 246–248, 428, 433, 437, 449, 450
Lonsurf, 362
loperamide, 226
lorazepam, 593
lung cancer, 513–522
Lupron, 244
LV5FU2, 474, 479
LVEF. *See* left ventricular ejection fraction
LY231514, 314
lymphoma, 522–538
Lynparza, 288
Lysodren, 265

M

M-BACOD, 530
MACOP-B, 530
maculopapular skin rash, 26, 193
magrath protocol, 532–533
MAID, 564
maintenance therapy, 501
malignant melanoma, 538–541
malignant mesothelioma, 541–542
mantle cell lymphoma, 536
MAO. *See* monoamine oxidase (MAO) inhibitors
Matulane, 328
MCV, 447
MDS. *See* myelodysplastic syndrome
MDX-1106, 279
mechlorethamine, 249–251, 428, 433, 437
medroxyprogesterone, 25
Megace, 251
megestrol, 463, 486
megestrol acetate, 251–253, 428, 433, 437
Mekinist, 386
melanoma, 121
melphalan, 253–255, 428, 433, 437, 524, 542, 545, 547
meperidine, 329
mercaptopurine, 255–257, 372
mesna, 469, 495, 503, 531, 534, 549, 564, 567–569
mesoridazine, 395
mesothelioma, 315
metastatic breast cancer, 28, 78, 142, 186, 379, 389
metastatic castration-resistant, 152
metastatic colorectal cancer, 47, 78, 296, 331, 417
metastatic gastric/gastroesophageal junction adenocarcinoma, 389
methadone, 395

methotrexate, 33, 98, 115, 182, 258–262, 407, 428, 434, 437, 447, 453, 458, 497, 501–504, 530, 532, 533–534, 536, 537, 549, 550
methylprednisolone, 503, 531
metoclopramide, 404, 590, 592, 593
metoprolol, 307
mini-BEAM, 524
Mitomycin, 262
mitomycin-C, 146, 262–265, 410, 428, 434, 437, 442–443, 448, 478, 479
mitotane, 265–267, 428, 434, 437, 442
mitoxantrone, 179, 267–269, 428, 434, 437, 506, 526–529, 532, 558
MK-3475, 312
monoamine oxidase (MAO) inhibitors, 24
MOPP, 523
moxifloxacin, 395
MP, 542–543
MPL, 543
MPT, 543
MTX, 258
mucositis, 261, 301
Multiple myeloma, 149, 542–548
Mustargen, 249
Mutamycin, 262
MVAC, 447
myelodysplastic syndrome (MDS), 41, 136, 548–549
myelosuppression, 24
myelosuppressive agents, 82, 375
Myleran, 68

N

N-methylhydrazine, 328
nab-paclitaxel, 514, 518, 556
nabilone, 593
nasopharyngeal cancer, 497
nausea/vomiting, 297
navelbine, 409, 458, 461, 565
nebivolol, 307
necitumumab, 270–272
nefazodone, 19, 38, 72, 109, 119, 310, 335, 354, 384, 398, 401
nelarabine, 272–274, 428, 434, 437, 504
nelfinavir, 19, 38, 72, 109, 119, 310, 354, 384, 398, 401
neoadjuvant chemotherapy, 2
nephrotoxic drugs, 351
nephrotoxicity, 99
netupitant, 591, 592
neuroendocrine tumors, 467–468
neurologic toxicity, 34
neurotoxicity, 10, 14, 24, 274, 296, 408, 411
neutropenia, 411
Nexavar, 347
Nilandron, 277

nilotinib, 274–276, 434, 493, 504, 511
nilutamide, 277–278, 428, 434, 437, 561
Ninlaro, 230
nitrogen mustard, 249, 523
nivolumab, 279–281, 520, 539, 564
Nolvadex, 358
non-Hodgkin's lymphoma, 45, 87, 101, 111,
    115, 268, 526–536
non-small cell lung cancer (NSCLC), 82, 97,
    142, 191, 315, 513–520
nonsteroidal anti-inflammatory drugs
    (NSAIDs), 16, 259, 316, 326
nonsteroidal antiandrogen agent, 52
Novantrone, 267
NSAIDs. See nonsteroidal anti-inflammatory
    drugs

O

obinutuzumab, 282–284, 509
octreotide, 467
octreotide LAR, 467
ocular toxicity, 100
ofatumumab, 284–287, 429, 434, 438, 510
olanzapine, 591, 593
olaparib, 287–289, 553
omacetaxine, 512
omacetaxine mepesuccinate, 290–292
Oncovin, 406
ondansetron, 590, 591, 593
Onivyde, 224
Ontak, 139
Opdivo, 279
oral bioavailability, 105, 302
oral capsules, 164
OSI-774, 159
osimertinib, 292–294
osteogenic sarcoma, 549–550
ovarian cancer, 23, 97, 149, 191, 377
    epithelial, 550–553
    germ cell, 554
oxaliplatin, 48, 294–297, 335, 429, 434,
    438, 444, 445, 466, 472–481,
    488–492, 532, 556
oxygen, 55

P

P-glycoprotein inhibitors, 341, 413
paclitaxel, 13, 47, 48, 78, 82, 98, 298–301,
    407, 429, 434, 438, 447, 452, 454, 455,
    457–460, 464, 466, 468–470, 484–489,
    488, 492, 494–495, 500, 513–515, 518,
    521, 522, 551–552, 558–560, 568, 569
palbociclib, 301–303, 462
palmar-plantar erythrodysesthesia. *See*
    hand-foot syndrome
palonosetron, 591, 592
pancreatic cancer, 160, 191, 192, 554–557
pancreatitis, 34

panitumumab, 303–305, 429, 434, 477,
    481, 483
panobinostat, 306–308, 544
Paraplatin, 81
paronychial inflammation, 93
paroxetine, 360
pazopanib, 308–311, 429, 434, 438, 563,
    566, 570
PC, 514
PCB, 514–515
PCE, 465
PCR, 508
PCV, 449
PD 0332991, 301
PD, 544
PEB, 466, 566
peg-interferon α-2b, 538
pegasparaginase, 429, 434
peginterferon α-2b, 214
pembrolizumab, 312–314, 540
pemetrexed, 314–317, 429, 434, 438, 449, 470,
    471, 514, 517–519, 542, 552, 553
penicillins, 259, 326
pentamidine, 395
pentostatin, 438, 508, 510, 512
performance scales, 421
peripheral neuropathy, 73, 83, 99, 144
peripheral sensory neuropathy, 62, 67
peripheral T-cell lymphoma, 536
Perjeta, 317
perphenazine, 307, 360
pertuzumab, 317–319, 429, 434, 438, 451,
    456, 460
PF, 495, 496
phenobarbital, 11, 19, 24, 25, 38, 51, 64, 69,
    74, 89, 95, 106, 109, 119, 128, 146, 160,
    171, 173, 189, 206, 208, 212, 215, 222,
    225, 229, 231, 234, 239, 243, 275, 288,
    292, 299, 302, 307, 310, 323, 335, 341,
    346, 354, 367, 379, 384, 395, 398, 401
phenothiazines, 395
Phenylalanine mustard, 253
phenytoin, 106, 109, 109, 112, 19, 25, 38, 51,
    64, 69, 72, 74, 79, 87, 89, 95, 98, 119,
    121, 128, 146, 152, 160, 171, 173, 206,
    208, 212, 213, 222, 225, 234, 239,
    243, 266, 275, 288, 292, 299, 302, 307,
    310, 323, 335, 341, 346, 351, 354, 367,
    379, 384, 395, 398, 401, 404, 407, 410
pimozide, 360, 395
Platinol, 96
platinum-based chemotherapy, 518
Plavix, 243
PLX4032, 397
pomalidomide, 319–322, 429, 434, 438, 544
Pomalyst, 319
POMALYST REMS, 321
ponatinib, 322–325, 429, 434, 438, 512
Portrazza, 270
posaconazole, 64, 323, 395

pralatrexate, 325–327, 429, 434, 438, 536
prednisone, 32, 501–504, 508, 510, 523–530, 532, 533, 543, 545, 558–559, 561
pregnancy, teratogenic potential and use in, 439
prepitant, 593
primary induction chemotherapy, 2
probenecid, 203, 259, 326
procainamide, 395
procarbazine, 327–330, 429, 434, 438, 449, 450, 523, 524, 537
prochlorperazine, 589, 590, 593
progressive multifocal leukoencephalopathy (PML), 67
Proleukin, 15
ProMACE/CytaBOM, 530
prostate cancer, 142, 268, 557–562
proton pump inhibitors, 64, 260, 413
Provenge, 343
pruritus, 305
pulmonary toxicity, 10, 12, 20, 56, 88, 93, 248, 305
Purinethol, 255
PVB, 567
PXD101, 42
pyridoxine, 24

Q

QT prolongation, 157
quinidine, 360, 395, 401

R

R-CHOP-14, 528–529
R-CHOP, 527
R-FCM, 527
R-GemOx, 532
R-MPV, 537
RAD001, 170
radiation therapy, 55, 91, 92, 98, 442–443, 449, 468, 471, 472, 486–487, 494, 496, 513, 537, 554, 555
ramucirumab, 331–333, 429, 435, 438, 482, 492, 518
ranolazine, 401
rapamycin, 366
receptor tyrosine kinases (RTKs), 18
regimen A, 533
regimen B, 533
regorafenib, 334–337, 429, 435, 438, 484, 494
renal cell cancer, 16, 48, 280, 562–564
renal toxicity, 34, 41, 248, 261
reserpine, 370
retinoic acid syndrome, 392
RevAssist^SM program, 237
reversible posterior leukoencephalopathy syndrome (RPLS), 39, 63, 75
Revlimid, 236
RICE, 532

rifampin, 11, 19, 38, 51, 64, 74, 89, 106, 109, 119, 128, 160, 171, 173, 189, 206, 212, 222, 225, 229, 231, 234, 239, 243, 275, 288, 292, 302, 307, 310, 323, 335, 341, 346, 354, 367, 384, 395, 398, 401
Risk Evaluation and Mitigation Strategy (REMS), 219
ritonavir, 19, 38, 72, 109, 119, 310, 341, 354, 384, 398, 401
Rituxan, 337
rituximab, 337–340, 429, 435, 438, 508–510, 527–530, 532, 535, 537
RMPT, 545
Roferon Interferon-α2b, 214
rolapitant, 591, 592
romidepsin, 340–342, 536
RPLS. *See* reversible posterior leukoencephalopathy syndrome
RTOG chemoradiation regimen, 554
Rubidomycin, 130
RVD, 544

S

salvage regimen, 567, 568
saquinavir, 19, 38, 72, 109, 119, 310, 354, 384, 395, 398, 401
scopolamine, 593
seizures, 95
selective noradrenergic reuptake inhibitors (SNRIs), 360
selective serotonin reuptake inhibitors (SSRIs), 360
semisynthetic taxane, 141
sertraline, 360
serum bilirubin levels, 9
serum electrolytes, 30
serum estradiol levels, 27
SGN-35, 65
sipuleucel-T, 343–344, 561
6-mercaptopurine, 146, 255, 428, 433, 437, 501–502
6-thioguanine (6-TG), 371, 503
SKI-606, 63
skin
    hyperpigmentation of, 69
    toxicity, 12, 150, 336, 371, 388
small cell lung cancer, 377, 520–522
small steady-state volume of distribution, 133
SN-38, 224
SNRIs. *See* selective noradrenergic reuptake inhibitors
sodium thiosulfate, 250
soft tissue sarcomas, 564–566
sonidegib, 444
sorafenib, 347–350, 429, 435, 438, 494, 499, 507, 562, 570
sotalol, 395
sparfloxacin, 395
Sprycel, 127

SSRIs. *See* selective serotonin reuptake inhibitors

St. John's wort, 11, 19, 38, 61, 64, 89, 106, 109, 119, 128, 152, 160, 171, 173, 189, 206, 212, 222, 223, 225, 227, 229, 231, 234, 239, 243, 275, 288, 292, 302, 307, 310, 323, 335, 341, 346, 354, 367, 384, 395, 398, 401

stage III colon cancer, 78

stanford regimen, 533–534

stanford V, 523

steroids, 254, 266, 351

STI571, 210

Stivarga, 334

streptozocin, 350–352, 429, 435, 438, 442, 467

Streptozotocin, 350

SU11248, 352

sulfamethoxazole, 326

sulfinpyrazone, 203

sunitinib, 352–355, 429, 435, 438, 468, 494, 519, 562, 570

Sutent, 352

Sylatron, 214

Synribo, 290

T

T-cell acute lymphoblastic leukemia (T-ALL), 273

T-cell lymphoblastic lymphoma (T-LBL), 273

T-cell prolymphocytic leukemia, 21

T-vec, 356

TAC, 453

Tafinlar, 118

Tagrisso, 292

talimogene laherparepvec, 356–358

tamoxifen, 358–361, 378, 379, 429, 435, 438, 456, 463

Tarceva, 159

Targretin, 50

TAS-102, 362–363, 484

Tasigna, 274

taxanes, 389, 403, 406, 409

Taxol, 298

Taxotere, 141

TC, 452

TCH, 455, 461

Tecentriq, 34

telithromycin, 19, 38, 72, 109, 119, 310, 335, 354, 384, 398, 401

Temodar, 364

temozolomide, 364–366, 429, 435, 438, 450, 467, 538–540

temozolomide radiation therapy, 449

temsirolimus, 366–368, 438, 486, 563

teniposide, 501

teratogenic effect, 370

terfenadine, 360, 395

testicular cancer, 97, 165, 168, 566–568

thalidomide, 320, 369–371, 429, 435, 438, 539, 543, 545, 547

Thalomid, 369

theophylline, 25

thiazide diuretics, 379

thiethylperazine, 590

thioguanine, 371–373, 430, 435, 438

Thioplex, 374

thioridazine, 360, 395

thiotepa, 373–375, 430, 435, 438

thrombocytopenia, 192, 231, 329

thymidine, 176, 182, 260, 315, 326

thymoma, 568–569

thyroid cancer, 239, 569–570

thyroid function tests, 51

TIC, 495

ticagrelor, 401

ticlopidine, 360

TIP, 494, 568

tolterodine, 307

topotecan, 48, 376–378, 430, 435, 438, 468, 471, 486, 521, 522, 538, 553, 569

toremifene, 378–380, 463

Torisel, 366

tositumomab, 380–383

TPF, 494

trabectedin, 383–385

trametinib, 386–388, 430, 435, 438, 539, 541

transient asymptomatic sinus bradycardia, 301

trastuzumab, 146, 388–390, 430, 435, 438, 451, 455, 460–461, 463, 491

Treanda, 44

tretinoin, 391–393, 430, 435, 505, 507

triazine, 23

tricyclic antidepressants, 329

trifluridine, 362

trimethoprim/sulfamethoxazole (Bactrim DS), 527, 530, 531

trimethroprim, 326

trimetrexate, 182

Trisenox, 29

troleandomycin, 395

tumor lysis syndrome, 45, 59, 67, 339

26S proteasome, 60

2-amino-9-β-D-arabinofuranosyl-6-methoxy-9H-purine, 272

2-chlorodeoxyadenosine (2-CdA), 100

2-fluoro-ara-adenosine (F-ara-A), 178

2-fluoro-ara-AMP, 178

Tykerb, 233

U

UGT1A1 inhibitor, 335, 349

UGT1A9, 348

V

VAB-6, 567

VAD, 543

vandetanib, 394–397, 570
vascular endothelial growth factor (VEGF), 46
vascular leak syndrome, 17, 140
vasopressor, 339
VCR, 406
Vectibix, 303
VEGF. *See* vascular endothelial growth factor
VeIP, 567
Velban, 403
Velcade, 60
vemurafenib, 397–399, 430, 438, 541
Venclexta, 400
venetoclax, 399–402
venlafaxine, 307
VePesid, 164
verapamil, 64, 171, 228, 392
Vesanoid, 391
Vidaza, 40
vinblastine, 402–405, 430, 435, 438, 447, 500, 513–514, 522, 558, 567
vincristine, 33, 405–409, 430, 435, 438, 449, 499, 501–503, 507, 521, 523, 533, 537, 543, 544, 565, 569
vinorelbine, 409–411, 430, 435, 438, 464, 469, 497, 500, 513, 516–517, 525, 542, 553
VIP, 569
vismodegib, 412–414, 444
vistonuridine (PN401), 176, 182
vitamin A supplements, 392
vitamin A toxicity, 392
vitamin B6 (pyridoxine), 24
vitamin B6, 80
voriconazole, 19, 38, 64, 72, 109, 119, 310, 323, 335, 341, 354, 384, 398, 401
vorinostat, 414–416, 430, 435, 438, 535
Votrient, 309

VP-16, 164
VP, 497

W

warfarin, 12, 25, 53, 106, 119, 160, 165, 168, 184, 189, 201, 206, 209, 212, 213, 234, 243, 256, 259, 266, 277, 292, 323, 341, 359, 379, 401, 415
white blood cells (WBCs), 31

X

Xalkori, 108
Xeloda, 76
XELOX, 444, 472
XP, 491

Y

Yervoy, 217
Yondelis, 383

Z

Zaltrap, 417
Zanosar, 350
ZD1839, 188
Zelboraf, 397
Zevalin, 197
ziv-aflibercept, 417–419, 438, 482
Zoladex, 193
zoledronic acid, 456
Zolinza, 414
Zydelig, 205
Zykadia, 89
Zytiga, 5